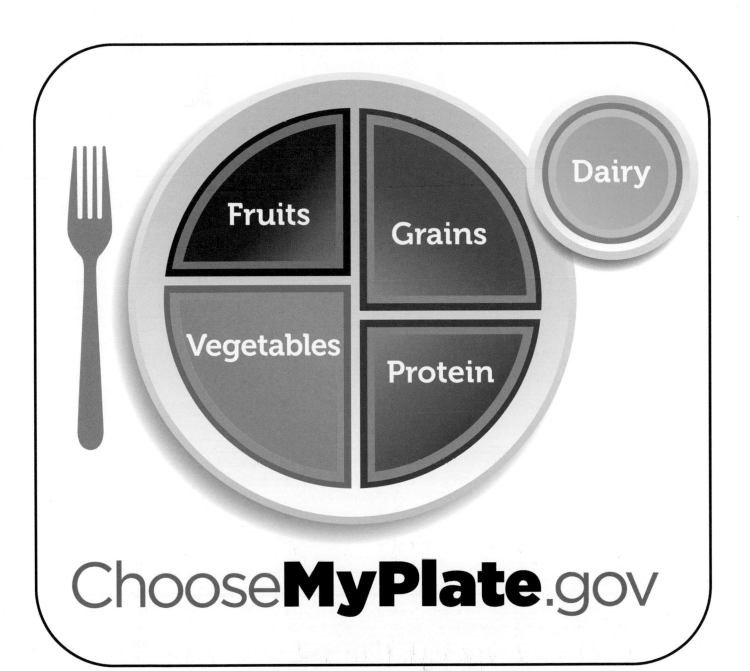

ChooseMyPlate.gov

Criteria and Dietary Reference Intake Values: FOR ENERGY BY ACTIVE INDIVIDUALS BY LIFE STAGE GROUP[a]

Life Stage Group	Criterion	Active PAL EER[b] (kcal/d) Male	Female
0 through 6 mo	Energy expenditure plus energy deposition	570	520 (3 mo)
7 through 12 mo	Energy expenditure plus energy deposition	743	676 (9 mo)
1 through 2 y	Energy expenditure plus energy deposition	1,046	992 (24 mo)
3 through 8 y	Energy expenditure plus energy deposition	1,742	1,642 (6 y)
9 through 13 y	Energy expenditure plus energy deposition	2,279	2,071 (11 y)
14 through 18 y	Energy expenditure plus energy deposition	3,152	2,368 (16 y)
>18 y	Energy expenditure	3,067[c]	2,403[c] (19 y)
Pregnancy			
14 through 18 y	Adolescent female EER plus change in Total Energy Expenditure (TEE) plus pregnancy energy deposition		
1st trimester			2,368 (16 y)
2nd trimester			2,708 (16 y)
3rd trimester			2,820 (16 y)
19 through 50 y	Adult female EER plus change in TEE plus pregnancy energy deposition		
1st trimester			2,403[c] (19 y)
2nd trimester			2,743[c] (19 y)
3rd trimester			2,855[c] (19 y)
Lactation			
14 through 18 y	Adolescent female EER plus milk energy output minus weight loss		
1st 6 mo			2,698 (16 y)
2nd 6 mo			2,768 (16 y)
19 through 50 y	Adult female EER plus milk energy output minus weight loss		
1st 6 mo			2,733[c] (19 y)
2nd 6 mo			2,803[c] (19 y)

[a]For healthy active Americans and Canadians. Based on the cited age, an active physical activity level, and the reference heights and weights cited in Table 1-1. Individualized EERs can be determined by using the equations in Chapter 5.

[b]PAL = Physical Activity Level, EER = Estimated Energy Requirement. The intake that meets the average energy expenditure of individuals at the reference height, weight, and age (see Table 1-1).

[c]Subtract 10 kcal/d for males and 7 kcal/d for females for each year of age above 19 years.

Dietary Reference Intakes (DRIs): DIETARY ALLOWANCES AND ADEQUATE INTAKES, TOTAL WATER AND MACRONUTRIENTS

Food and Nutrition Board, Institute of Medicine, National Academies

Life-Stage Group	Total Water (L/d)	Protein RDA/AI g/day[a]	AMDR[b]	Carbohydrate RDA/AI g/day	AMDR	Fiber RDA/AI g/day	AMDR[b]	Fat RDA/AI g/day	AMDR[b]	n-6 Polyunsaturated fatty acids (α-linoleic acid) RDA/AI g/day	AMDR[b]	n-3 Polyunsaturated fatty acids (α-linoleic acid) RDA/AI g/day	AMDR[d]
Infants													
0-6 mo	0.7*	9.1	ND[c]	60	ND	ND	ND	31		4.4*	ND	0.5*	ND
7-12 mo	0.8*	**11.0**	ND	95	ND	ND	ND	30		4.6*	ND	0.5*	ND
Children													
1-3 yr	1.3*	13	5-20	130	45-65	19*	ND	ND	30-40	7*	5-10	0.7*	0.6-1.2
4-8 yr	1.7*	19	10-30	130	45-65	25*	ND	ND	25-35	10*	5-10	0.9*	0.6-1.2
Males													
9-13 yr	2.4*	34	10-30	130	45-65	31*	ND	ND	25-35	12*	5-10	1.2*	0.6-1.2
14-18 yr	3.3*	52	10-30	130	45-65	38*	ND	ND	25-35	16*	5-10	1.6*	0.6-1.2
19-30 yr	3.7*	56	10-35	130	45-65	38*	ND	ND	20-35	17*	5-10	1.6*	0.6-1.2
31-50 yr	3.7*	56	10-35	130	45-65	38*	ND	ND	20-35	17*	5-10	1.6*	0.6-1.2
51-70 yr	3.7*	56	10-35	130	45-65	30*	ND	ND	20-35	14*	5-10	1.6*	0.6-1.2
>70 yr	3.7*	56	10-35	130	45-65	30*	ND	ND	20-35	14*	5-10	1.6*	0.6-1.2
Females													
9-13 yr	2.1*	34	10-30	130	45-65	26*	ND	ND	25-35	10*	5-10	1.0*	0.6-1.2
14-18 yr	2.3*	46	10-30	130	45-65	26*	ND	ND	25-35	11*	5-10	1.1*	0.6-1.2
19-30 yr	3.7*	46	10-35	130	45-65	25*	ND	ND	20-35	12*	5-10	1.1*	0.6-1.2
31-50 yr	3.7*	46	10-35	130	45-65	25*	ND	ND	20-35	12*	5-10	1.1*	0.6-1.2
51-70 yr	3.7*	46	10-35	130	45-65	21*	ND	ND	20-35	11*	5-10	1.1*	0.6-1.2
>70 yr	3.7*	46	10-35	130	45-65	21*	ND	ND	20-35	11*	5-10	1.1*	0.6-1.2
Pregnant													
≤18 yr	3.0*	71	10-35	175	45-65	28*	ND	ND	20-35	13*	5-10	1.4*	0.6-1.2
19-30 yr	3.0*	71	10-35	175	45-65	28*	ND	ND	20-35	13*	5-10	1.4*	0.6-1.2
31-50 yr	3.0*	71	10-35		45-65	28*	ND	ND	20-35	13*	5-10	1.4*	0.6-1.2
Lactating													
≤18 yr	3.8*	71	10-35	210	45-65	29*	ND	ND	20-35	13*	5-10	1.3*	0.6-1.2
19-30 yr	3.8*	71	10-35	210	45-65	29*	ND	ND	20-35	13*	5-10	1.3*	0.6-1.2
31-50 yr	3.8*	71	10-35	210	45-65	29*	ND	ND	20-35	13*	5-10	1.3*	0.6-1.2

Dietary cholesterol, trans fatty acids, saturated fatty acids: As low as possible while consuming a nutritionally adequate diet.

Added sugars: Limit to no more than 25% of total energy.[e]

Data from Dietary reference intakes for energy, carbohydrate, fiber, fat, fatty acids, cholesterol, protein, and amino acids. Washington, DC: The National Academies Press, 2002.

NOTE: This table represents Recommended Dietary Allowances (RDAs) in **bold type** and Adequate Intakes (AIs) in ordinary type. RDAs and AIs may both be used as goals for individual intake. RDAs are set to meet the needs of almost all (97%-98%) individuals in a group. For healthy breastfed infants, the AI is the mean intake. The AI for other life-stage and gender groups is believed to cover the needs of all individuals in the group, but lack of data prevents being able to specify with confidence the percentage of individuals covered by this intake.

[a]Based on 1.5 g/kg/day for infants, 1.1 g/kg/day for 1-3 yr; 0.95 g/kg/day for 4-13 yr; 0.85 g/kg/day for 14-18 yr; 0.8 g/kg/day for adults, and 1.1 g/kg/day for pregnant (using prepregnancy weight) and lactating women.

[b]Acceptable Macronutrient Distribution Range (AMDR) is the range of intake for a particular energy source that is associated with reduced risk of chronic disease while providing intakes of essential nutrients. If an individual has consumed in excess of the AMDR, there is a potential of increasing the risk of chronic diseases and insufficient intakes of essential nutrients.

[c]ND 5 Not determinable due to lack of data of adverse effects in this age group and concern with regard to lack of ability to handle excess amounts. Source of intake should be from food only to prevent high levels of intake.

[d]Approximately 10% of the total can come from longer-chain, n-3 fatty acids.

[e]Not a recommended intake. A daily intake of added sugars that individuals should aim for to achieve a healthful diet was not set.

Dietary Reference Intakes (DRIs): RECOMMENDED DIETARY ALLOWANCES AND ADEQUATE INTAKES, VITAMINS

Food and Nutrition Board, Institute of Medicine, National Academies

Life Stage Group	Vitamin A (µg/d)[a]	Vitamin C (mg/d)	Vitamin D (µg/d)[b,c]	Vitamin E (mg/d)[d]	Vitamin K (µg/d)	Thiamin (mg/d)	Riboflavin (mg/d)	Niacin (mg/d)[e]	Vitamin B6 (mg/d)	Folate (µg/d)[f]	Vitamin B12 (µg/d)	Pantothenic Acid (mg/d)	Biotin (µg/d)	Choline (mg/d)[g]
Infants														
0-6 mo	400*	40*	13	4*	2.0*	0.2*	0.3*	2*	0.1*	65*	0.4*	1.7*	5*	125*
7-12 mo	500*	50*	15	5*	2.5*	0.3*	0.4*	4*	0.3*	80*	0.5*	1.8*	6*	150*
Children														
1-3 y	300	15	15	6	30*	0.5	0.5	6	0.5	150	0.9	2*	8*	200*
4-8 y	400	25	15	7	55*	0.6	0.6	8	0.6	200	1.2	3*	12*	250*
Males														
9-13 y	600	45	15	11	60*	0.9	0.9	12	1.0	300	1.8	4*	20*	375*
14-18 y	900	75	15	15	75*	1.2	1.3	16	1.3	400	2.4	5*	25*	550*
19-30 y	900	90	15	15	120*	1.2	1.3	16	1.3	400	2.4	5*	30*	550*
31-50 y	900	90	15	15	120*	1.2	1.3	16	1.3	400	2.4	5*	30*	550*
51-70 y	900	90	15	15	120*	1.2	1.3	16	1.7	400	2.4[h]	5*	30*	550*
>70 y	900	90	20	15	120*	1.2	1.3	16	1.7	400	2.4[h]	5*	30*	550*
Females														
9-13 y	600	45	15	11	60*	0.9	0.9	12	1.0	300	1.8	4*	20*	375*
14-18 y	700	65	15	15	75*	1.0	1.0	14	1.2	400[i]	2.4	5*	25*	400*
19-30 y	700	75	15	15	90*	1.1	1.1	14	1.3	400[i]	2.4	5*	30*	425*
31-50 y	700	75	15	15	90*	1.1	1.1	14	1.3	400[i]	2.4	5*	30*	425*
51-70 y	700	75	15	15	90*	1.1	1.1	14	1.5	400	2.4[h]	5*	30*	425*
>70 y	700	75	20	15	90*	1.1	1.1	14	1.5	400	2.4[h]	5*	30*	425*
Pregnancy														
14-18 y	750	80	15	15	75*	1.4	1.4	18	1.9	600[j]	2.6	6*	30*	450*
19-30 y	770	85	15	15	90*	1.4	1.4	18	1.9	600[j]	2.6	6*	30*	450*
31-50 y	770	85	15	15	90*	1.4	1.4	18	1.9	600[j]	2.6	6*	30*	450*
Lactation														
14-18 y	1,200	115	15	19	75*	1.4	1.6	17	2.0	500	2.8	7*	35*	550*
19-30 y	1,300	120	15	19	90*	1.4	1.6	17	2.0	500	2.8	7*	35*	550*
31-50 y	1,300	120	15	19	90*	1.4	1.6	17	2.0	500	2.8	7*	35*	550*

SOURCES: Dietary Reference Intakes for Calcium, Phosphorous, Magnesium, Vitamin D, and Fluoride (1997); Dietary Reference Intakes for Thiamin, Riboflavin, Niacin, Vitamin B6, Folate, Vitamin B12, Pantothenic Acid, Biotin, and Choline (1998); Dietary Reference Intakes for Vitamin C, Vitamin E, Selenium, and Carotenoids (2000); Dietary Reference Intakes for Vitamin A, Vitamin K, Arsenic, Boron, Chromium, Copper, Iodine, Iron, Manganese, Molybdenum, Nickel, Silicon, Vanadium, and Zinc (2001); Dietary Reference Intakes for Water, Potassium, Sodium, Chloride, and Sulfate (2005); and Dietary Reference Intakes for Calcium and Vitamin D (2011). These reports may be accessed via www.nap.edu.

NOTE: This table (taken from the DRI reports, see www.nap.edu) presents Recommended Dietary Allowances (RDAs) in **bold type** and Adequate Intakes (AIs) in ordinary type followed by an asterisk (*). An RDA is the average daily dietary intake level; sufficient to meet the nutrient requirements of nearly all (97-98 percent) healthy individuals in a group. It is calculated from an Estimated Average Requirement (EAR). If sufficient scientific evidence is not available to establish an EAR, and thus calculate an RDA, an AI is usually developed. For healthy breastfed infants, an AI is the mean intake.
The AI for other life stage and gender groups is believed to cover the needs of all healthy individuals in the groups, but lack of data or uncertainty in the data prevent being able to specify with confidence the percentage of individuals covered by this intake.

[a] As retinol activity equivalents (RAEs). 1 RAE = 1 µg retinol, 12 µg β-carotene, 24 µg α-carotene, or 24 µg β-cryptoxanthin. The RAE for dietary provitamin A carotenoids is two-fold greater than retinol equivalents (RE), whereas the RAE for preformed vitamin A is the same as RE.

[b] As cholecalciferol. 1 µg cholecalciferol = 40 IU vitamin D.

[c] Under the assumption of minimal sunlight.

[d] As α-tocopherol. α-Tocopherol includes RRR-α-tocopherol, the only form of α-tocopherol that occurs naturally in foods, and the 2R-stereoisomeric forms of α-tocopherol (RRR-, RSR-, RRS-, and RSS-α-tocopherol) that occur in fortified foods and supplements. It does not include the 2S-stereoisomeric forms of α-tocopherol (SRR-, SSR-, SRS-, and SSS-α-tocopherol), also found in fortified foods and supplements.

[e] As niacin equivalents (NE). 1 mg of niacin = 60 mg of tryptophan; 0-6 months = preformed niacin (not NE).

[f] As dietary folate equivalents (DFE). 1 DFE = 1 µg food folate = 0.6 µg of folic acid from fortified food or as a supplement consumed with food = 0.5 µg of a supplement taken on an empty stomach.

[g] Although AIs have been set for choline, There are few data to assess whether a dietary supply of choline is needed at all stages of the life cycle, and it may be that the choline requirement can be met by endogenous synthesis at some of these stages.

[h] Because 10 to 30 percent of older people may malabsorb food-bound B12, it is advisable for those older than 50 years to meet their RDA mainly by consuming foods fortified with B12 or a supplement containing B12.

[i] In view of evidence linking folate intake with neural tube defects in the fetus, it is recommended that all women capable of becoming pregnant consume 400 µg from supplements or fortified foods in addition to intake of food folate from a varied diet.

[j] It is assumed that women will continue consuming 400 µg from supplements or fortified food until their pregnancy is confirmed and they enter prenatal care, which ordinarily occurs after the end of the periconceptional period—the critical time for formation of the neural tube.

Dietary Reference Intakes (DRIs): RECOMMENDED DIETARY ALLOWANCES AND ADEQUATE INTAKES, ELEMENTS

Food and Nutrition Board, Institute of Medicine-National Academies

Life Stage Group	Calcium (mg/d)	Chromium (µg/d)	Copper (µg/d)	Fluoride (mg/d)	Iodine (µg/d)	Iron (mg/d)	Magnesium (mg/d)
Infants							
0-6 mo	200*	0.2*	200*	0.01*	110*	0.27*	30*
7-12 mo	260*	5.5*	220*	0.5*	130*	11	75*
Children							
1-3 y	700*	11*	340	0.7*	90	7	80
4-8 y	1000*	15*	440	1*	90	10	130
Males							
9-13 y	1,300*	25*	700	2*	120	8	240
11-18 y	1,300*	35*	890	3*	150	11	410
19-30 y	1,000*	35*	900	4*	150	8	400
31-50 y	1,000*	35*	900	4*	150	8	420
51-70 y	1,200*	30*	900	4*	150	8	420
>70 y	1,200*	30*	900	4*	150	8	420
Females							
9-13 y	1,300*	21*	700	2*	120	8	240
14-18 y	1,300*	24*	890	3*	150	15	360
19-30 y	1,000*	25*	900	3*	150	18	310
31-50 y	1,000*	25*	900	3*	150	18	320
51-70 y	1,200*	20*	900	3*	150	8	320
>70 y	1,200*	20*	900	3*	150	8	320
Pregnancy							
≤18 y	1,300*	29*	1,000	3*	220	27	400
19-30 y	1,000*	30*	1,000	3*	220	27	350
31-50 y	1,000*	30*	1,000	3*	220	27	360
Lactation							
≤18 y	1,300*	11*	1,300	3*	290	10	360
19-30 y	1,000*	15*	1,300	3*	290	9	310
31-50 y	1,000*	45*	1,300	3*	290	9	320

SOURCES: Dietary Reference Intakes for Calcium, Phosphorous, Magnesium, Vitamin D, and Fluoride (1997); Dietary Reference Intakes for Thiamin, Riboflavin, Niacin, Vitamin B6, Folate, Vitamin B12, Pantothenic Acid, Biotin, and Choline (1998); Dietary Reference Intakes for Vitamin C, Vitamin E, Selenium, and Carotenoids (2000); Dietary Reference Intakes for Vitamin A, Vitamin K, Arsenic, Boron, Chromium, Copper, Iodine, Iron, Manganese, Molybdenum, Nickel, Silicon, Vanadium, and Zinc (2001); Dietary Reference Intakes for Water, Potassium, Sodium, Chloride, and Sulfate (2005); and Dietary Reference Intakes for Calcium and Vitamin D (2011). These reports may be accessed via www.nap.edu.

Dietary Reference Intakes (DRIs): ESTIMATED AVERAGE REQUIREMENTS
Food and Nutrition Board, Institute of Medicine, National Academies

Life Stage Group	Calcium (mg/d)	CHO (g/kg/d)	Protein (g/d)	Vit A (µg/d)[a]	Vit C (mg/d)	Vit D (µg/d)	Vit E (mg/d)[b]	Thiamin (mg/d)	Riboflavin (mg/d)	Niacin (mg/d)[c]	Vit B6 (mg/d)	Folate (µg/d)[d]	Vit B12 (µg/d)	Copper (µg/d)	Iodine (µg/d)	Iron (mg/d)	Magnesium (mg/d)	Molybdenum (µg/d)	Phosphorus (mg/d)	Selenium (µg/d)	Zinc (mg/d)
Infants																					
0-6 mo																					
7-12 mo			1.0													6.9					2.5
Children																					
1-3 y	500	100	0.87	210	13	10	5	0.4	0.4	5	0.4	120	0.7	260	65	3.0	65	13	380	17	2.5
4-8 y	800	100	0.76	275	22	10	6	0.5	0.5	6	0.5	160	1.0	340	65	4.1	110	17	405	23	4.0
Males																					
9-13 y	1,100	100	0.76	445	39	10	9	0.7	0.8	9	0.8	250	1.5	540	73	5.9	200	26	1,055	35	7.0
14-18 y	1,100	100	0.73	630	63	10	12	1.0	1.1	12	1.1	330	2.0	685	95	7.7	340	33	1,055	45	8.5
19-30 y	800	100	0.66	625	75	10	12	1.0	1.1	12	1.1	320	2.0	700	95	6	330	34	580	45	9.4
31-50 y	800	100	0.66	625	75	10	12	1.0	1.1	12	1.1	320	2.0	700	95	6	350	34	580	45	9.4
51-70 y	800	100	0.66	625	75	10	12	1.0	1.1	12	1.4	320	2.0	700	95	6	350	34	580	45	9.4
>70 y	1,000	100	0.66	625	75	10	12	1.0	1.1	12	1.4	320	2.0	700	95	6	350	34	580	45	9.4
Females																					
9-13 y	1,100	100	0.76	420	39	10	9	0.7	0.8	9	0.8	250	1.5	540	73	5.7	200	26	1,055	35	7.0
14-18 y	1,100	100	0.71	485	56	10	12	0.9	0.9	11	1.0	330	2.0	685	95	7.9	300	33	1,055	45	7.3
19-30 y	800	100	0.66	500	60	10	12	0.9	0.9	11	1.1	320	2.0	700	95	8.1	255	34	580	45	6.8
31-50 y	800	100	0.66	500	60	10	12	0.9	0.9	11	1.1	320	2.0	700	95	8.1	265	34	580	45	6.8
51-70 y	1,000	100	0.66	500	60	10	12	0.9	0.9	11	1.3	320	2.0	700	95	5	265	34	580	45	6.8
>70 y	1,000	100	0.66	500	60	10	12	0.9	0.9	11	1.3	320	2.0	700	95	5	265	34	580	45	6.8
Pregnancy																					
14-18 y	1,000	135	0.88	530	66	10	12	1.2	1.2	14	1.6	520	2.2	785	160	23	335	40	1,055	49	10.5
19-30 y	800	135	0.88	550	70	10	12	1.2	1.2	14	1.6	520	2.2	800	160	22	290	40	580	49	9.5
31-50 y	800	135	0.88	550	70	10	12	1.2	1.2	14	1.6	520	2.2	800	160	22	300	40	580	49	9.5
Lactation																					
14-18 y	1,000	160	1.05	885	96	10	16	1.2	1.3	13	1.7	450	2.4	985	209	7	300	35	1,055	59	10.9
19-30 y	800	160	1.05	900	100	10	16	1.2	1.3	13	1.7	450	2.4	1,000	209	6.5	255	36	580	59	10.4
31-50 y	800	160	1.05	900	100	10	16	1.2	1.3	13	1.7	450	2.4	1,000	209	6.5	265	36	580	59	10.44

SOURCES: Dietary Reference Intakes for Calcium, Phosphorous, Magnesium, Vitamin D, and Fluoride (1997); Dietary Reference Intakes for Thiamin, Riboflavin, Niacin, Vitamin B6, Folate, Vitamin B12, Pantothenic Acid, Biotin, and Choline (1998); Dietary Reference Intakes for Vitamin C, Vitamin E, Selenium, and Carotenoids (2000); Dietary Reference Intakes for Vitamin A, Vitamin K, Arsenic, Boron, Chromium, Copper, Iodine, Iron, Manganese, Molybdenum, Nickel, Silicon, Vanadium, and Zinc (2001); Dietary Reference Intakes for Energy, Carbohydrate, Fiber, Fat, Fatty Acids, Cholesterol, Protein, and Amino Acids (2002/2005); and Dietary Reference Intakes for Calcium and Vitamin D (2011). These reports may be accessed via www.nap.edu.

NOTE: An Estimated Average Requirement (EAR) is the average daily nutrient intake level estimated to meet the requirements of half of the healthy individuals in a group. EARs have not been established for vitamin K, pantothenic acid, biotin, choline, chromium, fluoride, manganese, or other nutrients not yet evaluated via the DRI process.

[a]As retinol activity equivalents (RAEs). 1 RAE = 1 µg retinol, 12 µg β-carotene, 24 µg α-carotene, or 24 µg β-cryptoxanthin. The RAE for dietary provitamin A carotenoids is two-fold greater than retinol equivalents (RE), whereas the RAE for preformed vitamin A is the same as RE.

[b]As α-tocopherol. α-Tocopherol includes RRR-α-tocopherol, the only form of α-tocopherol that occurs naturally in foods, and the 2R-stereoisomeric forms of α-tocopherol (RRR-, RSR-, RRS-, and RSS-α-tocopherol) that occur in fortified foods and supplements. It does not include the 2S-stereoisomeric forms of α-tocopherol (SRR-, SSR-, SRS-, and SSS-α-tocopherol), also found in fortified foods and supplements.

[c]As niacin equivalents (NE). 1 mg of niacin = 60 mg of tryptophan.

[d]As dietary folate equivalents (DFE). 1 DFE = 1 µg food folate = 0.6 µg of folic acid from fortified food or as a supplement consumed with food = 0.5 µg of a supplement taken on an empty stomach.

Mahan LK, Escott-Stump S, Raymond JL: Krause's food and the nutrition care process, ed 13, St. Louis, 2012, Saunders.

Dietary Reference Intakes (DRIs): TOLERABLE UPPER INTAKE LEVELS, VITAMINS
Food and Nutrition Board, Institute of Medicine, National Academies

Life Stage Group	Vitamin A (µg/d)[a]	Vitamin C (mg/d)	Vitamin D (µg/d)	Vitamin E (mg/d)[b,c]	Vitamin K	Thiamin	Riboflavin	Niacin (mg/d)[c]	Vitamin B6 (mg/d)	Folate (µg/d)[c]	Vitamin B12	Pantothenic Acid	Biotin	Choline (g/d)	Carotenoids[d]
Infants															
0-6 mo	600	ND[e]	25	ND	ND	ND	ND	ND	ND	ND	ND	ND	ND	ND	ND
7-12 mo	600	ND	38	ND	ND	ND	ND	ND	ND	ND	ND	ND	ND	ND	ND
Children															
1-3 y	600	400	63	200	ND	ND	ND	10	30	300	ND	ND	ND	1.0	ND
4-8 y	900	650	75	300	ND	ND	ND	15	40	400	ND	ND	ND	1.0	ND
Males															
9-13 y	1,700	1,200	100	600	ND	ND	ND	20	60	600	ND	ND	ND	2.0	ND
14-18 y	2,800	1,800	100	800	ND	ND	ND	30	80	800	ND	ND	ND	3.0	ND
19-30 y	3,000	2,000	100	1,000	ND	ND	ND	35	100	1,000	ND	ND	ND	3.5	ND
31-50 y	3,000	2,000	100	1,000	ND	ND	ND	35	100	1,000	ND	ND	ND	3.5	ND
51-70 y	3,000	2,000	100	1,000	ND	ND	ND	35	100	1,000	ND	ND	ND	3.5	ND
>70 y	3,000	2,000	100	1,000	ND	ND	ND	35	100	1,000	ND	ND	ND	3.5	ND
Females															
9-13 y	1,700	1,200	100	600	ND	ND	ND	20	60	600	ND	ND	ND	2.0	ND
14-18 y	2,800	1,800	100	800	ND	ND	ND	30	80	800	ND	ND	ND	3.0	ND
19-30 y	3,000	2,000	100	1,000	ND	ND	ND	35	100	1,000	ND	ND	ND	3.5	ND
31-50 y	3,000	2,000	100	1,000	ND	ND	ND	35	100	1,000	ND	ND	ND	3.5	ND
51-70 y	3,000	2,000	100	1,000	ND	ND	ND	35	100	1,000	ND	ND	ND	3.5	ND
>70 y	3,000	2,000	100	1,000	ND	ND	ND	35	100	1,000	ND	ND	ND	3.5	ND
Pregnancy															
14-18 y	2,800	1,800	100	800	ND	ND	ND	30	80	800	ND	ND	ND	3.0	ND
19-30 y	3,000	2,000	100	1,000	ND	ND	ND	35	100	1,000	ND	ND	ND	3.5	ND
31-50 y	3,000	2,000	100	1,000	ND	ND	ND	35	100	1,000	ND	ND	ND	3.5	ND
Lactation															
14-18 y	2,800	1,800	100	800	ND	ND	ND	30	80	800	ND	ND	ND	3.0	ND
19-30 y	3,000	2,000	100	1,000	ND	ND	ND	35	100	1,000	ND	ND	ND	3.5	ND
31-50 y	3,000	2,000	100	1,000	ND	ND	ND	35	100	1,000	ND	ND	ND	3.5	ND

SOURCES: Dietary Reference Intakes for Calcium, Phosphorous, Magnesium, Vitamin D, and Fluoride (1997); Dietary Reference Intakes for Thiamin, Riboflavin, Niacin, Vitamin B6, Folate, Vitamin B12, Pantothenic Acid, Biotin, and Choline (1998); Dietary Reference Intakes for Vitamin C, Vitamine E, Selenium, and Carotenoids (2000); Dietary Reference Intakes for Vitamin A, Vitamin K, Arsenic, Boron, Chromium, Copper, Iodine, Iron, Manganese, Molybdenum, Nickel, Silicon, Vanadium, and Zinc (2001); and Dietary Reference Intakes for Calcium and Vitamin D (2011). These reports may be accessed via www.nap.edu.

NOTE: A Tolerable Upper Intake Level (UL) is the highest level of daily nutrient intake that is likely to pose no risk of adverse health effects to almost all individuals in the general population. Unless otherwise specified, the UL represents total intake from food, water, and supplements. Due to a lack of suitable data, ULs could not be established for vitamin K, thiamin, riboflavin, vitamin B12, pantothenic acid, biotin, and carotenoids. In the absence of a UL, extra caution may be warranted in consuming levels above recommended intakes. Members of the general population should be advised not to routinely exceed the UL. The UL is not meant to apply to individuals who are treated with the nutrient under medical supervision or to individuals with predisposing conditions that modify their sensitivity to the nutrient.

[a]As preformed vitamin A only.

[b]As α-tocopherol; applies to any form of supplemental α-tocopherol.

[c]The ULs for vitamin E, niacin, and folate apply to synthetic forms obtained from supplements, fortified foods, or a combination of the two.

[d]β-Carotene supplements are advised only to serve as a provitamin A source for individuals at risk of vitamin A deficiency.

[e]ND = Not determinable due to lack of data of adverse effects in this age group and concern with regard to lack of ability to handle excess amounts. Source of intake should be from food only to prevent high levels of intake.

Dietary Reference Intakes (DRIs): TOLERABLE UPPER INTAKE LEVELS, ELEMENTS

Food and Nutrition Board, Institute of Medicine, National Academies

Life Stage Group	Arsenic[a]	Boron (mg/d)	Calcium (mg/d)	Chromium	Copper (µg/d)	Fluoride (mg/d)	Iodine (µg/d)	Iron (mg/d)	Magnesium (mg/d)[b]	Manganese (mg/d)	Molybdenum (µg/d)	Nickel (mg/d)	Phosphorus (g/d)	Selenium (µg/d)	Silicon[c]	Vanadium (mg/d)[d]	Zinc (mg/d)	Sodium (g/d)	Chloride (g/d)
Infants																			
0-6 mo	ND[e]	ND	1,000	ND	ND	0.7	ND	40	ND	ND	ND	ND	ND	45	ND	ND	4	ND	ND
7-12 mo	ND	ND	1,500	ND	ND	0.9	ND	40	ND	ND	ND	ND	ND	60	ND	ND	5	ND	ND
Children																			
1-3 y	ND	3	2,500	ND	1,000	1.3	200	40	65	2	300	0.2	3.0	90	ND	ND	7	1.5	2.3
4-8 y	ND	6	2,500	ND	3,000	2.2	300	40	110	3	600	0.3	3.0	150	ND	ND	12	1.9	2.9
Males																			
9-13 y	ND	11	3,000	ND	5,000	10	600	40	350	6	1,100	0.6	4.0	280	ND	ND	23	2.2	3.4
14-18 y	ND	17	3,000	ND	8,000	10	900	45	350	9	1,700	1.0	4.0	400	ND	ND	34	2.3	3.6
19-30 y	ND	20	2,500	ND	10,000	10	1,100	45	350	11	2,000	1.0	4.0	400	ND	1.8	40	2.3	3.6
31-50 y	ND	20	2,500	ND	10,000	10	1,100	45	350	11	2,000	1.0	4.0	400	ND	1.8	40	2.3	3.6
51-70 y	ND	20	2,000	ND	10,000	10	1,100	45	350	11	2,000	1.0	4.0	400	ND	1.8	40	2.3	3.6
>70 y	ND	20	2,000	ND	10,000	10	1,100	45	350	11	2,000	1.0	3.0	400	ND	1.8	40	2.3	3.6
Females																			
9-13 y	ND	11	3,000	ND	5,000	10	600	40	350	6	1,100	0.6	4.0	280	ND	ND	23	2.2	3.4
14-18 y	ND	17	3,000	ND	8,000	10	900	45	350	9	1,700	1.0	4.0	400	ND	ND	34	2.3	3.6
19-30 y	ND	20	2,500	ND	10,000	10	1,100	45	350	11	2,000	1.0	4.0	400	ND	1.8	40	2.3	3.6
31-50 y	ND	20	2,500	ND	10,000	10	1,100	45	350	11	2,000	1.0	4.0	400	ND	1.8	40	2.3	3.6
51-70 y	ND	20	2,000	ND	10,000	10	1,100	45	350	11	2,000	1.0	4.0	400	ND	1.8	40	2.3	3.6
>70 y	ND	20	2,000	ND	10,000	10	1,100	45	350	11	2,000	1.0	3.0	400	ND	1.8	40	2.3	3.6
Pregnancy																			
14-18 y	ND	17	3,000	ND	8,000	10	900	45	350	9	1,700	1.0	3.5	400	ND	ND	34	2.3	3.6
19-30 y	ND	20	2,500	ND	10,000	10	1,100	45	350	11	2,000	1.0	3.5	400	ND	ND	40	2.3	3.6
31-50 y	ND	20	2,500	ND	10,000	10	1,100	45	350	11	2,000	1.0	3.5	400	ND	ND	40	2.3	3.6
Lactation																			
14-18 y	ND	17	3,000	ND	8,000	10	900	45	350	9	1,700	1.0	4.0	400	ND	ND	34	2.3	3.6
19-30 y	ND	20	2,500	ND	10,000	10	1,100	45	350	11	2,000	1.0	4.0	400	ND	ND	40	2.3	3.6
31-50 y	ND	20	2,500	ND	10,000	10	1,100	45	350	11	2,000	1.0	4	400	ND	ND	40	2.3	3.6

SOURCES: Dietary Reference Intakes for Calcium, Phosphorous, Magnesium, Vitamin D, and Fluoride (1997); Dietary Reference Intakes for Thiamin, Riboflavin, Niacin, Vitamin B6, Folate, Vitamin B12, Pantothenic Acid, Biotin, and Choline (1998); Dietary Reference Intakes for Vitamin C, Vitamin E, Selenium, and Carotenoids (2000); Dietary Reference Intakes for Vitamin A, Vitamin K, Arsenic, Boron, Chromium, Copper, Iodine, Iron, Manganese, Molybdenum, Nickel, Silicon, Vanadium, and Zinc (2001); Dietary Reference Intakes for Water, Potassium, Sodium, Chloride, and Sulfate (2005); and Dietary Reference Intakes for Calcium and Vitamin D (2011). These reports may be accessed via www.nap.edu.

NOTE: A Tolerable Upper Intake Level (UL) is the highest level of daily nutrient intake that is likely to pose no risk of adverse health effects to almost all individuals in the general population. Unless otherwise specified, the UL represents total intake from food, water, and supplements. Due to a lack of suitable data, ULs could not be established for vitamin K, thiamin, riboflavin, vitamin B12, pantothenic acid, biotin, and carotenoids. In the absence of a UL, extra caution may be warranted in consuming levels above recommended intakes. Members of the general population should be advised not to routinely exceed the UL. The UL is not meant to apply to individuals who are treated with the nutrient under medical supervision or to individuals with predisposing conditions that modify their sensitivity to the nutrient.

[a] Although the UL was not determined for arsenic, there is no justification for adding arsenic to food or supplements.

[b] The ULs for magnesium represent intake from a pharmacological agent only and do not include intake from food and water.

[c] Although silicon has not been shown to cause adverse effects in humans, there is no justification for adding silicon to supplements.

[d] Although vanadium in food has not been shown to cause adverse effects in humans, there is no justification for adding vanadium to food and vanadium supplements should be used with caution. The UL is based on adverse effects in laboratory animals and this data could be used to set a UL for adults but not children and adolescents.

[e] ND = Not determinable due to lack of data of adverse effects in this age group and concern with regard to lack of ability to handle excess amounts. Source of intake should be from food only to prevent high levels of intake.

Body Mass Index Table

Normal: BMI 19–24 · Overweight: BMI 25–29 · Obese: BMI 30–39 · Extreme Obesity: BMI 40–54

Body Weight (pounds)

Height (inches) / BMI	19	20	21	22	23	24	25	26	27	28	29	30	31	32	33	34	35	36	37	38	39	40	41	42	43	44	45	46	47	48	49	50	51	52	53	54
58	91	96	100	105	110	115	119	124	129	134	138	143	148	153	158	162	167	172	177	181	186	191	196	201	205	210	215	220	224	229	234	239	244	248	253	258
59	94	99	104	109	114	119	124	128	133	138	143	148	153	158	163	168	173	178	183	188	193	198	203	208	212	217	222	227	232	237	242	247	252	257	262	267
60	97	102	107	112	118	123	128	133	138	143	148	153	158	163	168	174	179	184	189	194	199	204	209	215	220	225	230	235	240	245	250	255	261	266	271	276
61	100	106	111	116	122	127	132	137	143	148	153	158	164	169	174	180	185	190	195	201	206	211	217	222	227	232	238	243	248	254	259	264	269	275	280	285
62	104	109	115	120	126	131	136	142	147	153	158	164	169	175	180	186	191	196	202	207	213	218	224	229	235	240	246	251	256	262	267	273	278	284	289	295
63	107	113	118	124	130	135	141	146	152	158	163	169	175	180	186	191	197	203	208	214	220	225	231	237	242	248	254	259	265	270	278	282	287	293	299	304
64	110	116	122	128	134	140	145	151	157	163	169	174	180	186	192	197	204	209	215	221	227	232	238	244	250	256	262	267	273	279	285	291	296	302	308	314
65	114	120	126	132	138	144	150	156	162	168	174	180	186	192	198	204	210	216	222	228	234	240	246	252	258	264	270	276	282	288	294	300	306	312	318	324
66	118	124	130	136	142	148	155	161	167	173	179	186	192	198	204	210	216	223	229	235	241	247	253	260	266	272	278	284	291	297	303	309	315	322	328	334
67	121	127	134	140	146	153	159	166	172	178	185	191	198	204	211	217	223	230	236	242	249	255	261	268	274	280	287	293	299	306	312	319	325	331	338	344
68	125	131	138	144	151	158	164	171	177	184	190	197	203	210	216	223	230	236	243	249	256	262	269	276	282	289	295	302	308	315	322	328	335	341	348	354
69	128	135	142	149	155	162	169	176	182	189	196	203	209	216	223	230	236	243	250	257	263	270	277	284	291	297	304	311	318	324	331	338	345	351	358	365
70	132	139	146	153	160	167	174	181	188	195	202	209	216	222	229	236	243	250	257	264	271	278	285	292	299	306	313	320	327	334	341	348	355	362	369	376
71	136	143	150	157	165	172	179	186	193	200	208	215	222	229	236	243	250	257	265	272	279	286	293	301	308	315	322	329	338	343	351	358	365	372	379	386
72	140	147	154	162	169	177	184	191	199	206	213	221	228	235	242	250	258	265	272	279	287	294	302	309	316	324	331	338	346	353	361	368	375	383	390	397
73	144	151	159	166	174	182	189	197	204	212	219	227	235	242	250	257	265	272	280	288	295	302	310	318	325	333	340	348	355	363	371	378	386	393	401	408
74	148	155	163	171	179	186	194	202	210	218	225	233	241	249	256	264	272	280	287	295	303	311	319	326	334	342	350	358	365	373	381	389	396	404	412	420
75	152	160	168	176	184	192	200	208	216	224	232	240	248	256	264	272	279	287	295	303	311	319	327	335	343	351	359	367	375	383	391	399	407	415	423	431
76	156	164	172	180	189	197	205	213	221	230	238	246	254	263	271	279	287	295	304	312	320	328	336	344	353	361	369	377	385	394	402	410	418	426	435	443

SOURCE: Adapted from Clinical Guidelines on the Identification, Evaluation, and Treatment of Overweight and Obesity in Adults: The Evidence Report.

edition **4**

The Dental Hygienist's Guide to
Nutritional
CARE

Cynthia A. Stegeman, RDH, EdD, RDN, LD, CDE
Ohio Delegate to the Academy of Nutrition and Dietetics
Associate Professor, Dental Hygiene Program
University of Cincinnati
Cincinnati, Ohio

Judi Ratliff Davis, MS, RDN
Former Quality Assurance Nutrition Consultant
Women, Infants and Children (WIC) Program
Texas Department of State Health Services
Austin, Texas

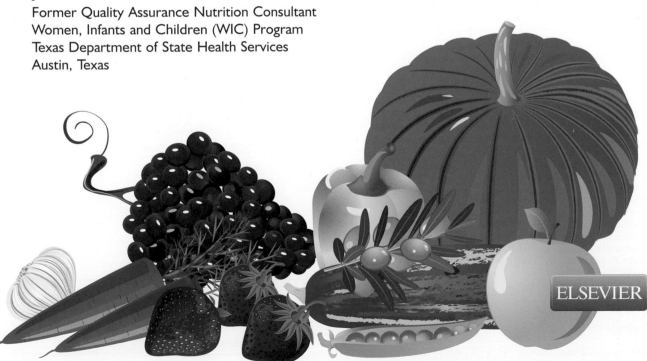

ELSEVIER

3251 Riverport Lane
St. Louis, Missouri 63043

Notices

Knowledge and best practice in this field are constantly changing. As new research and experience broaden our understanding, changes in research methods, professional practices, or medical treatment may become necessary.

Practitioners and researchers must always rely on their own experience and knowledge in evaluating and using any information, methods, compounds, or experiments described herein. In using such information or methods they should be mindful of their own safety and the safety of others, including parties for whom they have a professional responsibility.

With respect to any drug or pharmaceutical products identified, readers are advised to check the most current information provided (i) on procedures featured or (ii) by the manufacturer of each product to be administered, to verify the recommended dose or formula, the method and duration of administration, and contraindications. It is the responsibility of practitioners, relying on their own experience and knowledge of their patients, to make diagnoses, to determine dosages and the best treatment for each individual patient, and to take all appropriate safety precautions.

To the fullest extent of the law, neither the Publisher nor the authors, contributors, or editors, assume any liability for any injury and/or damage to persons or property as a matter of products liability, negligence or otherwise, or from any use or operation of any methods, products, instructions, or ideas contained in the material herein.

Library of Congress Cataloging-in-Publication Data

Stegeman, Cynthia A., author.
 The dental hygienist's guide to nutritional care / Cynthia A. Stegeman, Judith Ratliff Davis.—Edition 4.
  p. ; cm.
 Includes bibliographical references and index.
 ISBN 978-1-4557-3765-9 (pbk. : alk. paper)
 I. Davis, Judi Ratliff, author.   II. Title.
 [DNLM: 1. Nutritional Requirements.   2. Oral Health.   3. Dental Hygienists.   WU 113.7]
 RK60.7
 617.6'01—dc23
                                                                          2013042535

Vice President and Publisher: Linda Duncan
Executive Content Strategist: Kathy Falk
Content Strategist: Kristin Wilhelm
Content Development Specialist: Joslyn Dumas
Publishing Services Manager: Julie Eddy
Senior Project Manager: Celeste Clingan
Design Direction: Karen Pauls

Working together
to grow libraries in
developing countries

www.elsevier.com • www.bookaid.org

Printed in China

Last digit is the print number: 9 8 7 6 5 4 3 2

This 4th edition is dedicated to all of the dental hygiene students, faculty and practitioners throughout the world who use this text. Your curiosity and desire to gain evidence-based information regarding the role of nutrition in oral health continues to guide this text.

Cyndee and Judi

and

To my husband, son, family and dental hygiene and dietetic colleagues for their encouragement, support, visions and humor.

Cyndee

and

To my family, especially my 5 granddaughters: Riley, Avery, Ellie, Maggie, and Callie.

Judi

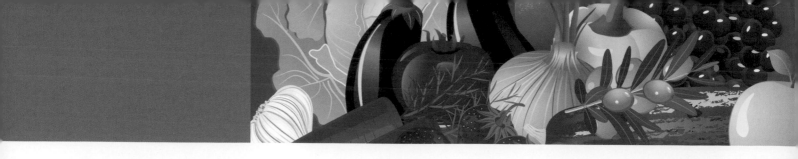

Preface

The study of nutrition is an interesting and rewarding topic for dental hygiene students, not only as it relates to patient education, but also for how it can affect the dental hygienist's own health. *The Dental Hygienist's Guide to Nutritional Care* is designed to show both dental hygiene students and practicing professionals how to apply sound nutrition principles when assessing, diagnosing, planning, implementing, and evaluating the total care of patients, as well as to help them contribute to the nutritional well-being of patients. *The Academy of Nutrition and Dietetics, American Dental Hygienists' Association and American Dental Association* each recognize nutrition as an integral component of oral health. The dental professional should be able to assess the oral cavity in relation to the patient's nutrition, dietary habits, and overall health status. A holistic approach to dietary management of a disease by all members of the healthcare team is especially appropriate to coordinate managed health care.

Since the subject of nutrition is a top priority in today's world, the consumer is challenged to comprehend and apply the overwhelming amount of nutritional information that can be confusing and conflicting. As the health source that patients may see most often, the dental professional should be able to knowledgeably and authoritatively discuss nutritional practices with his or her patients or provide appropriate referrals as needed.

NEW TO THIS EDITION

In this expertly revised edition you will find information on the most recent developments in the field including:

- *2010 Dietary Guidelines for Americans* and *MyPlate*
- Role of biochemistry in dental hygiene and nutrition with an expanded version located in Evolve
- Recent research surrounding vitamin D, a prevalent vitamin deficiency in the United States
- Recent research on Recommended Dietary Allowance (RDA) and Tolerable Upper Intake Level (UL) for calcium
- Health Applications in all chapters: **Gluten, Human Papillomavirus, Genetically Modified Foods, Smoking Cessation and Health Literacy**
- **Motivational Interviewing** for effectively communicating nutrition information to dental patients

Also included with the fourth edition is the addition of new and expanded **Evolve** resources. A complete listing of the material available on Evolve can be found in the *About Evolve* section of the preface.

ORGANIZATION

Part I, Orientation to Basic Nutrition, deals with basic principles of nutrition. A basic understanding of fundamental nutrition facts enables the dental hygienist to make wise judgments about eating habits, educate patients about needed dietary changes, and evaluate the flood of new information available. Nutrient deficiencies and excesses are addressed in sections entitled *Hyper-States* and *Hypo-States*, terms that are more congruent with real-life occurrences. Chapters addressing vitamins and minerals are arranged separately to cover the specific nutrients involved in oral calcified structures or oral soft tissues. A new chapter, *Concepts in Biochemistry*, introduces a basic understanding of biochemistry, the foundation for understanding and applying principles of nutrition. This chapter serves as a valuable resource throughout the textbook.

Part II, Considerations of Clinical Nutrition, addresses problems specifically involved in the application of basic nutrition principles through the lifespan and within ethnic groups. This helps the dental hygienist to recognize that food choices different from his or her own food patterns may actually be nutritionally healthy. By approaching any necessary modifications with sensitivity and respect, patients are more likely to make suggested changes. Alterations in nutritional requirements and eating patterns affected by various stages of life, specifically females, infants and children, and older adults, are discussed.

Part III, Nutritional Aspects of Oral Health, looks at factors involved in oral problems and the nutritional treatment of these problems. In these chapters, *Dental Considerations* and *Nutritional Directions* boxes provide specific information to consider during an assessment and educational dialogue by the dental professional including: (1) *physical* status and *dietary* habits; (2) *interventions*, or factors that need to be considered when caring for the patient; and (3) *evaluations* concerning the patient's ability or motivation to make changes based on what he or she has learned during the appointment with the dental hygienist. A nutritional assessment is a basic essential for the nutritional well-being of all patients and this involves performing a medical and dental assessment, evaluating dietary intake/history, and educating patients about recommended changes in food choices. Many conditions or their outcome are improved by encouraging patients to eat a wide variety of foods and beverages in appropriate portion sizes or to make minor changes in food choices to improve their health.

A variety of features throughout the text help to enhance the learning experience:

- **Student Learning Outcomes**: A list of outcomes accompanies each chapter to provide a guide to the important information to acquire from the chapter.
- **Key Terms**: A list of unfamiliar terms for each chapter; terms are **bolded and blue** in the text where they are defined and are also compiled in the **Glossary** for easy reference.
- **Test Your NQ** (nutrition quotient): An initial true-false pretest stimulates interest in the reading assignment; answers are conveniently located in the back of the book and on Evolve.
- **Dental Considerations**: Practical information that can affect the patient's care or nutritional status.
- **Nutritional Directions**: Information the patient should know or be taught to improve oral health and overall health status. The educational information can be used when discussing improvement of oral health, food choices, and/or overall health status with the patient.
- **Health Applications**: Each chapter covers current "hot topics" in nutrition including the ways a vegetarian can obtain an adequate balance of nutrients, causes and treatment of obesity, and use of vitamin and mineral supplements.
- **Case Application**: Potential patient situations describing a clinical situation and providing the five-step care plan to help "pull it all together."
- **Student Readiness:** Questions at the end of each chapter help students determine their comprehension of the subject.
- **Case Studies:** Practice case studies help students test their ability to make sound judgments when faced with real-life patient scenarios.

ABOUT EVOLVE

The expanded Evolve website offers a variety of additional learning tools that greatly enhances the text for both students and instructors.

For the Student

Evolve Student Resources offers the following:

- **Practice Quizzes.** Approximately 400 National Board Dental Hygiene Examination-style questions separated by chapter with instant-feedback answers, rationales, and page number references for remediation.
- **Illustrated Case Studies.** Written scenarios with accompanying photographs and follow-up questions present situations that may be encountered in practice. An excellent review source for the National Board Dental Hygiene Examination.
- **Nutritrac Nutrition Analysis Version 5.0**: An online tool that allows users to analyze specifics of food intake and

energy expenditure, manage weight loss and gain goals, and analyze nutrition and weight status.

- **Food Pyramids and Guides from Around the World.** Food pyramids and guides from a variety of countries including Mexico, Puerto Rico, the Philippines, Korea, China, Canada, Great Britain, Germany, Australia, Portugal, and Sweden. Also included are the Native American Food Pyramid and the Healthy Eating Plate (©Harvard University), Vegetarian Food Pyramid, My Vegan Plate, and MyPlate for Older Adults (©Tufts University).
- **Food Diary and Food Analysis Forms.** Printable versions of the forms needed to complete the Personal Assessment Project. Also included are printable versions of the Carbohydrate Intake Analysis and Menu Planning Record.
- **MNA Mini Nutritional Assessment.** A validated nutrition screening tool that can assess for malnutrition in patients 65 years and older.
- **Weblinks.** A variety of weblinks provide additional means of study and research.
- **Supplemental Material.** Reference material for additional education in a printable format.

For the Instructor

Evolve Instructor Resources offers the following:

- **Testbank.** An extensive testbank makes the creation of quizzes and exams much easier.
- **PowerPoint Presentations.** Presentations that provide ready-made lectures compliant with the content found in the text.
- **Image Collection.** An image collection that includes all the illustrations from the textbook, making it easy to incorporate a photo or drawing into a lecture or quiz.
- **Personal Assessment Project.** A classroom learning activity designed to help students objectively assess their own personal dietary patterns, practice the process of recording and analyzing food intake for its nutritive and cariogenic value, and use nutritional and dental knowledge to contribute to better general and oral health for self and patients.
- **Classroom Learning Activities.** A variety of interactive learning activities that can be incorporated into class to stimulate discussion and teamwork.

NOTE FROM THE AUTHORS

With a better understanding of the importance of food choices, the members of a multidiscipline healthcare team can complement each other and provide optimal care for the patient. Even though specific amounts of nutrients are mentioned, the intent of this text is not for prescriptive use. Instead, its purpose is to provide dental hygiene students and practicing dental professionals with a relative idea of the amounts of various nutrients needed so viable food sources can be recommended.

Cynthia A. Stegeman
Judi Ratliff Davis

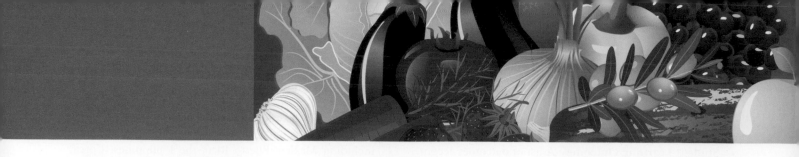

Acknowledgements

Because of the diversity of subjects presented in a general nutrition textbook, a compilation of the work of many people, whether direct or indirect, is necessary to present current and evidence-based information. Whether the aid was in the area of a research study or was verbal or written communications, each person's help and support is truly appreciated.

Our sincere thanks to Barbara Altshuler, Assistant Professor Emeritus, Caruth School of Dental Hygiene, Baylor College of Dentistry, who "birthed" this nutrition textbook for dental hygienists and took this baby to W.B. Saunders to develop a resource for dental hygienists to assess the nutritional status of their patients. While your "early retirement" is a true loss to the dental hygiene profession, we hope you are enjoying your family time.

It takes a team of experts to complete a textbook. We would like to acknowledge the hard work of Dr. Scott Tremain, Assistant Professor in the Department of Chemistry at the University of Cincinnati for creating a practical and usable chapter in biochemistry. Condensing complex information into one chapter is quite a feat. Another valuable and new contributor to this edition of the textbook is Dr. Amy Sullivan, RDH, Associate Professor and Dental Hygiene Admissions Chair at the University of Mississippi Medical Center. She worked diligently to improve Chapters 18 to 21. Beside her knowledge in dental issues, her excellent photos provide a wonderful addition to the text. We also thank her dental hygiene students for their participation in the photos to demonstrate various education concepts. Special thanks to the dental hygiene faculty, staff, and students at the University of Cincinnati for their encouragement, expertise, and provision of research. Their consistent support and praise make the monumental task of updating a nutrition textbook easier and rewarding

A special thanks to the librarians at the Texas Department of State Health Services, Carolyn Medina and David McLellan, who were superb at locating scientific references for "dramatic findings" publicized by the press. In addition to those listed, there are countless other friends and relatives to whom we wish to express our gratitude for their encouragement and support.

Objective critiques from reviewers are invaluable to a good publication. We appreciate the insight, perspective, words of encouragement, and valuable ideas of the following reviewers: Lisa F. Harper Mallonee, BSDH, MPH, RD, LD, Baylor College of Dentistry, Dallas, Texas, and Jodi Olmsted, RDH, Ph.D, School of Health Care Professions, University of Wisconsin, Stevens Point.

In addition, we appreciate the editing "eagle eye" of Luke Burroughs, RDH, a graduate of the University of Cincinnati dental hygiene program. He is currently working on a Master of Public Health at New Mexico State University.

We also wish to thank the many staff at Elsevier who worked so tirelessly in the various phases of planning and producing this book. We are especially grateful to Kristin Wilhelm, Content Strategist, and Joslyn Dumas, Content Development Strategist, for their helpful ideas and for seeing us through this project.

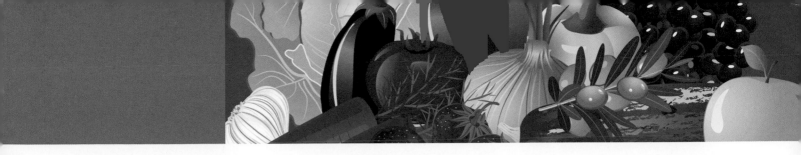

About the Authors

Cynthia A. Stegeman, RDH, EdD, RDN, LD, CDE is an Associate Professor in the Dental Hygiene Program at the University of Cincinnati. She has taught Nutrition and Health Education for over 25 years. Dr. Stegeman has been a dental hygienist for over 30 years and a long-time member of the American Dental Hygienists' Association and the Academy of Nutrition and Dietetics. She is currently the Ohio delegate to the Academy of Nutrition and Dietetics. She is also a Certified Diabetes Educator and practices as a dietitian in diabetes education. In addition, she speaks to numerous community and professional groups and has written over 80 publications on nutrition and dentistry. Dr. Stegeman received an Associate of Applied Science in Dental Hygiene from the University of Cincinnati; Bachelor of Science in Public Health Dentistry from Indiana University Purdue University at Indianapolis; Master of Education in Nutrition from the University of Cincinnati; Dietetic internship from The Christ Hospital in Cincinnati; and Doctorate of Education in Instructional Design and Technology from the University of Cincinnati.

Judi Ratliff Davis, MS, RDN lives in Austin, Texas, and retired from the Texas Department of State Health Services as a Quality Assurance Nutrition Consultant for the Women, Infants and Children (WIC) program. She is very active in service organizations in her community—Lake Travis Crisis Ministry, Healthcare Volunteer Associates Clinic, Lake Travis Mobile Meals, and Austin Disaster Relief Network. She has been an active member of the Academy of Nutrition and Dietetics for 47 years. She has had a variety of experiences in the field of nutrition, including teaching, clinical dietitian, and consultant. She has taught various nutrition and food service courses at Tarrant County College in Fort Worth, Texas. Her roles as a clinical dietitian include Home-Based Community Support, Tarrant County Mental Health Mental Retardation; Rehabilitation Hospital of North Texas, Arlington, Texas; Fort Worth State School, Fort Worth, Texas; Rex Hospital in Raleigh, North Carolina; and Baptist Memorial Hospital in San Antonio, Texas. She has also worked as a nutrition consultant for nursing homes and mental health facilities in western Virginia, San Antonio, and the Dallas-Fort Worth area, for the Greenhouse, a health spa in Arlington, Texas, and the Sugar Association. She is also the author of the nursing textbook *Applied Nutrition and Diet Therapy for Nurses*. She received her Bachelor of Science degree from the University of Texas in Foods and Nutrition, Austin; Master of Science degree in Nutrition from Texas Woman's University, Denton; and completed a dietetic internship at Indiana University Medical Center, Indianapolis.

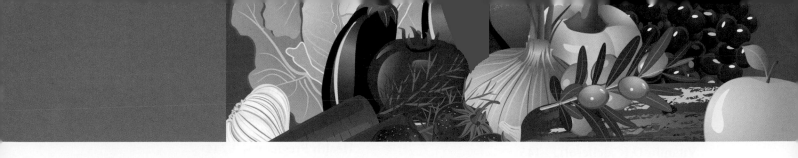

Contents

Part 1 Orientation to Basic Nutrition

1 Overview of Healthy Eating Habits, 2
  Basic Nutrition, 3
  Physiological Functions of Nutrients, 4
  Basic Concepts of Nutrition, 4
  Government Nutrition Concerns, 5
  Nutrient Recommendations: Dietary Reference
    Intakes, 5
  Food Guidance Systems for Americans, 6
  Dietary Guidelines for Americans, 2010, 7
  Myplate System, 16
  Other Food Guides, 20
  Nutrition Labeling, 21
  Health Application 1—Obesity, 28

2 Concepts in Biochemistry, 34
  What is Biochemistry?, 35
  Fundamentals of Biochemistry, 35
  Principle Biomolecules in Nutrition, 36
  Summary of Metabolism, 45
  Health Application 2—Lactose
    Intolerance, 48

3 The Alimentary Canal: Digestion
  and Absorption, 50
  Physiology of the Gastrointestinal
    Tract, 51
  Oral Cavity, 52
  Esophagus, 56
  Gastric Digestion, 56
  Small Intestine, 57
  Large Intestine, 60
  Health Application 3—Gluten-Related
    Disorders, 62

4 Carbohydrate: The Efficient Fuel, 66
  Classification, 67
  Physiological Roles, 71
  Requirements, 74
  Sources, 74
  Hyperstates and Hypostates, 77
  Nonnutritive Sweeteners/Sugar
    Substitutes, 80
  Health Application 4—High-Fructose
    Corn Syrup, 82

5 Protein: The Cellular Foundation, 86
  Amino Acids, 87
  Classification, 88
  Physiological Roles, 89
  Requirements, 90
  Sources, 91
  Underconsumption and Health-Related
    Problems, 93
  Overconsumption and Health-Related
    Problems, 95
  Health Application 5—Vegetarianism, 95

6 Lipids: The Condensed Energy, 101
  Classification, 102
  Chemical Structure, 103
  Characteristics of Fatty Acids, 104
  Compound Lipids, 104
  Cholesterol, 105
  Physiological Roles, 105
  Dietary Fats and Dental Health, 107
  Dietary Requirements, 108
  Sources, 108
  Overconsumption and Health-Related
    Problems, 113
  Underconsumption and Health-Related
    Problems, 114
  Fat Replacers, 115
  Health Application 6—Hyperlipidemia, 116

7 Use of the Energy Nutrients: Metabolism
  and Balance, 121
  Metabolism, 122
  Role of the Liver, 122
  Role of the Kidneys, 122
  Carbohydrate Metabolism, 123
  Protein Metabolism, 124
  Lipid Metabolism, 124
  Alcohol Metabolism, 125
  Metabolic Interrelationships, 125
  Metabolic Energy, 126
  Basal Metabolic Rate, 127
  Total Energy Requirements, 128
  Energy Balance, 129
  Inadequate Energy Intake, 131
  Health Application 7—Diabetes Mellitus, 132

8   Vitamins Required for Calcified
     Structures, 139
     Overview of Vitamins, 140
     Vitamin A (Retinol, Carotene), 141
     Vitamin D (Calciferol), 145
     Vitamin E (Tocopherol), 151
     Vitamin K, 152
     Vitamin C (Ascorbic Acid), 154
     Health Application 8—Antioxidants, 156

9   Minerals Essential for Calcified
     Structures, 160
     Bone Mineralization and Growth, 161
     Formation of Teeth, 161
     Introduction to Minerals, 161
     Calcium, 162
     Phosphorus, 167
     Magnesium, 168
     Fluoride, 170
     Health Application 9—Osteoporosis, 175

10   Nutrients Present in Calcified
     Structures, 178
     Copper, 179
     Selenium, 180
     Chromium, 181
     Manganese, 182
     Molybdenum, 183
     Ultratrace Elements, 183
     Health Application 10—Alzheimer
        Disease, 185

11   Vitamins Required for Oral Soft Tissues and
     Salivary Glands, 189
     Physiology of Soft Tissues, 190
     Thiamin (Vitamin B_1), 192
     Riboflavin (Vitamin B_2), 194
     Niacin (Vitamin B_3), 195
     Pantothenic Acid (Vitamin B_5), 197
     Vitamin B_6 (Pyridoxine), 198
     Folate/Folic Acid, 200
     Vitamin B_{12} (Cobalamin), 203
     Biotine (Vitamin B_7), 205
     Other Vitamins, 205
     Health Application 11—Vitamin, Mineral, and
        Herbal supplements, 206

12   Fluids and Minerals Required for Oral Soft
     Tissues and Salivary Glands, 213
     Fluids, 214
     Electrolytes, 223
     Sodium, 223
     Chloride, 228
     Potassium, 228
     Iron, 230
     Zinc, 232
     Iodine, 234
     Health Application 12—Hypertension, 236

Part II Application of Nutrition Principles

13   Nutritional Requirements Affecting Oral Health
     in Women, 243
     Health Pregnancy, 244
     Lactation, 255
     Oral Contraceptive Agents, 257
     Menopause, 259
     Health Application 13—Fetal Alcohol
        Spectrum Disorder, 260

14   Nutritional Requirements During Growth and
     Development and Eating Habits Affecting
     Oral Health, 265
     Infants, 266
     Dietary Recommendations and Guidelines
        for Growth (Children Older Than 2 Years
        of Age), 274
     Toddler and Preschool Children, 277
     Attention-Deficit/Hyperactivity
        Disorders, 280
     Children with Special Needs, 281
     School-Age Children (7 to
        12 Years Old), 281
     Adolescents, 282
     Health Application 14—Childhood and
        Adolescent Obesity, 285

15   Nutritional Requirements for Older Adults and
     Eating Habits Affecting Oral Health, 292
     General Health Status, 293
     Physiological Factors Influencing Nutritional
        Needs and Status, 294
     Socioeconomic and Psychological
        Factors, 297
     Nutrient Requirements, 298
     Eating Patterns, 301
     MyPlate for Older Adults, 301
     Health Application 15—Genomics, 303

16   Food Factors Affecting Health, 308
     Healthcare Disparities, 309
     Food Patterns, 309
     Working with Patients with Different
        Food Patterns, 310
     Food Budgets, 311
     Maintaining Optimal Nutrition During
        Food Preparation, 316
     Food Fads and Misinformation, 323
     Referrals for Nutritional Resources, 329
     Role of Dental Hygienists, 332
     Health Application 16—Food Insecurity in the
        United States, 333

17   Effects of Systemic Disease on Nutritional
     Status and Oral Health, 339
     Effects of Chronic Disease on Intake, 340
     Anemias, 342

Other Hematological Disorders, 344
Gastrointestinal Problems, 345
Cardiovascular Conditions, 346
Skeletal System, 348
Metabolic Problems, 348
Neuromuscular Problems, 352
Neoplasia, 354
Acquired Immunodeficiency Disease, 355
Mental Health Problems, 357
Health Application 17—Human
    Papillomavirus, 360

Part III Nutritional Aspects of Oral Health

18   Nutritional Aspects of Dental Caries: Causes,
    Prevention, and Treatment, 364
    Major Factors in the Dental Caries
        Process, 365
    Other Factors Influencing
        Carcinogenicity, 369
    Dental Plan, 371
    Health Application 18—Genetically
        Modified Foods, 377

19   Nutritional Aspects of Gingivitis and
    Periodontal Disease, 381
    Physical Effects of Food on
        Periodontal Health, 383
    Nutritional Considerations for
        Periodontal Patients, 383
    Gingivitis, 383

Chronic Periodontitis, 384
Necrotizing Periodontal Disease, 388
Health Application 19—Tobacco
    Cessation, 390

20   Nutritional Aspects of Alterations in the
    Oral Cavity, 393
    Orthodontics, 394
    Xerostomia, 394
    Root Caries and Dentin Hypersensitivity, 396
    Dentition Status, 397
    Oral and Maxillofacial Surgery, 398
    Loss of Alveolar Bone, 399
    Glossitis, 399
    Temporomandibular Disorder, 400
    Health Application 20—Functional
        Foods, 400

21   Nutritional Assessment and Education for
    Dental Patients, 406
    Evaluation of the Patient, 407
    Assessment of Nutritional Status, 408
    Identification of Nutritional Status, 413
    Formation of Nutrition Treatment Plan, 415
    Facilitative Communication Skills, 418
    Health Application 21—Health Literacy, 419

Glossary, 423

Answers to Nutritional Quotient Questions, 434

Index, 439

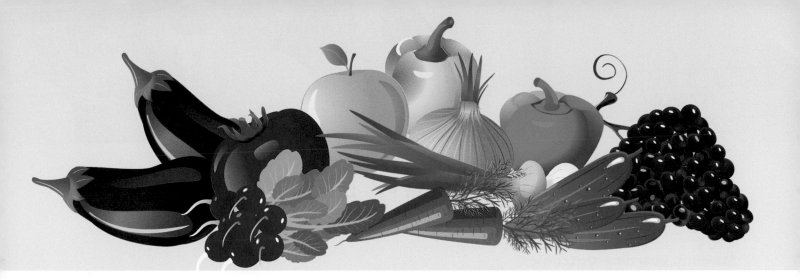

PART I
Orientation to Basic Nutrition

1   **Overview of Healthy Eating Habits, 2**
2   **Concepts in Biochemistry, 34**
3   **The Alimentary Canal: Digestion and Absorption, 50**
4   **Carbohydrate: The Efficient Fuel, 66**
5   **Protein: The Cellular Foundation, 86**
6   **Lipids: The Condensed Energy, 101**
7   **Use of the Energy Nutrients: Metabolism and Balance, 121**
8   **Vitamins Required for Calcified Structures, 139**
9   **Minerals Essential for Calcified Structures, 160**
10   **Nutrients Present in Calcified Structures, 178**
11   **Vitamins Required for Oral Soft Tissues and Salivary Glands, 189**
12   **Fluids and Minerals Required for Oral Soft Tissues and Salivary Glands, 213**

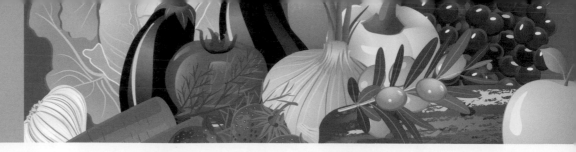

Chapter 1

Overview of Healthy Eating Habits

Student Learning Outcomes

Upon completion of this chapter, the student will be able to achieve the following student learning outcomes:

- Describe the general physiological functions of the six nutrient classifications of foods.
- Identify factors that influence patients' food habits.
- Name the food groups on *MyPlate*.
- Determine the amounts needed from each of the food groups on *MyPlate* for a well-balanced 2000 kilocalorie diet.
- Identify significant nutrient contributions of each food group, and assess their implications for a patient's oral health.

- Describe the *Dietary Guidelines for Americans* and their purpose.
- Assess dietary intake of a patient, using the *Dietary Guidelines for Americans* and *MyPlate*.
- Motivate a patient to improve food choices.
- Explain the different purposes of dietary reference intakes (DRIs), *MyPlate*, and reference daily intakes (RDIs).
- Apply basic nutritional concepts to help patients with nutrition-related problems.

Key Terms

Acceptable macronutrient distribution ranges (AMDRs)
Adequate intake (AI)
Bariatric surgery
Body mass index (BMI)
Calorie
Daily reference value (DRV)
Daily value (DV)
Dietary reference intakes (DRIs)
Dietetic Technician, Registered (DTR)
Energy
Enrichment
Estimated average requirement (EAR)
Estimated energy requirement (EER)
Fortification
Ghrelin
Health claim
Hypertension
Kilocalorie (kcal)
Low nutrient density

Macronutrients
Micronutrients
Nutrient content claims
Nutrient-dense
Nutrients
Nutrition
Nutrition Facts label
Nutritionist
Obesity
Overweight
Precursor
Qualified health claims
Recommended dietary allowances (RDAs)
Reference daily intake (RDI)
Registered dietitian (RD)/registered dietitian nutritionist (RDN)
Satiety
Tolerable upper intake level (UL)
Unqualified health claims
Whole grains

Test Your NQ

1. **T/F** Milk is a perfect food for everyone.
2. **T/F** According to the *Dietary Guidelines for Americans,* consumption of all sugars should be reduced.
3. **T/F** Water is the most important nutrient.
4. **T/F** Dietary reference intakes (DRIs) are required daily intakes essential for all patients to be healthy.
5. **T/F** Good nutrition is possible regardless of a patient's cultural habits.
6. **T/F** Based on *MyPlate*, two to four servings daily are needed from the fruit and vegetable group.
7. **T/F** The *Dietary Guidelines for Americans* were written for healthy people to help reduce their risk of developing chronic diseases.
8. **T/F** Sugar is the leading cause of chronic health problems.
9. **T/F** The goal of *MyPlate Food Guidance System* is to convey the importance of variety, moderation, and proportion.
10. **T/F** The only nutrients that provide energy are carbohydrates, fats, and vitamins.

The dental hygiene profession continues to grow and rapidly move into the forefront of health care. To function as valuable members of today's healthcare team, the dental hygienist must be knowledgeable in various aspects of health care. Because of the lifelong synergistic bidirectional relationship between oral health and nutritional status, dental hygienists and registered dietitians and nutritionists need to be competent in assessing and providing basic education to patients, and provide referrals to each other to effect comprehensive patient care.

All registered dietitians and some nutritionists are considered experts in the field of food nutrition, but their training prepares them for slightly different areas. A **nutritionist** may have a 4-year degree in foods and nutrition and usually works in a public health setting assisting people in the community, such as pregnant teenagers or older individuals, with diet-related health issues. In many states, a nutritionist is legally defined and is licensed or certified. Nutritionists work in local or state health departments and in the extension service of a land-grant university. A **registered dietitian (RD)** or **registered dietitian nutritionist (RDN)** has completed a minimum of a bachelor's degree in foods and nutrition with training in normal and clinical nutrition, food science, food service management, research, and medical nutrition therapy. A new credential established by the Academy of Nutrition and Dietetics is the RDN. An RDN must pass a national registration examination and receive continuing education. RDNs working in hospitals, long-term care facilities, healthcare providers' offices, and pharmaceutical companies may be more involved with Medical Nutrition Therapy, or specialized diets. RDNs may also work in settings dealing principally with basic nutrition, such as in schools, community and research settings, wellness and fitness centers, public health and community programs, educational institutions, and health and wellness preventive programs. The addition of the term "nutritionist" helps identify the type of work performed. Actually, all registered dietitians are nutritionists but not all nutritionists are registered dietitians.

A **Dietetic Technician, Registered (DTR)** has completed a 2-year degree program in a dietetic technician program or has a 4-year degree from an approved (Accreditation Council for Education in Nutrition and Dietetics) program. A DTR, like the RDN, must pass a national registration examination and receive continuing education. The DTR normally works under the supervision of an RDN in such practice areas as hospitals, clinics, and nursing homes, but they may also work independently to provide general nutrition education to healthy populations.

Dental professionals typically see patients on a more regular basis than other healthcare professionals; this allows observation of many physical signs, particularly oral signs, of a nutrient deficiency or medical condition that affects nutritional status before it is diagnosed. Recognition of abnormal conditions and early referral to an appropriate healthcare professional can lead to positive health outcomes for patients. Assessment of dietary information obtained from a patient can also uncover habits detrimental to oral health that can be addressed in the dental office. Additionally, compromised oral health may affect food choices. For example, patients with missing dentition or ill-fitting dentures may avoid foods that are hard to chew and reduce the quality and variety of their diets.

Finally, dental hygienists can follow up on the goals established by patients to evaluate their understanding and compliance. Overall, the dental hygienist is committed to prevention of oral disease as well as the promotion of health and wellness. All healthcare professionals must work together to enhance patient care. This textbook provides the dental professional with the nutrition information that can realistically be applied to and practiced with patients in the dental setting.

BASIC NUTRITION

Nutrition is the process by which living things use food to obtain nutrients for energy, growth and development, and maintenance. **Energy** is the ability or power to do work. **Nutrients** are biochemical substances that can be supplied only in adequate amounts from an outside source, normally from food. One aspect of nutrition is the integration of physiological and biochemical reactions within the body: (a) digesting food to make nutrients available, (b) absorbing and delivering nutrients to the cells where they are used, and (c) eliminating waste products.

Nutrition is a relatively new science and still an evolving discipline. People want science to be definitive; they become confused and concerned when scientific research challenges what the public assumes to be factual. In nutrition, something that is considered to be true today may be disrupted by future research refuting established beliefs. In many cases, the media exacerbates this situation by highlighting findings from a new research study that cannot be reproduced in further research. The pace of research has quickened; this text is based on current, well-established, and evidence-based nutrition advice. Everyone in the healthcare field must continue to stay abreast of ongoing research to be able to respond to questions from patients.

Americans are interested in food and health issues and are concerned about their diet, their physical activity, and substances in foods they eat. More than half of Americans find it easier to do their own taxes than to choose a balanced diet that provides their nutrient needs.[1] This may be related to the fact that nutrition information is ever-changing.

Psychological and social factors that enter into frequent decisions concerning food choices are also important aspects of nutrition. Freedom of choice and variety in consumption are important components of an individual's personal and social life. Tastes, budget, environment, and cultural attitudes influence food choices. The systemic and environmental effects of nutrients, which are determined by these food choices, affect dental health.

PHYSIOLOGICAL FUNCTIONS OF NUTRIENTS

Physiologically, foods eaten are used for energy, tissue building, maintenance and replacement, and obtaining or producing numerous regulatory substances. The classes of macronutrients and micronutrients obtained from foods are the following:
1. Water
2. Proteins
3. Carbohydrates
4. Fats
5. Minerals
6. Vitamins

Of the above-listed nutrients, only proteins, carbohydrates, and fats provide energy. Alcohol also provides calories and limited or no nutrients. The potential energy value of foods within the body is expressed in terms of the kilocalorie, more frequently referred to as the **calorie**. A **kilocalorie (kcal)** is a measure of heat equivalent to 1000 calories.

Nutrients work together and interact in complex metabolic reactions. Proteins, carbohydrates, and fats provide energy that the body needs for metabolic processes. However, the body cannot use energy from these caloric-containing components of food without adequate amounts of vitamins and minerals. Vitamins and minerals, along with protein and water, are essential for the body to build and maintain body tissues and to regulate essential body processes.

BASIC CONCEPTS OF NUTRITION

Foods differ in the amount of nutrients they furnish. Any individual food can be compatible with good nutrition but should be evaluated in the context of the patient's physiological needs, the food's nutrient content, and other food choices. The premise of nutritional care is that, in any cultural or environmental circumstance or for any personal taste or preference, good nutrition is possible. The total diet or overall pattern of food intake is the most important focus of healthy eating.[2]

Increasing the variety of foods consumed reduces the probability of developing isolated nutrient deficiencies, nutrient excesses, and toxicities resulting from non-nutritive components or contaminants in any particular food. A dietary change to eliminate or increase intake of one specific food component or nutrient usually alters the intake of other nutrients. For instance, because red meats are an excellent source of iron and zinc, decreasing cholesterol intake by limiting these meats can reduce dietary iron and zinc intake.

Essential nutrients are needed throughout life on a regular basis; only the amounts of nutrients require change. The patient's consumption of foods and beverages, stage of growth and development, sex, body size, weight, physical activity, and state of health influence nutrient requirements.

Some nutrients can be converted by the body to meet physiological needs. Nonessential nutrients can be used by the body, but either are not required or can be synthesized from dietary precursors. **Precursors** are substances from which an active substance is formed. An example is carotene, found in fruits and vegetables, which the liver can convert into an active form of vitamin A.

Water is the most important nutrient. After water, nutrients of highest priority are those that provide energy, which must be provided from foods or can be supplied from quantities stored in the body. The human body has adaptive mechanisms that allow toleration of modest ranges in nutrient intakes. For instance, the metabolic rate usually decreases as a result of decreased caloric intake.

Dental Considerations

- Because nutrients work interdependently, a lack or excess of one can interfere with or prevent use of another. Asking the patient to record food and beverage intake for the past 24 to 72 hours allows assessment of nutrient intake.
- Evaluation of the patient's intake of macronutrients and micronutrients can help determine whether intake is adequate or excessive.

Nutritional Directions

- No single food contains all the essential nutrients in amounts needed for optimal health.
- Nutritional intake can either improve or adversely affect health.

GOVERNMENT NUTRITION CONCERNS

Before 1977, nutritional efforts focused on ensuring that the U.S. food supply provided adequate nutrients to prevent deficiency diseases. The U.S. government recognized health and nutritional problems related to food choices in 1977 with the *United States Dietary Goals,* which addressed excessive consumption of some nutrients. In 1988, the Surgeon General issued a report confirming that 5 of the 10 leading causes of death (coronary heart disease [CHD], certain types of cancer, stroke, diabetes mellitus, and atherosclerosis) were associated with dietary intake. These reports provided comprehensive science-based objectives to improve the health of the U.S. population and to establish national objectives for promoting health and preventing disease.

Healthy People Nutrition Objectives

Healthy People 2000: National Health Promotion and Disease Prevention Objectives, initially issued in 1990 by the U.S. Department of Health and Human Services (USDHHS), established objectives and goals to measure progress in specific areas. *Healthy People 2020*[4] *(HP2020)* identifies emerging public health priorities and aligns them with health promotion strategies driven by the best evidence available. HP 2020 is organized into 42 topic areas with about 600 measurable objectives to be accomplished by 2020. It targets 22 objectives related to nutrition and weight, and 17 objectives related to oral health. The objectives for *Healthy People* focus on (a) increasing the quality and years of healthy life, (b) eliminating health disparities among racial and ethnic groups, (c) creating social and physical environments that promote good health for everyone, and (d) promoting quality of life, healthy development, and healthy behaviors of all age groups. Ongoing monitoring indicates progress in reducing the number of deaths from CHD, stroke, certain cancers, and in other areas, but there has been an increase in the number of overweight and obese Americans, and little to no progress in the area of reducing health disparities for minority and low-income groups. In the area of oral health objectives, dental caries in primary teeth of children aged 2 to 4 years, and the proportion of adults age 35 to 44 years with untreated dental decay increased.[3]

Based on progress made on objectives, new goals were set for 2010 and again for 2020. Oral health objectives from HP 2010 that were met included a reduction of gingivitis and an increase in the percentage of long-term care residents who receive dental treatment. Many of the 10-year national objectives were continued if they had not been met and/or goals were adjusted. HP 2020 decreased the goal to reduce the prevalence of childhood obesity among youth ages 2 to 19 years from 16.2% to 14.6%. An oral health objective continuing from HP 2010 to HP 2020 is to increase the percentage of the U.S. population served by community water systems that are optimally fluoridated. New topics continue to be added as needed. One new 2020 oral health objective is to increase the proportion of children who have received dental sealants. Other relevant objectives are referenced throughout this text. The website (http://www.healthypeople.gov/2020/default.aspx) is updated frequently, providing consumers and healthcare providers the opportunity to monitor progress.

NUTRIENT RECOMMENDATIONS: DIETARY REFERENCE INTAKES

Recommendations for the amounts of required nutrients have undergone significant changes over the years, and the revised sets of nutrient-based reference values are collectively called the dietary reference intakes (DRIs) (see front matter, pp. i to iv). In 1993, the Food and Nutrition Board of the Institute of Medicine (IOM) undertook this major project, which was completed in 2004. The government publishes the DRIs that are established by an expert group of scientists and RDNs from the United States and Canada. These groups of experts base their recommendations on available scientific evidence from different types of studies on the nutrients.

Previous recommended dietary allowances (RDAs) focused on amounts of nutrients necessary to prevent deficiency diseases. The current DRIs additionally attempt to (a) estimate amounts of required nutrients to improve the long-term health and well-being of people by reducing the risk of chronic diseases, e.g., heart disease, osteoporosis, and cancer, affected by nutrition; and (b) establish maximum safe levels of tolerance. The four categories of nutrient-based reference values are relevant for various stages of life. The DRIs were intended for planning and assessing diets of healthy Americans and Canadians. The DRIs are inappropriate for malnourished individuals or patients whose requirements are affected by a disease state.

Estimated Average Requirement

The estimated average requirement (EAR) is the amount of a nutrient that is estimated to meet the needs of half of the healthy individuals in a specific age and gender group. This set of values is useful in assessing nutrient adequacy or planning intakes of population groups, not individuals.

Recommended Dietary Allowance

The new RDA is generally higher than the EAR and provides a sufficient amount of a nutrient to meet the requirements of nearly all (97% to 98%) healthy individuals. These recommendations provide a generous margin of safety and are intended as a goal for achieving adequate intakes. No health benefits are established for consuming intakes greater than the RDA.

Adequate Intakes

If sufficient scientific evidence was unavailable to determine an EAR or RDA, an **adequate intake (AI)** was established, based on scientific judgments. An AI, which is derived from mean nutrient intakes by groups of healthy people, is the average amount of a nutrient that seems to maintain a defined nutritional state. An AI is expected to exceed average requirements of virtually all members of a life stage/gender group, but is more tentative than an RDA. AI values were established for various life stages for several nutrients, including fluoride, because of uncertainties about the scientific data to determine EAR and RDA values that would reduce the risk of chronic disease.

Tolerable Upper Intake Level

A **tolerable upper intake level (UL)** is the maximum daily level of nutrient intake that probably would not cause adverse health effects or toxic effects for most individuals in the general population. The potential risk of adverse effects increases as intake exceeds the UL. The term *tolerable intake* was selected to avoid implying that these higher levels would result in beneficial effects. These values are especially helpful because of increased consumption of nutrients in the form of dietary supplements or from enrichment and fortification. This recommendation pertains to habitual daily use and is based on the combined intake of food, water, dietary supplements, and fortified foods with a few exceptions: the UL for magnesium applies only to intake from nonfood sources; the ULs for vitamin E, niacin, and folate apply only to fortified foods or supplement sources; and the UL for vitamin A only applies to intake of preformed retinol, regardless of the source.

Acceptable Macronutrient Distribution Ranges

Acceptable macronutrient distribution ranges (AMDRs) were established for the macronutrients, fat, carbohydrate, protein, and two polyunsaturated fatty acids, to ensure sufficient intakes of essential nutrients, while reducing risk of chronic disease. **Macronutrients** are energy-providing nutrients needed in larger amounts than **micronutrients**, e.g., vitamins and minerals. The AMDR is a range of intakes for food components that provide kilocalories; these are expressed as a percentage of total energy intake because the intake of each depends on intake of the others or of the total energy requirement of the individual. Increasing or decreasing one energy source while consuming a set amount of kilocalories affects the intake of the other sources of energy. For instance, if an individual who routinely consumes 2000 kcal decides to reduce fat intake, either protein or carbohydrate intake would need to increase to provide the 2000 kcal. Consuming amounts outside of the ranges increases risk of insufficient intake of essential nutrients. Recommended ranges for carbohydrates, fats, and proteins allow more flexibility in dietary planning for healthy individuals and development of eating plans to meet an individual's preferences.

Estimated Energy Requirement

The **estimated energy requirement (EER)** is defined as dietary energy intake that is predicted to maintain energy balance in healthy, normal-weight individuals of a defined age, gender, weight, height, and physical activity level consistent with good health. The EER is similar to the EAR, and no RDA was established because consuming more kilocalories than are needed would result in weight gain. Because energy requirement depends on activity level, four different activity levels are provided.

Summary of Dietary Reference Intakes

Because nutrient requirements are influenced by age and sexual development, the DRIs are listed for 16 groups, separating gender groups after 10 years of age. Separate levels are established for three categories of pregnant and lactating women. Also, two age groups for the older American population are available.

These guidelines apply to average daily intakes. Meeting the recommendations for every nutrient on a daily basis is very difficult and unnecessary. These nutrient goals are intended to be met by consuming a variety of foods whenever possible.

Dental Considerations

- Use of DRIs as an assessment guide is for healthy patients only.
- An individual's exact requirement for a specific nutrient is not known for certain.
- The ULs may be used to warn patients that excessive intake of nutrients from nutritional supplements could lead to adverse effects if taken on a regular basis.

Nutritional Directions

- The DRIs are general guidelines for good health, rather than specific requirements.
- Generally, specific foods or food groups, rather than nutrients, should be discussed with patients.
- If an individual's food consumption is below the RDA for a nutrient over several days, more food choices containing that particular nutrient should be encouraged.

FOOD GUIDANCE SYSTEM FOR AMERICANS

Identification of nutrients and knowledge of their physiological function are significant developments. However, patients eat and think in terms of food, not nutrients. Nutrient requirements and information must be interpreted into the "food" language patients understand. The USDHHS and the U.S. Department of Agriculture (USDA) released the seventh edition of the *Dietary Guidelines for Americans*

(Dietary Guidelines) in 2010. These *Dietary Guidelines* are based on scientific knowledge to promote health and reduce risk for major chronic disease through diet, physical activity, and food safety. They are designed to help Americans choose foods that will meet nutrient requirements, promote health, support active lives, and reduce risks of chronic disease. The *Dietary Guidelines* are the foundation for *MyPlate* (www.ChooseMyPlate.gov), released in 2011 to help consumers become healthier by making better food choices.

Another helpful tool is the food label that helps consumers determine what kind and how much food to eat. Nutrition labeling, required for most packaged foods, provides information on certain nutrients. The Nutrition Facts label provides information on nutrient content of food and the number of servings in the package. Knowing how to interpret labels enables consumers to accurately apply *Dietary Guidelines* messages that correspond to the nutrients and other information on the label.

DIETARY GUIDELINES FOR AMERICANS, 2010

Because of new scientific information related to nutrient requirements and changing health status of Americans, these guidelines have been revised every 5 years since 1980. The content of the *Dietary Guidelines* has not changed much over the past 30 years, but more specific guidelines and recommendations provide useful information tailored for the general public and special populations.

The *Dietary Guidelines* address diet, physical activity and other issues related to food intake and energy expenditure with an ultimate goal of improving Americans' health by promoting healthy eating, which includes food safety. They reflect the preponderance of scientific evidence based on current nutrition-related health problems and summarize information regarding individual nutrients and food components. The guidelines contain technical information involving key health issues. Integrated recommendations are developed for eating patterns that can be adopted (see Fig. 1-1) as part of an overall healthy eating pattern. They are primarily oriented for policymakers, nutrition educators, nutritionists and healthcare providers, rather than the general public. Government nutrition programs utilize the guidelines to determine funding for research, nutrition labeling, and to develop nutrition education information for the public. *MyPlate*, which replaces the well-known *Food Guide Pyramid*, translates the *Dietary Guidelines* into a consumer-friendly form for the public.

Based on food intake surveys, the typical American diet is below the recommended amounts for whole grains, vegetables, fruits, dairy, seafood, oils, fiber, potassium, vitamin D, and calcium. But solid fats and added sugars (soda), refined grains, sodium, and saturated and *trans* fats are consumed in amounts above the recommended limits.[5] The guidelines specifically address the nutrients or food groups providing these nutrients.

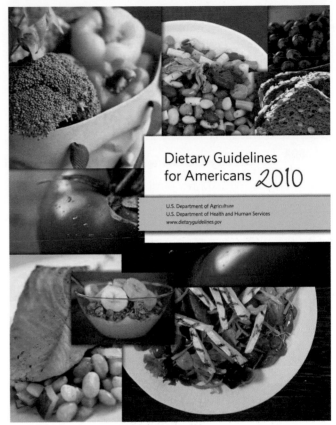

FIGURE 1-1 *Dietary Guidelines for Americans* 2010. (From the U.S. Department of Agriculture and U.S. Department of Health and Human Services: *Dietary guidelines for Americans, 2010*, 7th ed, Washington, DC, December 2010, U.S. Government Printing Office. Available at: http://health.gov/dietaryguidelines/dga2010/DietaryGuidelines2010.pdf.)

The guidelines promote use of foods to meet physiological needs. In addition to the array of nutrients provided by food, hundreds of other naturally-occurring substances present in food, especially antioxidants, may protect against chronic health conditions. In some cases, fortified foods are advisable sources of nutrients that otherwise might be consumed in less than recommended amounts, such as folic acid. Supplements, recommended if a specific nutrient cannot or is not otherwise being met by food intake, cannot replace a healthful diet. Food is the ideal source of nutrients.

Kilocalorie control and daily physical activity are the cornerstones of the 2010 *Dietary Guidelines* designed particularly to curtail the U.S. epidemic of overweight and obesity. These *Dietary Guidelines* encompass two dominant concepts: (a) maintain kilocalorie balance over time to achieve and sustain a healthy weight, and (b) focus on consuming nutrient-dense foods and beverages. Nutrient-dense foods provide substantial amounts of vitamins and minerals, but relatively few kilocalories. When more foods or beverages are chosen that have a low nutrient density (containing high fat, alcohol, or sugar content), consuming enough nutrients without gaining weight is more difficult. The consumption of excessive kilocalories from fats, added sugars, and refined grains reduces intake of nutrient-dense foods and beverages.

Many Americans need to decrease their caloric intake and increase caloric expenditure to curb the obesity epidemic and improve their health. A healthy eating pattern emphasizes vegetables, fruits, whole grains, fat-free or low-fat milk and milk products, seafood, lean meats and poultry, eggs, beans and peas, and nuts and seeds. Healthy food choices promote health, reduce the risk of chronic disease, and also prevent foodborne illness. Key recommendations from the 2010 *Dietary Guidelines for Americans* are listed in Box 1-1. The guidelines support healthy eating habits to improve health and quality of life, as shown in the sample menu in Fig. 1-2.

BOX 1-1   Dietary Guidelines for Americans Executive Summary, 2010: Key Recommendations

Balancing Calories to Manage Weight
- Prevent and/or reduce overweight and obesity through improved eating and physical activity behaviors.
- Control total calorie intake to manage body weight. For people who are overweight or obese, this will mean consuming fewer calories from foods and beverages.
- Increase physical activity and reduce time spent in sedentary behaviors.
- Maintain appropriate calorie balance during each stage of life—childhood, adolescence, adulthood, pregnancy and breastfeeding, and older age.

Foods and Food Components to Reduce
- Reduce daily sodium intake to less than 2300 mg and further reduce intake to 1500 mg among persons who are 51 and older and those of any age who are African American or have hypertension, diabetes, or chronic kidney disease. The 1500 mg recommendation applies to about half of the U.S. population, including children, and the majority of adults.
- Consume less than 10 percent of calories from saturated fatty acids by replacing them with monounsaturated and polyunsaturated fatty acids.
- Consume less than 300 mg per day of dietary cholesterol.
- Keep *trans* fatty acid consumption as low as possible by limiting foods that contain synthetic sources of *trans* fats, such as partially hydrogenated oils, and by limiting other solid fats.
- Reduce the intake of calories from solid fats and sugars.
- Limit the consumption of foods that contain refined grains, especially refined grain foods that contain solid fats, added sugars, and sodium.
- If alcohol is consumed, it should be consumed in moderation—up to one drink per day for women and two drinks per day for men—and only by adults of legal drinking age.*

Foods and Nutrients to Increase
Individuals should meet the following recommendations as part of a healthy eating pattern while staying within their calorie needs.
- Increase vegetable and fruit intakes.
- Eat a variety of vegetables, especially dark-green and red and orange vegetables and beans and peas.
- Consume at least half of all grains as whole grains. Increase whole-grain intake by replacing refined grains with whole grains.
- Increase intake of fat-free or low-fat milk and milk products, such as milk, yogurt, cheese, or fortified soy beverages.†

- Choose a variety of protein foods, which include seafood, lean meat and poultry, eggs, beans and peas, soy products, and unsalted nuts and seeds.
- Increase the amount and variety of seafood consumed by closing seafood in place of some meat and poultry.
- Replace protein foods that are higher in solid fats with choices that are lower in solid fats and calories and/or are sources of oils.
- Use oils to replace solid fats where possible.
- Choose foods that provide more potassium, dietary fiber, calcium, and vitamin D, which are nutrients of concern in American diets. These foods include vegetables, fruits, whole grains, and milk and milk products.

Recommendations for Specific Population Groups
Women capable of becoming pregnant‡
- Choose foods that supply heme iron, which is more readily absorbed by the body, additional iron sources, and enhancers of iron absorption such as vitamin C-rich foods.
- Consume 400 mcg per day of synthetic folic acid (from fortified foods and/or supplements) in addition to food forms of folate from a varied diet.§

Women who are pregnant or breastfeeding‡
- Consume 8 to 12 ounces of seafood per week from a variety of seafood types.
- Due to their high methyl mercury content, limit white (albacore) tuna to 6 ounces per week and do not eat the following four types of fish: tilefish, shark, swordfish, and king mackerel.
- If pregnant, take an iron supplement, as recommended by an obstetrician or other health care provider.

Individuals ages 50 years and older
- Consume foods fortified with vitamin B_{12}, such as fortified cereals, or dietary supplements.

Building Healthy Eating Patterns
- Select an eating pattern that meets nutrient needs over time at an appropriate calorie level.
- Account for all foods and beverages consumed and assess how they fit within a total healthy eating pattern.
- Follow food safety recommendations when preparing and eating foods to reduce the risk of foodborne illness.

From U.S. Department of Agriculture and U.S. Department of Health and Human Services: *Dietary guidelines for Americans, 2010,* 7th ed, Washington, DC, U.S. Government Printing Office, December 2010.
*There are many circumstances when people should not drink alcohol.
†Fortified soy beverages have been marketed as "soymilk," a product name consumers could see in supermarkets and consumer materials. However, FDA regulations do not contain provisions for the use of the term soymilk. Therefore, in this document, the term "fortified soy beverage" includes products that may be marketed as soymilk.
‡Includes adolescent girls.
§"Folic acid" is the synthetic form of the nutrient; whereas, "folate" is the form found naturally in foods.

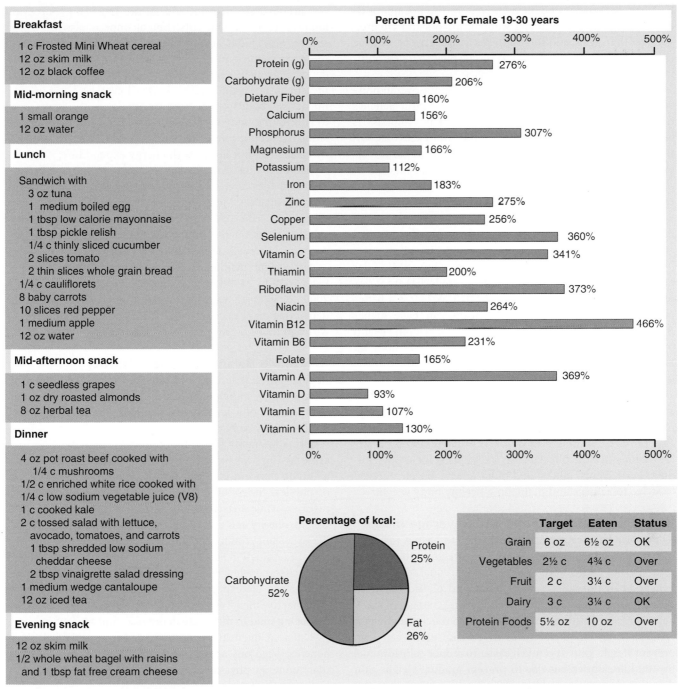

Breakfast

1 c Frosted Mini Wheat cereal
12 oz skim milk
12 oz black coffee

Mid-morning snack

1 small orange
12 oz water

Lunch

Sandwich with
  3 oz tuna
  1 medium boiled egg
  1 tbsp low calorie mayonnaise
  1 tbsp pickle relish
  1/4 c thinly sliced cucumber
  2 slices tomato
  2 thin slices whole grain bread
1/4 c cauliflorets
8 baby carrots
10 slices red pepper
1 medium apple
12 oz water

Mid-afternoon snack

1 c seedless grapes
1 oz dry roasted almonds
8 oz herbal tea

Dinner

4 oz pot roast beef cooked with
  1/4 c mushrooms
1/2 c enriched white rice cooked with
1/4 c low sodium vegetable juice (V8)
1 c cooked kale
2 c tossed salad with lettuce,
  avocado, tomatoes, and carrots
  1 tbsp shredded low sodium
    cheddar cheese
  2 tbsp vinaigrette salad dressing
1 medium wedge cantaloupe
12 oz iced tea

Evening snack

12 oz skim milk
1/2 whole wheat bagel with raisins
  and 1 tbsp fat free cream cheese

Percent RDA for Female 19-30 years

Nutrient	Percent
Protein (g)	276%
Carbohydrate (g)	206%
Dietary Fiber	160%
Calcium	156%
Phosphorus	307%
Magnesium	166%
Potassium	112%
Iron	183%
Zinc	275%
Copper	256%
Selenium	360%
Vitamin C	341%
Thiamin	200%
Riboflavin	373%
Niacin	264%
Vitamin B12	466%
Vitamin B6	231%
Folate	165%
Vitamin A	369%
Vitamin D	93%
Vitamin E	107%
Vitamin K	130%

Percentage of kcal:

Protein 25%
Fat 26%
Carbohydrate 52%

	Target	Eaten	Status
Grain	6 oz	6½ oz	OK
Vegetables	2½ c	4¾ c	Over
Fruit	2 c	3¼ c	Over
Dairy	3 c	3¼ c	OK
Protein Foods	5½ oz	10 oz	Over

FIGURE 1-2 Sample menu based on the *Dietary Guidelines for Americans* and *MyPlate*.

Balancing Kilocalories to Manage Weight

Weight management is difficult for most Americans because of copious amounts of highly palatable foods and lack of physical activity. Body weight should be evaluated in relation to a person's height using the body mass index (BMI) to determine health risks that increase at higher levels of overweight and obesity. Currently, **body mass index (BMI)** is the preferred method of defining healthy weight because it correlates more closely with actual body fat than height and weight tables. BMI can be determined by using the table on p. v, or this mathematical formula: divide weight (in pounds) by height (in inches), divide that number by height (in inches) again, and then multiply the answer by 703. A BMI of less than 25 is generally considered a healthy weight, as chronic disease risk increases in most people who are above this level. A BMI of 25 or greater indicates **overweight**; a BMI of 30 or greater indicates **obesity**. A study of more than 75,000 people found that those with a high BMI (over 30) had a 26% greater risk of developing CHD.[6] A BMI above 25 in almost 1.5 million white adults was associated with increased all-cause mortality.[7] BMI reflects overall fat distribution and can be calculated quickly and inexpensively. BMI is not appropriate for pregnant and nursing women, infants and children younger than age 2, and some athletes with a large percentage of muscle. The Evolve website has special tables for determining BMI for children 2 to 20 years old.

A BMI is a number that reveals little about overall body composition. It is a starting point in assessing a patient's health status and risks. Athletes usually have high BMIs because of their increased muscle mass, not excess fat. On the other hand, a frail or inactive person with a normal-range BMI may have excess body fat and not appear out of shape. Additional muscle tissue aids body functions, but excessive fat interferes with normal metabolism. A desirable weight depends on the amount and location of body fat and other health indicators, e.g., blood pressure, glucose, and cholesterol and triglyceride levels.

Major ethnic differences exist regarding BMI.[8] For example, Asian Americans or Indians (from India) are at risk of health problems at a lower BMI (18.5 to 23.9 is a better range) than whites; African Americans can have higher BMIs (28) than other populations without developing health problems. Older people can tolerate a little more body fat and tend to have a better survival rate with a BMI in the upper range of normal.

Overweight and obesity have increased significantly among both adults and children during the last two decades in the United States. Two-thirds of adults and one-third of children are overweight or obese.[9] Overweight and obesity are serious health concerns. All individuals, including children, adolescents, adults, and older adults, are encouraged to strive to achieve and maintain a healthy body weight.

Kilocalorie Balance: Food and Beverage Intake

Kilocalorie balance over time is the key to weight management. For a person to maintain a set weight, energy consumed from foods and beverages must equal kilocalories expended in normal body functions and physical activity. Because weight loss is a challenge requiring changes in many behaviors and patterns, prevention of too much weight gain is ideal. Even small decreases in caloric intake can help prevent weight gain. It is much easier to reduce caloric intake by 100 kilocalories per day to prevent gradual weight gain than to reduce daily intake by 500 kilocalories to lose weight. In general, the best choice for weight loss involves a change in lifestyle, both in diet and physical activity.

Americans have increased consumption of all major categories of foods and most beverages. American's average intake of 2195 kcal/day during 2009-2010 was a slight decline from a record 2269 kcal/day in 2003-2004, but still remained above the 1971-1975 level of 1955 kcal/day.[10] Added fats and oils, grains, milk and milk products, and caloric sweeteners contributed to the increased caloric intake.[11] Snacking frequency increased, providing about one-third of all daily caloric intake from solid fats and added sugars.[12] Supersized portions require special attention. Studies show that controlling portion sizes helps limit energy intake, especially when eating foods high in kilocalories. Portion sizes should be consistent with a person's activity level.

Carbohydrate, protein, and fat are the main sources of kilocalories from nutrients, but alcohol is also a caloric source. Most foods and beverages contain combinations of these macronutrients in varying amounts. There is little evidence that any individual caloric food group (carbohydrate, protein, or fat) or individual food or beverage, has a unique impact on body weight. Caloric intake is the key factor to controlling body weight—accomplished not by manipulating the proportions of fat, carbohydrates, and protein, but by balancing kilocalories with energy expenditure.

Although most Americans are consuming more kilocalories than they use, intake is only one side of the energy balance equation. Many Americans spend most of their time engaged in sedentary behaviors that expend minimal kilocalories. Consequently, many children and adults routinely consume more kilocalories than they expend.

For weight maintenance, caloric needs typically range from 1600 to 2400 kilocalories daily for adult women and 2000 to 3000 kilocalories for adult men, with variances depending on physical activity. The metabolic rate decreases with age, thus lowering caloric requirements for older adults.

Kilocalorie Balance: Physical Activity

Regular physical activity and physical fitness are important factors for an individual's health, sense of well-being, and maintenance of a healthy body weight. Physical activity is defined as any body movement produced by skeletal muscles resulting in energy expenditure. Physical activity is not the same as physical fitness. Physical fitness is related to the ability to perform physical activity. People with high levels of physical fitness are at lower risk of developing chronic diseases, while a sedentary lifestyle increases risk for overweight, obesity and many chronic diseases. After comparing life expectancy values from the National Health and Nutritional Examination Surveys (NHANES) with U.S. Life Tables, researchers concluded that somewhat-active and active white men have a life expectancy approximately 2.4 years longer than inactive men.[13] Furthermore, physical activity can aid in managing mild to moderate depression and anxiety.

Different intensities and types of exercise yield distinct benefits. Vigorous activity improves physical fitness more than moderate physical activity, also burning more kilocalories per unit of time. Resistance exercise increases muscular strength and endurance and maintains or increases muscle mass. Weight-bearing exercise increases peak bone mass during growth, maintains peak bone mass during adulthood, and reduces the rate of bone loss during aging; this may reduce the risk of osteoporosis. Also, regular exercise can help prevent falls, common sources of injury and disability in older adults.

Physical activity may be accomplished in short bouts (10-minute periods) of moderate-intensity activity performed three to six times during the course of a day; it is the cumulative total that improves health status and increases caloric expenditure.[14] The higher a person's physical activity level, the more kilocalories can be consumed without gaining weight. This makes it easier to plan a daily food intake pattern that meets recommended nutrient requirements.

In addition to physical activity, a high-quality diet that does not provide excess kilocalories is needed to enhance the health of most Americans. Many Americans need to change their eating patterns by choosing healthy foods that include nutrient-dense foods and beverages they enjoy, that also meet nutrient requirements within their kilocalorie needs. In general, individuals should become more conscious of what they eat and what they do.

Key Recommendations

- Women are encouraged to achieve and maintain a healthy weight before becoming pregnant.
- Adults ages 65 years and older who are overweight are encouraged not to gain additional weight. Intentional weight loss may be beneficial, resulting in improved quality of life and reduction of chronic diseases and associated disabilities.
- To maintain body weight in a healthy range, balance kilocalories consumed from foods and beverages with kilocalories expended.
- Kilocalories from alcoholic beverages should be limited.
- To prevent gradual weight gain over time, make small decreases in kilocalories from foods and beverages and increase physical activity.
- Engage in regular physical activity and reduce sedentary activities to promote health, psychological well-being, and a healthy body weight.
  - For adults to reduce the risk of chronic disease: Engage in at least 30 minutes of moderate-intensity physical activity, beyond usual activity, on most days of the week.
  - To help adults manage body weight and prevent gradual unhealthy body weight gain: Engage in approximately 60 minutes of moderate- to vigorous-intensity activity on most days of the week while not exceeding caloric intake requirements.
  - For adults to sustain weight loss: participate in at least 60 to 90 minutes of daily moderate-intensity physical activity while not exceeding caloric intake requirements. (Some people may need to consult a healthcare provider before participating in this level of activity).
  - For most adults, greater health benefits can be obtained by engaging in physical activity of more vigorous intensity or longer duration. Achieve physical fitness by including cardiovascular conditioning, stretching exercises for flexibility, and resistance exercises or calisthenics for muscle strength and endurance.

Foods and Food Components to Reduce

Some food components and certain foods that are consumed in excessive amounts may increase risk of several chronic diseases. These include sodium, solid fats (major sources of saturated and *trans* fatty acids), added sugars and refined grains. In addition, some people consume too much alcohol. These items generally replace nutrient-dense foods, so consuming adequate amounts of recommended nutrients within caloric needs is impossible. Even if a person is at an ideal weight, consuming too much sodium, solid fats, saturated and *trans* fatty acids, cholesterol, added sugars, and alcohol increases the risk of chronic diseases e.g., CHD, diabetes, and certain types of cancer. Foods that can be suggested are noted in Table 1-1.

Sodium

Sodium is an essential nutrient, but the body normally requires relatively small quantities available from naturally-occurring sodium in foods without added amounts. Most Americans consume more sodium than they need; therefore, decreasing sodium intake is advisable for all. In general, high sodium intake is associated with **hypertension** (high blood pressure). Hypertension increases an individual's risk of CHD, stroke, congestive heart failure, and kidney disease. To prevent the development of high blood pressure with increasing age, lifestyle changes are recommended. Reducing sodium intake, increasing potassium intake, losing excess body weight, increasing physical activity, and eating an overall healthful diet are encouraged.

The natural sodium content of food accounts for only approximately 10% of total intake; discretionary sodium (e.g., salt added at the table or in cooking) provides another 5% to 10% of intake. More than 75% is added to prepared foods by manufacturers and food establishments. Because most of the sodium consumed is from processed foods, the goal should concentrate primarily on reducing sodium added during food processing, and on changing food selections to more fresh foods and fewer processed items. Caloric intake is associated with sodium intake (i.e., the more foods and beverages consumed, the more sodium is consumed). Therefore, by reducing kilocalorie intake, sodium intake is lowered somewhat.

Fats

Although fats and oils are important in a healthful diet, heart health is affected by the type and total amount of fat. Usually, high fat intake (more than 35% of kilocalories) is associated with a higher intake of saturated fat, *trans* fatty acid and cholesterol, and with consumption of excess kilocalories. People have no dietary requirement for saturated fatty acids, *trans* fatty acids, or cholesterol which may raise low-density lipoproteins (LDLs, [undesirable blood lipids]). On the other hand, if fat intake is less than 20% of kilocalories, inadequate intakes of vitamin E and essential fatty acids may lead to unfavorable changes in high-density lipoproteins ("good" type of cholesterol, HDLs) and triglycerides (TGs) in the blood.

Saturated fatty acids should provide less than 10% of kilocalories and should be replaced with monounsaturated and polyunsaturated fatty acids. The recommendation is to limit cholesterol to less than 300 mg/day. *Trans* fatty acid consumption should be as low as possible.

Solid fats are solid at room temperature and usually contain a high percentage of saturated and/or *trans* fatty acids. Solid fats are consumed as a food or as ingredients in foods (e.g., shortening in a cake or hydrogenated oils in fried foods). These fats, abundant in the American diet, contribute significantly to excess caloric intake.

Table 1-1	Frequency of use of foods for implementing dietary guidelines		
Food Groups	**Choose More Often**	**Choose Less Often**	**Major Contributions**
Fats	Corn, cottonseed, olive, sesame, soybean, safflower, sunflower, peanut, canola oils Mayonnaise or salad dressing (made from olive oils) Avocado Olives	Butter, lard Margarine made from hydrogenated or saturated fats Coconut or palm oil Hydrogenated vegetable shortening Bacon Meat/fat drippings, gravy, sauces	Vitamin A, kilocalories, essential fatty acids
Soups	Lightly salted soups with fat skimmed Cream-style soups (with low-fat milk)	Commercially prepared soups and mixes	Fluid, kilocalories (may contain a variety of vitamins, minerals, and proteins, depending on type)
Sweets and desserts	Desserts that have been sweetened lightly or contain only moderate fat, such as puddings made from skim milk, angel food cake, fruit-based desserts	Desserts high in sugar or fats, candy, pastries, cakes, pies, whole-milk puddings, cookies	Kilocalories (fats, carbohydrates)
Beverages	Water Unsweetened soft drinks Decaffeinated drinks	Sweetened beverages Caffeine-containing beverages Alcoholic beverages	Fluid, kilocalories (unless sugar-free)
Milk and milk products	Low-fat or skim milk Low-fat cheese Low-fat yogurt	Whole-milk Whole-milk cheeses Whole-milk yogurt Ice cream	Kilocalories, calcium, protein, phosphorus, vitamins A and D, riboflavin
Vegetables, including starchy vegetables	Fresh, frozen, or canned; potatoes—baked or boiled Include one dark green or deep orange vegetable daily	Deep-fried vegetables, chips Pickled vegetables Highly salted vegetables or juices	Kilocalories, vitamins A and C, dietary fiber, potassium, zinc, cobalt, folic acid
Fruits	Unsweetened fruits or juices Include one citrus fruit/juice or one tomato juice daily	Sweetened fruits or juices Coconut Avocado	Kilocalories, dietary fiber, vitamins A and C
Breads, starches, and cereals	Whole-grain breads or cereals Muffins, bagels, tortillas Enriched pasta, rice, grits or noodles	Snack chips or crackers Sweetened cereals Pancakes, doughnuts, and biscuits	Kilocalories, B-complex vitamins, magnesium, copper, iron, dietary fiber
Meats or substitutes	Lean meats, fish, shellfish, poultry without skin Low-fat cheese (e.g., cottage cheese and part skim mozzarella) Peanut butter Soybeans, tofu Dry beans and peas	Fried or fatty meats/fish Fried poultry or poultry with skin High-fat cheeses (e.g., cheddar and processed cheese) Eggs Nuts	Kilocalories, protein, iron, zinc, copper, B-complex vitamins
Miscellaneous	Herbs, spices, flavorings	Salt and salt/spice combinations	Sodium

From Peckenpaugh NJ: *Nutrition essentials and diet therapy*, 11th ed, Philadelphia, 2010, Saunders.

Added Sugars

Sugars, whether they are naturally present or added to the food, and grains supply physiological energy in the form of glucose. The body does not respond differently to sugars added to food than it does to those naturally present, but added sugars supply kilocalories with few or no nutrients. Consumption of foods containing large amounts of added sugars increases the difficulty of obtaining adequate nutrients without weight gain. Additionally, the frequency and duration of sugars and refined grain consumption are important factors in caries risk because they increase exposure to cariogenic substrates.

Refined Grains

Carbohydrates or starchy foods are essential for a healthful diet. Americans generally consume adequate amounts of grains, but most are refined that are frequently high in solid fats and added sugars. When whole grains are refined, vitamins, minerals, and dietary fiber are lost in the process. Most refined grains are enriched with some of the nutrients lost in the process, but dietary fiber and some vitamins and minerals are not routinely added back in the enrichment process. Enrichment is the process of restoring iron, thiamin, riboflavin, folic acid, and niacin removed during processing to approximately their original levels. This process is controlled by the U.S. Food and Drug Administration (FDA), which establishes the quantity of nutrients that can be added.

Despite the fact that enriched grains have a positive role in providing some vitamins and minerals, excessive amounts can result in excess kilocalories being consumed. The recommended amount of refined grains is less than 3 servings daily; most refined grains should be replaced with whole grains.

Alcohol

Alcohol consumption can have beneficial or harmful effects depending on the amount consumed, age and other characteristics of the person consuming the alcohol, and other circumstances. Fewer Americans consume alcohol today compared to 50 or 100 years ago. Estimated mean daily intake is 1.2 drinks for men and 0.4 for women.[15]

The risks of heavy alcohol consumption include increased potential for liver cirrhosis, hypertension, cancers of the upper gastrointestinal tract, injury, violence, and death. Because alcoholic beverages supply kilocalories with few nutrients, adequate nutrient intake without weight gain is difficult with excessive alcohol consumption.

In moderation, alcohol may have beneficial effects for middle-aged and older adults, but not for young people. Adults who consume one to two alcoholic beverages a day appear to have a lower risk of CHD. Alcohol use among young adults is associated with a higher risk of traumatic injury and death. A distinct disadvantage of alcohol consumption (even one drink per day) significantly increases risk for oral and pharyngeal cancers.[16]

An alcoholic beverage is defined as 12 oz of regular beer, 5 oz of wine, or 1.5 oz of distilled spirits (80 proof). Moderation is not intended as an average over several days, but rather as the amount consumed on any single day. Because of adverse effects of alcohol consumption for many individuals, other lifestyle changes (healthy diet, physical activity, avoidance of smoking, and maintenance of a healthy weight) reduce risk of CHD and are more advisable than recommending alcohol intake.

Key Recommendations

- Consume less than 2300 mg of sodium (approximately 1 tsp of salt) per day. People of ages 51 years and older, all African Americans, and people with hypertension, diabetes, or chronic kidney disease, should further reduce intake to 1500 mg sodium per day.
- Read nutrition labels and choose and prepare foods with less sodium.

- Avoid processed foods like hot dogs and deli meats, and choose fresh or frozen vegetables over canned versions.
- For 2000 kcal/day intake, solid fats and added sugars should comprise less than 13% of the kilocalories, or approximately 258 kcal.
- Replace foods containing saturated fatty acids with foods containing monounsaturated and polyunsaturated fatty acids.
- Consume less than 300 mg per day of dietary cholesterol.
- Avoid processed foods containing synthetic sources of *trans* fats such as partially hydrogenated oils.
- Limit the consumption of refined grains to three servings a day, especially those that also contain solid fats, added sugars, and sodium.
- Reduce the incidence of dental caries by practicing good oral hygiene and consuming sugar- and starch-containing foods and beverages less frequently.
- Adults of legal drinking age should consume alcoholic beverages in moderation—up to one drink daily for women and two drinks per day for men.
- Excessive drinking is an important health problem and is not limited to college-age individuals.
- Alcoholic beverages should not be consumed by some individuals, including those who cannot limit their alcohol intake; women of childbearing age who may become pregnant, pregnant and lactating women; children and adolescents; individuals taking prescription or over-the-counter medications that can interact with alcohol, engaging in activities that require attention, skill, or coordination (e.g., driving or operating machinery), and those with specific medical conditions (e.g., liver disease, hypertriglyceridemia, and pancreatitis).

Foods and Nutrients to Increase

Despite an abundance of nutritious foods available in the United States, many individuals do not choose a variety of foods that provide all their nutrient requirements and, especially, that enable them to remain within their kilocalorie needs. Intake of vegetables, fruits, whole grains, milk and milk products, and oils are lower than recommended for most Americans. These food groups provide desirable amounts of potassium, magnesium, calcium, dietary fiber, and vitamins D and folate, which are frequently lacking in American diets. (Physiological roles and sources of various nutrients are listed in the chapters where the nutrient is discussed.) The *Dietary Guidelines* recommend an increased intake of nutrient-dense foods that are lean or low in solid fats, and minimize or exclude added solid fats, added sugars and refined starches. Vegetables, fruits, whole grains, fat-free or low-fat milk and milk products, seafood, lean meats and poultry, eggs, beans and peas (legumes), and nuts and seeds prepared without added solid fats, sugars, starches, and sodium, are nutrient-dense.

Fruits and Vegetables

People who consume more fruits and vegetables have a reduced risk of chronic diseases, including stroke and other

CHDs, type 2 diabetes, and certain cancers (oral cavity and pharynx, larynx, lung, esophagus, stomach, and colon-rectum), and a longer lifespan. Fruits and vegetables, because of their high water content, are more filling with fewer kilocalories. Many fruits and vegetables provide high levels of potassium that can lower blood pressure. Fruit juice can be part of a healthful diet, but even if it is 100% fruit juice, it lacks dietary fiber and excess amounts can contribute extra kilocalories.

Whole Grains

Whole grains are grains and grain products made from the entire grain seed, usually called the kernel, which consists of bran, germ, and endosperm. If the kernel has been cracked, crushed, or flaked, it must retain nearly the same relative proportions of bran, germ, and endosperm as the original grain in order to be called whole grain. When selecting whole grains, the first or second ingredient listed on the ingredient panel should be "whole grain." Many, but not all, whole grains are also a good source of dietary fiber. At least half the recommended grain servings should be whole-grain foods to meet the fiber recommendation.

Whole grains are a poor source of folic acid, so when an individual relies exclusively on whole grains, some cereal products fortified with folic acid should be included. This is especially important for women who are capable of becoming pregnant. Fortification is the process of adding nutrients not present in the natural product or increasing the amount above that in the original product. Most processed breakfast cereals undergo fortification to achieve nutrient levels higher than those occurring naturally in the grain. Serious birth defects may occur during early pregnancy if adequate amounts of folic acid are not consumed by the mother. Table 1-2 shows the nutrient differences between whole grain, whole wheat, and enriched breads.

Dietary fiber has a number of beneficial effects on health, including decreased risk of CHD, constipation, and type 2 diabetes. Consuming at least three servings of whole grains daily may help with weight maintenance and lower risk for other chronic diseases.

Milk and Milk Products

Moderate evidence shows that intake of milk and milk products is linked to improved bone health and a reduced risk of CHD and type 2 diabetes, and lower blood pressure in adults. Americans are choosing whole (full-fat) or reduced fat (2%) milk rather than the recommended fat-free (skim) or low-fat (1%) milk. Cheese is a frequently chosen milk product; most cheeses are high in fat. Fat-free or low-fat milk and milk products provide the same nutrients with less fat and fewer kilocalories. Children who establish the habit of drinking milk are more likely to drink milk as adults.

Protein Foods

Seafood, meat, poultry, eggs, beans, peas, soy products, nuts, and seeds are all classified as protein foods. The fatty portions of meat (beef and pork), poultry, and eggs are

Table 1-2	Comparison of nutrient values of selected whole-grain and enriched breads			
Nutrients	Enriched White	Whole Wheat	Whole Grain	Rye
Protein (g)	2.56	3.63	3.47	2.72
Total dietary fiber (g)	0.8	1.9	1.9	1.9
Thiamin (mg)	0.149	0.099	0.073	0.139
Riboflavin (mg)	0.68	0.060	0.034	0.107
Niacin (mg)	1.338	1.320	1.051	1.218
Vitamin B_6 (mg)	0.024	0.059	0.068	0.024
Total folate (mcg)	48	14	20	48
Iron (mg)	1.01	0.68	0.65	0.91
Zinc (mg)	0.24	0.50	0.44	0.36
Calcium (mg)	73	30	27	23
Phosphorus (mg)	29	57	59	40
Magnesium (mg)	7	23	20	13

Data from U.S. Department of Agriculture, Agricultural Research Service. 2012. *USDA National Nutrient Database for Standard Reference, Release 25,* 2012. Accessed January 16, 2013. Available at: http://www.ars.usda.gov/nutrientdata

considered solid fats; fats in seafood, nuts, and seeds are considered oils. Beans and peas do not contain significant quantities of fat. To decrease intake of saturated fats, lean cuts of meat and poultry (without skin) should be chosen, and seafood, nuts, and seeds should replace some of the protein foods. Moderate evidence indicates that eating peanuts, walnuts, almonds, and pistachios reduces risk factors for CHD when they are part of a nutritionally adequate diet and within kilocalorie needs. Nuts and seeds are high in kilocalories; thus small portions should replace other protein foods (meat or poultry) to avoid increasing caloric intake. Additionally, unsalted nuts and seeds are recommended to control sodium intake.

Seafood includes all edible marine animals from the sea and freshwater lakes and rivers including fish, such as salmon, tuna, trout and tilapia, and shellfish, such as shrimp, crab, and oysters. The adult recommendation is approximately 20% of total intake of protein foods. Moderate evidence shows that 8 or more ounces of seafood per week from a variety of seafood sources, provides omega-3 fatty acids associated with prevention of CHD. Pregnant or breastfeeding women are warned to avoid fish high in mercury—tilefish, shark, swordfish, and king mackerel—and to limit white tuna to 6 ounces per week.

Oils

Oils are liquid at room temperature and contain a high percentage of monounsaturated and polyunsaturated fatty acids. They contribute essential fatty acids and vitamin E, so replacing some saturated fatty acids with oils lowers both total cholesterol and LDL blood lipid levels.

Nutrients of Concern

Vegetable, fruit, whole grain, milk and milk products, and seafood consumption is so low that scientists composing the

Dietary Guidelines are concerned about the adequacy of intake of potassium, dietary fiber, calcium, and vitamin D for most Americans. Iron and folate intake are of concern for young women, especially those capable of becoming pregnant. Because of reduced absorption of vitamin B_{12}, older Americans are encouraged to include foods fortified with vitamin B_{12}. These nutrients are discussed in subsequent chapters.

Key Recommendations

- Consume a sufficient amount of fiber-rich fruits and vegetables while staying within energy needs. Two cups of fruit and 2.5 cups of vegetables per day are recommended for a reference 2000 kcal intake, with higher or lower amounts depending on the kilocalorie level.

- Choose a variety of fruits and vegetables each day. In particular, select from all five vegetable subgroups (dark green, orange and red, legumes, starchy vegetables, and other vegetables) several times a week.

- Adding more fruits, vegetables, whole grains, and fat-free or low-fat milk and milk products may have beneficial health effects and provide good sources of nutrients commonly lacking in American diets.

- Consume three or more servings of whole-grain products per day, with the rest of the recommended grains coming from enriched products. In general, at least half the grains should come from whole grains.

- Replace most refined grain food choices with whole-grain foods that are nutrient-dense (low in added sugars and fats) to keep total kilocalorie intake within limits.

- Consume a variety of nutrient-dense foods and beverages within and among the basic food groups while choosing foods that limit intake of saturated and *trans* fats, cholesterol, added sugars, salt, and alcohol.

- Because fruit juices contain little or no fiber, whole fruits (fresh, frozen, canned, or dried) are wiser choices.

- Protein-containing foods are important, but most Americans consume adequate amounts, so for most, an increase is not recommended.

- Keep total fat intake between 20% and 35% of kilocalories, with most fats coming from sources of polyunsaturated and monounsaturated fatty acids, such as fish, nuts, and vegetable oils.

- When selecting and preparing meat, poultry, dry beans, and milk or milk products, choose products that are lean, low-fat or fat-free.

- Limit intake of fats and oils high in saturated and/or *trans* fatty acids, and choose products low in such fats and oils.

- Choose fiber-rich fruits, vegetables, and whole grains often.

Building Healthy Eating Patterns

Principles for Achieving a Healthy Eating Pattern

Many traditional eating patterns provide health benefits; no one specific eating pattern has a monopoly on providing short and long-term health benefits. Research studies conducted on some of these eating patterns measuring specific health outcomes or health-related risk factors led to their endorsement by the USDA and USDHHS. In addition to the recommended *MyPlate* eating pattern, the DASH (Dietary Approaches to Stop Hypertension) diet (discussed in Chapter 12), and the Mediterranean-style eating patterns have undergone considerable research on health outcomes and nutrient and food group composition to the extent they are deemed beneficial. They contain common components recommended in the *Dietary Guidelines*. Average American eating patterns currently bear little resemblance to these dietary recommendations.

Focus on Nutrient-Dense Foods

Because of our sedentary lifestyle, most individuals can accommodate only a limited number of kilocalories from solid fats and added sugars. Nutrient-dense foods are essential to avoid excessive kilocalories.[17]

Remember Beverages Count

Beverages provide necessary fluid intake, but many beverages add kilocalories without providing essential nutrients. Beverage choices should be planned in the context of total caloric intake. Fruit juices and fluid milk provide essential nutrients along with kilocalories, but their intake also must be considered in view of their caloric content. Beverages such as water and unsweetened coffee and tea contribute to total water intake without additional kilocalories.

Follow Food Safety Principles

The food safety guideline is designed to reduce risks from foods contaminated with harmful bacteria, viruses, parasites, toxins, and chemical and physical contaminants. Healthful eating requires a safe food supply provided by farmers, food producers, markets, food service establishments, and other food handlers. The *Dietary Guidelines* address simple food-handling principles to implement when preparing, serving and storing food to minimize risk of foodborne illness. This topic is further addressed in Chapter 16.

Key Recommendations

- Meet recommended intakes with energy needs by adopting a balanced eating pattern, such as *MyPlate*, Mediterranean-style patterns, or the DASH Eating Plan (discussed in Chapter 12, *Health Application 12*).

- Choose and prepare foods and beverages with little added sugars or caloric sweeteners. Drinking fluoridated water and/or using fluoride-containing dental products helps reduce the risk of dental caries. Most bottled water is not fluoridated, so its use should be considered in context of the fluoride content of tap water in the area where it is bottled.

- Avoid raw (unpasteurized) milk or any products made from unpasteurized milk, raw or partially cooked eggs or foods containing raw eggs, raw or undercooked meat and poultry, unpasteurized juices, and raw sprouts.

- To avoid microbial foodborne illness:
  - Clean hands, food contact surfaces, and fruits and vegetables. Meat and poultry should not be washed or rinsed.
  - Separate raw, cooked, and ready-to-eat foods while shopping, preparing, or storing foods.
  - Cook foods to a safe temperature to kill microorganisms.
  - Chill (refrigerate) perishable food promptly and defrost foods properly.

Dental Considerations

- The *Dietary Guidelines* do not necessarily apply to patients with conditions that interfere with normal nutrition and require a special diet or for children younger than 2 years of age.
- Nutrient-dense foods provide substantial amounts of vitamins and minerals and relatively few kilocalories. Foods that can be suggested to patients are noted in Table 1-1.
- Fats provide energy and essential fatty acids, and are important for absorption of fat-soluble vitamins A, D, E, and K, and carotenoids.
- Processed foods and oils provide approximately 80% of *trans* fats with the remainder coming from natural sources or animal foods. "*Trans*" fats from natural sources are not considered detrimental.
- Provide the patient with a definition or example of moderation (e.g., ¼ tsp salt per day or 5 oz glass of wine for a woman per day).

Nutritional Directions

- Nutritional advice should include diets that follow the *Dietary Guidelines* and provide all the nutrients needed for growth and health.
- Encourage patients to consume more dark green and orange-red vegetables, legumes, fruits, whole grains, and low-fat milk and milk products.
- Encourage patients to consume less refined grains, total fats (especially saturated and *trans* fats), added sugars, and kilocalories.
- Read food labels when choosing foods high in fiber or low in fats to check if the kilocalories or grams of sugar have increased.
- A patient needing 2000 kcal daily should limit saturated fat intake to 20 g or less.
- Carbohydrate-containing foods—fruits, vegetables, grains, and milk—are important sources of many nutrients, but these selections should be chosen wisely, within the context of a kilocalorie-controlled diet.
- By reducing frequency and duration of oral exposure to fermentable carbohydrate intake and optimizing oral hygiene practices, such as drinking fluoridated water, brushing and flossing, dental caries can be minimized.
- A person's preference for salt is not fixed; the desire for salty foods tends to decrease after consuming foods lower in salt for a period of time.
- The recommended dietary fiber intake is 14 g per 1000 kcal consumed.
- Residual moisture on produce may promote survival and growth of microbes. Drying the food is critical if the item will not be eaten or cooked immediately.
- Dietetic, sugar-free, or reduced fat products may not be low in kilocalories; this is dependent on other ingredients in the food.

MYPLATE SYSTEM

MyPlate is part of a comprehensive communications initiative to promote healthful food choices. The new *MyPlate* icon (Fig. 1-3), replaces the well-known *MyPyramid* symbol. *MyPlate* food guidance system provides assistance in implementing the recommendations of the *Dietary Guidelines* and the DRIs. *MyPlate* is a system that includes interactive websites and educational modules.

The key tool of this guidance system is the website, *www.chooseMyPlate.gov*. This new food guidance system is revolutionary for a number of reasons. The website is an interactive nutrition education tool intended to help consumers apply personalized dietary guidance to achieve a healthful lifestyle through better eating and increased physical activity.

MyPlate continues with the principles embodied in the previous *MyPyramid* icon but is more specific in certain areas. *MyPlate* serves as a simple, research-based icon that sends a clear message on proportionality and exemplifies what should be on a plate of healthy foods. The tools, particularly the graphics, are designed to help Americans make food choices that are adequate for meeting nutritional standards. They also promote food choices moderate in energy level (kilocalories) and in food components or nutrients often consumed in excess (fats, added sugars, and sodium). Foods providing similar kinds of nutrients are grouped together, and as a rule, foods in one group cannot replace those in another (Table 1-3). *MyPlate* is intended to be used as food guidance for the U.S. general public and not a therapeutic diet for any specific health condition.

MyPlate (see Fig. 1-3) is designed to convey the same message of balance, variety, moderation, and adequate nutrients. The *MyPlate* icon is divided into four quadrants, each section is a different color that represents a food type: fruits are red; vegetables, green; protein foods, purple; and whole grains, brown. A smaller blue circle next to the plate represents a dairy product, especially fat-free or skim milk.

The quadrants indicate the recommended proportions on the plate for protein (approximately 5 oz a day for an average person), grain (preferably whole grain), fruit, and vegetables at each meal. This icon does not, however, indicate specific amounts to eat. Portion equivalents, in relation to items patients can relate to, are shown in Box 1-2. The main message of the plate to consumers is: (a) fruits and vegetables should fill half the plate; (b) lean protein foods such as lean red meats, poultry, seafood, nuts and seeds, beans, and soy products, should be chosen in moderation (approximately 5 oz/day), occupying one-fourth of the plate; (c) whole grains should occupy about one-fourth of the plate; and (4) milk products, especially fat-free or low-fat (1%), should also be chosen.

The ChooseMyPlate.gov website (also available in Spanish, choosemyplate.gov/en-espanol.html) provides numerous materials and useful information for both consumers and health professionals. Six tabs at the top provide links to a wealth of nutritional and physical activity information to clarify any questions: *MyPlate*, Weight Management &

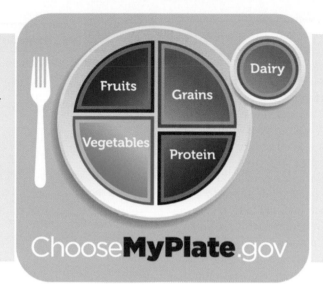

Balancing Calories

- Enjoy your food, but eat less.
- Avoid oversized portions.

Foods to Increase

- Make half your plate fruits and vegetables.
- Make at least half your grains whole grains.
- Switch to fat-free or low-fat (1%) milk.

Foods to Reduce

- Compare sodium in foods like soup, bread and frozen meals--and choose the foods with lower numbers.
- Drink water instead of sugary drinks.

FIGURE 1-3 *My Plate.* (From United Stated Department of Agriculture: ChooseMyPlate.gov, 2011.)

Table 1-3	Principal nutrient contributions of each food group				
Nutrients	**Vegetable**	**Fruit**	**Meat**	**Milk**	**Grain**
Protein			X	X	X
Vitamin A	X	X			
Vitamin D				X*	
Vitamin E	X				
Vitamin C	X	X			
Thiamin			X		X†
Riboflavin				X	X†
Niacin			X		X†
Vitamin B$_6$			X	X	
Folate/folic acid	X	X			X†
Vitamin B$_{12}$			X‡	X‡	
Calcium				X	
Phosphorus			X	X	X
Magnesium	X			X	X§
Iron			X		X†
Zinc			X	X	X
Fiber	X	X			X§

*If fortified.
†If enriched.
‡Only animal products.
§Whole grains.

BOX 1-2	What Counts as a Portion Equivalent?

- 3 oz meat—deck of cards or the size of your palm
- 2 oz meat—small chicken drumstick or thigh
- 1 oz meat—about 3 tbsp
- 1 cup vegetables—size of a fist
- Medium apple, orange, peach—size of a tennis ball
- ¼ cup dried fruit—golf ball
- ½ cup fruit or vegetable—half of a baseball
- 1 cup broccoli—light bulb
- Medium potato—computer mouse
- ½ cup cooked pasta—ice cream scoop or half a baseball
- 1 bagel—diameter of a compact disc (CD)
- 1 oz cheese—2 dominos or 2 dice
- 2 tbsp peanut butter—ping-pong ball
- 1 tsp butter or margarine—tip of thumb

Calories, Physical Activity, SuperTracker & Other Tools, Printable Materials & Ordering, and Healthy Eating Tips. Some of the valuable in-depth nutritional data and resources in the *MyPlate* tab include: foods included in each group and subgroup; pictures of the foods in blue font; amounts of each group needed daily for various stages of life; amount, portion, or equivalent of a serving; health benefits and nutrients; tips for choosing foods from each group; portion (or ounce equivalent); information about kilocalories and tips for weight management; and healthy eating tips for the general public as well as for special groups—pregnant and breastfeeding women and preschoolers. Five major media companies will be using the *MyPlate* icon on recipes to take the guesswork out of finding healthy recipes. A new Pinterest page (http://www.pinterest.com/MyPlaterecipes) and the Food and Nutrition Service (http://www.fns.usda.gov/fncs-recipe-box) provide healthy recipes (based on *MyPlate* and *Dietary Guidelines)* for all types of cooks (consumers, schools, and child care providers).

The physical activity tab has links that discuss the what, why, and how much physical activity, as well as tips for increasing physical activity and tools for calculating how many kilocalories different physical activities burn. The "SuperTracker" can help an individual plan, analyze, and track food intake and physical activity and provides resources for kilocalories, fat, portions, and food labels. It allows an individual to (a) create a customized appropriate, caloric allowance with a corresponding food group plan based on the individual's gender, age, activity level and weight goals; (b) self-monitor or journal food intake with the "My Journal" feature; (c) track what and how much is eaten to compare the current diet with a customized plan; (d) monitor the intensity and duration of daily activities with the Physical Activity Tracker feature; and (e) interact with a virtual coach, receiving "how-to" tips and feedback related to the individual's goals. The program evaluates foods based on the recommended number of servings for the individual from each food group. A database of 8,000 foods provides information about a specific food (kilocalories, serving size, and food group). Additionally 600 types of physical activity are available for planning 12 different caloric levels of food intake (ranging from 1000 to 3200 kcal per day) designed to help individuals find the caloric balance that will help achieve a healthier weight. The website allows individuals to maintain a record of their food intake and physical activity for up to one year. It evaluates physical activity status and provides related energy expenditure information and educational messages.

Many of the USDA materials (brochures, tip sheets, graphics, and archived material), available in English or Spanish, can be accessed from the "Printable Materials & Ordering" tab or the links at the bottom of the *MyPlate* homepage, "Resources for Nutrition & Health."

Make Half Your Plate Fruits and Vegetables

Fruit Group

The key message, "Make half your plate fruits and vegetables" can be better understood in terms of quantity recommended daily or weekly. The daily recommendation for fruit is 1.5 to 2 cups, but most adults eat less than 1.5 cups daily.[18] Snacks provide about one-third of the total daily fruit intake for adults.[19]

Any fruit or 100% fruit juice counts as part of the fruit group. Fruits are naturally low in fat, sodium, and kilocalories, and do not contain cholesterol. They are also important sources of potassium, dietary fiber, vitamin C, and folate. Fresh, frozen, canned, or dried fruits are recommended for their fiber content, but fruit juice should be minimized because it does not contain fiber.

Vegetable Group

Two to 3 cups of vegetables are recommended for adults daily, to include a weekly amount of 1.5 to 2 cups dark green vegetables, 4 to 6 cups red and orange vegetables, 1.5 to 2 cups dry beans and peas, 4 to 6 cups starchy vegetables, and 4 to 5 cups other vegetables. (Specific amounts for different genders and age groups are available on the ChooseMyPlate.com website). The total amount of red, orange, and dark-green vegetables recommended per week is 7 cups, but dietary-intake surveys show most Americans eat only about 3.5 cups per week.[20]

Vegetables are primary sources of the required nutrients dietary fiber, vitamin A (carotenoids), vitamin C, folic acid, and potassium (Table 1-4). Most vegetables are low in fat in their natural state and are cholesterol free. Because of their high water and fiber content, most vegetables are relatively low in kilocalories. Dark-green vegetables provide calcium, iron, magnesium and riboflavin. Beans are unusual because

Table 1-4	Contributions of selected fruits and vegetables		
Fruit/Vegetable	Vitamin A[1,2]	Vitamin C[3,4]	Fiber[5,6]
Acorn squash	X	X	X
Apple			X
Avocado		X	XX
Banana		X	X
Bell pepper		XX	
Bok choy	XX	XX	N/A
Broccoli, cooked	XX	XX	X
Brussels sprouts	X	XX	X
Cabbage		XX	X
Cantaloupe	XX	XX	
Carrot	XX	X	X
Cauliflower		XX	
Celery			X
Collard greens	XX	XX	
Grapefruit	XX	X X	
Iceberg lettuce	X		
Kale	XX	XX	
Kiwi		XX	X
Kohlrabi		XX	X
Mango	XX	XX	
Orange		XX	
Papaya	XX	XX	
Pear			X
Prune, dried	X		XX
Romaine lettuce	XX		
Spinach	XX	X	
Strawberry		XX	
Sweet potato	XX	XX	X
Swiss chard	XX	XX	
Tomato	X	XX	

1. X = Good source: 500-950 IU/100 g
2. XX = Excellent source: ≥ 950 IU/100 g
3. X = Good source: 6-11.4 mg/100 g
4. XX = Excellent source: ≥11.4 mg/100 g
5. X = Good source: 2.5-4.75 g/100 g
6. XX = Excellent source: ≥4.75 g/100 g

Data from U.S. Department of Agriculture, Agricultural Research Service. *USDA National Nutrient Database for Standard Reference, Release 25.* Nutrient Data Laboratory, 2012. Accessed January 16, 2013. Available at: http://www.ars.usda.gov/ba/bhnrc/ndl

they are in both the vegetable and protein groups. Beans contain protein, fiber, calcium, folic acid, and potassium.

Grains Group

Five to 8 oz of grains are recommended daily for adults with a goal of choosing at least half (or a minimum of 3) of the total recommended servings as whole grains. All whole-grain, refined and enriched, or fortified-grain products are included in this group, e.g., barley, buckwheat, bulgur, corn, millet, rice, rye, oats, sorghum, wheat, and wild rice. A variety of whole-grain products should be selected, including wheat, rice, oats, and corn. Whole-grain products contribute more fiber, magnesium, phosphorous, and zinc than do enriched products (see Table 1-3). Enriched breads and cereals are fortified with folic acid, which is important for women who may become pregnant.

Most Americans (61%) believe they are consuming adequate amounts of whole grains, but the Dietary Guidelines Advisory Committee estimates that 95% of Americans do not reach guideline amounts.[21] The difficulty in identifying whole grains is a major barrier. Labels like "100% wheat," "stone-ground," and "multigrain" do not guarantee that the food contains whole grain. Whole grains differ from a nutritional perspective, with significant variations in levels and effects of the fiber. Multiple conflicting definitions exist for identifying whole grain products, causing confusion for consumers. Color is a poor indicator of whole grains because molasses or caramel food coloring may be added. As a result of the *Dietary Guidelines*, food manufacturers have introduced more processed foods with higher whole-grain content. Based on the FDA guidelines, "whole grain" includes "cereal grains that consist of the intact and unrefined, ground, cracked, or flaked fruit of the grains whose principal components—the starchy endosperm, germ, and bran—are present in the same relative proportions as they exist in the intact grain."

Milk and Milk Products Group

The recommendation for this group is 3 cups for all age groups, except children younger than 9 years of age. Children 2 to 3 years old need 2 cups, and 4- to 8-year-olds need 2.5 cups of milk. Milk products provide calcium and potassium, and may be a good source of vitamin D. Fortified milk products are important sources of vitamin D. However, many milk substitutes (cheese, yogurt, and ice cream) are not fortified with vitamin D (unless made with fortified milk). Whole milk and many cheeses are high in saturated fat and can have negative health implications. Low-fat or fat-free milk products provide little or no fat and should be chosen most often to avoid consuming more kilocalories than needed. Whole milk consumption has dropped, and reduced-fat milk intake has remained stable, resulting in less overall milk consumption. The dairy group does not include high-fat products, such as butter and cream, because they are not high in calcium, riboflavin, and protein.

The consumption of milk and milk products can help children and adolescents achieve peak bone mass and reduce the risk of low bone mass and osteoporosis. In terms of oral health, two studies indicate that higher dairy product consumption is associated with decreased prevalence and severity of periodontal disease.[22,23]

Protein Group

This group includes all high-protein foods, including meat, poultry, fish, dry beans or peas, eggs, nuts, and seeds. Lean or low-fat meat and poultry selections are recommended. Fish, nuts, and seeds contain a healthy type of fat, so they should be chosen more often than meat or poultry. Dry beans and peas, such as kidney beans, pinto beans, lima beans, black-eyed peas, and lentils, are included in this group, as well as in the vegetable group.

The daily recommendation for foods from the protein group is 5 to 6.5 ounces. These foods are also important

Table 1-5	Outstanding contributions of various protein foods
Protein Food	**Nutrient**
Lean red meats	Iron B vitamins Zinc
Pork	Thiamin Zinc
Poultry	Potassium Niacin
Liver and egg yolks	Vitamin A Iron Zinc
Dry peas and beans, soybeans, and nuts	Magnesium Fiber Zinc

sources of protein, B vitamins (niacin, thiamin, riboflavin, and B_6), vitamin E, iron, zinc, and magnesium. A variety of foods from this group should be included, as each food has distinct nutritional advantages (Table 1-5). By varying choices and including fish, nuts, beans, and seeds, the intake of healthful fats, such as monounsaturated fatty acids and polyunsaturated fatty acids, is increased. Dry beans and peas are excellent sources of plant protein and dietary fiber, and contribute other nutrients also found in meats, poultry, and fish. Whether they are counted as a vegetable or a meat, several cups a week are recommended. Vegetarians can choose eggs, beans, nuts, nut butters, peas, and soy products to obtain adequate amounts of protein (see Chapter 5).

Current scientific evidence indicates that the amount of protein intake is not a public health concern for adults and children older than 4 years of age, but leaner types of protein foods need to be chosen more often. Most Americans consume approximately twice as much protein as they need. Although this may not be harmful, high-fat meats may be an undesirable source of kilocalories, cholesterol, and/or saturated fatty acids. Protein supplements promoted to increase muscle mass do not contain nutrients important for health other than what foods provide. These should be used only after consulting a healthcare provider or the RDN.

Dental Considerations

- Many patients understand the general concepts of healthy eating, but they lack specific knowledge or motivation to help implement the recommendations. Most questions or misunderstandings are related to servings and food group placement.
- Dental hygienists should be knowledgeable enough to provide foundational information about whole grains, types of fats, and physical activity.
- Assess each patient's diet to determine nutrient adequacy or inadequacy. (For example, if a patient eliminates fruits and vegetables, vitamin A and C deficiencies may develop; if milk and other milk products are eliminated, calcium and vitamin D deficiencies may develop).

Continued

Dental Considerations—cont'd

- Ensure patients are aware of the number and size of servings recommended from each food group daily to obtain adequate nutrients.
- Although consumers are getting the message that they need to make positive dietary and lifestyle changes, putting that advice into practice is challenging and confusing for many (Fig. 1-4).
- A large proportion of Americans, regardless of their weight, are malnourished in terms of vitamins and mineral intake. However, they should not be told to eat less food, but to choose more nutrient-dense foods.

Nutritional Directions

- Within each food group, individual foods can vary widely in the number of kilocalories furnished; therefore knowledge about serving sizes is important.
- If nutrient-dense foods are selected from each food group in the amounts recommended, a small amount of discretionary kilocalories can be consumed as added fats or sugars, alcohol, or other foods.
- Dairy products are poor sources of iron and vitamin C, but they are good sources of protein, calcium, and riboflavin.
- Caloric consumption can be decreased by substituting low-fat or skim milk for whole milk. The nutrient content is the same for whole milk and low-fat milk, except for the amount of fat and kilocalories. Skim milk (1%) or fat-free milk is recommended for all healthy Americans older than age 2 years.
- Foods in the grains group are economical as well as nutritious; they may be staple items for those in lower socioeconomic groups. However, whole-grain products may be more expensive, so encourage patients to increase these food choices as much as possible.
- Cholesterol occurs naturally in all foods of animal origin.
- Elimination or reduction of one or more food groups will reduce the variety of food intake, thereby reducing the number or amount of nutrients consumed.
- Adults watching their weight should choose minimal amounts of servings from all groups and limit portion sizes.

American diets are out of balance with dietary recommendations

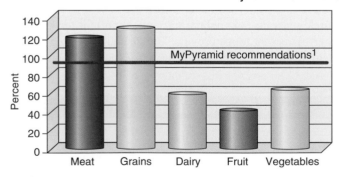

[1]2009 data based on a 2,000 calorie diet

Note: Food availability data serve as proxies for food consumption
Source: USDA, ERS

FIGURE 1-4 American diets are out of balance with dietary recommendations. (From the U.S. Department of Agriculture and Economic Research Center. Available at http:// webarchives.cdlib.org/wayback.public/UERS _ag_1/20120208040825/ http://www.ers.usda.gov/Briefing/ DietQuality/charts/balance_diets_ers.jpg.)

OTHER FOOD GUIDES

Not all healthcare professionals agree that *MyPlate* is the ideal method to promote health and wellness. However, the recommendations in *MyPlate* are remarkably consistent with other population-based recommendations designed to control obesity, diabetes, CHD and stroke, hypertension, cancer, and osteoporosis. Although different guides were derived from different types of nutrition research and for different purposes, they share consistent messages: eat more fruits, vegetables, legumes, and whole grains; eat less added sugar and saturated fat; and emphasize plant oils. Primary differences are in the types of recommended vegetables and protein sources, and the amount of recommended dairy products and total oil/fats. Overall nutrient values are also similar for most nutrients.

The recommendations in *MyPlate* are similar to the recommendations of the DASH eating plan (discussed in Chapter 12), the American Heart Association (discussed in Chapter 6), the American Diabetes Association (discussed in Chapter 7), the National Cholesterol Education Program Expert Panel on Detection, Evaluation and Treatment of High Blood Cholesterol in Adults (Adult Treatment Panel III), and the American Cancer Society. Calculated nutrient intakes associated with following any of these guidelines are generally within the ranges of nutrient recommendations of the *Dietary Guidelines*.

Healthy Eating Plate

One alternative food guide is the Healthy Eating Plate created by nutrition faculty at Harvard School of Public Health (Fig. 1-5). The goal of this plate is to help people stay healthy by choosing a healthy diet. The legend outside the plate describes what types of food should be chosen at a typical meal— colorful fruits and vegetables, whole grains, low-fat meats— with a reminder to choose healthy oils like olive and canola. Water, tea, or coffee (with little or no sugar) are good choices for some meals, limiting low-fat milk to 2 servings/day. "Stay active!" is a reminder to stay active to facilitate weight control. The plate should be a moderate size to meet the individual's energy needs.

Canada's Food Guide

Canada has also developed a pictorial food guide to help Canadians choose food wisely (Fig. 1-6). The *Food Guide* rainbow encourages consumers to find their own healthy lifestyle—a pot of gold. The website (http://www.hc-sc.gc.ca/ fn-an/food-guide-aliment/myguide-monguide/index- eng.php) is interactive, allowing consumers to personalize the food guide, providing recipes, tips for healthy eating and physical activity, and other educational materials.

Other Nations' Guides

Many nations eat very differently than Americans. No one food is essential for good health. People in many countries are healthy (sometimes healthier than Americans) despite eating very different types of foods. This is further discussed

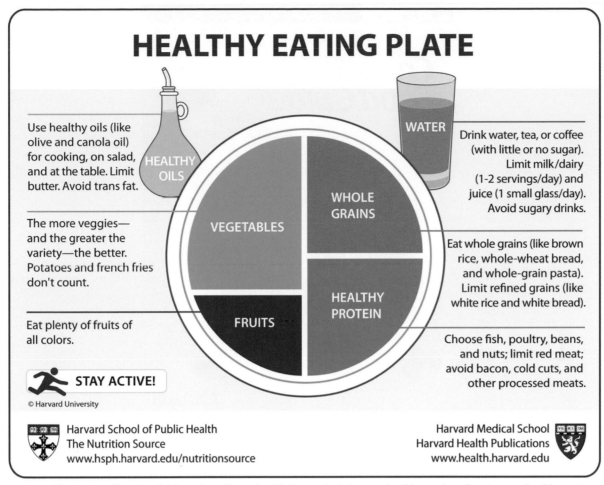

FIGURE 1-5 Healthy Eating Plate. Available at: http://www.health.harvard.edu/images/healthy-eating-plate-images/healthy-eating-plate.pdf. (Copyright © 2011, Harvard University. For more information about The Healthy Eating Plate, please see The Nutrition Source, Department of Nutrition, Harvard School of Public Health, and Harvard Health Publications, www.health.harvard.edu.)

in Chapter 16; food guides from other countries are shown on the inside of the back cover.

NUTRITION LABELING

Nutrition Facts Label

Two categories of claims currently can be used on foods in the United States: nutrient content claims and health claims. Nutrient content claims describe the percentage of a nutrient in a product relative to the daily value. Health claims describe a relationship between a food or food component and reduced risk of a disease or health-related condition. These claims are based on a very high standard of scientific evidence with significant agreement.

In a concerted effort by the USDA and FDA to improve the health and well-being of the American people by enhancing nutritional knowledge, the Nutrition Facts label was designed as a graphic tool to inform consumers about nutrient content of foods available in the supermarket (Fig. 1-7). Nutrition labels on product packaging help health educators and consumers know what nutrients are in a food, enabling them to compare nutritional values of various products.

These labels provide nutrition information regarding general recommendations for most adults. Consumers are more likely to read nutrition labels to compare similar products or when they are considering purchasing a new item.

The labeling policy requires that approximately 90% of all foods provide nutritional information based on the nutrients provided in a single serving. In 2012, the USDA's Food Safety and Inspection Service began requiring packages of ground or chopped meat and poultry, and the most popular whole, raw cuts of meat and poultry (such as chicken breast or steak), to have nutritional information either on the package labels or on display for consumers. These nutrition labels differ from the Nutrition Facts label required by the FDA; they list the number of calories and grams of total fat and saturated fat in a product. For foods that are not packaged, the information must be displayed at the point of purchase (e.g., in a counter card, sign, or booklet).

The FDA established standardized serving portions for food labels (based on a reference amount) in an effort to educate and provide the consumer with information about how foods fit into a healthy diet. The number of servings in a container is expressed to the nearest whole number. One

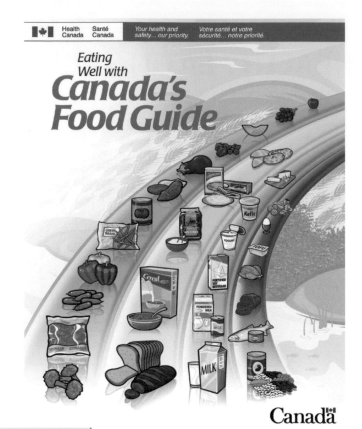

FIGURE 1-6 Eating well with Canada's food guide. (From *Canada's Guide*. Last modified: May 23, 2012. © Her Majesty the Queen in Right of Canada, represented by the Minister of Health Canada, 2011. This publication may be reproduced without permission. No changes permitted. HC Pub.: 4651 Cat.: H164-38/1-2011E-PDF ISBN: 978-1-100-19255-0. Available at http://www.hc-sc.gc.ca/fn-an/food-guide-aliment/order-commander/index-eng.php.)

Make each Food Guide Serving count...
wherever you are – at home, at school, at work or when eating out!

▸ **Eat at least one dark green and one orange vegetable each day.**
- Go for dark green vegetables such as broccoli, romaine lettuce and spinach.
- Go for orange vegetables such as carrots, sweet potatoes and winter squash.

▸ **Choose vegetables and fruit prepared with little or no added fat, sugar or salt.**
- Enjoy vegetables steamed, baked or stir-fried instead of deep-fried.

▸ **Have vegetables and fruit more often than juice.**

▸ **Make at least half of your grain products whole grain each day.**
- Eat a variety of whole grains such as barley, brown rice, oats, quinoa and wild rice.
- Enjoy whole grain breads, oatmeal or whole wheat pasta.

▸ **Choose grain products that are lower in fat, sugar or salt.**
- Compare the Nutrition Facts table on labels to make wise choices.
- Enjoy the true taste of grain products. When adding sauces or spreads, use small amounts.

▸ **Drink skim, 1%, or 2% milk each day.**
- Have 500 mL (2 cups) of milk every day for adequate vitamin D.
- Drink fortified soy beverages if you do not drink milk.

▸ **Select lower fat milk alternatives.**
- Compare the Nutrition Facts table on yogurts or cheeses to make wise choices.

▸ **Have meat alternatives such as beans, lentils and tofu often.**

▸ **Eat at least two Food Guide Servings of fish each week.***
- Choose fish such as char, herring, mackerel, salmon, sardines and trout.

▸ **Select lean meat and alternatives prepared with little or no added fat or salt.**
- Trim the visible fat from meats. Remove the skin on poultry.
- Use cooking methods such as roasting, baking or poaching that require little or no added fat.
- If you eat luncheon meats, sausages or prepackaged meats, choose those lower in salt (sodium) and fat.

Enjoy a variety of foods from the four food groups.

Satisfy your thirst with water!
Drink water regularly. It's a calorie-free way to quench your thirst. Drink more water in hot weather or when you are very active.

* Health Canada provides advice for limiting exposure to mercury from certain types of fish. Refer to www.healthcanada.gc.ca for the latest information.

Advice for different ages and stages...

Children
Following *Canada's Food Guide* helps children grow and thrive.

Young children have small appetites and need calories for growth and development.

- Serve small nutritious meals and snacks each day.
- Do not restrict nutritious foods because of their fat content. Offer a variety of foods from the four food groups.
- Most of all... be a good role model.

Women of childbearing age
All women who could become pregnant and those who are pregnant or breastfeeding need a multivitamin containing **folic acid** every day. Pregnant women need to ensure that their multivitamin also contains **iron**. A health care professional can help you find the multivitamin that's right for you.

Pregnant and breastfeeding women need more calories. Include an extra 2 to 3 Food Guide Servings each day.

Here are two examples:
- Have fruit and yogurt for a snack, or
- Have an extra slice of toast at breakfast and an extra glass of milk at supper.

Men and women over 50
The need for **vitamin D** increases after the age of 50.

In addition to following *Canada's Food Guide*, everyone over the age of 50 should take a daily vitamin D supplement of 10 µg (400 IU).

Eat well and be active today and every day!

The benefits of eating well and being active include:
- Better overall health.
- Lower risk of disease.
- A healthy body weight.
- Feeling and looking better.
- More energy.
- Stronger muscles and bones.

Be active
To be active every day is a step towards better health and a healthy body weight.

Canada's Physical Activity Guide recommends building 30 to 60 minutes of moderate physical activity into daily life for adults and at least 90 minutes a day for children and youth. You don't have to do it all at once. Add it up in periods of at least 10 minutes at a time for adults and five minutes at a time for children and youth.

Start slowly and build up.

Eat well
Another important step towards better health and a healthy body weight is to follow *Canada's Food Guide* by:

- Eating the recommended amount and type of food each day.
- Limiting foods and beverages high in calories, fat, sugar or salt (sodium) such as cakes and pastries, chocolate and candies, cookies and granola bars, doughnuts and muffins, ice cream and frozen desserts, french fries, potato chips, nachos and other salty snacks, alcohol, fruit flavoured drinks, soft drinks, sports and energy drinks, and sweetened hot or cold drinks.

Read the label
- Compare the Nutrition Facts table on food labels to choose products that contain less fat, saturated fat, trans fat, sugar and sodium.
- Keep in mind that the calories and nutrients listed are for the amount of food found at the top of the Nutrition Facts table.

Limit trans fat
When a Nutrition Facts table is not available, ask for nutrition information to choose foods lower in trans and saturated fats.

Take a step today...
✓ Have breakfast every day. It may help control your hunger later in the day.
✓ Walk wherever you can – get off the bus early, use the stairs.
✓ Benefit from eating vegetables and fruit at all meals and as snacks.
✓ Spend less time being inactive such as watching TV or playing computer games.
✓ Request nutrition information about menu items when eating out to help you make healthier choices.
✓ Enjoy eating with family and friends!
✓ Take time to eat and savour every bite!

For more information, interactive tools, or additional copies visit Canada's Food Guide on-line at:
www.healthcanada.gc.ca/foodguide

or contact:
Publications
Health Canada
Ottawa, Ontario K1A 0K9
E-Mail: publications@hc-sc.gc.ca
Tel.: 1-866-225-0709
Fax: (613) 941-5366
TTY: 1-800-267-1245

Également disponible en français sous le titre :
Bien manger avec le Guide alimentaire canadien

This publication can be made available on request on diskette, large print, audio-cassette and braille.

Nutrition Facts		
Per 0 mL (0 g)		
Amount		% Daily Value
Calories 0		
Fat 0 g		0 %
Saturates 0 g		0 %
+ Trans 0 g		
Cholesterol 0 mg		
Sodium 0 mg		0 %
Carbohydrate 0 g		0 %
Fibre 0 g		0 %
Sugars 0 g		
Protein 0 g		
Vitamin A 0 %	Vitamin C	0 %
Calcium 0 %	Iron	0 %

How do I count Food Guide Servings in a meal?

Here is an example:

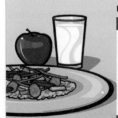

Vegetable and beef stir-fry with rice, a glass of milk and an apple for dessert		
250 mL (1 cup) mixed broccoli, carrot and sweet red pepper	=	**2 Vegetables and Fruit** Food Guide Servings
75 g (2½ oz.) lean beef	=	**1 Meat and Alternatives** Food Guide Serving
250 mL (1 cup) brown rice	=	**2 Grain Products** Food Guide Servings
5 mL (1 tsp) canola oil	=	part of your **Oils and Fats** intake for the day
250 mL (1 cup) 1% milk	=	**1 Milk and Alternatives** Food Guide Serving
1 apple	=	**1 Vegetables and Fruit** Food Guide Serving

FIGURE 1-6, cont'd

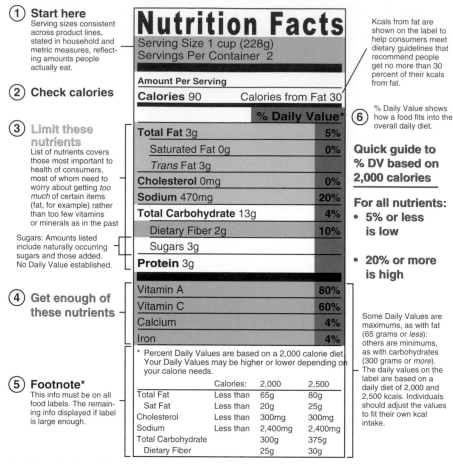

FIGURE 1-7 An example of the food label format that currently is mandatory in the United States. (From How to understand and use the nutrition facts label. Department of Health and Human Services, FDA, June 2000; updated July 22, 2011. Available at http://www.fda.gov/Food/ResourcesForYou/Consumers/NFLPM/ucm274593.htm.)

of the main issues with nutrition labeling is that rules for labeling portions can be confusing for consumers and are complicated further by the fact that Americans usually eat larger portions. For example, a 12-oz can of soda has 140 kcal and is legally considered a single serving, but a 20-oz bottle lists 100 kcal per serving because a single serving in a larger container is 8 oz. Per FDA regulations, a serving of bagel is about 2 oz, which is one-fourth the size of most bagels. Misleading serving sizes may be a reason consumers are eating far more kilocalories than they think.

Nutrients provided on the nutrition label include total kilocalories; total kilocalories from fats; total fat and saturated fat (g); *trans* fat (g); cholesterol (g); total carbohydrates, complex carbohydrates, and sugars (g); dietary fiber (g); protein (g); sodium (mg); and vitamins and minerals (%). **Daily reference values (DRVs)** provide information for nutrients important for making wise food choices, i.e., total fat, saturated fat, protein, cholesterol, carbohydrate, fiber, and sodium. A product's nutrient profile is based on the percentage of DRVs (Table 1-6), but the term **daily value (DV)** is used on the label. DVs for protein, fat, saturated and *trans* fatty acids, cholesterol, sodium and potassium, total carbohydrate, and dietary fiber are based on various scientific documents written between 1987 and 1991, extracting

Table 1-6	Daily reference values (DRVs)*
Food Component	**DRV**
Protein	50 g†
Carbohydrate	300 g
Total fat	<65 g
Saturated fat	<20 g
Cholesterol	<300 mg
Sodium	<2400 mg
Potassium	>3500 mg
Fiber	25 g

From Kurtzweil P: "Daily values" encourage healthy diet. In *FDA consumer: focus on food labeling*, Washington, DC, 1993, Department of Health and Human Services.

*Daily reference values (DRVs) do not appear on the nutrient label. The term *daily value* appears on the label for ease of understanding and reflects the DRV and the DRI standards to encourage a healthy diet.

†Protein amount is for adults and children older than 4 years of age only. The RDI for protein has been established for certain groups: children 1-4 years, 16 mg; infants <1 year, 14 g; pregnant women, 60 g; nursing mothers, 65 g.

Table 1-7	Reference daily intakes
Nutrient	**Amount**
Vitamin A	5000 IU
Vitamin C	60 mg
Thiamin	1.5 mg
Riboflavin	1.7 mg
Niacin	20 mg
Calcium	1 g
Iron	18 mg
Vitamin D	400 IU
Vitamin E	30 IU
Vitamin B_6	2 mg
Folic acid	400 mcg
Vitamin B_{12}	6 mcg
Phosphorus	1 g
Iodine	150 mcg
Magnesium	400 mg
Zinc	15 mg
Copper	2 mg
Biotin	0.3 mg
Pantothenic acid	10 mg

recommended intakes to establish a basis for DVs for nutrients without RDAs.

For ease of standardizing the label, 2000 kcal is the reference amount for calculating the percentage of the DV provided in a serving. The vitamin and mineral content of a product is listed only in terms of percent DV (%DV). This rough guide indicates whether the food contains a small or large amount of a nutrient and is useful in comparing nutrient content of various products. Foods that provide 20% or more of the DV are considered high in a nutrient. Although nutrient label information uses the term *daily value,* the amounts for the nutrients are based on the **reference daily intake (RDI),** which is usually larger than the RDA for a specific age/gender group (Table 1-7). No %DV has been established for *trans* fats, sugars, and protein. Information regarding sugars and *trans* fats can be used to limit their intake. DVs are not the recommended intake for an individual or population group and are not meant to be used for planning diets. They are merely reference numbers used to compare various foods and to provide a perspective on daily nutrient needs, not to assess nutritional adequacy of a diet.

The requirement to label products has resulted in food manufacturers reformulating foods to provide products consumers feel are healthier. As a result of consumer preferences, a significant number of foods have been reformulated to contain less sugar, high fructose corn syrup, and *trans* fats, and more fiber.

The FDA expects to issue a proposal for changes to the Nutrition Facts label in the near future, but they have not discussed the scope of the proposed rule; they are expected to address serving sizes, daily values, adjustments to label formats, and additional nutrient declarations.

Health Claims

A label cannot include an explicit or implied nutrient content claim unless it uses terms that have been defined by the FDA, such as "free," "low," "more," or "reduced." Box 1-3 defines some of the established terms and definitions used on food labels.

Only health claims that have been approved and authorized by the FDA can be used on food products and dietary supplements. Health claims allowed by the FDA include statements dealing with the relationship between a specific nutrient and its ability to reduce the risk of disease or health-related conditions, as listed in Box 1-4. If a food is labeled with such a claim, it must meet specific criteria regarding the amount of that specific nutrient and sometimes other nutrients in the product. Products making a claim are required to use the FDA's exact wording.

Health claims on foods are limited and regulated in an effort to protect consumers from false or misleading claims. **Unqualified health claims** must be supported by qualified experts agreeing that scientific evidence is available determining a relationship between a nutrient and a specific disease. **Qualified health claims** are supported by some evidence, but do not meet the scientific standard; thus their claim must be accompanied by a disclaimer as specified by the FDA. Since 2002, when the FDA began allowing companies to petition for qualified health claims, 12 qualified health claims have been permitted on food labels. A health claim must use the exact wording specified by the FDA. For instance, the first qualified claim allowed by the FDA was the association between nuts and heart disease; verbiage on the package must read[24]: "Scientific evidence suggests but does not prove 1.5 ounces per day of most nuts such as (insert name of specific nut) as part of a diet low in saturated fat and cholesterol may reduce the risk of heart disease."

Additional Nutrition Labels

Many consumers are confused by the Nutrition Facts panel and prefer information in a quicker and easier to read format. Research shows consumers can more easily interpret and select healthier products with nutrient-specific front-of-package nutrition labels that incorporate text and symbolic colors to indicate nutrient levels rather than nutrient-specific labels that emphasize numeric information, as is currently displayed on the Nutrition Facts label.[25] Food manufacturers, supermarket chains, trade associations, and health organizations have developed comprehensive mechanisms to provide information about the nutritional quality of foods and beverages either on product packaging or shelf tags in retail settings nutrition labeling systems. In these programs, foods are rated based on their nutritional profiles for containing healthy ingredients (fiber and whole grains) and less of nutrients that are considered unhealthy (saturated and *trans* fats). These ratings allow consumers to compare different types of the same food within a category. Fact-based systems list kilocalories and/or nutrient amounts and sometimes the percent daily values from the Nutrition Facts

---

BOX 1-3   Food Label Terminology

Calories
- *Calorie free*: Fewer than 5 calories per serving
- *Low calorie*: 40 calories or less per serving, or per 50 g of the food
- *Reduced or fewer calories*: At least 25% fewer calories per serving than reference food

Fat
- *Fat-free*: Less than 0.5 g of fat per serving
- *Saturated fat–free*: Less than 0.5 g per serving, and the level of *trans* fatty acids does not exceed 1% of total fat
- *Low fat*: 3 g or less per serving, or per 50 g of the food
- *Low saturated fat*: 1 g or less per serving and not more than 15% of calories from saturated fatty acids
- *Reduced or less fat*: At least 25% less per serving than reference food
- *Reduced or less saturated fat*: At least 25% less per serving than reference food

Cholesterol
- *Cholesterol-free*: Less than 2 mg of cholesterol and 2 g or less of saturated fat per serving
- *Low cholesterol*: 20 mg or less or 2 g or less of saturated fat per serving, or per 50 g of the food
- *Reduced or less cholesterol*: At least 25% less and 2 g or less of saturated fat per serving than reference food

Sodium
- *Sodium-free*: Less than 5 mg per serving
- *Low sodium*: 140 mg or less per serving, or per 50 g of the food
- *Very low sodium*: 35 mg or less per serving, or per 50 g of the food
- *Reduced or less sodium*: At least 50% less per serving than reference food

Fiber
- *High fiber*: 5 g or more per serving (foods with high-fiber claims must meet the definition for low fat, or the level of total fat must appear next to the high-fiber claim)

- *Good source of fiber*: 2.5 to 4.9 g per serving
- *More or added fiber*: At least 2.5 g more per serving than reference food

Sugar
- *Sugar free*: Less than 0.5 g per serving
- *No added sugar, without added sugar, or no sugar added*:
  - No sugars are added during processing or packaging, including ingredients that contain sugars (e.g., fruit juices, applesauce, or dried fruit)
  - Processing does not increase the sugar content to an amount higher than is naturally present in the ingredients (a functionally insignificant increase in sugars is acceptable from processes used for purposes other than increasing sugar content)
  - The food that resembles it and for which it substitutes normally contains added sugars
  - If it does not meet the requirements for a low- or reduced-calorie food, that product bears a statement that the food is not low calorie or reduced calorie, and directs consumers' attention to the nutritional panel for additional information on sugars and calorie content
- *Reduced sugar*: At least 25% less sugar per serving than reference food

Healthy
Products using the term "healthy" in the product name or as a claim on the label must contain, per serving, no more than 3 g of fat, 1 g of saturated fat, 350 mg of sodium, or 60 mg of cholesterol. They must supply at least 10% of the daily value for at least one of six nutrients: vitamins A and C, calcium, iron, protein, and fiber. Raw meat, poultry, and fish can be labeled "healthy" if they contain, per serving, no more than 5 g of fat, 2 g of saturated fat, and 95 mg of cholesterol.

U.S. Food and Drug Administration: *Food labeling guide*. September 1994; revised October 2009. Accessed January 17, 2013: http://www.fda.gov/Food/GuidanceComplianceRegulatoryInformation/GuidanceDocuments/FoodLabelingNutrition/FoodLabelingGuide/default.htm.

BOX 1-4   Claims Authorized by the U.S. Food and Drug Administration

- Calcium and reduced risk of osteoporosis
- Sodium and increased risk of hypertension
- Dietary fat and increased risk of cancer
- Saturated fat and cholesterol and increased risk of heart disease
- Fiber-containing grain products, fruits, and vegetables, and reduced risk of cancer
- Fruits, vegetables, and grain products that contain fiber, particularly soluble fiber, and reduced risk of heart disease
- Fruits and vegetables and reduced risk of cancer
- Folic acid and reduced risk of neural tube defects during pregnancy
- Noncariogenic carbohydrate sweeteners and reduced risk of dental caries

- Soluble fiber from certain foods and reduced risk of heart disease
- Soy protein and reduced risk of heart disease
- Plant sterol/stanol esters and reduced risk of heart disease
- Whole-grain foods and reduced risk of heart disease and certain cancers
- Potassium and reduced risk of hypertension and stroke
- Fluoride and decreased risk of dental caries
- Saturated fat, cholesterol, and *trans* fats and increased risk of heart disease
- Substitute of saturated fat with unsaturated fatty acids and decreased risk of heart disease

panel on the front of the product or on a shelf tag. Examples of this system include Nutrition at a Glance (Kellogg Company), What's Inside (Mars, Inc.), and Nutrition Highlights (General Mills).

Better-for-You programs translate nutrient information into a symbol signifying that the product meets the criteria established by the sponsoring organization. Since 1985, the American Heart Association has tried to make heart-healthy grocery shopping easier with its heart check symbol. A food has to meet certain criteria to qualify to use this symbol. The Whole Grain Council has different stamps indicating two different levels of whole grain in a serving. Produce for Better Health Foundation's More Matters icon, Kraft's Sensible Solutions, and Sara Lee's Nutritional Spotlight, are several other programs that have been developed. These food rating programs can help individuals make better food choices, but the Nutrition Facts panel still needs to be reviewed. Furthermore, in order to make wise choices, food should be selected within the context of the whole diet.

The FDA is concerned that these different labeling programs could mislead consumers about the health benefits of the food. They fear that multiple systems may create more confusion, and that these systems' criteria may not be stringent enough or consistent with the *Dietary Guidelines*. Another concern is that they may encourage consumers to choose highly processed foods and refined grains rather than fruits, vegetables, and whole grains. The FDA is currently working on criteria that products must meet to display front-of-the-package nutrition claims. The FDA has asked the IOM to consider developing a single standardized guidance system for front-of-package labels. Whether all nutrition and health claims from the front of processed food packages will be eliminated or the Nutrition Facts label will be revised to provide nutrition in a less confusing format is yet to be determined.

Dental Considerations

- The dental hygienist must ensure the appropriate RDIs are used for the patient's age or grouping (e.g., when talking to a pregnant patient, the RDI for pregnancy should be used).
- To prevent confusion, the acronyms RDI and DRV are not used on labels; however, dental hygienists need to be aware of the basis for the information presented.
- The number of teaspoons of sugar in a food product can be determined from the label (see Fig. 1-7). Four grams of sugar is equivalent to 1 level teaspoon of sugar. A product containing 16 g of sugar has 4 tsp of sugar. Measuring the number of teaspoons of sugar in a product is a valuable visual aid for patients.

- To determine the percentage of sugar in a serving of a food, (a) multiply the number of grams of sugar in a product by 4 (kcal/g), (b) divide this number by the total number of kilocalories per serving, and (c) multiply by 100 to establish the percentage of calories as sugar. Using the example of the label shown in Fig. 1-7:

$$5 \text{ g sugar} \times 4 \text{ kcal/g} = 20 \text{ kcal from sugar}$$

$$20 \text{ kcal sugar} \div 250 \text{ kcal/serving} = 0.08 \times 100\% = 8\%$$

Nutritional Directions

- Read labels carefully. Ingredients are listed in order of quantity (by weight). Choose products that have less fat or oils or in which fats are listed last.
- Food labels are a useful tool to compare nutrient values of foods and learn valuable sources of nutrients. Review a label together with the patient and family. Ask the patient to bring in several labels of commonly used foods in the household for you to discuss with the patient.
- Fortified foods and supplements should not be purchased in an attempt to meet 100% of the RDIs because this may result in greater nutrient consumption than is needed, especially for young children. Concerns should be addressed to a healthcare provider or RDN.
- Because portion sizes between products can vary, remind patients to compare these when comparing products.

- Encourage patients to keep portion sizes consistent with activity level.
- On a label, point out the DVs that indicate kilocalories (carbohydrate, fat, and protein), those indicating they should be limited (fat, saturated and *trans* fat, cholesterol, and sodium), and how to determine whether a product contains a small or large amount of a nutrient (see Fig. 1-7).
- Unsweetened juices and milk contain significant amounts of sugars because of the natural content of simple carbohydrates. This may be confusing for some patients because both are encouraged in appropriate amounts. Looking at "sugars" on the label may be misleading, whereas the total carbohydrate in the product more closely reflects actual carbohydrate content. Soluble fiber is included in the total carbohydrate kilocalories, but not insoluble fiber.

HEALTH APPLICATION I   Obesity

The U.S. population is leading the rest of the world in obesity, but this health problem has become a global issue. Americans comprise 5% of the world's population, yet the United States accounts for almost one-third of the world's weight because of obesity. Obesity is a threat to the world's future food security.[26]

Although the prevalence of obesity is showing signs of leveling off, obesity remains at unacceptably high levels. During the past 20 years, the heaviest BMI groups have been increasing at the fastest rates.[27] In 2010, approximately 6.6% of adults were severely obese (more than 100 pounds over a healthy weight), up from 3.9% in 2000. More alarming is the forecast that the prevalence of obesity may reach 51% by 2030.[28] Additionally, the statistics are very discouraging in ethnic groups (i.e., Hispanics, African Americans, Native Americans, and Alaska Natives) because the prevalence of obesity is markedly higher than in white Americans.

The *Healthy People 2010* goals of 15% obesity among adults were not met. The goals of *Healthy People 2020* nutritional objectives include increasing the proportion of adults who are at a healthy weight to 33.9% compared with the current level of 30.8% in 2005-2008, and reducing the proportion of adults who are obese to 30.5% compared with 33.9% who were obese in 2005-2008.[29] The 2020 goals related to the objectives to attain a healthy weight include increasing the proportion of adults who engage in leisure-time physical activity, meeting federal physical activity guidelines for aerobic physical activity and muscle-strengthening activity (adults and adolescents), and increasing the proportion of trips made by walking or bicycling. Thirteen states currently have adult obesity rates above 30% whereas 20 years ago, no state had an obesity rate above 15%. If rates continue to increase at the current pace, adult obesity rates could exceed 60% in 13 states by 2030.[30]

Maintaining a healthy weight is a major goal to reduce the burden of illness and its consequent reduction in quality of life and life expectancy. Obesity and overweight in adulthood go hand-in-hand with chronic diseases. These include hypertension, osteoarthritis, elevated blood cholesterol or triglyceride levels, heart disease, diabetes, gallbladder disease, sleep apnea and respiratory problems, and many cancers–esophageal, colon and rectum, breast (after menopause), endometrial (lining of the uterus), and kidney.[31] In addition to major health risks associated with obesity, researchers have found it affects other physiological functions related to quality of life and diseases: reduced sense of smell,[32] greater feelings of drowsiness and fatigue,[33] and decreased levels of fertility (lower level of testosterone in males).[34] Overweight takes a toll on the joints, especially knees, and overweight people are at increased risk of sleep apnea and asthma. Most of these conditions are associated with significant decreases in life expectancy, but also impact quality of life. Obesity affects many other aspects of life: education, income, employability, and social position. Obesity also impacts psychological and social factors related to negative attitudes that affect interpersonal interactions.

Because overweight and obesity seem to contribute to other health problems, their economic impact on the healthcare system is immense. Current estimates suggest that the yearly medical cost of adult obesity today is between $147 billion and $210 billion[35] (16.5% of the total national medical bill)[36] and is projected to increase by $48 to $66 billion/year in the United States by 2030.[37] Reducing obesity could save billions of dollars for the healthcare industry.

Weight distribution is also a factor in predicting health risk. Excess fat in the abdominal area (the "apple-shaped" body), known as android obesity, is characteristic of men, but some women also tend to accumulate more fat around the waist, especially after menopause. Accumulation of fat in the hips or thighs (the "pear-shaped body"), called gynecoid obesity, is typical of women. Any amount of upper body obesity or increased abdominal fat increases health risks. In contrast, lower body or gynecoid obesity has been thought to be relatively benign. A recent study found that gluteal adipose tissue is associated with a prediabetic condition.[38] Patients with this pattern of obesity have more difficulty losing weight and maintaining a healthy weight.

Larger waist measurements indicate accumulating fat stores and are associated with increased health risks. Having a proportionately large waist is associated with an accumulation of fat around the heart, liver, and other internal organs. Women greater than 5 feet in height whose waist measurement is more than 34 to 35 inches have more health risks. For men, risk increases at a waist measurement of 39 or 40 inches, and becomes even more serious with measurements greater than 40 inches.[39]

Two inexpensive, quick ways to help determine fat accumulation in the abdominal area, thereby determining overall health risks, are waist-to-height ratio (compares the waist measurement to height) and waist-to-hip ratio (compares waist measurement to hip measurement). The waist measurement should be less than half of the person's height. A high BMI is associated with a higher mortality risk, but waist to height ratio appears to be a more accurate indicator of mortality risk.[40] Researchers worldwide are studying which method is best for different genders and nationalities. Gold standard methods that determine body fat more accurately, such as magnetic resonance imagings (MRIs), dual-energy x-ray absorptiometry (DEXA) scans, and bioelectrical impedance scales, are significantly more expensive and require specialized equipment.

Obesity is the result of consistent caloric overconsumption in excess of energy expenditure. The Centers for Disease Control and Prevention (CDC) estimates that average daily energy intake increased almost 7% for men and approximately 22% for women between 1971 and 2010.[41] American men consume an average of 2600 kcal, and women consume approximately 1850 kcal. This increased intake reflects a consumption level that is conducive for weight gain in inactive individuals.

Genetic influence is a significant factor contributing to obesity. Body weight is affected by genes, metabolism, hormones, food choices, behavior, environment, culture, and socioeconomic status. Although genetics and the environment may increase the risk of weight gain, the foods an individual chooses significantly affect body weight.

The United States has cultivated an environment with an abundance of foods containing hidden fats and sugars that can promote obesity. Many factors in the American culture have made food more accessible, including fast food restaurants, prepackaged food, and soft drinks. Fast foods account for 11.3% of total daily kilocalories.[42] Portion sizes have also increased, and more people are eating at home less often. When people eat out, they tend to consume more kilocalories—an additional 100-200 kcal per meal.[43] Contrary to popular

HEALTH APPLICATION 1   Obesity—cont'd

belief, pizza, burgers, chicken, and french fries from restaurants and fast food establishments account for less energy than breads, grain-based desserts, pasta, and soft drinks from stores.[44] In some cases, understanding physiological benefits of weight loss can be motivating for patients. Weight loss is highly desirable in individuals with certain risk factors and advisable for others. A 10% weight loss is associated with a decrease in serum glucose, cholesterol, systolic blood pressure, and uric acid. Other physical symptoms that can be expected to improve with weight loss include shortness of breath, easy fatigability, fluid retention, gastric disorders, headaches, decreased energy level, decreased sexual interest, joint pains, muscle cramps, elevated pulse rate, sleeping disorders, urinary infection, and varicose veins.

Treatment of obesity has a high level of noncompliance and failure. Because weight loss is so difficult, prevention of weight gain should be strongly emphasized. The incidence of obesity needs to be approached on four levels: (a) individuals should be accountable for their food choices; (b) families must assume responsibility for foods available to their children, with parents acting as role models for healthful diet and exercise habits; (c) communities should provide opportunities for exercise (parks, sidewalks, sports programs) and schools should provide healthy food choices; and (d) more research should be conducted in this area to discover optimal, effective ways of weight management.

Weight management is very difficult for most individuals. It is a lifelong commitment to change one's lifestyle—regular exercise, wise food choices, and behavior modifications. Weight loss should be motivated by internal rather than external reasons ("I am doing this for myself," rather than "I will lose weight for my son's wedding"). Any treatment for weight loss should always be a serious undertaking with a high level of motivation and long-term commitment. Such an approach increases the likelihood both of successful weight loss and maintaining a healthy weight.

One pound of fat equals 3500 kcal. Losing weight can be accomplished by eating fewer kilocalories, increasing activity, or a combination of both. A 0.5- to 2-lb per week weight loss is recommended to lose body fat while minimizing muscle loss. To accomplish this goal, food intake must be 500 kcal less than needed per day, which results in loss of 1 lb per week. An additional energy expenditure of 500 kcal per day is recommended to lose an additional pound of weight. When weight loss is achieved slowly, it is usually more effective and is maintained for a longer period.

Numerous strategies have been implemented to treat overweight and obesity. No one treatment is best for everyone; each modality varies in effectiveness, risk, and cost. Drugs and surgical procedures currently being used for weight loss are beyond the scope of this text. A realistic goal regarding the rate and amount of weight loss must be established for each individual trying to reduce weight.

Millions of obese individuals have chosen **bariatric surgery** (surgical procedure on the stomach or small intestine or both for weight reduction), which usually results in greater, sustained weight loss than conventional methods; reduced incidence of diabetes, cardiovascular events, and hypertension; and a longer life.[45-47] This drastic but effective measure has many drawbacks and side effects, including absorption of many nutrients, pulmonary embolism, and some postoperative deaths.

Popular weight-reduction diets devised for weight loss are abundant (see the Evolve website). Although many different plans "guarantee" weight loss, no guaranteed easy cure exists for maintaining a healthy weight. A weight reduction diet needs to be followed for an extended time; and it must be appealing, flexible, and affordable for the individual trying to lose weight. It can be balanced in terms of nutrients, yet hypocaloric. Reducing caloric intake to less than 1200 kcal for women and 1400 kcal for men is not recommended because adequate amounts of nutrients are not provided.

Popular diets vary in their nutritional adequacy and consistency with guidelines for risk reduction. The low-carbohydrate, high-protein diet has come into a favorable light as a result of numerous studies indicating that low-carbohydrate, high-protein diets are more effective in promoting weight loss and reducing blood lipid levels. A dietary regimen that stresses meat and high-fat foods but eliminates sugar and most carbohydrates may be more successful at helping people lose weight because high-protein foods provide greater **satiety** (feeling of fullness).

Higher-protein diets appear to have small to moderate improvements in weight loss, BMI, waist circumference, lean body mass, and a slightly negative effect on body fat storage.[48,49] Proteins may suppress **ghrelin** (an appetite-stimulating hormone) production better than carbohydrates and lipids.[50] Diets that are considered high-fat may cause undesirable cholesterol levels to increase, but weight loss as a result of inadequate kilocalorie intake itself usually improves blood lipid levels regardless of the macronutrient composition. Reviews about various popular diets are available from the Academy of Nutrition and Dietetics at http://www.eatright.org/dietreviews/#.UPXCiGegERg and healthy tips for losing weight are available at http://www.eatright.org/Public/content.aspx?id=6849#.UPXBy2egERg.

Different diets work for different people; all components of energy balance, including energy intake from carbohydrates, protein, and fat, and expenditure, interact with one another to impact body weight. A change to any one aspect will correspond to profound changes in the other side of the equation. Unreasonable expectations and unrealistic predictions are frequently made about the weight-loss benefits of exercise and dietary interventions by making only minor adjustments. A diet that totally eliminates one category (fat or carbohydrate) or a specific group of foods (fruits or meats) is not advisable.

Indispensable to any weight-loss program is a preplanned food allotment with specified times for eating throughout the day to lessen feelings of deprivation and to eliminate excessive food intake. The total amount of food should be divided into at least three feedings. Eating only once or twice a day is associated with consuming more kilocalories,[51] impulsive snacking, and increased adipose tissue and serum cholesterol. Some "free" foods or beverages (foods containing less than 20 kcal per serving) may be available for snack periods, but regular mealtimes are important. A diet that requires the least amount of change in usual dietary patterns has better long-term success. A 1200- to 1500-kcal diet is relatively safe; when accompanied by an exercise program, the rate of weight loss is augmented, and muscle mass is maintained.

A weight-reduction diet should satisfy the following criteria: (a) meets all nutrient needs except energy, (b) suits tastes and habits, (c) minimizes hunger and fatigue, (d) is accessible

Continued

HEALTH APPLICATION I   Obesity—cont'd

and socially acceptable, (e) encourages a change in eating pattern, and (f) favors improvement in overall health. Box 1-5 provides some questions to help determine the validity of a weight-reduction diet. Common reasons indicated for discontinuing a weight-loss regimen: (a) trouble controlling food choices, (b) difficulty motivating oneself to eat appropriately, and (c) using food as a reward.

Treatment of obesity is improved when increased energy expenditure occurs along with decreased caloric intake. Exercise alone has a modest effect on weight loss; it positively affects energy metabolism. Initiation of an exercise regimen may lead to weight gain in the form of muscle mass, but the health benefits are significant, including improved cardiovascular fitness, improved plasma lipoprotein profile, improved carbohydrate metabolism, increased energy expenditure, and enhanced psychological well-being.

Behavior modification for weight control refers to getting in touch with the reality of which foods are being consumed and in what quantity, and when and why eating occurs. One of the most important components of an effective weight control program is learning new ways of dealing with old habits. Comprehensive behavior-modification programs include diet and exercise programs individually tailored for patients. A team approach including a healthcare provider, a psychologist, an RDN, and family members is effective in helping the individual make necessary long-lasting changes in food choices and lifestyle behaviors. A food diary for recording amounts and types of food eaten, emotional status, and environmental factors helps provide new insights to devise strategies for dealing with eating habits.

Although behavior-modification approaches to weight control are helpful, maintaining weight loss remains a major problem. Studies indicate that programs need to be approximately 20 to 24 weeks long and more comprehensive, including relapse prevention training and use of social support systems.

BOX 1-5   Evaluating Weight Loss Diets or Programs

The program should evaluate the individual's BMI, and whether the weight is principally from increased fat stores or increased muscle mass and possible contributing factors.

The cost of the program should be realistic and reasonable.

The program should be adaptable for various lifestyles and something an individual can continue indefinitely.

Tips for Evaluating Safety and Effectiveness of Reduction Diets
1. Stay current with scientific research. Nutrition is a relatively new science, and new developments are still evolving to increase our knowledge base.
2. Evaluate diet trends and claims for effects on overall health.
3. Compare recommendations with known nutrition science and recommendations such as *MyPlate* and *Dietary Guidelines for Americans*.
4. Calculate nutritional requirements of the individual considering the diet, and determine what nutrients would be lacking.
5. Evaluate diets using the following principles:
   - What is the weight loss recommendation?
   - What is the success rate of the program?
   - What is the basis for advertisements and endorsements?

- Has any scientific research been done to evaluate the safety and effectiveness of the diet?
- What is the cost of the program? Are special foods or nutrient supplements required, and what do they cost? Are there other additional fees?
- Is the program medically supervised?
- Are any major food groups excluded?
- Are the foods appealing to the individual? Does the program allow occasional consumption of favorite foods?
- Is it permissible to eat in restaurants and other people's homes at least occasionally?
- Are certain foods avoided because they cause specific problems?
- Are certain foods used to "cure"?
- Are dramatic statements made that contradict well-established nutrition principles or reputable scientific organizations?
- Are exercise and behavior modification included?
- Can an individual live on the program for a lifetime?
- Is there a maintenance plan?
- Does it promote good food habits?

Case Application for the Dental Hygienist

A young healthy mother who has a 3-year-old son at home comes to the dental office for a 6-month recare appointment. She expresses concern about foods she should be eating and feeding her husband and son to improve and maintain their overall health for optimal growth and development of the child. She has learned a little about the food groups, the *Dietary Guidelines for Americans*, and nutrition labels from the press, but does not know how to implement them.

Nutritional Assessment
- Willingness to seek nutritional information
- Desire for increased control of nutritional health habits
- Knowledge of community resources
- Cultural or religious influences
- Knowledge regarding the *Dietary Guidelines*, food labels, and *MyPlate*
- Definition of optimal nutrition

Case Application for the Dental Hygienist—cont'd

Nutritional Diagnosis
Health-seeking behaviors related to lack of knowledge concerning optimal nutrition and current standards.

Nutritional Goals
The patient verbalizes correct information concerning the *Dietary Guidelines* and food labels, and can name the food groups, the number of servings needed, and portion sizes from each group of *MyPlate*.

Nutritional Implementation
Intervention: Ask the patient to write down everything she ate yesterday from the time she got up yesterday until this morning when she got up.
Rationale: This will help you tailor the information you provide to the patient's needs.
Intervention: Encourage variety of food intake, using *MyPlate*. Review the number of servings needed and serving size.
Rationale: The total balance of food intake matters, and the best balance incorporates variety to promote optimal nutrition. Providing the minimal number of servings prevents nutritional deficiencies in healthy individuals.
Intervention: (a) Suggest that the mother and her husband have their blood lipid profiles checked if not recently done; (b) emphasize a decreased intake of fats, saturated and *trans* fats, and cholesterol by trimming excess fat and eating smaller servings of meat (about the size of a fist or a deck of cards).
Rationale: Decreasing fats, saturated and *trans* fats, and cholesterol helps reduce the risk of heart disease.
Intervention: (a) Stress the importance of eating vegetables, fruits, and grains, and (b) explain that complex carbohydrates are not fattening.
Rationale: Dietary fiber is important for healthy bowel functioning and can reduce symptoms of chronic constipation, diverticular disease, and hemorrhoids, and decrease the risk of developing obesity, cancer, and diabetes.
Intervention: (a) Explain how to read labels for sugar. The name of most sugars end in "-ose." (b) Emphasize moderation of sugar intake. (c) Explain that "dietetic" and "sugar-free" do not mean that the product is low in kilocalories. (d) Explain the relationship between sugar and tooth decay, and emphasize the importance of proper oral hygiene after sugar consumption.
Rationale: Refined sugar contains kilocalories and no other nutrients, but is acceptable when used in items that contain appreciable amounts of other nutrients (e.g., a pudding would provide more nutrients than a gelatin dessert or carbonated beverages).
Intervention: (a) Stress using sodium and salt in moderation; (b) emphasize that "no salt added" does not mean that the product is low in sodium.
Rationale: Good habits that do not foster a high level of salt preference are recommended.
Intervention: Emphasize that any alcohol intake should be in moderation (one drink a day for women and two drinks a day for men), if at all.
Rationale: Alcohol is high in kilocalories and contains few, if any, nutrients.
Intervention: (a) Review an entire label with the mother to help her understand how to interpret it. (b) Determine a serving size. (c) Explain the types of carbohydrates. (d) Determine the percentage of fat in a product by multiplying the grams of fat by 9, and compare this number with the total kilocalories; if the amount is more than 30%, do not consume that product every day. (e) Look at cholesterol levels. (f) Emphasize that "no cholesterol" does not indicate that the product contains no saturated or *trans* fat. (g) Point out the sodium level, and if it is greater than 400 mg, encourage its use in moderation.
Rationale: Knowledge increases compliance and allows informed choices regarding food choice.
Intervention: Refer the patient to county extension agencies or to a registered dietitian.
Rationale: These agencies and nutritional professionals provide practical guidelines via newsletters, workshops, and written materials for healthy patients wanting to improve health.

Evaluation
To determine effectiveness of care, the patient reads labels and chooses the best buy for the nutrient content. The patient states the basic guidelines for nutrition; the hygienist explains to her that serving sizes for her son are different than the standard serving size (available on *ChooseMyPlate* website). Additionally, the patient should be able to plan a menu using recommended foods, and to state how to obtain and use community information/support. The patient should be able to indicate how changes in food choices would not only improve overall health, but also maintain health of the oral cavity and ensure optimal growth of her son with minimal or no problems in the oral cavity.

STUDENT READINESS

1. A patient asks you the difference between food and nutrition. What would you say?
2. Locate an advertisement in a popular magazine or newspaper for a weight reduction product or program, and list the merits of the product or program stated in the ad. Then list information about the product or program that might have been omitted or should be questioned. Evaluate the product or program using information from Box 1-5.
3. Discuss popular weight reduction diets (see the Evolve website) and how they may have adverse effects.
4. Distinguish between nutrient recommendations and requirements.
5. Keep a record of all the foods you eat for 24 hours. Was your intake adequate as evaluated by *MyPlate?* In what areas did you do well? Where can you improve? Provide specific recommendations for making changes.
6. Collect nutrition labels for three similar products. Compare the nutrient values to determine which is a better source of nutrients. Which is a better buy for the amount of nutrients it contains?
7. List the *Dietary Guidelines for Americans*. In which areas do you do well? In which areas would you like to improve your choices? Do you believe you have enough information to make knowledgeable changes?
8. Discuss the pros and cons of allowing nutritional claims on products.

9. If a food label indicates that one serving of the product has 23 g of carbohydrate and 15 g of sugar with 140 kcal (total), how many teaspoons of sugar does the product contain? What percentage of carbohydrate does this product contain?

References

1. International Food Information Council Foundation: *2012 Food & Health Survey–Consumer Attitudes Toward Food Safety, Nutrition and Health.* May 2012. Accessed August 14, 2013: http://www.foodinsight.org/Content/3840/2012%20IFIC%20Food%20and%20Health%20Survey%20Report%20of%20Findings%20%28for%20website%29.pdf.

2. Freeland-Graves JH, Nitzke S: Position of the Academy of Nutrition and Dietetics: total diet approach to healthy eating. *J Acad Nutr Diet* 113(2):307–317, 2013.

3. U.S. Department of Health and Human Services: *Final Review Healthy People 2010, Final Review. Oral Health, Topic 21.* Accessed August 14, 2013: http://www.cdc.gov/nchs/data/hpdata2010/hp2010_final_review_focus_area_21.pdf.

4. U.S. Department of Health and Human Services: *Healthy People 2020*: Last updated December 17, 2012. Accessed August 14, 2013: http://www.healthypeople.gov/2020/default.aspx.

5. U.S. Department of Agriculture; U.S. Department of Health and Human Services: *Dietary Guidelines for Americans, 2010*, ed 7, Washington, DC, 2010, U.S. Government Printing Office.

6. Nordestgaard BG, Palmer TM, Benn M, et al: The effect of elevated body mass index on ischemic heart disease risk: causal estimates from a Mendelian randomisation approach. *PLoS Med* 2012 May 1:31001212. doi:10.1371/journal.pmed. Accessed August 14, 2013: http://www.plosmedicine.org/article/info%3Adoi%2F10.1371%2Fjournal.pmed.1001212.

7. Berrington de Gonzalez A, Hartge P, Cerhan JR, et al: Body-mass index and mortality among 1.46 million white adults. *N Engl J Med* 363(23):2211–2219. 2010.

8. Kam K: Why your BMI doesn't tell the whole story. *Web MD Feature* 2012. Accessed August 14, 2013: http://www.webmd.com/diet/features/bmi-drawbacks-and-other-measurements.

9. Centers for Disease Control and Prevention: *Fast stats—obesity and overweight.* Updated October 10, 2012. Accessed August 14, 2013: http://www.cdc.gov/nchs/fastats/overwt.htm.

10. Ford ES, Dietz WH: Trends in energy intake among adults in the United States: findings from NHANES. *Am J Clin Nutr* 97(4):848–853, 2013.

11. USDA Economic Research Service: *U.S. food supply: nutrients and other food components, per capita per day.* Accessed August 14, 2013: http://www.ers.usda.gov/data-products/food-availability-%28per-capita%29-data-system.aspx.

12. Moshfegh AJ: *Monitoring the U.S. population's diet: the third step—the national "What We Eat in America" survey.* March 2012. Accessed August 14, 2013: http://www.ars.usda.gov/is/AR/archive/mar12/diet0312.htm?pf=1.

13. Janssen I, Carson V, Lee IM, et al: Years of life gained due to leisure-time physical activity in the U.S. *Am J Prev Med* 44(1):23–29, 2013.

14. Loprinzi PD, Cardinal BJ: Association between biologic outcomes and objectively measured physical activity accumulated in ≥10-minute bouts and <10-minute bouts. *Am J Health Promot* 27(3):143–151, 2013.

15. Guenther PM, Ding EL, Rimm EB: Alcoholic beverage consumption by adults compared to Dietary Guidelines: results of the National Health and Nutrition Examination survey, 2009-2010. *J Acad Nutr Diet* 113(4):546–550, 2012.

16. Tarvainen L, Kyyrönen P, Kauppinen T, et al: Cancer of the mouth and pharynx, occupation and exposure to chemical agents in Finland 1971-95. *Int J Cancer* 123(3):653–659, 2008.

17. Britten P, Cleveland LE, Koegel KL, et al: Impact of typical rather than nutrient-dense food choices in the U.S. Department of Agriculture food patterns. *J Acad Nutr Diet* 112(10):1560–1569, 2012.

18. Moshfegh AJ: Monitoring the U.S. population's diet the third step—the national "What We Eat in America" survey. *Agric Res* 60(3):16–21, 2012.

19. Moshfegh AJ: Monitoring the U.S. population's diet the third step—the national "What We Eat in America" survey. *Agric Res* 60(3):16–21, 2012.

20. Moshfegh AJ: Monitoring the U.S. population's diet the third step—the national "What We Eat in America" survey. *Agric Res* 60(3):16–21, 2012.

21. U.S. Department of Agriculture; U.S. Department of Health and Human Services: *Dietary Guidelines for Americans, 2010*, ed 7, Washington, DC, 2010, U.S. Government Printing Office.

22. Shimazaki Y, Shirota T, Uchida K, et al: Intake of dairy products and periodontal disease: the Hisayama study. *J Periodontal* 79(1):131–137, 2008.

23. Al-Zahrani MS: Increased intake of dairy products is related to lower periodontitis prevalence. *J Periodontol* 77(2):289–294, 2006.

24. U.S. Food and Drug Administration (FDA): *Qualified health claims: letter of enforcement discretion—nuts and coronary heart disease.* 2003 Jul 14. Accessed August 14, 2013: http://www.fda.gov/Food/IngredientsPackagingLabeling/LabelingNutrition/ucm072926.htm.

25. Hersey JC, Wohlgenant KC, Arsenault JE, et al: Effects of front-of-package and shelf nutrition labeling systems on consumers. *Nutr Rev* 71(1):1–14, 2013.

26. Walpole SC, Prieto-Merino D, Edwards P, et al: The weight of nations: an estimation of adult human biomass. *BMC Public Health* 12:439, 2012.

27. Sturm R: *People who are severely overweight remain fastest increasing group of obese Americans.* RAND Health, October 1, 2012. Accessed August 14, 2013: http://www.rand.org/news/press/2012/10/01/index1.html.

28. Finkelstein EA, Khavjou OA, Thompson H, et al: Obesity and severe obesity forecasts through 2030. *Am J Prev Med* 42(6):563–570, 2012.

29. U.S. Department of Health and Human Services: *Office of Disease Prevention and Health Promotion. Healthy People 2020.* Washington, DC. Accessed August 14, 2013: http://www.healthypeople.gov/2020/topicsobjectives2020/objectiveslist.aspx?topicId=29.

30. Levi J, Segal L, Laurent R: *F as in Fat: How Obesity Threatens America's Future 2012*, Washington, D.C., 2012, Trust for America's Health.

31. National Cancer Institute, National Institutes of Health: *Fact Sheet: Obesity and cancer risk.* Updated January 03, 2012. Accessed: August 14, 2013: http://www.cancer.gov/cancertopics/factsheet/Risk/obesity.

32. Palouzier-Paulignan B, Lacroix MC, Aimé P, et al: Olfaction under metabolic influences. *Chem Senses* 37(9):769–797, 2012.

33. Fernandez-Mendoza J, Vgontzas AN, Liao D, et al: Insomnia with objective short sleep duration and incident hypertension: the Penn State cohort. *Hypertension* 60(4):929–935, 2012.

34. Mogri M, Dhindsa S, Quattrin T, et al: Testosterone concentrations in young pubertal and post-pubertal obese males. *Clin Endocrinol (oxf)* 78(4):593–599, 2013.

35. Cawley J, Meyerhoefer C: *The medical care costs of obesity: an instrumental variables approach.* National Bureau of Economic Research, NBER Working Paper No. 16467. October 18 2010. Accessed on August 14, 2013: http://www.nber.org/papers/w16467.

36. Cawley J, Meyerhoefer C: *The medical care costs of obesity: an instrumental variables approach.* National Bureau of Economic

Research, NBER Working Paper No. 16467. October 18 2010. Accessed on August 14, 2013: http://www.nber.org/papers/w16467.

37. Wang YC, McPherson K, Marsh T, et al: Health and economic burden of the projected obesity trends in the USA and the UK. *Lancet* 378(9793):815–825, 2011.

38. Jialal I, Devaraj S, Kaur H, et al: Increased chemerin and decreased omentin-1 in both adipose tissue and plasma in nascent metabolic syndrome. *J Clin Endocrinol Metab* 98(3):E514–E517, 2013.

39. Kam K: Why your BMI doesn't tell the whole story. *Web MD Feature*, 2012. Accessed August 14, 2013: http://www.webmd.com/diet/features/bmi-drawbacks-and-other-measurements.

40. Ashwell M, Gunn P, Gibson S: Waist-to-height ratio is a better screening tool than waist circumference and BMI for adult cardiometabolic risk factors: systematic review and meta-analysis. *Obesity Reviews* 13(3):275–286, 2012.

41. U.S. Department of Agriculture, Economic Research Service: *Food Availability (per capita) data system.* Accessed August 14, 2013: http://www.ers.usda.gov/data-products/food-availability-%28per-capita%29-data-system.aspx.

42. Fryar CD, Ervin RB: *Caloric intake from fast food among adults: United States, 2007-2010.* NCHS Data Brief No. 114, February 2013. Accessed August 14, 2013: http://www.cdc.gov/nchs/data/databriefs/db114.htm.

43. Todd J, Mancino L: Eating out increases daily calorie intake. *Amber Waves* 8(2), 2010. Accessed August 8, 2013: http://www.ers.usda.gov/amber-waves/2010-june/eating-out-increases-daily-calorie-intake.aspx#.UghF6W3nKIU.

44. Drewnowski A, Rehm CD: Energy intakes of US children and adults by food purchase location and by specific food source. *Nutr J* 12:59, 2013. doi:11.1186/1475-2891-12-59.

45. Neovius M, Narbro K, Keating C, et al: Health care use during 20 years following bariatric surgery. *JAMA* 308(11):1132–1141, 2012.

46. Adams TD, Davidson LE, Litwin SE, et al: Health benefits of gastric bypass surgery after 6 years. *JAMA* 308(11):1122–1131, 2012.

47. Colquitt JL, Picot J, Loveman E, et al: Surgery for obesity. *Cochrane Database Syst Rev* (2):CD003641, 2009. Accessed August 14, 2013: http://onlinelibrary.wiley.com/doi/10.1002/14651858.CD003641.pub3/abstract.

48. Santesso N, Akl EA, Bianchi M, et al: Effects of high- versus lower-protein diets on health outcomes: a systematic review and meta-analysis. *Eur J Clin Nutr* 66(7):780–788, 2012.

49. Bray GA, Smith SR, de Jonge L, et al: Effect of dietary protein content on weight gain, energy expenditure, and body composition during overeating, a randomized controlled trial. *JAMA* 307(1):47–55, 2012.

50. Lomenick JP, Melguizo MS, Mitchell SL, et al: Effects of meals high in carbohydrate, protein, and fat on ghrelin and peptide YY secretion in prepubertal children. *J Clin Endocrinol Metab* 94(11):4463–4471, 2009.

51. Bachman JL, Phelan S, Wing RR, et al: Eating frequency is higher in weight loss maintainers and normal-weight individuals than in overweight individuals. *J Am Diet Assoc* 111(11):1730–1734, 2011.

ⓔ EVOLVE RESOURCES

Please visit http://evolve.elsevier.com/Stegeman/nutritional for additional practice and study support tools.

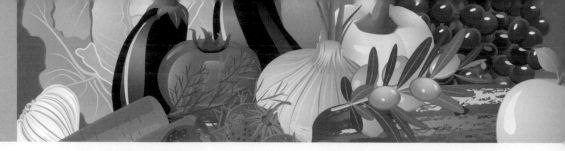

Chapter 2

Concepts in Biochemistry

Scott M. Tremain, PhD

Student Learning Outcomes

Upon completion of this chapter, the student will be able to achieve the following outcomes:

- Explain the role of biochemistry in dental hygiene and nutrition.
- Assign biomolecules according to functional group.
- Compare and contrast the structure, function, and properties of the four major classes of biomolecules (carbohydrates, proteins, nucleic acids, and lipids).
- Outline the structure, function, and property of monosaccharides, disaccharides, and polysaccharides.
- Outline the structure, function, and property of amino acids and proteins.
- Compare and contrast the roles of enzymes, coenzymes, and vitamins in nutrition.
- Outline the structure, function, and property of nucleotides and nucleic acids.
- Outline the structure, function, and property of fatty acids, triglycerides, and steroids.
- Differentiate catabolism from anabolism. Explain connections between metabolic pathways in carbohydrate, protein, and lipid metabolism.

Key Terms

Active site
Adenosine 5′-triphosphate (ATP)
Adipose tissue
Aerobic
Amino acids
Amphiphilic
Amylase
Anabolism
Anhydrous
Antioxidants
Biomolecule
Carbohydrates
Catabolism
Chemical bonds
Cholesterol
Coenzymes
Condensation reaction
Covalent bond
Disaccharide
Enzymes
Epinephrine
Essential amino acids (EAAs) or indispensable amino acids
Fatty acids (FAs)
Flavin adenine dinucleotide (FAD/FADH$_2$)
Functional group
Genome
Glucagon

Glycogen
Glucogenic amino acids
Gluconeogenesis
Glycolysis
Glycosidic bond
Hormone
Hydrocarbon
Hydrogenation reaction
Hydrolysis reaction
Hydrophilic
Hydrophobic
Hydroxyapatite
Insulin
Ionic bond
Ketogenic amino acids
Ketone bodies
Linoleic acid
Lipase
Lipids
Lipoproteins
Melting point
Metabolism
Mitochondria
Molecule
Monomer
Monosaccharide
Monounsaturated fatty acid (MUFA)
Nicotinamide adenine dinucleotide (NAD$^+$/NADH)

Nonessential amino acids (NEAAs) or dispensable
    amino acids
Nucleic acids
Nucleotides
Oils
Oxidation
Oxidation-reduction reactions
Oxidative phosphorylation
Peptide bond
Photosynthesis
Polymer
Polypeptide
Polysaccharide
Polyunsaturated fatty acid (PUFA)

Precursor
Protease
Proteins
Redox coenzymes
Reduction
Respiration
Side chain (R group)
Saturated fatty acids
Substrate
Sugar alcohol
Tricarboxylic acid cycle (TCA cycle)
Triglyceride (TG)
Unsaturated fatty acids
Vitamins

Test Your NQ

1. **T/F** A hydrolysis reaction produces water as a product, while a condensation reaction requires water as a reactant.
2. **T/F** Nucleotides are the building blocks of proteins.
3. **T/F** Hydrophilic molecules dissolve readily in water.
4. **T/F** Sucrose is a disaccharide containing glucose and galactose.
5. **T/F** A substrate binds the enzyme active site and is converted into product.
6. **T/F** When the hydrogen atoms are on opposite sides of the double bond, the structure is a *trans* isomer.

7. **T/F** An unsaturated fatty acid with 16 carbons has a lower melting temperature than a saturated fatty acid with 16 carbons.
8. **T/F** Catabolism involves the reduction of carbohydrates into carbon dioxide and water.
9. **T/F** Insulin activates glycogen degradation to regulate carbohydrate and lipid metabolism.
10. **T/F** Humans lack the enzymes to synthesize essential (indispensable) amino acids, so they must be obtained from foods.

It is essential for dental professionals to have a basic understanding of biochemistry because it is the foundation for understanding and applying the concepts of nutrition. An overview of the biochemical concepts relevant to nutrition will serve as a wonderful resource as the learner goes through this textbook. A comprehensive review of chemistry and biochemistry concepts can be found online at Evolve.

WHAT IS BIOCHEMISTRY?

Biochemistry is the study of life at the molecular level. The three major areas of biochemistry are structure, metabolism, and information. Structure describes the three-dimensional arrangement of atoms in a molecule, the smallest particle of a substance that retains all the properties of the substance. Important for life, the structure of a biomolecule determines its function. A biomolecule is any molecule that is produced by a living cell or organism, which would include carbohydrates, proteins, nucleic acids, and lipids, as well as other organic compounds found in living organisms; in contrast, a nutrient is a substance required by the body that must be supplied by an outside source which is usually food.

Metabolism involves the production and use of energy. In metabolism, energy can be extracted from dietary carbohydrates, proteins, and lipids and used to create the biomolecules required for life. This highly regulated system ensures that energy is not wasted. Information involves the transfer of biological information from deoxyribonucleic acid (DNA) to ribonucleic acid (RNA) to protein. The blueprint for life is stored in DNA and the resulting proteins carry out all the processes required for life.

FUNDAMENTALS OF BIOCHEMISTRY

Atoms in a compound are held together by chemical bonds. There are two types of chemical bonds that form. An ionic bond forms between a positively charged metal ion and a negatively charged nonmetal ion. Hydroxyapatite in tooth enamel is composed of ionic bonds between calcium ions (Ca^{2+}), phosphate ions (PO_4^{3-}), and hydroxide ions (OH^-). A covalent bond forms when electrons are equally shared between two nonmetals. Ultimately, the biomolecules responsible for life are based on carbon (C) because of carbon's ability to form stable covalent bonds to itself and many other atoms, forming long chains and rings. In addition to carbon, the combination of different atoms, like hydrogen (H), oxygen (O), nitrogen (N), sulfur (S), and phosphorus (P), into biomolecules provides for great variety in chemical structure, properties and reactivity in biological systems. One way to organize this variety in chemical structure is the classification of molecules into functional groups. A **functional group** is a group of atoms that gives a family of molecules its characteristic chemical and physical properties. Molecules that have similar functional groups have similar properties. Figure 2-1 defines and exemplifies a few functional groups found in biochemistry.

Functional groups can be converted into other functional groups via chemical reactions such as oxidation-reduction, condensation, and hydrolysis. **Oxidation-reduction** reactions are important in metabolism as biomolecules are degraded or synthesized. **Oxidation** can be defined as a loss of electrons, an increase in charge, a gain of O atoms, or a loss of H atoms. **Reduction** can be defined as a gain of electrons, a decrease in charge, a loss of O atoms, or a gain of H atoms. In metabolism, energy is extracted from glucose ($C_6H_{12}O_6$) by completely oxidizing it to carbon dioxide (CO_2). Condensation and hydrolysis reactions are important in digestion and metabolism. In general, a **condensation** reaction creates a new molecule by forming a bond between two smaller molecules, while a **hydrolysis** reaction breaks a larger molecule into two smaller molecules. When carbohydrates, proteins, and lipids are digested, these biomolecules are hydrolyzed into smaller building blocks for absorption in the digestive system.

PRINCIPLE BIOMOLECULES IN NUTRITION

As shown in Table 2-1, the four major classes of biomolecules are carbohydrates, proteins, nucleic acids, and lipids. These biomolecules are characterized by the type of polymer, and monomer they contain as well as by their general function. A **polymer** is a large molecule containing numerous repeating units called monomers. A **monomer** is the smallest repeating unit present in a polymer.

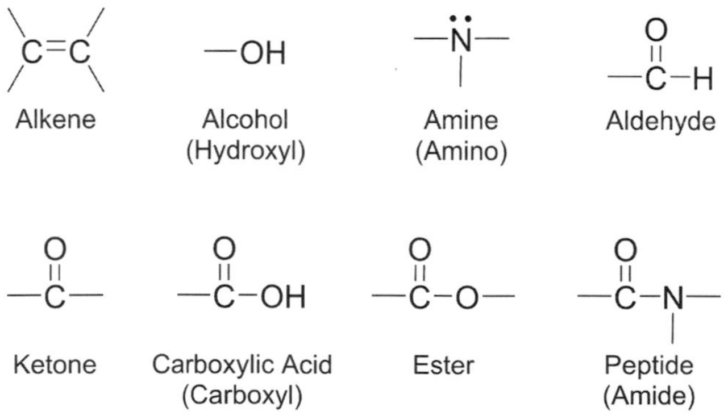

Carbohydrate Structure and Function

The biological function of **carbohydrates** involves energy metabolism and storage. As shown in Figure 2-2, plants use photosynthesis to make oxygen (O_2) and glucose ($C_6H_{12}O_6$), the carbohydrate from which animals acquire the energy required for life. Via the process of **respiration**, animals degrade the carbohydrate glucose ($C_6H_{12}O_6$) into CO_2 and water (H_2O), and plants use these products for photosynthesis.

Carbohydrates are classified as monosaccharides, disaccharides, and polysaccharides, depending on the number of sugar monomers present (one, two, or many). **Monosaccharides** are composed of a single monomeric unit with the molecular formula $C_n(H_2O)_n$, where n is 3 to 8. Figure 2-3 shows the linear structures of the most common monosaccharides. Monosaccharides undergo oxidation-reduction reactions. When a monosaccharide is reduced, the aldehyde functional group changes to a **sugar alcohol** (e.g., sorbitol).

In aqueous solution, linear monosaccharides spontaneously form cyclic structures. When two monosaccharides combine, a **disaccharide** is formed. This involves the formation of a **glycosidic bond**. As shown in Figure 2-4, two glucose monomers can combine via a condensation reaction to form maltose. Maltose is a disaccharide that results from

FIGURE 2-1 Common functional groups in biochemistry.

Table 2-1	The four major classes of biomolecules	
Polymer	**Monomer**	**Function**
Carbohydrates (polysaccharides)	Monosaccharides	Energy source, energy storage form and structure
Proteins	Amino acids	Structure and biocatalysts (enzymes)
Nucleic acids	Nucleotides	Genetic information transfer and energy
Lipids		Energy source, energy storage form, and biological membranes

$$6\ CO_2 + 6\ H_2O + \textit{Energy} \underset{\text{degradation}}{\overset{\text{photosynthesis}}{\rightleftharpoons}} C_6H_{12}O_6 + 6\ O_2$$

FIGURE 2-2 The carbon cycle. Plants utilize photosynthesis (use solar energy) to produce glucose ($C_6H_{12}O_6$) and oxygen (from *left* to *right*), while animals utilize respiration to degrade glucose ($C_6H_{12}O_6$) for energy (from *right* to *left*).

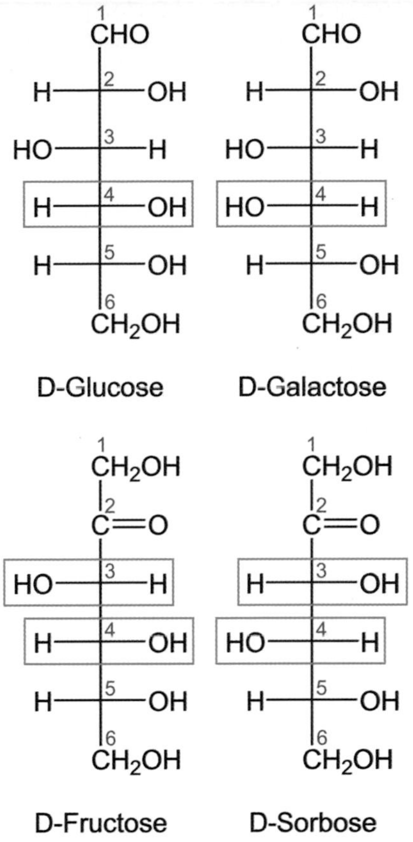

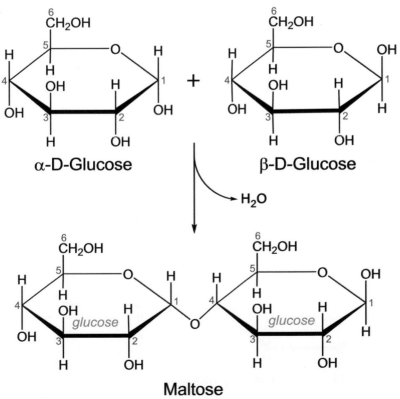

FIGURE 2-3 The linear structures of common monosaccharides. Monosaccharides are classified as aldoses and ketoses. Aldoses contain an aldehyde functional group, while ketoses contain a ketone functional group. D-glucose ($C_6H_{12}O_6$) is an aldohexose because it contains an aldehyde (represented by CHO at carbon 1) and six carbons. D-Fructose ($C_6H_{12}O_6$) is a ketohexose because it contains a ketone (at carbon 2) and six carbons.

FIGURE 2-4 Formation of the disaccharide maltose from two glucose molecules. Water (H_2O) is released as a product in this condensation reaction.

the degradation of starch and is used in brewing alcoholic beverages. When glucose and fructose combine, the disaccharide sucrose is formed (Figure 2-5). This disaccharide is table sugar and one of the sweetest carbohydrates. When the two monosaccharides galactose and glucose combine, the disaccharide lactose is formed (Figure 2-5). This disaccharide is found in milk and dairy products.

Many monosaccharides combine to form a polysaccharide. As shown in Table 2-2, polysaccharides can be characterized by the monosaccharide monomer present and overall function. One of the most important dietary polysaccharides is starch, the storage form of energy in plants. Starch is composed of two different polysaccharides (α-amylose and amylopectin). Figure 2-6 shows the linear structure of the polysaccharide α-amylose. Figure 2-7 shows the branched structure of the polysaccharide amylopectin. Important for

the storage of energy in animals, glycogen also is a branched polysaccharide containing glucose monomers. The highly branched structure of glycogen allows its rapid degradation into glucose when energy is needed.

Protein Structure and Function

In an organism, proteins are essential for almost every physiological function, such as providing structure, helping muscles contract, transporting and storing substances, catalyzing reactions, regulating metabolism, and providing protection. Proteins are composed of building blocks or monomer units called amino acids. As shown in Figure 2-8, the general structure of an amino acid consists of an amino group ($-NH_3^+$), a carboxyl group ($-COO^-$), and a side chain (R group) that varies from one amino acid to another. The classification of the 20 common amino acids is based on the

Table 2-2	Summary of common polysaccharides	
Name	**Monomer**	**Biological Function**
Amylose (in starch)	Glucose	Nutrient storage (plants)
Amylopectin (in starch)	Glucose	Nutrient storage (plants)
Glycogen	Glucose	Nutrient storage (animals)
Dextran	Glucose	Nutrient storage (yeast and bacteria)
Inulin	Fructose	Nutrient storage (plants)
Cellulose	Glucose	Structure in plants
Pectin	Galacturonic acid	Structural rigidity in plants and gelling agent in yogurt and jelly
Lignin	Coniferyl alcohol	Structural rigidity in plant cell walls

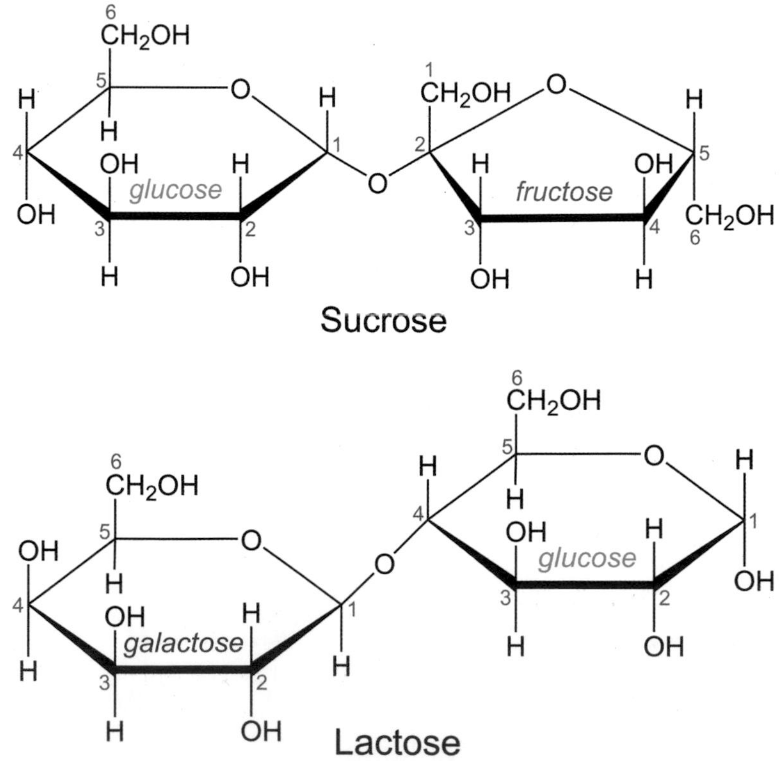

FIGURE 2-5 The structures of the disaccharides sucrose and lactose.

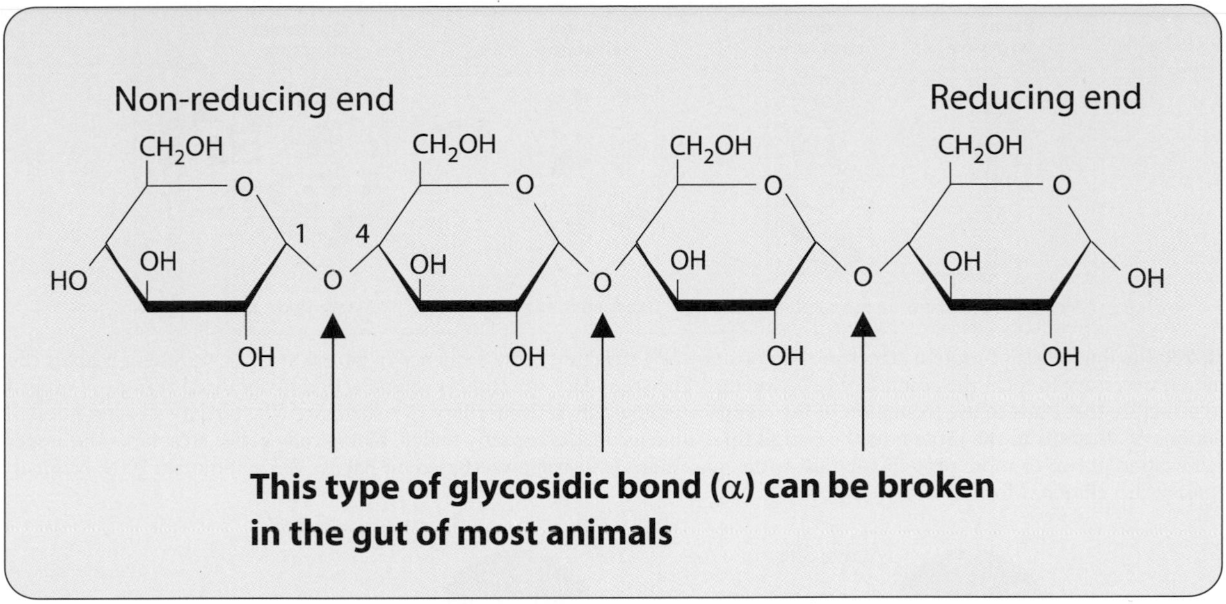

Non-reducing end / Reducing end

This type of glycosidic bond (α) can be broken in the gut of most animals

FIGURE 2-6 The linear structure of the polysaccharide α-amylose, a component of starch containing glycosidic linkages that are easily digested. (Batmanian L, Worral S, Ridge J: *Biochemistry for health professionals,* ©2011, Sydney, Elsevier Australia.)

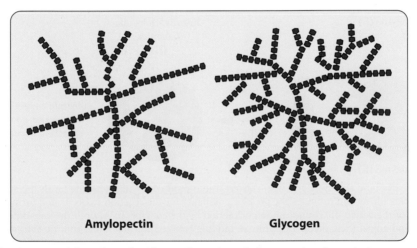

Amylopectin   **Glycogen**

FIGURE 2-7 The branched structures of the polysaccharides amylopectin and glycogen. Amylopectin is a component of starch (the storage form of energy in plants) containing glucose monomers. Glycogen is the storage form of energy in animals containing glucose monomers. (Batmanian L, Worral S, Ridge J: *Biochemistry for health professionals,* ©2011, Sydney, Elsevier Australia.)

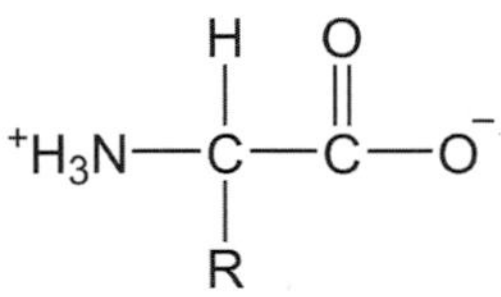

FIGURE 2-8 Structure of an amino acid. At neutral pH, the amino group ($-NH_3^+$) is positively charged, while the carboxyl group ($-COO^-$) is negatively charged.

structure of their side chain. Amino acids polymerize to form long chains called **polypeptides** through the formation of strong covalent **peptide bonds**. Proteins can consist of as few as 50 to as many as millions of amino acid monomers in one or more polypeptides arranged in a biologically functional way. As shown in Figure 2-9, a protein will become biologically active when it folds into its distinct compact three-dimensional structure.

Enzymes Catalyze Biochemical Reactions

Enzymes catalyze all biochemical reactions. Enzymes begin the process of digesting dietary proteins (**proteases**), carbohydrates (**amylases**), and lipids (**lipases**). They also carry out all the metabolic reactions involving the degradation and biosynthesis of the biomolecules required for life.

As shown in Figure 2-10, enzymes catalyze reactions by specifically binding a **substrate** and converting it into a product. The **active site** is the region of an enzyme that selectively binds a substrate and contains the amino acids that directly participate in the chemical transformation that converts a substrate into a product. Many enzymes need additional help to complete a specific biochemical reaction. **Coenzymes** are nonprotein organic substances that assist enzymes in converting a substrate into a product and are

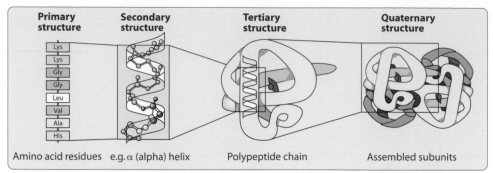

FIGURE 2-9 The four levels of protein structure. The primary (1°) structure is the sequence of amino acids in a protein; it holds the information necessary to form the secondary (2°) structure. The secondary structure is characterized by localized regions of repeating ordered structure that leads to the formation of the compact, biologically active tertiary (3°) structure. The tertiary structure describes the positions of all atoms in the protein or the overall three-dimensional, compactly folded, biologically active structure. The association and organization of two or more protein subunits is the quaternary (4°) structure. (Based on Baynes & Dominiczak, 2009. *Medical Biochemistry,* 3rd edition. Mosby.)

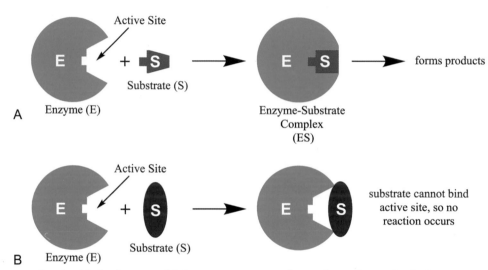

FIGURE 2-10 Enzyme active sites bind substrate and help convert it into product. When substrate binds the active site, an intermediate enzyme-substrate (ES) complex forms and provides the greatest possibility for the reaction to occur and form products. A substrate that neither fits nor induces a fit in the active site cannot undergo reaction by the enzyme. In **A,** both the substrate (S) and the active site of the enzyme (E) are flexible and adjust their shape for optimum binding between the active site and the substrate. In **B,** the substrate (S) does not fit the enzyme (E) active site, so a reaction will not occur and product will not form. (Based on Baynes & Dominiczak, 2009. *Medical Biochemistry,* 3rd edition. Mosby.)

regenerated at the end of a reaction. Many vitamins are converted into biologically active coenzymes.

Vitamins or "vital amines" are essential nutrients required in the diet because they cannot be synthesized by the organism itself. Many water-soluble vitamins are precursors of coenzymes. As shown in Table 2-3, water-soluble vitamins from foods may need to be converted into a biologically active form (a coenzyme) before binding an enzyme active site. Lipid-soluble or fat-soluble vitamins accumulate in fat deposits and cell membranes in the body. Lipid-soluble vitamins obtained from dietary sources are not involved as coenzymes, but they are converted into a biologically active form.

Nucleic Acid Structure and Function

The biological functions of nucleic acids like DNA and RNA are to store and transfer genetic information. The genetic information in an organism, the genome, contains all the information needed for the complete development of a living organism. The central dogma shown in Figure 2-11 describes biological information transfer within cells (DNA→RNA→Protein). Messenger RNA carries the message from DNA to the ribosome, the site of protein synthesis. The ribosome is composed of protein and ribosomal RNA. Transfer RNA carries an amino acid to the ribosome for incorporation into the growing polypeptide chain.

Nucleic acids are composed of building blocks called nucleotides. As shown in Figure 2-12, the general structure of a nucleotide consists of sugar attached to a nitrogenous base and phosphate. The sugar is ribose in RNA or deoxyribose in DNA.

Lipid Structure and Function

Lipids have many different structures and biological functions. They are involved in energy metabolism and storage,

Table 2-3	**Common vitamins and coenzymes**	
Water-Soluble Vitamins	**Coenzyme**	**Function**
Thiamine (vitamin B$_1$)	Thiamine pyrophosphate (TPP)	Decarboxylation
Riboflavin (vitamin B$_2$)	Flavin adenine dinucleotide (FAD) and flavin mononucleotide (FMN)	Electron transfer (oxidation-reduction)
Niacin (vitamin B$_3$)	Nicotinamide adenine dinucleotide (NAD$^+$); nicotinamide adenine dinucleotide phosphate (NADP$^+$)	Electron transfer (oxidation-reduction)
Pantothenic acid (vitamin B$_5$)	Coenzyme A (CoA)	Acetyl group transfer
Pyridoxine (vitamin B$_6$)	Pyridoxal phosphate (PLP)	Transamination
Cobalamin (vitamin B$_{12}$)	Methylcobalamin	Methyl group transfer
Ascorbic acid (vitamin C)	Ascorbic acid (vitamin C)	Collagen biosynthesis; healing of wounds
Biotin	Biocytin	Carboxylation
Folic Acid	Tetrahydrofolate (THF)	Methyl group transfer
Lipid-Soluble Vitamins	**Biologically Active Form**	**Function**
Vitamin A	Retinal	Formation of visual pigments
Vitamin D	1,25-Dihydroxycholecalciferol	Absorption of calcium and phosphate, bone development
Vitamin E	α-Tocopherol	Antioxidant; prevents oxidation of vitamin A and unsaturated fatty acids
Vitamin K	Phylloquinone (vitamin K$_1$) and menaquinone (vitamin K$_2$)	Synthesis of prothrombin for blood clotting

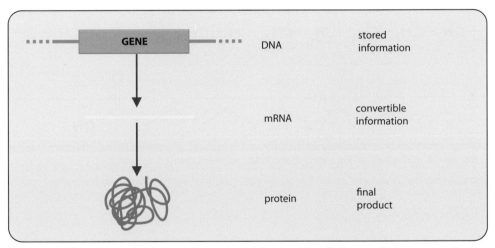

FIGURE 2-11 The central dogma of biological information transfer. DNA is composed of genes that are transcribed into messenger RNA (mRNA) and translated into protein. (Batmanian L, Worral S, Ridge J: *Biochemistry for health professionals,* ©2011, Sydney, Elsevier Australia.)

serve as structural components of biological membranes, provide insulation and protection, act as **hormones** that regulate the body, serve as vitamins, and act as detergents in digestion. In contrast to **hydrophilic** ("water loving") biomolecules, lipids are **hydrophobic** ("water fearing") compounds that do not readily combine with water.

Fatty acids (FAs) are a structural component present in more complex lipids, such as **triglycerides (TGs)**. TGs, also referred to as triacylglycerols, are the storage forms of FAs and considered the metabolic fuel for cells stored in **adipose** (fat) tissue. FAs are **amphiphilic** ("loving at both ends") possessing a hydrophilic carboxyl group "head" and hydrophobic **hydrocarbon** chain "tail" containing only carbon and

hydrogen atoms. The structure of a FA (e.g., lauric acid which has 12 carbon atoms) can be represented in a number of different ways, but the most common is the skeletal (line) structure as shown in Figure 2-13.

FAs can be classified according to the presence or absence of C=C (double) bonds. **Saturated fatty acids** like lauric acid, shown in Figure 2-13, contain only C–C (single) bonds, while **unsaturated fatty acids** are alkenes that contain one or more C=C bonds. As shown in Figure 2-14, **monounsaturated fatty acids (MUFAs)** like oleic acid contain just one C=C bond, while **polyunsaturated fatty acids (PUFAs)** like **linoleic acid** contain more than one C=C bond.

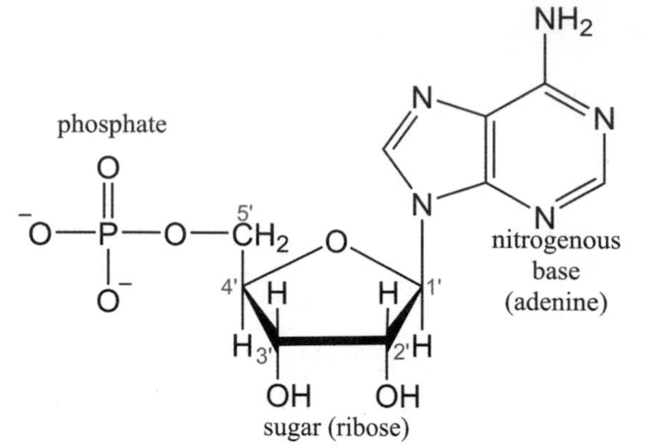

FIGURE 2-12 The structure of the nucleotide adenosine 5′-monophosphate (AMP). AMP consists of the sugar ribose, the nitrogenous base adenine, and a phosphate group.

FAs have common names and systematic names, but they also utilize an abbreviated symbol notation that depends on the total number of carbons and C=C bonds present. Table 2-4 summarizes the number of carbon atoms, common name, abbreviated symbol notation and typical lipid source for many common FAs. In contrast to the delta (Δ) numbering system, the omega (ω) numbering system indicates the position of a C=C bond by numbering the carbon chain from the methyl (–CH₃) end. Figure 2-15 shows how the omega (ω) numbering system is used in the PUFAs linolenic acid and linoleic acid.

In MUFAs and PUFAs, the C=C bond can either be a *cis* isomer or *trans* isomer. As shown in Figure 2-16, the *cis* isomer of oleic acid has the H atoms on the same side of the C=C bond, so there exists a significant bend, or "kink," in the long hydrocarbon tail. In the *trans* isomer of oleic acid,

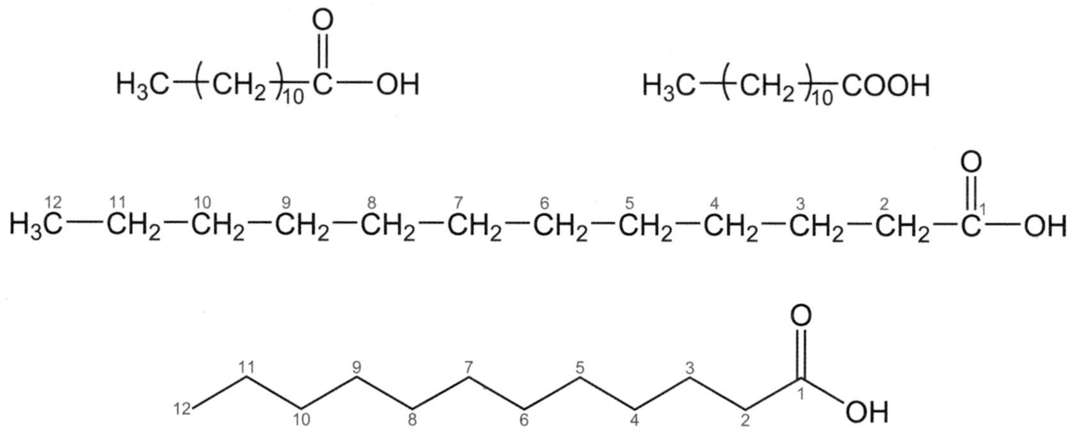

FIGURE 2-13 Four different structural representations of the fatty acid lauric acid. The skeletal (line) structure at the bottom is the most efficient way of representing the numerous carbon atoms in the long hydrocarbon chain.

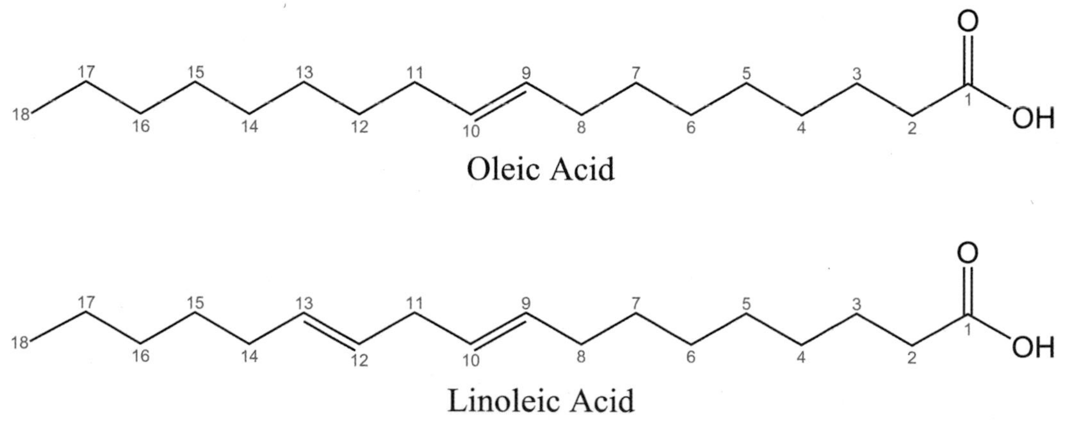

Oleic Acid

Linoleic Acid

FIGURE 2-14 Structure of unsaturated fatty acids. Oleic acid is a monounsaturated fatty acid (MUFA) with a C=C bond at carbon 9, while linoleic acid is a polyunsaturated fatty acid (PUFA) with C=C bonds at carbon 9 and carbon 12. For oleic acid, the abbreviated symbol notation is $(18:1)^{\Delta 9}$ where the first number corresponds to the total number of carbons (18), the second number corresponds to the total number of C=C bonds (1) and the superscript corresponds to the delta (Δ) locations of the C=C bonds between carbons 9 and 10 in the long carbon chain numbered starting from the carboxyl (–COOH) end. For linoleic acid, the abbreviated symbol notation is $(18:2)^{\Delta 9,12}$.

Table 2-4	Summary of common fatty acids		
Number of Carbon Atoms	**Common Name**	**Abbreviated Symbol Notation**	**Typical Lipid Source**
4	Butyric acid	(4:0)	Butterfat
8	Caprylic acid	(8:0)	Coconut oil
12	Lauric acid	(12:0)	Coconut oil, palm kernel oil
14	Myristic acid	(14:0)	Butterfat, coconut oil
16	Palmitic acid	(16:0)	Palm oil, animal fat
16	Palmitoleic acid	$(16:1)^{\Delta 9}$	Some fish oils, beef fat
18	Stearic acid	(18:0)	Cocoa butter, animal fat
18	Oleic acid	$(18:1)^{\Delta 9}$	Olive oil, canola oil
18	Linoleic acid	$(18:2)^{\Delta 9,12}$	Most vegetable oils; safflower, corn, soybean
18	Linolenic acid	$(18:3)^{\Delta 9,12,15}$	Soybean oil, canola oil, walnuts, wheat germ oil
20	Arachidic	(20:0)	Peanut oil
20	Arachidonic acid	$(20:4)^{\Delta 5,8,11,14}$	Lard, meats
20	Eicosapentaenoic acid (EPA)	$(20:5)^{\Delta 5,8,11,14,17}$	Fish oils, shellfish
22	Docosahexaenoic acid (DHA)	$(22:6)^{\Delta 4,7,10,13,16,19}$	Fish oils, shellfish

Adapted from Mahan LK, Escott-Stump S, Raymond JL: *Krause's food & the nutrition care process*, ed 13, St Louis, Saunders, 2012.

Linolenic Acid (ω-3 Fatty Acid)

Linoleic Acid (ω-6 Fatty Acid)

FIGURE 2-15 The omega (ω) numbering system for FAs. Linolenic acid is an ω-3 polyunsaturated fatty acid, while linoleic acid is an ω-6 polyunsaturated fatty acid.

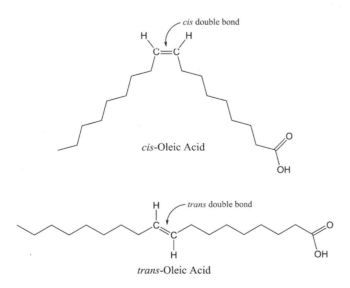

cis double bond

cis-Oleic Acid

trans double bond

trans-Oleic Acid

FIGURE 2-16 Structure of *cis-trans* isomers in MUFAs. Oleic acid is a MUFA with a C=C bond at carbon 9.

the H atoms are on opposite sides of the C=C bond and the long hydrocarbon tail remains straight and extended. *Cis* isomers predominate in nature.

The characteristics, properties and reactivity of a FA can be understood in terms of its structure. As the number of carbon atoms increases, the **melting point** of the FA increases because of stronger attractive forces. Moreover, the melting points of saturated FA are higher than unsaturated FAs. Saturated FAs exhibit stronger attractive forces as a result of the compact, tight packing of their long extended hydrocarbon tails, thus they are solids at room temperature. As shown in Figure 2-16, unsaturated FAs have "kinks" at the *cis* C=C bonds that prevent compact packing resulting in weaker attractive forces and lower melting points, thus they are liquids (**oils**) at room temperature.

TGs are the storage forms of FAs and are considered the metabolic fuel for cells stored in adipose tissue. As shown in Figure 2-17, a TG consists of a 3-carbon glycerol backbone with three FAs attached. The alcohol functional groups of the

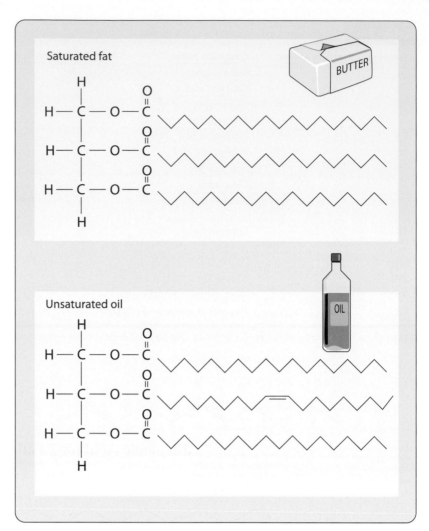

FIGURE 2-17 Comparison of TGs containing saturated FAs and unsaturated FAs. The solid fat found in butter is predominantly composed of TGs containing saturated FAs. The extended hydrocarbon tails of the saturated FAs pack together better, leading to stronger attractive forces. The liquid oil found in vegetable oils is predominantly composed of TGs containing unsaturated FAs. The "kinked" hydrocarbon tails of the unsaturated FAs do not pack well, leading to weaker attractive forces. (Batmanian L, Worral S, Ridge J: *Biochemistry for health professionals,* ©2011, Sydney, Elsevier Australia.)

glycerol backbone react with the carboxylic acid functional groups of three FAs to form a TG. In the resulting TG, an ester functional group links each FA to the glycerol backbone. The properties of a TG mirror those of the FAs present. A TG that is solid at room temperature is called a fat, whereas a TG that is liquid at room temperature is called an oil. TGs that are predominantly composed of saturated FAs are solid fats at room temperature, whereas those that are predominantly composed of unsaturated FAs are liquid oils at room temperature.

In TGs, unsaturated FAs that have C=C bonds can be the site of many different types of chemical reactions. A **hydrogenation reaction**, shown in Figure 2-18, involves the addition of a hydrogen molecule (H_2) to a C=C bond to form a saturated FA with C–C bonds. By controlling the amount of H_2 gas added, it is possible to control how many C=C bonds are converted into C–C bonds, thereby controlling the melting point of the resultant product. Partial hydrogenation of a liquid vegetable oil can be used to create soft semisolid fat products such as spreadable tub margarines and solid shortening. Partial hydrogenation of vegetable oil results in a small amount of the *cis* C=C bonds being converted into unwanted *trans* C=C bonds.

Another common, but unwanted, reaction involving C=C bonds is oxidation. Oxidation of unsaturated fats leads to rancidity, so **antioxidants**, like vitamins C and E, butylated hydroxyanisole (BHA), and butylated hydroxytoluene (BHT), are added to vegetable oils to prevent this.

Another class of lipids includes steroids. Steroids are a family of lipids containing a hydrophobic nucleus of four rings fused together. As shown in Figure 2-19, **cholesterol** is the most abundant steroid and is an important stabilizing component of biological membranes. Cholesterol is also the precursor of steroid hormones (progesterone, estradiol and testosterone), bile acids, and lipid-soluble vitamin D.

Lipids must be transported through the bloodstream to be stored, to be used for energy or to make hormones. However, lipids do not readily dissolve in blood. Therefore, they are transported via water-soluble complexes called lipoproteins. As shown in Figure 2-20, **lipoproteins** are spherical particles with a hydrophilic surface and a hydrophobic interior that can transport TGs, FAs, and cholesterol.

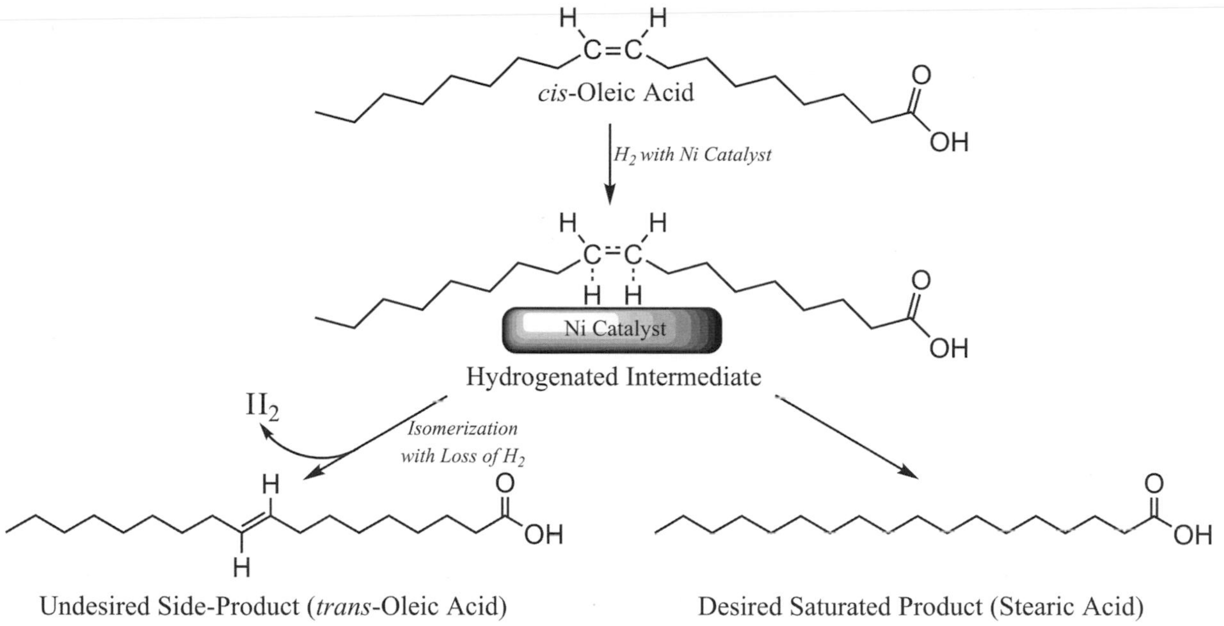

H   H
\\C=C//

cis-Oleic Acid

O

OH

H₂ with Ni Catalyst

H   H
\\C=C//
H   H

Ni Catalyst

Hydrogenated Intermediate

H₂

*Isomerization
with Loss of H₂*

H

H

O

OH

O

OH

Undesired Side-Product (*trans*-Oleic Acid)

Desired Saturated Product (Stearic Acid)

FIGURE 2-18 Hydrogenation of unsaturated FAs to form saturated FAs. In these hydrogenation reactions, a nickel (Ni) catalyst speeds up the reaction by providing a location for the H atoms to more easily react with the C=C bond. In the hydrogenation process, a slight possibility exists for the two H atoms to react with themselves and not the C=C bond. If this occurs, an undesired *trans* C=C bond results.

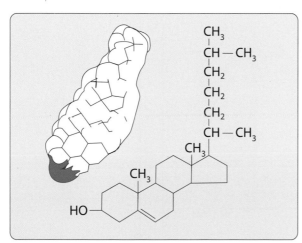

CH_3
$CH-CH_3$
CH_2
CH_2
CH_2
$CH-CH_3$
CH_3
CH_3
HO

FIGURE 2-19 Structure of cholesterol. Cholesterol consists of a hydrophobic fused ring structure with a single hydrophilic alcohol (–OH) at one end (indicated in red in the globular structure of cholesterol). (Based on Baynes & Dominiczak, 2009. *Medical Biochemistry,* 3rd edition. Mosby.)

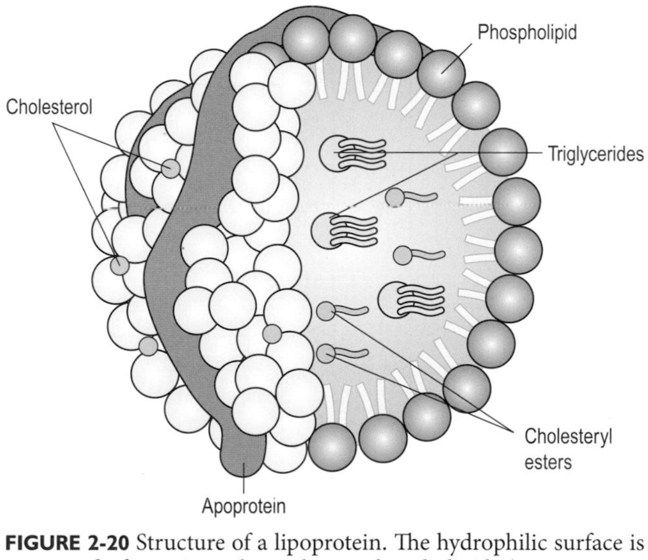

Phospholipid

Cholesterol

Triglycerides

Cholesteryl esters

Apoprotein

FIGURE 2-20 Structure of a lipoprotein. The hydrophilic surface is composed of protein and membrane phospholipids (or glycerophospholipids) while the hydrophobic core is composed of TGs and cholesterol esters. (From Baynes J, Dominiczak M: *Medical biochemistry,* ed 3, 2010, St Louis, Mosby.)

SUMMARY OF METABOLISM

Metabolism is how cells acquire, transform, store, and use energy. It is the sum total of all chemical reactions (organized into pathways) in an organism. It also includes the coordination, regulation, and energy requirements of those reactions. The three characteristics of catabolism are the production of energy, the degradation of more complex molecules into smaller molecules, and the oxidation of metabolites. In contrast, the three characteristics of anabolism are the requirement of energy input, the biosynthesis of more complex biomolecules from simple precursors, and the reduction of

metabolites. Figure 2-21 summarizes the flow of energy in the form of adenosine 5′-triphosphate (ATP) within catabolism and anabolism.

Figure 2-22 summarizes the complex processes involved in catabolism of proteins, carbohydrates, and lipids. Initially, proteins, carbohydrates, and lipids obtained in the diet are hydrolyzed into their simpler building blocks. Dietary protein is broken down into amino acids, dietary carbohydrates into monosaccharides like glucose, and dietary lipids into glycerol and FAs. Next, amino acids, glucose, and FAs

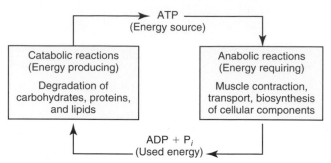

FIGURE 2-21 Energy flow in catabolism and anabolism. Energy is captured in catabolism to synthesize ATP from adenosine diphosphate (ADP) and phosphate (P_i). Energy for this process is extracted from the catabolism of carbohydrates, lipids, and proteins. ATP is used as an energy source in anabolism by being hydrolyzed to ADP and P_i. Muscle contraction, transport and the biosynthesis of cellular components requires energy in the form of ATP.

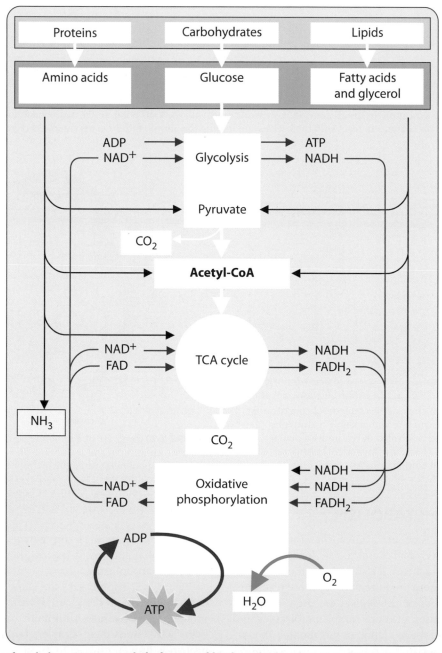

FIGURE 2-22 Summary of catabolism. Proteins, carbohydrates, and lipids are broken down into CO_2, H_2O, and NH_3 with the production of energy. The flow of C, H, O, and N atoms through catabolism are shown in white arrows and black arrows. The flow of energy as ATP and the flow of electrons as nicotinamide adenine dinucleotide (NAD^+/NADH) are shown in red arrows. (Based on Baynes & Dominiczak, 2009. *Medical Biochemistry*, 3rd edition. Mosby.)

Table 2-5	Hormonal regulation of metabolism	
Hormone	**Increased or Stimulated**	**Decreased or Inhibited**
Insulin	Entry of glucose into cells Glycolysis Glycogen biosynthesis Triglyceride biosynthesis	Gluconeogenesis Triglyceride hydrolysis Glycogen degradation Blood glucose levels
Glucagon	Glycogen degradation (liver) Gluconeogenesis (liver) Blood glucose levels	Glycogen biosynthesis Glycolysis (liver)
Epinephrine	Glycogen degradation (muscle) Glycolysis (muscle) Triglyceride hydrolysis Blood glucose levels	Glycogen biosynthesis

are converted into a common intermediate called acetyl-CoA. Acetyl-CoA then enters the **tricarboxylic acid cycle (TCA cycle)**, the central metabolic pathway also known as the citric acid cycle or Krebs cycle, and is oxidized to CO_2. As nutrients are oxidized in catabolism, electrons are released from the metabolic pathways of glycolysis and the TCA cycle. **Redox coenzymes** capture and transfer these electrons, leading to the conversion of O_2 into H_2O and the synthesis of ATP in the metabolic process called **oxidative phosphorylation**. One redox coenzyme called **nicotinamide adenine dinucleotide (NAD^+/NADH)** is derived from the vitamin niacin; NAD^+ is then reduced to NADH by accepting electrons. Another redox coenzyme called **flavin adenine dinucleotide (FAD/$FADH_2$)** is derived from the vitamin riboflavin; FAD is reduced to $FADH_2$ by accepting electrons. Ultimately, the end products of catabolism are CO_2, H_2O, and ammonia (NH_3).

Carbohydrate Metabolism

A major source of energy for the body comes from the degradation of carbohydrates. Complete **aerobic** oxidation of glucose ($C_6H_{12}O_6$) produces CO_2, H_2O, and energy captured as ATP.

$$C_6H_{12}O_6 + 6\,O_2 \rightarrow 6\,CO_2 + 6\,H_2O + 36\,ATP$$

As shown in Figure 2-22, the digestion of dietary carbohydrates begins in the mouth as amylase enzymes hydrolyze polysaccharides into monosaccharides. These monosaccharides enter the bloodstream and are transported to the tissues that need energy. Glucose oxidation begins with **glycolysis**, entering the TCA cycle with CO_2 being produced. As glucose is oxidized, electrons are captured by the reduced coenzymes NADH and $FADH_2$. NADH and $FADH_2$ transfer electrons to the **mitochondria**, the power source of the cell. In oxidative phosphorylation, these electrons ultimately reduce O_2 into H_2O and the energy is used to synthesize ATP.

When dietary glucose is in excess, it is stored as the polysaccharide glycogen in muscles and the liver. Later, when blood glucose levels decrease and the body needs energy again, glycogen is converted back into glucose. When glycogen is depleted, **gluconeogenesis** in the liver can convert pyruvate (and other simple noncarbohydrate precursors like lactate and amino acids) into glucose for energy.

Three hormones regulate carbohydrate metabolism to maintain constant blood glucose levels (Table 2-5). **Insulin** is a signal of the "fed" state and is secreted when blood glucose levels are high. It activates glycolysis and glycogen biosynthesis-metabolic pathways that lower blood glucose levels. **Glucagon** is a signal of the "starved" state and is secreted when blood glucose levels are low. It activates gluconeogenesis and glycogen degradation-metabolic pathways that raise blood glucose levels. **Epinephrine** is the "fight or flight" hormone secreted in time of immediate energy need. It activates glycogen degradation for energy.

Protein Metabolism

The major role of proteins is to provide amino acids for the synthesis of new proteins for the body. Amino acids are also a source of N for the synthesis of many biomolecules, such as hormones, heme, and nitrogenous bases. Even though carbohydrates and lipids are the preferred sources of energy, proteins can be an energy source of last resort under conditions of fasting and starvation.

As shown in Figure 2-22, the digestion of proteins begins when enzymes like proteases hydrolyze proteins into amino acids. When amino acid levels exceed requirements, the amino group is removed, releasing free NH_3. Because high levels of NH_3 are toxic, mammals use the urea cycle to convert excess NH_3 into urea for excretion. Amino acids are further degraded, entering the TCA cycle with CO_2 being produced. The degradation of amino acids for energy can be classified as either ketogenic or glucogenic. **Ketogenic amino acids** degrade into acetyl-CoA that can be converted into **ketone bodies**, soluble forms of lipids that can be used as fuel for the body. **Glucogenic amino acids** degrade into pyruvate and other TCA cycle intermediates that can be converted into glucose as a fuel for the body.

When amino acids are synthesized, they utilize common precursors found in metabolic pathways like glycolysis and the TCA cycle. Unfortunately, humans cannot synthesize all 20 common amino acids because they lack the

Table 2-6	Essential (indispensable) and nonessential (dispensable) amino acids
Essential (Indispensable)	**Nonessential (Dispensable)**
Arginine[a]	Alanine
Histidine[a]	Asparagine
Isoleucine	Aspartic acid
Leucine	Cysteine
Lysine	Glutamic acid
Methionine	Glutamine
Phenylalanine	Glycine
Threonine	Proline
Tryptophan	Serine
Valine	Tyrosine[b]

[a]Arg and His are essential (indispensable) in babies and young children but not adults.
[b]Tyr is synthesized from Phe.

necessary enzymes, so these essential amino acids (EAAs) or indispensable amino acids must be obtained in the diet. The body uses enzymes to synthesize nonessential amino acids (NEAAs) or dispensable amino acids. Table 2-6 lists the EAAs and NEAAs.

Lipid Metabolism

Another major source of energy for the body comes from the catabolism of lipids. Because of their structure, lipids can be oxidized to produce more energy than carbohydrates or proteins. Lipids are also anhydrous; therefore the energy per gram of lipids (9 kcal/g) is greater than that of carbohydrates (4 kcal/g). Lipids can be stored in adipose tissue in unlimited amounts.

As shown in Figure 2-22, the digestion of dietary lipids begins when enzymes like lipase hydrolyze TGs into free FAs and glycerol. FAs are degraded two carbons at a time, producing acetyl-CoA, which enters the TCA cycle and produces CO_2. In the degradation of FAs, electrons are captured by the reduced coenzymes NADH and $FADH_2$. Subsequently, ATP is synthesized in the mitochondria via oxidative phosphorylation.

Excess dietary lipids are stored as TGs in adipose cells. When blood glucose levels are low and glycogen stores are depleted, the utilization of TGs stored in adipose tissue is activated. As shown in Table 2-5, the hormone epinephrine activates TG hydrolysis yielding free FAs and glycerol for energy.

Under conditions of fasting, starvation, untreated diabetes and low-carbohydrate diets, excessive degradation of FAs produces too much acetyl-CoA. Excessive levels of acetyl-CoA and low levels of carbohydrates results in a bottleneck at the TCA cycle. Not all the acetyl-CoA can be degraded, so it is converted into ketone bodies and transported via the bloodstream to tissues that need energy, particularly the heart and brain, when blood glucose levels are low.

HEALTH APPLICATION 2   Lactose Intolerance

Some patients are unable to digest specific carbohydrates because of insufficient amounts of disaccharide degrading enzymes. When those carbohydrates are eaten, the disaccharide is fermented by intestinal bacteria rather than being broken down into simple sugars. This results in malabsorption of the disaccharide, accompanied by diarrhea, abdominal cramps, flatulence, and halitosis. The National Institutes of Health (NIH) consensus concluded most people with lactose malabsorption do not have clinical lactose intolerance and many who think they are lactose intolerant are not lactose malabsorbers.[1] Lactase, an intestinal enzyme responsible for lactose digestion, is the only disaccharidase whose activity is reduced in a significant proportion of older children and adults. Conversely, all infants of every racial and ethnic group can successfully digest the lactose in human milk and infant formulas.

Lactose intolerance primarily affects African Americans, Hispanic Americans, Native Americans, Asian Americans, Alaskan Natives, and Pacific Islanders. For most people, lactase deficiency appears to be genetically determined with gradual decreases in lactase activity after weaning. It may also be a temporary condition caused by gastrointestinal diseases or intestinal mucosa damage. Occasionally, an infant has a lactase deficiency at birth because of an inborn error of metabolism. Lactose intolerance can be diagnosed based on the results of a blood, breath, or stool test ordered by a healthcare provider.

Nutritional Care

Lactase deficiency is easily treated by reducing lactose-containing foods in one's diet. Because milk provides significant amounts of calcium, vitamin D, phosphorus, riboflavin, and sometimes protein, elimination is not advisable. The ability to digest lactose is not an all-or-nothing phenomenon; most patients with lactose intolerance can tolerate some lactose. The amount of dairy products is reduced to a patient's tolerance level (Box 2-1). Based on evidence available to the NIH, most adults and adolescents who have been diagnosed with lactose malabsorption can tolerate at least 12 g of lactose.[1] Milk is tolerated better when taken with a meal and limited to 8 oz at a time. Whole milk is better tolerated than skim milk.

Individuals who avoid dairy products may exacerbate their risk for osteoporosis. Calcium is necessary for adequate bone accretions and optimal peak bone mass. When children and teenagers' diets are deficient in calcium and/or vitamin D, bone accretion may be affected, and optimal peak bone mass may not occur. Patients should be taught the approximate calcium composition of milk products they tolerate (see Chapter 9, Table 9-2) so that they can try to consume adequate amounts.

HEALTH APPLICATION **2** **Lactose Intolerance—cont'd**

Fermented dairy products—especially yogurt, buttermilk, aged cheese, and sour cream—are often better tolerated by lactase-deficient individuals than other dairy products. Because it contains active lactase and less lactose, yogurt made with the organisms *Lactobacillus bulgaricus* or *Streptococcus thermophilus* is better tolerated than nonfermented dairy products. Most commercially available unflavored yogurt can be beneficial to lactose-intolerant patients. Pasteurization of frozen yogurts decreases the lactase activity and kills lactose-producing bacteria, so most frozen yogurts are not well tolerated by lactose-intolerant patients.

Commercially available lactase in tablet or liquid form can be beneficial. Lactase tablets, taken with a lactose-containing food, are effective in the stomach's acidic environment for approximately 45 minutes. Liquid lactase is effective in a neutral pH, and when added to milk, the lactose is hydrolyzed before ingestion. Specialized lactose-reduced products are also commercially available.

BOX 2-1 **Suggestions for Lactose-Intolerant Patients**

- Adequate amounts of calcium need to be provided when milk and milk products are avoided. Because of different tolerance levels, each patient needs to experiment to determine which method is most effective for providing necessary nutrients without discomfort. Consume small amounts of lactose-containing foods with meals several times a day.
- Consume fermented dairy products—yogurt,* kefir,† and buttermilk—that contain probiotics (live bacteria).
- Choose aged cheeses (e.g., Swiss, Colby, and Longhorn) that naturally contain less lactose.
- Try small amounts of whole-milk dairy products.
- Buy lactose-reduced or lactose-free products.
- Read ingredient labels for "hidden" lactose (whey, milk by-products, nonfat dry milk powder, malted milk, buttermilk, and dry milk solids). Also check for lactose in prescription and over-the-counter drugs.
- Drink or eat calcium-fortified foods, such as orange juice, soymilk, and cereals.
- Use over-the-counter lactase enzymes available in tablet or liquid form to hydrolyze the lactose in milk products or consume lactose-hydrolyzed commercially available milk.
- Increase consumption of other calcium-containing foods, such as salmon and sardines canned with bones, spinach, kale, broccoli, turnip and beet greens, molasses, tofu, almonds, orange, eggs, and shrimp.
- Consider commercially available nutrition supplements, such as Resource (Novartis/Sandoz Nutrition) and Boost and Sustacal (Nestle Health Science).
- If the previous suggestions are not feasible to maintain an adequate intake of 800 mg of calcium, consult a healthcare provider or dietitian for calcium supplements that are well absorbed. These supplements may also need to include vitamin D.

*Unflavored yogurt is usually best tolerated.
†Kefir is a fermented milk beverage that contains different bacteria than yogurt.

STUDENT READINESS

1. Explain how the three major areas of biochem-istry (structure, metabolism, and information) are different.
2. For each of the following functional groups, find an example in the textbook of a biomolecule containing that functional group: alkene, alcohol, amine, aldehyde, ketone, carboxylic acid, ester, and peptide (amide).
3. Compare and contrast the functions of carbohydrates, proteins, nucleic acids, and lipids.
4. Differentiate between monosaccharides, disaccharides, and polysaccharides. Give an example of each.
5. Compare and contrast the structure and function of lactose and sucrose.
6. What is the difference between starch and glycogen?
7. What is the difference between enzymes and coenzymes?
8. Explain the structural reason why lipids do not readily dissolve in water.
9. What are the differences between a saturated fatty acid and an unsaturated fatty acid in terms of structure and properties?
10. In your own words, explain the central dogma of biological information transfer (DNA→RNA→Protein).
11. Contrast catabolism and anabolism.
12. Draw your own diagram illustrating how proteins, carbohydrates, and lipids are degraded to make energy in metabolism. Indicate on your diagram where ATP is produced. What are the three end products of catabolism containing C, H, O, or N?
13. Compare and contrast the hormones insulin, glucagon, and epinephrine.

Reference

1. Shaukat A, Levitt MD, Taylor BC, et al: Systematic review: effective management strategies for lactose intolerance. *Ann Intern Med* 152(12):797–803, 2010.

ⓔ EVOLVE RESOURCES

Please visit http://evolve.elsevier.com/Stegeman/nutritional for additional practice and study support tools.

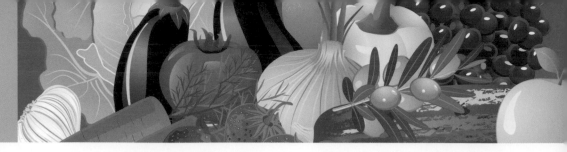

Chapter 3

The Alimentary Canal: Digestion and Absorption

Student Learning Outcomes

Upon completion of this chapter, the student will be able to achieve the following student learning outcomes:

- Discuss factors that influence food intake.
- Describe general functions of each digestive organ.
- Identify chemical secretions necessary for digestion of energy-containing nutrients and in what parts of the gastrointestinal tract they are secreted.
- Point out the nutrients that require digestion and the digested products that can be absorbed.
- Explain the role of gastrointestinal motility in digestion and absorption.
- Choose points in Nutritional Directions for educating dental patients.
- Describe how digestion and absorption may affect nutritional status and oral health.

Key Terms

Accessory organs
Alimentary canal
Alveolar process
Anorexia
Anosmia
Autoimmune disorder
Bile
Bolus
Cancellous bone
Chyme
Celiac disease
Constipation
Demineralization
Dysgeusia
Emulsification
Gluten
Gluten sensitivity
Gustatory
Hydrolysis
Hypergeusia
Hypogeusia
Iatrogenic
Large intestine
Lower esophageal sphincter
Lymphatic system
Mastication

Masticatory efficiency
Microflora
Microvilli
Olfactory nerves
Osmosis
Pancreatic enzymes
Papillae
Pathogenic
Peristalsis
Phantom taste
Portal circulation
Prebiotics
Probiotics
Proteolytic enzymes
Remineralize
Residue
Small intestine
Sphincter muscles
Symbiotics
Systemic condition
Taste buds
Trabecular bone
Valves
Wheat allergy
Xerostomia

⊙ Test Your NQ

1. **T/F** The alimentary tract is approximately 30 feet long.
2. **T/F** The hydrolysis of carbohydrate yields fatty acid and glycerol.
3. **T/F** Most absorption occurs in the stomach.
4. **T/F** Fat-soluble nutrients always enter the portal circulation.
5. **T/F** Taste disorders are often the result of problems in smell rather than taste.

6. **T/F** Lactose is the name of an enzyme.
7. **T/F** The digestive process begins in the oral cavity.
8. **T/F** Villi are located in the large intestine.
9. **T/F** Missing, decayed, or poorly restored teeth can affect food intake.
10. **T/F** Saliva aids in oral clearance of food.

Foods are composed of large chemical molecules that cannot be used unless they are broken down to an absorbable form. The digestive system is designed to (a) ingest foods; (b) digest or break down complex molecules into simple, soluble materials that can be absorbed; and (c) eliminate unused residues. Only energy-providing macronutrients (carbohydrate, protein, and fat) must be digested for absorption. Most vitamins, minerals, alcohol, and water can be absorbed as eaten.

The gastrointestinal tract can also be used to deliver complex chemical substances, such as oral medications. Medications frequently affect or can be affected by foods, modifying absorption, metabolism, or excretion of either the food or the drug. They may also affect nutritional status by altering taste or salivary flow; both of these conditions influence the amount and types of foods consumed. Dental hygienists need to become familiar with normal gastrointestinal processes because disturbances in the gastrointestinal tract may affect nutritional status and oral health of patients.

PHYSIOLOGY OF THE GASTROINTESTINAL TRACT

The digestive system includes the alimentary canal and several accessory organs (Fig. 3-1). The alimentary canal is a tubular structure approximately 30 feet long (five times the height of an average man). The **alimentary canal,** extending from the mouth to the anus, comprises all the body parts through which food passes. It includes the oral cavity, pharynx, esophagus, stomach, small intestine, and large intestine. The **small intestine** is comprised of the duodenum, jejunum, and ileum; the **large intestine** includes the cecum, colon, and rectum. **Accessory organs**—the salivary glands, liver, gallbladder, and pancreas—provide secretions essential for digestion and absorption. Digestion involves two basic types of action on food: (a) mechanical and (b) chemical. Mechanical actions include chewing and peristalsis, which break up and mix foods, permitting better blending of foodstuffs with digestive secretions. Chemical actions involve salivary enzymes and digestive juices, reducing foodstuffs to absorbable molecules.

Chemical Action

A large molecule can be split into smaller ones that are water-soluble and can be used by cells; this process is called hydrolysis. The hydrolysis of energy nutrients requires water. The following are basic hydrolysis reactions in food digestion:

$$Protein + H_2O \rightarrow amino\ acids$$

$$Fat + H_2O \rightarrow fatty\ acids + glycerol$$

$$Carbohydrate + H_2O \rightarrow monosaccharides$$

These reactions depend on enzymes. Enzymes are complex proteins that enable metabolic reactions to proceed at a faster rate without being exhausted themselves. In protein hydrolysis, the substrate for the enzyme is protein, and amino acids are basic end products. An enzyme forms a temporary chemical compound with the substrate. When the reaction is completed, the complex separates, releasing new chemical compounds and the enzyme.

Because the enzyme is reused, only small amounts are needed. Enzymes function comparable to keys: they are very specific and function on only one substrate, similar to a key fitting a particular lock, as shown in Chapter 2, Figure 2-10. The name for some enzymes is derived from the name of the substrate, with the suffix -*ase* (e.g., lactase is the enzyme produced to catalyze the breakdown of lactose).

Mechanical Action

The wall of the gastrointestinal tract is similar from the esophagus to the rectum (Fig. 3-2, *A*). A layer of muscles encircles the tube, allowing the diameter of the tube to expand and contract. Food particles are broken up and mixed by the churning action. The outer fibers of the muscular coat (longitudinal muscle) run lengthwise and are responsible for **peristalsis,** involuntary rhythmic waves of contraction traveling the length of the alimentary tract.

Doorlike mechanisms between the digestive segments, called **valves** or **sphincter muscles**, are designed to (a) retain food in each segment until completion of the mechanical actions and digestive juices, (b) allow measured amounts of food to pass into the next segment, and (c) prevent food from "backing up" into the preceding area. Regulation of these valves is complex, involving muscular function and different pressures on each side of the valve.

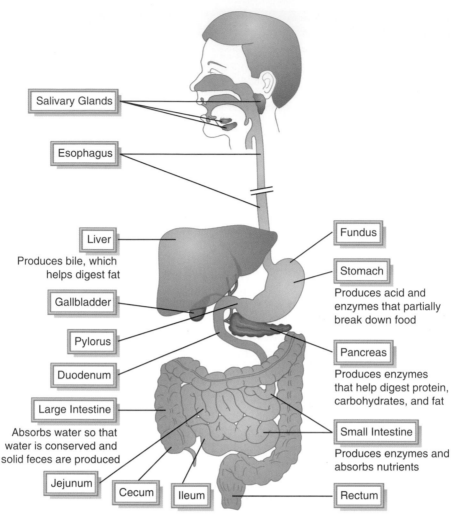

FIGURE 3-1 The digestive process. (From Peckenpaugh NJ: *Nutrition essentials and diet therapy*, ed 11, St Louis, 2010, Saunders Elsevier.)

 Dental Considerations

- Gurgling sounds, caused by air and fluid in the normal abdomen, indicate peristalsis is occurring.
- If the alimentary tract is not functioning properly, even with intake of adequate amounts, nutrients may not be absorbed as a result of alterations in digestion and absorption. The patient may be prone to nutrient deficiencies, poor healing, or fecal impactions.
- Loss of motility in the stomach and small intestine results in impaired gastric and intestinal emptying. This allows excessive growth of bacteria, which may injure the surface of the intestine, cause diarrhea, and interfere with nutrient absorption. Patients who are immobile (because of injury, trauma, or debilitating illness) or patients with uncontrolled diabetes are more prone to these disorders.
- Food–drug interactions have the potential to cause nutritional problems or erratic drug responses. Knowledge of common drugs, (including over-the-counter medications, herbals, and supplements), and understanding how they interact with food is important. For example, consuming milk or milk products while taking tetracycline decreases the amount of tetracycline and calcium available to the body.

 Nutritional Directions

- Taking over-the-counter enzyme tablets may not be beneficial because enzymes are digested before they can be used. Prescription pancreatic enzymes have a special enteric coating preventing the enzyme from being exposed to gastric juices. Lactase, a nonprescription enzyme, is effective for lactose-intolerant individuals because it is either added to or taken with lactose-containing foods, allowing conversion of lactose into two monosaccharides before gastric juices can affect the enzyme (see *Health Application 2: Lactose Intolerance* in Chapter 2).
- Patients reporting gastrointestinal problems should be assessed for adequate nutrient intake using *MyPlate* or *Dietary Guidelines*. If intake is inadequate, the patient should be referred to the patient's primary care provider or an RDN.

ORAL CAVITY

Taste and Smell

Generally, food choices are influenced by three sensory perceptions: sight, smell, and taste. **Gustatory** (taste) sensations evoke pronounced feelings of pleasure or aversion; in the

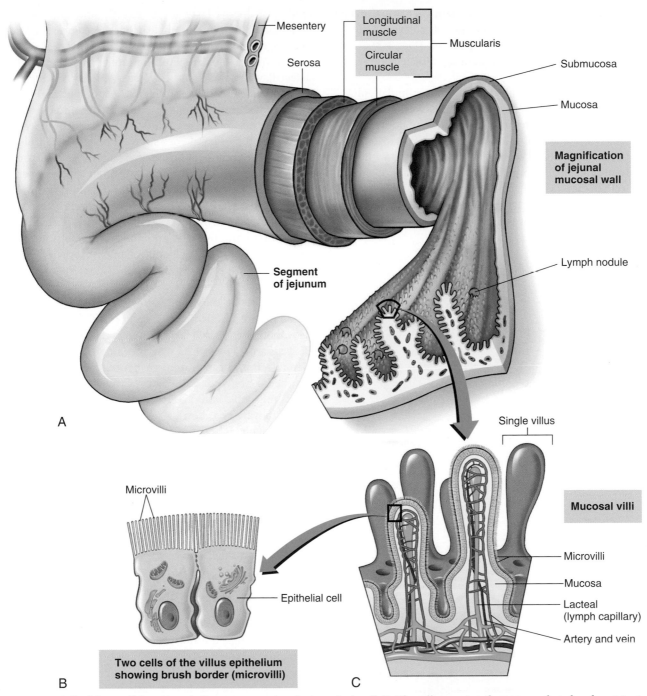

FIGURE 3-2 Wall of the small intestine. **A,** Layers composing the intestinal wall. **B,** The villi covering the mucosa that absorb nutrients. **C,** Further enlargement shows the brush border or microvilli enzymes that are available to hydrolyze nutrients further for absorption. (From Standring S: *Gray's anatomy: the anatomical basis of clinical practice,* ed 40, London, 2009, Churchill Livingstone.)

United States, taste is the primary determinant of food choices. The presentation of food, its color and aroma, may be the basis for acceptance or rejection. Food flavors are derived from characteristics of substances ingested, including taste, aroma, texture, temperature, and irritating properties. Approximately 75% of flavor is derived from odors.

The mouth, or oral cavity, plays an important role in the digestive system. It is the "port of entry" where receptors for sense of taste, or **taste buds,** are located. A taste bud consists of 30 to 100 cells embedded in the surrounding epithelium,

termed **papillae.** Taste papillae appear on the tongue as little red dots, or raised bumps, and are most numerous on the dorsal epithelium. These cells replace themselves every 3 to 10 days; disease, drugs, nutritional status, radiation, and age can affect them. As food is chewed, gustatory receptors come into contact with chemicals dissolved in saliva.

Nerve cells carry messages to the brain, which interprets flavors as sweet, sour, salty, or bitter. These four basic tastes reflect specific constituents of food. Taste buds for all four sensations are located throughout the mouth, but specific kinds of buds are concentrated in certain (but overlapping) areas. Taste buds also are found on the soft palate, epiglottis, larynx, and posterior wall of the pharynx (Fig. 3-3). Taste and smell are essential for maintaining sufficient intake to meet physiological needs.

Food stimulates taste buds, and aromas stimulate **olfactory nerves**, receptors for smell. In contrast to the four basic tastes, an almost unlimited number of unique odors can be detected. No tactile sensation indicates the origin of odor sensations. Food-related aromas may be confused with taste sensations, and taste disorders often result from problems in smell rather than taste. Prevalence of olfactory impairment is high in older adults with the problem increasing with age. This is most likely the reason an elderly patient will state that food "just doesn't taste good." Exactly how and why taste preferences shift remains unclear, but preferences are known to change significantly with aging.

Loss of smell, or **anosmia**, results in limited capacity to detect flavor of food and beverages. Ability to smell food being prepared and eaten influences food selection. Smell is also a protective mechanism; odors are used to help determine whether foods are harmful or spoiled. Upper respiratory infections, nasal or sinus problems, neurological disorders, endocrine abnormalities, aging, or head trauma may cause anosmia. A common cold often impairs a person's sense of smell, causing loss of appetite and limiting the ability to "taste" and enjoy food. The rate of the continuous renewal process undergone by olfactory receptor cells is depressed in malnutrition and by some antibiotics. Some of these disorders are self-limited; however, chemosensory losses from chemotherapy, upper respiratory infection, and aging may be irreversible.[1,2]

Dysgeusia is persistent, abnormal distortion of taste, including sweet, sour, bitter, salty, or metallic tastes. Dysgeusia without identifiable taste stimuli is called **phantom taste**. Dysgeusia may be caused by a previous viral upper respiratory infection, head trauma, a neurological or psychiatric disorder, a **systemic condition** (a disease or disorder that affects the whole body), **xerostomia** (dry mouth from inadequate salivary secretion), a severe nutritional deficiency, an invasive dental procedure resulting in nerve damage, an oral bacterial or fungal infection, or burning mouth syndrome,[3] or it may have an iatrogenic causation. **Iatrogenic** refers to an adverse condition resulting from medical treatment, e.g., medications, irradiation, surgery. These conditions may also cause **hypogeusia** or loss of taste, and **hypergeusia** or heightened taste acuity. Dysgeusia may also result from breathing through the mouth. The dental hygienist is frequently the first healthcare provider to detect a patient's taste disorder. Hyperkeratinization of the epithelium causing blockage of taste buds and affecting dietary intake may be observed during an oral examination.

Gustatory and olfactory disorders, whether caused by disease or drugs, are not mere inconveniences or neurotic symptoms. They affect food choices and dietary habits. A poor appetite, also called **anorexia**, may occur when medications cause loss of taste acuity. Taste stimulants affect salivary and pancreatic secretions, gastric contractions, and intestinal motility. Therefore, gustatory disorders can also affect digestion.

Because gustatory and olfactory disorders can result in deterioration of a patient's general condition or nutritional status, these abnormalities must always be considered in dental and nutritional care. Potentially adverse compensatory habits may develop (e.g., decreased sweet or salty perceptions may result in excessive usage of sweets or salts, which may be potentially harmful, especially for patients with diabetes or hypertension). Also, addition of sugar can increase the incidence of caries. Persistent taste distortions can lead to inadequate caloric intake, resulting in unintentional weight loss or malnutrition.

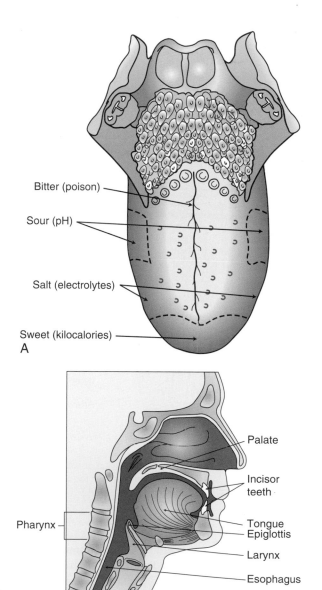

Bitter (poison)

Sour (pH)

Salt (electrolytes)

Sweet (kilocalories)

A

Palate

Incisor teeth

Pharynx

Tongue
Epiglottis

Larynx

Esophagus

B

FIGURE 3-3 A, Regions of taste on the tongue. **B**, The oropharyngeal cavity showing the regions that contain taste buds, which include the epiglottis, soft palate, laryngeal pharynx, and oral pharynx.

Saliva

Adequate saliva flow is essential for oral health which includes maintenance of soft tissues in the oral cavity, including taste buds. Saliva, secreted by salivary glands, is essential in taste sensations, functioning to (a) lubricate oral tissues for chewing, swallowing, and digestion; (b) remove debris and microorganisms; (c) provide antibacterial action; (d) neutralize, dilute, and buffer bacterial acids; (e) **remineralize** (restoration or renewal of calcium, phosphates, and other minerals to areas that have been damaged by incipient caries, abrasion, or erosion); (f) prevent plaque accumulation; (g) facilitate taste; and (h) promote ease of speech. An average of 1 to 2 mL/min of this complex fluid helps maintain integrity of teeth against physical, chemical, and microbial insults.

Saliva is supersaturated with calcium phosphates that allow demineralized areas of hydroxyapatite in enamel to be remineralized. **Demineralization** occurs when calcium, phosphate, and other minerals are lost from tooth enamel, causing tooth enamel to dissolve. This occurs because of acids produced by fermentable carbohydrates combining with acidogenic bacteria (see Chapter 18); it is not caused by insufficient calcium. Genetic variations of saliva, especially amylase, affect food preferences and intake by influencing oral sensory properties of food.[4]

Acidic, sour, or bitter tastes stimulate salivary flow. Saliva production is also stimulated by consumption of tasty foods and gum chewing. An increase in oral clearance rate decreases risk of caries formation (for more information, see Chapter 18). Saliva blends with food particles to moisten foods so they are more easily manipulated and prepared for swallowing.

Some chemical action or hydrolysis of nutrients begins in the mouth. Table 3-1 shows the functions of the different constituents in saliva. Because food is normally in the mouth briefly, ptyalin, or salivary amylase, initiates starch digestion. If a carbohydrate food, such as a cracker, is chewed and held in the mouth for a few seconds, it will begin to taste sweet, indicating that some starch is being hydrolyzed to dextrin and maltose.

Dry mouth from inadequate salivary flow, also called xerostomia, leads to diminished gustatory function (see Chapter 20 for additional details). Xerostomia may result in frequent oral ulcerations, increased sensitivity of the tongue to spices and flavors, and increased risk of dental caries. Many drugs, including diuretics, cause xerostomia. Diuretics, prescribed to help the body eliminate fluids, also cause a decrease in salivary flow. Increasing fluid intake to 8 to 10 cups daily is important to compensate for these losses.

Teeth

Teeth play a major role in digestion by crushing and grinding food into smaller pieces, a process known as **mastication**. In contrast to bone, neither tooth enamel nor dentin can be repaired or replaced in significant amounts by any natural process. Only small amounts of enamel and dentin are

Table 3-1	Digestive functions of saliva	
Saliva Component	**Classification**	**Function**
Mucin	Glycoprotein	Lubricates food for easier passage and protects the lining of the gastrointestinal tract
Ptyalin (amylase)	Enzyme	Initiates hydrolysis of complex carbohydrates to simple sugars
Lysozyme (antibody)	Enzyme	Breaks down cell walls of some ingested bacteria

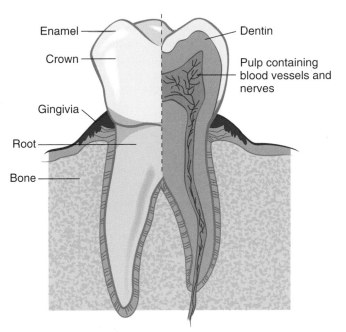

FIGURE 3-4 Diagram of a tooth.

repaired or replaced through enamel remineralization and through secondary dentin deposition around the pulp chamber of the tooth (Fig. 3-4). Mineral deposition and resorption affect the bone that supports the dentition. This supporting bone, known as alveolar bone, is primarily **trabecular bone** (bony spikes forming a meshwork of spaces) and **cancellous bone** (bone within the spaces created by the network of trabecular bone, which appears spongy and contains bone marrow in small hollows). Negative calcium balance increases susceptibility to resorption and bone loss in the **alveolar process** (comprised of the maxillary and mandibular crest and serves as the bony investment for the teeth). The maxilla and mandible to some extent depend on the presence of teeth and occlusal forces associated with chewing to prevent calcium resorption. Chewing firm foods helps maintain proper balance between alveolar bone resorption and new bone formation. Teeth and supporting bone structures are affected by adequate nutrient intake, digestive function, and hormonal balance.

Mastication reduces food particle size. Inability to masticate food adequately may result in larger chunks of food being swallowed. Larger pieces of food increase potential for food obstruction in the airway. Food asphyxiation, which may result in sudden death, occurs in many individuals with defective, incomplete, or poorly fitting dentures. Loss of even one permanent molar may decrease masticatory efficiency, or how well a patient prepares food for swallowing. Even after patients become fully adjusted to well-fitted dentures, masticatory efficiency is less than when they had their natural teeth.

Digestion of food is facilitated by increasing its surface area. Whether or not particle size affects its digestibility is uncertain. However, when elderly patients have digestive problems, masticatory efficiency is usually a factor. Frequently, when masticatory efficiency declines, people either choose foods that require less chewing or use techniques to soften foods, e.g., stewing meats, steaming vegetables, or dunking cookies or toast in fluids. In many circumstances, hypersensitive, poorly restored, decayed, abscessed, or periodontally-involved teeth affect food choices and limit the variety of foods chosen.

ESOPHAGUS

The swallowing reflex moves a bolus, or the swallowed mass of food, into the esophagus where it is transported to the stomach by peristalsis and gravity. The esophagus is a continuous tube approximately 10 inches (25 to 30 cm) long that connects the pharynx with the stomach. It penetrates the diaphragm through an opening called the esophageal hiatus. The lower esophageal sphincter comprises a group of very strong circular muscle fibers located just above the stomach. The lower esophageal sphincter relaxes to permit food into the stomach, but contracts tightly to prevent regurgitation, or "backwashing," of stomach contents.

Dental Considerations

- Assess nutritional status of patients with gustatory or olfactory disorders for changes in dietary habits and appetite that may lead to a dietary deficiency, increased use of spices (especially salt and sugar), food textures, and development of food cravings or dislikes.[5]
- Patients commonly complain about "taste" or "flavor" of food when olfactory as well as gustatory sensations are impaired.
- Assess patients for possible dietary deficiencies (niacin, vitamins A and B_{12}, zinc, copper, nickel) because these can be a factor in gustatory abnormalities.
- Zinc depletion may decrease taste acuity but is not the reason for all cases of hypogeusia. Currently, no tests can accurately assess marginal zinc status in humans.[6]
- Xerostomia may compound nutritional intake problems related to taste loss and may make chewing and swallowing more difficult.
- Patients with difficulty chewing are likely to lose taste acuity; monitor food intake.

- Edentulous patients or patients with ill-fitting dentures should be monitored because quality and quantity of food intake may be compromised.
- Dentures may cause alterations in taste, either caused by altered masticatory efficiency or by the appliance covering the palatal taste buds. Patients with complete dentures exhibit poorer taste and texture tolerance compared with patients with partial dentures or compromised natural dentition.
- Postmenopausal women with low dental bone mass may have decreased levels of total bone mass. Carefully assess an older woman's mandibular bone density, which could result in early diagnosis or detection of osteoporosis.
- Although food intake often decreases when patients initially receive a set of dentures, after an initial adjustment period, food intake usually increases with improved ability to chew.
- Carefully evaluate anecdotal reports or studies involving limited numbers of patients to support a beneficial effect of vitamins or minerals on dysgeusia.
- Refer patients with persistent gustatory, masticatory, or swallowing difficulties to a healthcare provider or RDN to determine types of foods needed to obtain adequate nutrients.

Nutritional Directions

- Natural teeth are more efficient for chewing and biting than any prosthesis.
- Tooth loss is not inevitable; most people can maintain their natural dentition throughout life with consistent, preventive dental measures.
- For xerostomia, increase fluid intake with meals to facilitate oral clearance. Nutrient-dense foods in a liquid or semiliquid form are beneficial.
- No proven intervention enhances diminished taste acuity or ameliorates dysgeusia. Encourage experimentation with texture, spiciness, and temperature. Enhance visual presentation of food and serve in a calm, relaxing environment.
- To improve nutrient intake when mastication is less efficient, special cooking techniques (e.g., stewing meats), chewing longer, and choosing soft foods are preferable to pureeing foods. For example, cream-style corn can replace corn on the cob, and applesauce can replace raw apples.
- Particularly for new denture wearers, herbs and spices and contrasting food flavor combinations (e.g., sweet and sour) can enhance taste perception.
- New denture wearers may slow the rate of alveolar resorption by taking calcium and vitamin D supplements. Refer the patient to a healthcare provider or RDN for a nutritional assessment.

GASTRIC DIGESTION

A bolus entering the stomach is mixed with gastric secretions by peristaltic contractions, producing chyme, a semifluid material produced by gastric juices on ingested food. Gastric secretions include mucus, hydrochloric acid, enzymes, and a component called intrinsic factor.

The low pH of stomach contents (approximately 1.5 to 3.0) is beneficial for several reasons: (a) kills or inhibits growth of most food bacteria, (b) denatures proteins and facilitates hydrolysis to amino acids, (c) activates gastric enzymes, (d) hydrolyzes some carbohydrates, and (e) increases solubility and absorption of calcium and iron.

Two major enzymes are found in gastric juice: pepsin and lipase. Pepsin is capable of hydrolyzing large protein molecules to smaller fragments. Gastric lipase is involved in digestion of short- and medium-chain triglycerides (e.g., triglycerides found in butterfat). Mucus forms an alkaline coating on the lining of the stomach to protect the stomach against digestion by pepsin. Intrinsic factor, secreted in the stomach, is essential for absorption of vitamin B_{12} in the small intestine.

Normal gastric secretion is regulated by nerves and hormonal stimuli. Visual, olfactory, and gustatory senses stimulate gastric secretions. Fear, sadness, pain, and depression are generally accompanied by decreased secretions; anger, stress, and hostility may increase secretions.

An adult stomach functions as a reservoir to hold an average meal for 3 to 4 hours. The stomach empties at different rates depending on the size of the stomach and composition of the chyme. The rate of passage through the stomach (fastest to slowest) is liquids, carbohydrates, proteins, and fats. When a mixture of foods is presented, this pattern is not as well defined. The smaller the stomach capacity, the more rapidly the stomach empties. (This is exemplified in infants, who must be fed frequently until the stomach size expands.) Fats remain in the stomach longer, providing greater satiety than proteins or carbohydrates. Small amounts of chyme are released from the stomach through the pyloric sphincter to allow for adequate digestion and absorption in the small intestine.

Very little absorption occurs in the stomach because few foods are completely hydrolyzed to nutrients the body can use at this stage. Nutrients that can be absorbed from the stomach include some water, alcohol, and a few water-soluble substances (e.g., amino acids and glucose).

Dental Considerations

- Dietary constituents that increase hydrochloric acid and pepsin secretions are proteins, calcium, caffeine, coffee, and alcohol. These may need to be limited in patients with ulcers or certain gastrointestinal tract disorders.
- Because gravity facilitates movement of food down the esophagus, patients who are in a supine position may have some difficulty swallowing and may reflux gastric contents, especially after eating. Aspiration of acid reflux into the lungs is possible. To prevent an emergency situation, place the patient in a semisupine position for treatment. If possible, schedule the appointment 3 hours after a meal to minimize reflux.

Nutritional Directions

- Vomiting is one of the body's methods of eliminating toxins from contaminated foods.
- Vomiting can also be stimulated by rapid changes in body motion or by drugs.
- Heartburn is a result of regurgitation (reflux) of the stomach contents into the esophagus. Acidic gastric secretions produce discomfort or pain, which may be relieved if the patient remains in an upright position after eating.
- Eating in a calm, relaxing atmosphere helps reduce gastric secretions.
- Over an extended period, chronic problems with vomiting or reflux can result in sensitive teeth and varying degrees of tooth erosion, especially on lingual and occlusal surfaces.

SMALL INTESTINE

Most of the energy-providing nutrients are completely hydrolyzed and absorbed within the small intestine. Most vitamins and minerals are also absorbed in the small intestine. The small intestine is specially designed to perform these tasks with juices secreted by the accessory organs and its complex luminal wall (Fig. 3-5). The small intestine is approximately 15 feet long, and foods are retained therein for 3 to 10 hours.

Digestion

Throughout the walls of the small intestine are villi, finger-like projections rising out of the mucosa into the intestinal lumen (see Fig. 3-2, B, C). These villi increase the surface area of the alimentary tract to approximately 3000 square feet. Each villus is also covered with a layer of epithelial cells containing microvilli, which collectively form the brush border cells. Microvilli are minute cylindrical processes located on the surface of intestinal cells, which greatly increase the intestinal absorptive surface area. The pH change and motility in the small intestine inhibit bacterial growth.

Acidic chyme entering the intestine stimulates hormones to release pancreatic juices into the duodenum. Cholecystokinin, a hormone released in response to the presence of fat in chyme, stimulates the gallbladder to contract and release bile. Bile is produced and secreted by the liver and is stored in the gallbladder. The action of bile salts allows insoluble molecules to be divided into smaller particles, a process called emulsification. This process allows greater exposure of fats to intestinal and pancreatic lipases. Peristalsis also facilitates mixing and the emulsification process by bile.

Pancreatic enzymes enter the duodenum through the pancreatic duct and function best in neutralized chyme. Pancreatic enzymes hydrolyze carbohydrates, proteins, and fats. Proteolytic enzymes, which hydrolyze proteins, are produced and stored in the pancreas in an inactive form.

Specific digestive enzymes lining the brush border of the microvilli are responsible for completing hydrolysis of carbohydrates, proteins, and fats. Not everything in foods can

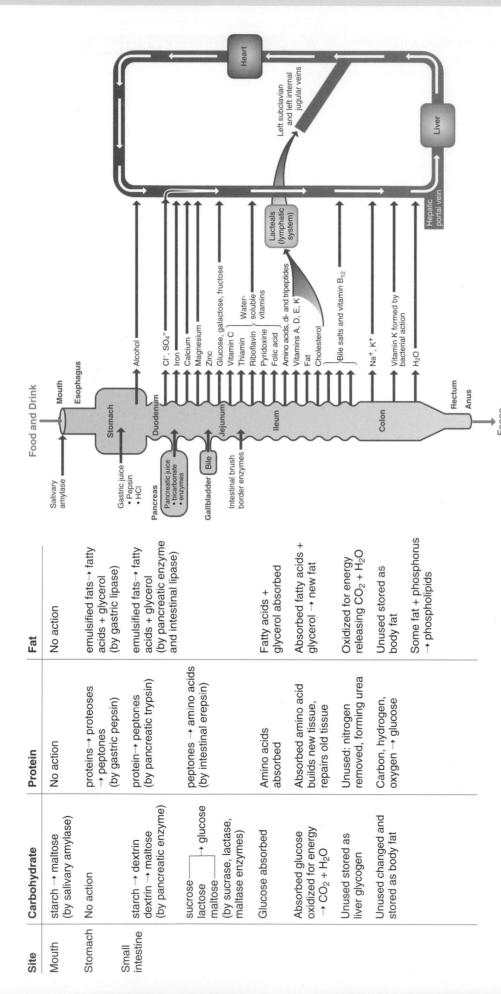

FIGURE 3-5 Digestive process of carbohydrate, protein, and fat. Cl⁻, chloride; CO_2, carbon dioxide; HCl, hydrochloric acid; H_2O, water; K⁺, potassium; Na⁺, sodium; SO_4, sulfate. (From Peckenpaugh NJ: *Nutrition essentials and diet therapy*, ed 11, Philadelphia, 2010, Saunders Elsevier. Modified from Mahan LK, et al: *Krause's food and the nutrition care process*, ed 13th, St Louis, 2012, Saunders Elsevier.)

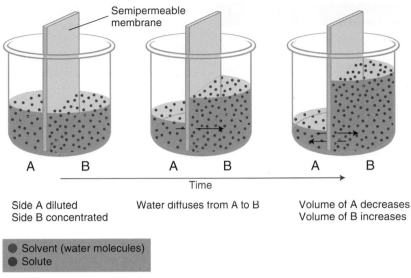

Semipermeable
membrane

Time

Side A diluted   Water diffuses from A to B   Volume of A decreases
Side B concentrated   Volume of B increases

● Solvent (water molecules)
● Solute

FIGURE 3-6 Osmotic pressure.

be completely digested. For example, the human body lacks enzymes that can digest cellulose, a carbohydrate found in plants. Other factors affecting digestion and absorption are as important to nutritional status as adequate intake, i.e., (a) amount of the nutrient consumed; (b) physiological need; (c) condition of the digestive tract, (the amount of secretions, motility, and absorptive surface); (d) level of circulating hormones; (e) presence of other nutrients or drugs ingested at the same time that enhance or interfere with absorption; and (f) presence of adequate amounts of digestive enzymes.

Absorption of Nutrients

Only after absorption of the nutrient into the intestinal mucosa is it considered to be "in" the body. Generally, absorption of nutrients occurs by passive diffusion or active transport mechanisms. Passive diffusion is the passage of a permeable substance from a more concentrated solution to an area of lower concentration. Active transport occurs when absorption is from a region of lower concentration to one of a higher concentration; this mechanism requires a carrier and cellular energy. Approximately 80% to 90% of fluid intake is absorbed in the small intestine by osmosis. **Osmosis** is the passage of water through a semipermeable membrane to equalize osmotic pressure exerted by ions in solutions (Fig. 3-6). Water moves freely in both directions across the intestinal mucosa. Absorbable nutrients pass through the microvilli and enter the portal vein if they are water soluble and through the lymphatic system if they are fat soluble.

Absorption Into Portal Circulation

Most nutrients (monosaccharides, amino acids, glycerol, water-soluble vitamins, minerals, and short- and medium-chain fatty acids) are absorbed through the mucosa of the small intestine into the **portal circulation** (absorption of nutrients from the gastrointestinal tract and spleen into the

bloodstream and through the portal vein to the liver). Metabolism of the nutrients then is initiated in the liver.

Absorption of Fat-Soluble Nutrients

The absorption process for long-chain fatty acids is complex because the molecules are large and insoluble. Long-chain fatty acids are broken apart to allow passage through the intestinal wall into the lymphatic system. The **lymphatic system** is comprised of lymph (plasmalike tissue fluid), the lymph nodes, and lymph vessels that are not connected to the blood system. Nutrients are carried through the thoracic duct and flow into the venous blood via the left subclavian vein. Absorption of the four fat-soluble vitamins—A, D, E, and K—is not as complex. Bile salts and lipases increase their water solubility so these vitamins are absorbed along with other fats in the lymphatic system.

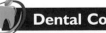

Dental Considerations

- An enzymatic deficiency in the gastrointestinal tract results in some nutrients not being digested, thus preventing their absorption. The most prevalent enzyme deficiency is lactase deficiency, which is discussed in Chapter 2, *Health Application 2: Lactose Intolerance.*
- Unless preventive care is taken, patients with large portions of the gastrointestinal tract removed, as in bariatric surgery, may develop nutritional deficiency symptoms because digestive secretions or absorptive areas are removed (see Fig. 3-5).
- If motility is increased, as in diarrhea, nutrients are not exposed to digestive secretions and absorptive surfaces long enough for maximum absorption. Severe or prolonged diarrhea may result in numerous deficiencies, the most rapid being a fluid deficit or dehydration.

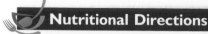

LARGE INTESTINE

Small amounts of chyme remaining in the ileum are released through the ileocecal valve into the cecum. Only about 5% of ingested foods and digestive secretions continue to the large intestine. For most adults, it takes 16 to 24 hours for foodstuffs to travel the full length of the gut.

Functions

The large intestine, so named because of its large diameter, has little or no digestive function. Its main functions are to reabsorb water and electrolytes (mainly sodium and potassium) and to form and store the residue (feces) until defecation. Residue in the intestinal tract is the total amount of fecal solids, including undigested or unabsorbed food, and metabolic (bile pigments) and bacterial products. Chyme entering the large intestine with 500 to 1000 mL of water is excreted as feces containing only 100 to 200 mL of fluid. Essentially, all absorption occurs in the proximal half of the colon.

The inner lining of the large intestine is smooth, lacking the numerous villi found in the small intestine. Its only important secretion is mucus, which protects the intestinal wall, aids in holding particles of fecal matter together, and helps to control the pH in the large intestine.

Undigested Residues

Fiber, obtained from fruits, vegetables, and whole-grain products, results in increased residue and has a water-holding capacity, contributing to bulkier feces. Dietary fiber is not digestible and works as a laxative. Foods may contain other substances that increase fecal output. One example is prune juice, which yields no residue on chemical digestion, but is classified as a high-residue food because it contains a laxative that indirectly increases volume of the stool. Residue

has a beneficial side effect of stimulating peristalsis, resulting in improved muscle tone.

Microflora

Because of decreased peristalsis and a neutral pH, more than a trillion harmless bacteria thrive in the colon. Humans have more bacteria in the body than human cells. The 400 different species of microorganisms living in the large intestine are called microflora. Microflora have several important roles: (a) breaking down substances that human enzymes are unable to digest; (b) synthesizing vitamins needed by humans (vitamin K, vitamin B_{12}, biotin, thiamin, and riboflavin); (c) boosting the immune system to improve protection against infection; and (d) inhibiting pathogenic (harmful) bacteria. Types of food and medications ingested influence the type, activity, and relative numbers of bacteria. An imbalance of intestinal flora can impact overall health. Bacterial activity produces various gases contributing to flatus (gas) in the colon. Fecal odor is a result of compounds produced by these bacteria.

Some dietary components are not classified as nutrients, but they are considered protective nutrients because of health benefits they provide. Probiotics are living microorganisms (usually bacteria) that confer a health benefit on the host when administered in adequate amounts. Scientists do not know exactly how probiotics work; they may produce anti-microbial substances that destroy harmful microorganisms. Microflora must be identified and demonstrated to have a beneficial effect in controlled studies to be called probiotics. There is no established recommended intake, but supplements generally contain 10 billion to 20 billion active cultures per dose.

Each probiotic strain is unique, and the properties and effects of each strain must be assessed individually (Table 3-2). A bacterium's name has three parts: the genus (e.g., *Lactobacillus*), the species (e.g., *Acidophilus*), and the strain (such as LA-5). Strains can differ in what they do even within the same species. Sound research studies support only a small number of probiotic strains because of difficulty in identifying the function of each strain.

Probiotic studies in the scientific literature have reported the following effects: improved digestive function; reduced risk/shortened duration of certain acute common infectious

Table 3-2	Probiotics and prebiotics	
Class/Component	**Source***	**Potential Benefit**
Probiotics		
Certain species and strains of *Lactobacillus, Bifidobacterium,* yeast	Certain yogurts, other cultured dairy products, and nondairy applications	May improve gastrointestinal health and systemic immunity
Prebiotics		
Inulin, fructooligosaccharides, polydextrose, arabinogalactan, Polyols—lactulose, lactitol	Whole grains, onions, bananas, garlic, honey, leeks, artichokes, fortified foods and beverages, dietary supplements, and other food applications	May improve gastrointestinal health; may improve calcium absorption

Adapted from International Food Information Council Foundation: *Media guide on food safety and nutrition: 2004-2006.* Accessed August 15, 2013: http://www.ific.org/publications/factsheets/preprobioticsfs.cfm.
*Examples are not all-inclusive.

diseases; enhanced immune function; prevented and treated antibiotic-associated diarrhea and traveler's diarrhea; and improved tolerance to lactose.[7-10] Antibiotic treatment frequently disturbs gastrointestinal flora, sometimes resulting in *Clostridium difficile*-associated diarrhea. Scientific research indicates that probiotic treatment is effective in reducing in *C. difficile*–associated diarrhea.[11] Limited studies have reported that certain probiotics can help prevent allergies in children, decrease *Helicobacter pylori* colonization (a cause of ulcers) in the stomach, prevent recurrence of some inflammatory bowel conditions, and help in controlling oral yeast infections.[12] *Lactobacillus acidophilus* and *Bifidobacterium bifidus*, found in some yogurts and other fermented dairy products, have been shown to help prevent pathogenic bacteria from proliferating and healthy bacteria from becoming toxic.

Probiotics are considered food or dietary supplements in the United States. Probiotics are found in fermented dairy products, such as kefir, yogurt, and cheeses. New products have been introduced with probiotics added to bread, orange juice, infant formula, cereal, cookies and even chewing gum. Pasteurization can kill the bacteria. Probiotics are available in various forms, including capsules, powders, creams, and suppositories. Commercial products are generally safe with few side effects, relatively inexpensive, and readily available.

The U.S. government does not test the quality of probiotics or require companies to scientifically demonstrate health benefits before labeling the product as containing beneficial probiotics. With lax labeling regulations, it is difficult to know which products have proven health benefits and whether they contain what the label indicates. Not all probiotic products on the market meet the minimum criteria established for probiotics. These products do not usually disclose the levels or strain designations of added bacteria, so consumers do not know if the product has been shown to be efficacious for specific effects. Quality issues include (a) viability of organisms, (b) presence of contamination organisms, (c) protection of organisms from stomach acid, and (d) ability of a pill to properly break apart to release their ingredients.[13]

Research is expanding reliable knowledge and understanding of probiotics. Scientific research must continue to be interpreted cautiously, but evidence on the health benefits of probiotics continues to accumulate. Unfortunately, many products may have health benefits that have not been validated.

Prebiotics are nondigestible food ingredients that have beneficial effects on the host by selectively stimulating growth or activity, or both, of beneficial colonic microorganisms. Fiber, particularly fermentable fiber, is crucial for good health. Prebiotics are specialized ingredients that influence specific bacteria, their fermentation end products, and possible health effects on the host. Prebiotics increase mineral absorption (especially calcium and magnesium) from the foods containing them.

Prebiotics pass into the large intestine intact where they stimulate growth and activity of healthy bacteria; in contrast, probiotics influence the types of bacteria present. Simply put, prebiotics are food for probiotics. Probiotics together with prebiotics that support their growth are called symbiotics because they cooperatively promote probiotic benefits more efficiently. The benefits associated with probiotics are strain-specific and benefits of prebiotics are substance-specific.

Peristalsis

The purpose of peristalsis in the large intestine is to force feces into the rectum. These large waves occur only two to three times daily.

Constipation is a common problem for many people. The National Institute of Diabetes and Digestive and Kidney Diseases of the National Institutes of Health defines constipation as having a bowel movement fewer than three times per week with hard, dry, small, and difficult-to-pass stools.[14]

Dental Considerations

- Bowel habits, stress, exercise, and nutritional intake (especially the amount of fiber and fluid intake) affect gastrointestinal transit rate.
- Lengthy retention of feces in the large intestine allows more reabsorption of water, causing the feces to become hard and dry and leading to constipation.
- For most patients, microbes in probiotics are beneficial, but should be consumed in moderation. However, patients who have a poor immune response should consult a healthcare provider or RDN before using probiotics.
- Probiotics may be beneficial to treat traveler's diarrhea, prevent and treat urinary tract infections, irritable bowel disease, and other conditions.
- Specific probiotic strains have different biological activities and provide a variety of health benefits.
- Many patients may have symptoms of a chronic digestive problem, such as heartburn, abdominal pain, constipation, diarrhea, and gastroesophageal reflux disease. Some of these problems can be addressed with dietary or lifestyle changes.
- Antibiotic therapy normally kills bacteria in the colon and inhibits bacterial production of vitamins. Patients on long-term antibiotic therapy may develop vitamin K, vitamin B_{12}, and biotin deficiencies.

Nutritional Directions

- Constipation can be treated by increasing fluid intake or by gradually increasing nondigestible food components (fiber) in the diet, or both.
- Activity also affects gastrointestinal mobility. Active individuals who routinely choose high-fiber foods and drink adequate amounts of liquids are less likely to become constipated than sedentary people.
- The frequency of bowel movements varies from after each meal to once every 2 days.
- Probiotics as a dietary supplement may be beneficial in providing high levels of bacteria if the products are responsibly formulated and stored properly. These products should be purchased only from reputable companies and should contain the United States Pharmacopeia (USP) or the National Formulary (NF) symbol on their packaging.
- The presence of higher levels of bifidobacteria in the intestines of breastfed infants may be a reason why they are generally healthier than formula-fed infants.
- A probiotic should be able to survive and establish itself in the intestinal environment.

HEALTH APPLICATION 3   Gluten-Related Disorders

In 2012, in response to an insurgence of gluten-free products, a panel of 15 international experts recognized that gluten reactions are not limited to celiac disease. Three conditions related to the ingestion of gluten have become a concern: (a) an autoimmune disorder (celiac disease); (b) allergic reactions (wheat allergy), and (c) immune-mediated disorder (non-celiac gluten sensitivity or gluten sensitivity).[15] Although celiac disease, wheat allergy, and gluten sensitivity may be treated with similar diets, they are not the same condition. **Gluten** is a structural protein component of these grains: wheat, rye, barley, and triticale (cross-bred hybrid of wheat and rye). Gluten-containing grains were introduced into the human diet approximately 10,000 years ago with the advent of agriculture.

Celiac disease is an **autoimmune disorder** (condition that causes the body to form antibodies to one's own tissues) caused by a permanent sensitivity to gluten in genetically-susceptible individuals. If the condition is not diagnosed and treated, microvilli in the small intestine are damaged, ultimately impairing absorption of nutrients. Microvilli normally allow nutrients from food to be absorbed from the small intestine into the bloodstream. **Wheat allergy** is another adverse immunological reaction specific to wheat proteins. **Gluten sensitivity** involves neither allergic nor autoimmune mechanisms. Gluten-sensitive patients are unable to tolerate gluten and may develop gastrointestinal symptoms, but the overall clinical picture is generally less severe and the small intestine is not impaired.

Celiac disease is more common in countries predominantly populated by people of European origin, affecting approximately 1% of the U.S. population (about 3 million Americans). Less than 10% of the cases have been diagnosed. Recent studies indicate a rising prevalence of celiac disease during the last several decades.[16] More Americans may have gluten sensitivity than celiac disease.

For most individuals with celiac disease, fatigue is a major symptom. Other common signs and symptoms of the disease include diarrhea, abdominal pain, bloating, lactose intolerance, headaches, joint pain, skin rashes, depression, and short stature. A blistering rash, known as dermatitis herpetiformis, may be seen in patients with asymptomatic celiac disease. Without treatment, poor absorption of iron, folate, calcium, vitamin D, and other nutrients may result in anemia and osteoporosis. Other long-term serious health complications are neurological conditions; malignancies and lymphoid neoplasms; and squamous cell carcinoma of the mouth, oropharynx, and esophagus.

In the oral cavity, enamel defects and recurrent aphthous stomatitis are the most common symptoms.[17] Antibodies generated against gluten can react with a major protein enamel, causing enamel defects in developing teeth.[18] Eruption of teeth in children with celiac disease is delayed.[19] People with celiac disease must permanently exclude gluten to avoid long-term adverse consequences of this life-long chronic condition. The only course of treatment is a strict gluten-free diet.

Diagnosis of celiac disease begins with a blood test for specific antibodies. If this test is positive, the standard for diagnosis is a biopsy of the small intestine, unless the person is following a gluten-free diet. If the individual has been following a gluten-free diet prior to a biopsy, the lining of the small intestine will not show damage, so a definite diagnosis is very difficult.

The diagnosis of gluten sensitivity is made after celiac disease and wheat allergy have been excluded using gluten elimination or reduction. Gluten sensitivity can be unpleasant, but it is not harmful to long-term health; the overall clinical picture is less severe for those without concurrent autoimmune disease. Symptoms of gluten sensitivity include abdominal pain, eczema, headache, foggy mind, fatigue, diarrhea, depression, anemia, numbness in the extremities, and joint pain. Testing for wheat allergy includes a skin prick test to wheat.

For people who suspect they have gluten sensitivity, a diagnosis to rule out celiac disease is preeminent before initiating a gluten-free diet to obtain a valid diagnosis. A gluten-free diet should be the last resort when gluten sensitivity is suspected. If testing for celiac disease is negative, the individual should try a gluten-free diet for at least a week, but no longer than a month, to determine if symptoms are alleviated.

Many Americans who suffer from irritable bowel syndrome are probably sensitive to gluten and may benefit from a gluten-free diet. Patients with wheat allergy may also benefit from a gluten-free diet, but strict adherence may be less important. Experts have not determined how strictly or for how long the diet should be followed or what complications may arise by following it.

A gluten-free diet can initially be an overwhelming undertaking. Gluten is a thickener; many processed foods use gluten-containing grains, additives, or preservatives. Gluten is not only in food products, but beer, cosmetics, and postage stamps also contain gluten. All fresh fruits and vegetables, dairy products, and fresh meats—beef, chicken, fish, lamb, pork, are naturally gluten-free. The gluten-free diet can be well-balanced if foods are chosen wisely, (e.g., more legumes and foods with lower energy density). Consumption of more fruits and vegetables, gluten-free whole grains, nuts, and seeds can help improve the nutritional value. Recent evidence suggests that a gluten-free diet may lead to reductions in beneficial gut bacteria.[20] Probiotics can be especially helpful to increase gut bacteria and reduce symptoms of digestive irritation. Dietary fiber from whole foods, gluten-free sources (chia seeds, ground flaxseeds, rice bran, fruit and vegetables) help strengthen and soothe the gastrointestinal tract.

Many gluten-free foods are not fortified or enriched. Nutrients added in enrichment are lacking in whole grain cereals. The diet may be lacking iron, calcium, fiber, thiamin, riboflavin, niacin, folate, and vitamin D. Evidence strongly suggests that if patients are left on their own, a variety of macro- and micronutrient deficiencies can develop. Gluten-free products may become healthier overall as manufacturers develop ways to fortify them. Extra sugar and fat are added to simulate the texture and fluffiness that gluten imparts, making many gluten-free products higher in fat and sugar than other products.

New gluten-free products are introduced on the market almost daily. Food manufacturers are labeling foods "gluten-free" that are naturally free of gluten. In 2013, the U.S. Food and Drug Administration (FDA) published a regulation for voluntary labeling of "gluten free" foods. Foods bearing that label cannot contain more than 20 parts per million (ppm) of gluten. (Lower amounts could not be reliably detected).

In celiac disease, even gluten-containing crumbs can damage the intestinal mucosa. Certain grains, such as oats, can

<u>HEALTH APPLICATION</u> **3**   **Gluten-Related Disorders—cont'd**

be contaminated with wheat during growing and processing. Wheat flour can remain airborne for hours (especially in bakeries) and contaminate exposed preparation surfaces and utensils or uncovered gluten-free products such as fruits. Cross-contamination can also occur at home if foods are prepared on common surfaces or with appliances or utensils that are not thoroughly cleaned after being used to prepare gluten-containing foods, e.g., toaster, microwave, or flour sifter.

A large percentage of Americans are currently on a "gluten free" craze, following a gluten-free diet, either believing it is healthier or may help with weight loss. When patients with celiac disease go on a gluten-free diet, some gain, some lose, but for most, weights remain the same.[21-23] There is nothing inherently healthy about a gluten-free diet, and no evidence indicates that gluten is harmful to healthy people without a gluten-related disorder.

For most individuals, wheat gluten may impart some healthy benefits: (a) lower blood lipids and reduced risk of CHD; (b) lower blood pressure; (c) improved immune system; (d) healthier composition of colonic bacteria; and (e) protection from some cancers. Because gluten-free flours, such as rice flour and cornstarch, typically cause a higher rise in blood sugars compared to wheat-based flours, a gluten-free diet may exacerbate insulin resistance, weight gain, and glucose intolerance. A gluten-free diet may adversely affect gut health in those without celiac disease or gluten sensitivity. A gluten-free diet is necessary for those with celiac disease or gluten intolerance, but may not be healthy for people without those conditions.[24]

Case Application for the Dental Hygienist

Mr. A complains that he can hardly talk because his mouth is dry and sticky. Sores in his mouth make his dentures very uncomfortable. He states he does not leave his home often because he is unable to easily find liquids to prevent his tongue from sticking to the sides and roof of his mouth. He also complains that eating is difficult. Mr. A reports his healthcare provider prescribed a diuretic for his hypertension.

Nutritional Assessment
- Recent change in weight
- Dietary intake
- Preferred fluids, frequency of intake
- Food preparation techniques
- Medications taken
- Oral examination to determine the condition of the underlying tissues
- Fit of dentures
- Willingness to learn and to change habits

Nutritional Diagnosis
Knowledge deficit of the effects of diuretics on hydration of the body related to lack of information and understanding.

Nutritional Goals
The patient will continue taking the diuretic. His nutrient intake will improve to prevent further weight loss, and his fluid intake will increase to 8 to 10 glasses of fluid a day.

Nutritional Implementation
Intervention: Discuss the importance of adequate salivary flow for maintenance of soft tissues, taste functions, and teeth. If indicated and desired, suggest products designed to relieve xerostomia to provide temporary comfort as needed.
Rationale: Xerostomia has severe deleterious effects on a patient's ability to talk and on integrity of oral tissues.

Intervention: Review the importance of meticulous oral hygiene and periodically removing dentures.
Rationale: Xerostomia promotes plaque formation, which can lead to further gingival irritations for this patient. Removal of dentures allows underlying tissue to become healthy again.
Intervention: Discuss that although diuretics may cause this condition, they are important for his health.
Rationale: To prevent other health problems, Mr. A must continue the medication as prescribed by his healthcare provider.
Intervention: Discuss ways he can increase his fluid intake to 8 to 10 glasses daily: (a) drink more fluid with meals; (b) carry fluids with him in a large covered thermal container.
Rationale: To replace fluids excreted because of the diuretic, adequate fluid intake is essential.
Intervention: Encourage increased intake of nutrient-dense liquid or semiliquid foods, such as milkshakes, cream soups, gravies, and sauces.
Rationale: These foods contain larger proportions of nutrients, which will help Mr. A to consume adequate amounts of nutrients and will prevent weight loss.
Intervention: Recommend tips to relieve the dryness in his mouth, such as sugar-free mints and gum containing xylitol or ice chips.
Rationale: The patient's comfort will be enhanced if his mouth is moist; oral complications associated with xerostomia will be minimized. Use of chewing gum or mints containing xylitol will stimulate salivary flow, reduce caries-causing bacteria, and assist with remineralization of any early carious lesions.

Evaluation
If the patient continues to take the prescribed diuretic, consumes a well-balanced diet, increases fluid intake, uses correct oral hygiene practices, maintains body weight, and can state why he was having all these problems, dental hygiene care was effective.

STUDENT READINESS

1. Chart or diagram the gastrointestinal secretions, where they are produced, and their digestive actions on nutrients present in milk. Homogenized milk contains the following: lactose (a disaccharide), proteins, emulsified fats, calcium, riboflavin, and vitamins A and D. Where are the end products absorbed?

2. Define alimentary canal, hydrolysis, enzyme, and residue.

3. A patient has problems secreting too much hydrochloric acid. What types of food would you recommend a patient to avoid?

4. Cut a small hole (1 mm in diameter) in a piece of paper. Place the tip of your tongue through the hole. Looking in the mirror, count the number of taste buds. Compare your findings with other classmates of varying ages. Observe the number of taste buds on adolescent and older patients.

5. If caloric intake were equal, which of the following breakfasts would probably delay feelings of hunger longest? Explain your reason.
   a. Dry cereal with skim milk, toast with jelly, and coffee with sugar.
   b. Egg with ham, toast with butter, and coffee with cream.

6. What are absorbable products resulting from digestion of carbohydrates, proteins, and fats?

7. Within what section of the alimentary canal does most digestion and absorption take place?

8. Considering secretions and the functions of the gastrointestinal tract, discuss the fallacy of diets that claim only one type of food (e.g., fruits) should be eaten at a given time.

9. Could constipation be called a nutrient deficiency? Defend your answer.

10. What types of problems might be encountered when a patient does not chew his or her food well? Discuss dental issues that can lead to decreased ability to masticate food.

11. View http://www.foodinsight.org/Resources/Detail.aspx?topic=Foods_for_Health_Eating_for_Digestive_Health. Summarize the information from the video. What information can you personally use?

CASE STUDY

A 22-year-old Asian woman reports a history of lactose intolerance. She is concerned about her calcium intake because she has eliminated all dairy products from her diet.

1. What should be included in dietary recommendations made by the dental hygienist?
2. Can this patient consume dairy products?
3. Which dairy products are best tolerated by lactose-deficient individuals?
4. When should lactase tablets be taken?
5. What symptoms may the patient report that are associated with lactose intake?
6. Why should she include dairy products?

References

1. Kalogjera L, Dzepina D: Management of smell dysfunction. *Curr Allergy Asthma Rep* 2012 (Epub ahead of print).
2. Rombaux P, Martinage S, Huart C, et al: Post-infectious olfactory loss: a cohort study and update. *B-ENT* 5(Suppl 13):89–95, 2009.
3. Jääskeläinen SK: Pathophysiology of burning mouth syndrome. *Clin Neurophysiol* 127(1):71–77, 2012.
4. Mandel AL, Peyrot des Gachons C, Plank KL, et al: Individual differences in AMY1 gene copy number salivary a-amylase levels and the perception of oral starch. *PLoS ONE* 5(10):e13352, 2010.
5. Hutton JL, Baracos VE, Wismer WV: Chemosensory dysfunction is a primary factor in the evolution of declining nutritional status and quality of life in patients with advanced cancer. *J Pain Symptom Manage* 33(2):156–165, 2007.
6. Gruner T, Arthur R: The accuracy of the zinc taste test method. *J Altern Complement Med* 18(6):541–550, 2012.
7. Allen SJ, Martinez EG, Gregorio GV, et al: Probiotics for treating acute infectious diarrhea. *Cochrane Database Syst Rev* (2):CD003048, 2004.
8. Bernaola Aponte G, Bada Mancilla CA, Carreazo Pariasca NY, et al: Probiotics for treating persistent diarrhoea in children. *Cochrane Database Syst Rev* (11):CD007401, 2010.
9. Upadhyay N, Moudgal V: Probiotics: a review. *J Clin Outcomes Manag* 19(2):74–86, 2012.
10. Hempel S, Newberry SJ, Maher AR, et al: Probiotics for the prevention and treatment of antibiotic-associated diarrhea: a systematic review and meta-analysis. *JAMA* 307(18):1959–1969, 2012.
11. Johnston BC, Ma SS, Goldenberg JZ, et al: Probiotics for the prevention of *Clostridium difficile*-associated diarrhea: A systematic review and meta-analysis. *Ann Intern Med* 157(12):878–888, 2012.
12. Hatakka K, Ahola AJ, Yli-Knuuttila H, et al: Probiotics reduce the prevalence of oral candida in the elderly—a randomized controlled trial. *J Dent Res* 86(2):125–130, 2007.
13. Consumer Lab: *Product review: probiotics for adults, children and pets*. Initial posting: February 7, 2012. Accessed August 15, 2013: https://www.consumerlab.com/reviews/Probiotic_Supplements_Lactobacillus_acidophilus_Bifidobacterium/probiotics/.
14. National Institutes of Health, National Digestive Diseases Information Clearinghouse (NDDIC): *Constipation*. Accessed August 15, 2013: digestive.niddk.nih.gov/ddiseases/pubs/constipation/index.aspx.
15. Sapone A, Bai JC, Ciacci C, et al: Spectrum of gluten-related disorders: consensus on new nomenclature and classification. *BMC Med* 10:13, 2012.
16. Rubio-Tapia A, Ludvigsson JF, Brantner TL, et al: The prevalence of celiac disease in the United States. *Am J Gastroenterol* 107(10):1538–1544, 2012.
17. Shteyer E, Berson T, Lachmanovitz O, et al: Oral health status and salivary properties in relation to gluten free diet in children with celiac disease. *J Pediatr Gastroenterol Nutr* 57(1):49–52, 2013.
18. Muñoz F, Del Río N, Sóñora C, et al: Enamel defects associated with coeliac disease: putative role of antibodies against gliadin in pathogenesis. *Eur J Oral Sci* 120(2):104–112, 2012.
19. Cond R, Costacurta M, Maturo P, et al: The dental age in the child with celiac disease. *Eur J Paediatr Dent* 12(3):184–188, 2011.
20. Gaesser GA, Angadi SS: Gluten-free diet: imprudent dietary advice for the general population? *J Acad Nutr Diet* 112(9):1330–1333, 2012.
21. Ukkola A, Mäki M, Kurppa K, et al: Changes in body mass index on a gluten-free diet in coeliac disease. a nationwide study. *Eur J Intern Med* 23(4):384–388, 2012.

22. Valletta E, Fornaro M, Cipolli M, et al: Celiac disease and obesity: need for nutritional follow-up after diagnosis. *Eur J Clin Nutr* 64(11):1371–1372, 2010.

23. Cheng J, Brar PS, Lee AR, et al: Body mass index in celiac disease: beneficial effect of a gluten-free diet. *J Clin Gastroenterol* 44(4):267–271, 2010.

24. Gaesser GA, Angadi SS: Gluten-free diet: imprudent dietary advice for the general population? *J Acad Nutr Diet* 112(9):1330–1333, 2012.

EVOLVE RESOURCES

Please visit http://evolve.elsevier.com/Stegeman/nutritional for additional practice and study support tools.

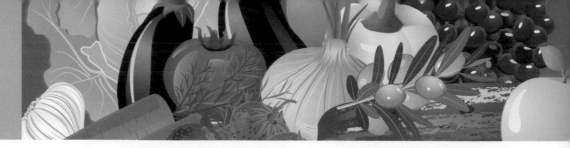

Chapter 4

Carbohydrate: The Efficient Fuel

Student Learning Outcomes

Upon completion of this chapter, the student will be able to achieve the following student learning outcomes:

- Identify major carbohydrates in foods and in the body.
- Outline ways glucose can be used by the body.
- Summarize the functions of dietary carbohydrates.
- Explain the importance of dietary carbohydrates.
- Identify dietary sources of lactose, other sugars, and starches.
- Summarize the role and sources of dietary fiber.
- Describe the role of carbohydrates in the caries process.
- Formulate recommendations for patients concerning carbohydrate consumption to reduce risk for dental caries.

Key Terms

Added sugars
Anticariogenic
Cariogenic
Cariostatic
Complex carbohydrates
Dental erosion
Dextrins
Dietary fiber
Evidence Analysis Library
Fermentable carbohydrate
Functional fiber
Hyperglycemia
Hypoglycemia
Ketones

Ketosis
Lipogenesis
Nondigestible
Nutrient density
Phenylketonuria
Plaque biofilm
Polyols
Resistant starch
Streptococcus mutans (S. mutans)
Sugar alcohols
Synergistic
Total fiber
Viscous fiber

Test Your NQ

1. **T/F** Raw sugar is nutritionally superior to white sugar.
2. **T/F** Fructose is the principal carbohydrate in honey.
3. **T/F** All caloric sugars can be metabolized by plaque biofilm.
4. **T/F** The desire for sweetness in the diet is an acquired taste.
5. **T/F** Fiber tends to regulate the rate of foods passing through the gastrointestinal tract.
6. **T/F** Carbohydrates are absorbed as monosaccharides.
7. **T/F** Excessive consumption of carbohydrates is the main cause of obesity.
8. **T/F** Glucose is the same as table sugar.
9. **T/F** Eliminating sucrose from the diet prevents development of dental caries.
10. **T/F** Natural sugars in foods can be just as cariogenic as added sugars.

Carbohydrates have been the major source of energy for people since the dawn of history. Worldwide, carbohydrates are the most important source of energy, furnishing 80% to 90% of kilocalories for some African and Asian nations. Nutrition experts from many countries recommend that carbohydrates should represent 50% of total energy intake,[1] yet only 40% to 50% of the American diet is from carbohydrates.[2] Carbohydrate foods add variety and palatability to the diet and are the most economical form of energy.

As discussed in Chapter 2, carbohydrates contain carbon, hydrogen, and oxygen. During photosynthesis, carbon dioxide and water result in formation of carbohydrates and the release of oxygen. Because glucose and other carbohydrates are essentially hydrogen (and oxygen) atoms bound to a carbon backbone, a carbohydrate could also be referred to as a "hydrated carbon." The popular belief that carbohydrates have some mysterious "fattening" power is unfounded. During the 1950s, carbohydrates acquired a bad reputation in the United States as best-selling books claimed Americans were victims of "carbohydrate poisoning." More recently, critics have labeled sugar as "toxic" and "addictive." Naturally, these unscientific statements affect food consumption patterns. Resurgence of the popular low-carbohydrate, high-protein, weight-reduction diets have caused the pendulum to again swing away from choosing carbohydrate foods. Many of these diets are nutritionally unbalanced, providing inadequate amounts of nutrients known to help protect against several chronic diseases.

As can be seen in Fig. 4-1, carbohydrate intake has fluctuated more than intake of any other macronutrient. In 1977, the U.S. Senate Select Committee on Nutrition and Human Needs released *Dietary Goals for the United States*, advising Americans of reduced risk of various chronic diseases by consuming more complex carbohydrates (fruits, vegetables, legumes, and whole-grain products). Food supply data indicate that 49% of total kilocalories come from carbohydrates for men, and 51.6% for women. Americans consume less than eight servings of grain products daily and less than one serving of whole grains.[3] Even if people are consuming an adequate number of servings from the whole grains and refined grains group, the types of foods chosen need to be adjusted to improve fiber intake and decrease added sugars (sugars added to foods during processing or at the table). Because most high-carbohydrate food choices are regular sodas, cakes, cookies, pastries, and pies, intake of fat and sugar is detrimentally affected. Mean intakes of caloric sweeteners decreased from 100.1 g per day in 1999-2000 to 76.7 g per day in 2007-2008.[4]

Misconceptions surrounding the intake of sugars are: (a) sugar is the cause of tooth decay, (b) food with a high sugar concentration is more dangerous to the teeth, and (c) avoidance of sticky sweets prevents tooth decay. The incidence of caries has decreased in industrialized countries with water fluoridation despite increased sugar consumption. Approximately 90% of all snack foods contain fermentable carbohydrates (i.e., carbohydrates that can be metabolized by bacteria in plaque biofilm, including all sugars and cooked or processed starches). The presence of sucrose and other carbohydrates in the mouth increases the volume and formation rate of plaque biofilm. Even low amounts of sucrose promote production of polysaccharides (glucans) by *Streptococcus mutans (S. Mutans)*, the bacteria that facilitate adherence of plaque biofilm to teeth. These glucans help provide a matrix, supporting communities of microorganisms collectively referred to as plaque biofilm. All dental practitioners must be knowledgeable about the effect of carbohydrates on soft and hard tissues in the oral cavity, and about chronic health problems caused by low-carbohydrate, high-fat diets. Dental professionals need to be able to educate patients about ways to modify carbohydrate consumption and intake patterns that are consistent with overall good health.

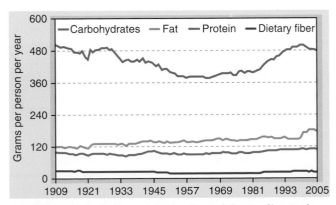

FIGURE 4-1 Carbohydrates, protein, fat, and dietary fiber in the U.S. food supply. Note carbohydrate intake fluctuation over time. (Data compiled by Economic Research Service using data from U.S. Department of Agriculture, Center for Nutrition Policy and Promotion.)

CLASSIFICATION

Chapter 2 and the Evolve website provide detailed biochemistry information regarding carbohydrates, including their structure and metabolism. Generally, the chemical components of carbohydrates are in these proportions: $C_n(H_2O)_n$. An empirical formula such as $C_6H_{12}O_6$ or $C_{12}H_{22}O_{11}$ can readily be identified as a carbohydrate. The number of carbon atoms in the molecule is used to classify carbohydrates. Monosaccharides are simple sugars containing two to six carbon atoms. Disaccharides are composed of two simple sugars joined together and contain 12 carbon atoms. Polysaccharides are complex carbohydrates containing a minimum of 10 units of various simple sugars.

Monosaccharides and disaccharides contribute to the palatability of a food because of their sweetness. Temperature, pH, and the presence of other substances influence the sweetness of a food. Relative sweetness of sugars is measured by subjective sensory tasting; sucrose is used as the standard of comparison (Table 4-1).

Monosaccharides

The simplest carbohydrates, monosaccharides, are absorbed without further digestion. The monosaccharides of greatest significance in foods and body metabolism are glucose, fructose, and galactose. Chapter 2, Fig. 2-3 identifies slight differences between these three six-carbon sugars and glucose.

Glucose

Also called dextrose or corn sugar, glucose is naturally abundant in many fruits, such as grapes, oranges, and dates, and in some vegetables, including fresh corn. It is prepared commercially as corn syrup or by special processing of starch. Glucose is the principal product formed by the digestion of disaccharides and polysaccharides. It provides energy for cells via the bloodstream. Glucose is the only sugar transported through the bloodstream that can nourish all cells in the body.

Fructose

Fructose, also known as levulose, is found naturally in honey and fruits. It is the sweetest of the monosaccharides and is a product of the digestion of sucrose. Fructose can be manufactured from glucose.

Table 4-1	Sugars and sweeteners: caloric value, relative sweetness, and cariogenicity		
Sugar or Sweetener	**Kcal/g**	**Relative Sweetness***	**Relative Cariogenicity***
Fructose	4	173	80-100
Honey (fructose and glucose)	3	130	100
Sucrose	4	100	100
Molasses (sucrose and invert sugar)	2.4	100	100
Brown sugar (sugar and molasses)	3.8	100	100
Dextrose/glucose (corn syrup)	4	74	‡N/A
Galactose	4	60	‡N/A
Maltose	4	50	‡N/A
Lactose	4	16	40-60
Reduced-Calorie Sweeteners††			
Xylitol	2.4	100	
Tagatose	1.5	92	0
Maltitol	2.1	90	0
Erythritol	0.2	70	0
Sorbitol	2.6	60	0
Mannitol	1.6	50	0
Hydrogenated starch hydrolysates	2.4	40-90	0
Isomalt	2	45-65‡‡	0
Trehalose	4	45	0
Lactitol	2	40	0
Nonnutritive Sweeteners††			
Acesulfame K	0	200	0
Aspartame	0	200	0
Cyclamate***	0	30	0
Dihydrochalcones†††	0	1500	Unknown
Lu han guo (monk fruit)	0	200	0
Neotame	0	7000-13,000	0
Rebaudioside A (Truvia, Stevia)	0	250-300	0
Saccharin	0	300	0
Sucralose	0	600	0
Thaumatin (Talin)***	0	2000-3000	Unknown

*Relative to sucrose (= 100).
‡Information not available.
††Data from Calorie Control Council, Copyright © 2012 Calorie Control Council. Accessed August 16, 2013: http://www.caloriecontrol.org/.
‡‡Accessed August 16, 2013: http://toxnet.nlm.nih.gov/cgi-bin/sis/search/a?dbs+hsdb:@term+@DOCNO+7969
***Not approved for use in the United States; approved for use in the European Union and Zimbabwe.
†††Not approved for use in the United States; approved for use in Canada, European Union, and more than 100 other countries.

Galactose

Galactose, another six-carbon sugar, is a product of lactose digestion (milk sugar). Galactose is rarely found free in nature. Physiologically, it is a constituent of nerve tissue and is produced from glucose during lactation.

Sugar Alcohols

Sugar alcohols, also called polyols, are formed from or converted to sugar. Sugar alcohols may appear naturally in foods or be added by a manufacturer. The most common polyols include sorbitol, xylitol, and mannitol.

For a given quantity, tagatose and xylitol add about the same amount of sweetness as glucose but furnish fewer kilocalories. Incomplete absorption of sugar alcohols produces a laxative effect—soft stools or diarrhea—by causing an osmotic transfer of water into the gastrointestinal tract. Advantages of sugar alcohols are that they do not cause sudden increases in blood glucose levels, and they do not contribute to tooth decay.

The benefit of sorbitol is that it is absorbed and metabolized more slowly than sucrose. Sorbitol, the most commonly used sugar alcohol, is the least expensive. Mannose is a six-carbon sugar found in some legumes. Mannitol, derived from mannose, is found in foods. Xylitol is a sweetener with approximately the same perceived sweetness and 40% less kilocalories than sugar. It is found in fruits and vegetables (lettuce, carrots, and strawberries). As a food additive, it is more expensive than other sugar alcohols, but has no aftertaste.

Disaccharides

Intact disaccharides cannot be metabolized by the body, but they contribute to body functions after they have been digested. All are hydrolyzed during digestion to their constituent monosaccharides for absorption.

Sucrose

Granulated table sugar is the most common form of sucrose, which is a combination of one molecule of glucose and one molecule of fructose, as shown in Chapter 2, Fig. 2-5. Commercially, sucrose is produced from sugar cane or sugar beets (not to be confused with red beets). It is also found in molasses, maple syrup, and maple sugar. Some fruits (apricots, peaches, plums, raspberries, honeydew, cantaloupe) and vegetables (beets, carrots, parsnips, winter squash, peas, corn, sweet potatoes) naturally contain varying amounts of sucrose.

Lactose

The sugar found in milk is lactose. Lactose, which contains galactose and glucose (see Chapter 2, Fig. 2-5) is unique to mammalian milk. In the fermentation of milk, some of the lactose is converted to lactic acid, giving buttermilk and yogurt their characteristic flavors.

Maltose

Maltose, shown in Chapter 2, Fig. 2-4, contains two molecules of glucose. Also called *malt sugar,* maltose does not occur naturally. It is created in bread making and brewing beer and is present in some processed cereals and baby foods.

Dental Considerations

- Assess patients with an increased risk of dental caries for frequency of sugar intake, including sources of natural and added sugars.
- Newborns exhibit a preference for sweetness, so it is not considered an acquired taste. Although infants and young children typically select the most intensely sweet tastes, the pleasure response to sweet taste is observed across individuals of all ages, races, and cultures.[5]
- A judgmental attitude or criticism by the dental hygienist is not beneficial in modifying a patient's use of carbohydrates or sugars.

Nutritional Directions

- All caloric sugars and starches, whether they are naturally occurring in foods or added to foods, have some cariogenic effect.
- Sugar alcohols are not fermented alcohols and do not need to be restricted by individuals suffering with alcoholism.
- All disaccharides contain the same caloric and nutrient content. The body cannot distinguish between natural honey, refined table sugar, or high-fructose corn syrup (see *Health Application 4*); all are absorbed and metabolized in the same manner as their component sugars.
- Encourage use of hard candies and chewing gum containing sugar alcohols (xylitol and sorbitol) to prevent caries. However, inform patients that using more than three to four pieces of sugar alcohol–containing items daily may cause gastrointestinal distress.

Polysaccharides or Complex Carbohydrates

Complex carbohydrates, also called polysaccharides, contain more than 10 monosaccharides (see Chapter 2, Fig. 2-7). Some polysaccharides have a role in energy storage and are digestible. Dietary fiber is largely indigestible by intestinal enzymes in humans.

Starch

Starches are composed of many glucose units that may be in long chains or branched. Most food sources of complex carbohydrates are in the form of starch from cereal grains, roots, vegetables, and legumes. The amount of starch present in a vegetable increases with its maturity. For example, corn tastes much sweeter immediately after it is picked than it does several days later because the simple sugars in corn have not developed into starch. In contrast, the amount of starch in fruit decreases as it ripens—that is, complex carbohydrates are broken down during the ripening process into simple sugars. In digestion, complex carbohydrates are broken down into dextrin molecules until the end product, glucose, is absorbed (Fig. 4-2).

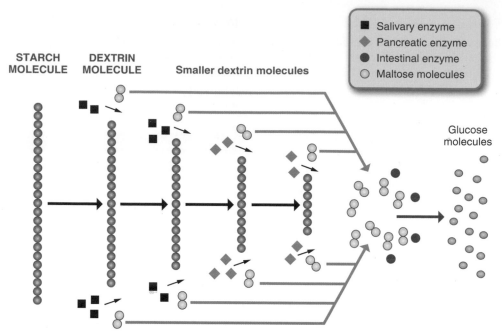

FIGURE 4-2 The gradual breakdown of large starch molecules into glucose by digestion enzymes. (From Mahan LK, Escott-Stump S, Raymond JL: *Krause's food and the nutrition care process*, ed 13, St Louis, 2012, Saunders Elsevier.)

The presence of the cell wall, or cellulose, surrounding the starch granule is the reason starches are insoluble in cold water. Cellulose is composed of long straight chains of glucose units bound together in a very strong bonding to provide great mechanical strength with limited flexibility. Cooking facilitates the digestive process by causing the granules to swell, rupturing the cell wall so that digestive enzymes have access to the starch inside the cell. In cooking, this swelling is referred to as thickening, as occurs in making gravy. Industrially, food starch is modified by chemicals to produce a better thickening agent.

Glucose Polymers

Industrially-produced carbohydrate supplements are composed of glucose, maltose, and dextrins. Dextrins are long glucose chains split into shorter ones or intermediate products of digestive enzymes on starch molecules. In the process of toasting bread, dextrins are produced (see Fig. 4-2). Consistent with other carbohydrate products, glucose polymers provide energy equivalent to 4 kcal/g.

Glycogen

Glycogen is the carbohydrate storage form of energy in humans (see Fig. 2-7). Stored in the muscle and liver, glycogen is readily available as a source of glucose and energy. Carbohydrates are frequently consumed in excess of immediate energy needs. Excess glucose is converted to glycogen until the limited glycogen storage capacity is filled; simultaneously, glucose is converted into fats and stored as adipose tissue. The total amount of glycogen stores is relatively small, only enough to meet energy demands for less than a day.

Dietary Fiber

Fiber refers to nondigestible components of food and has desirable health effects. Nondigestible means enzymes in the human gastrointestinal tract cannot digest and absorb the substance; plant cells remain largely intact through the digestive process. Foods contain soluble or insoluble fiber based on whether they become viscous (sticky, thick) in water. Insoluble and soluble fibers have different physiological functions in the body. Dietary fiber consists of several different types of nondigestible carbohydrates and lignin that occur naturally in plants.

Dietary fiber includes polysaccharides, lignin, and associated substances in plants, such as whole grains, legumes, vegetables, fruits, seeds, and nuts (Table 4-2). Sources of dietary fiber usually contain other macronutrients, such as digestible carbohydrate and protein normally found in foods. During food processing, many compounds are added that have the same physiological effect as naturally occurring fiber, but the food may not have other health benefits, such as vitamins and minerals or alter satiety.

Resistant starch is a form of dietary fiber that cannot be digested. It delivers some of the health benefits of soluble and insoluble fibers. Resistant starches are not absorbed, so they function as a prebiotic by providing fatty acids for bacteria in the colon. Resistant starches trap water and add bulk to the stool, helping with regularity.

Fiber added during the manufacturing process is called functional fiber. Functional fiber consists of isolated, nondigestible carbohydrates that have beneficial physiological effects in humans. Functional fibers may be modified from the natural state or commercially produced, as long as scientific research has shown beneficial physiological effects of

Table 4-2	Synopsis of total fibers				
				Physiological Response	
Type of Fiber	Dietary Fiber Sources	Laxation	Normalization of Blood Lipid Concentration	Attenuation of Blood Glucose Response	
Cellulose	Whole-wheat, whole rye, bran, cabbage family, peas/beans, apples, root vegetables, fresh tomatoes	Yes	Neutral	Neutral	
Gums and mucilages	Oats, dried beans, legumes, brown rice, barley, guar	Neutral	Yes	Yes	
Hemicellulose	Bran, cereals, whole grains, dried beans	Yes	Unknown	Unknown	
Lignin (noncarbohydrate)*	Fruits and edible seeds, mature vegetables, whole grains, flax seed	Yes	Unknown	Unknown	
Pectin	Apples, citrus fruits, berries, carrots	Somewhat	Yes	Yes	
Psyllium	Psyllium seeds, high-fiber cereals	Yes	Yes	Yes	

Data from Institute of Medicine of the National Academies: *Dietary reference intakes: energy, carbohydrate, fiber, fat, fatty acids, cholesterol, protein, and amino acids*, Washington, DC, 2002, National Academies Press.
*Also classified as a phytochemical.

the product. Manufacturers have isolated various types of fiber from carbohydrate sources because of their functional properties, such as thickening or emulsifying. Many of these substances, including carrageenan and guar gum, are common food additives.

Total fiber is the sum of dietary fiber and functional (added) fiber. Many fibers can be classified either as dietary fiber or functional fiber, depending on whether they are a natural component of the food or added to the food during processing. Plant-based foods are a good source of dietary fiber, but commercially developed functional fibers for use in processed foods also have a beneficial role in health. Various types of fibers have distinct properties resulting in different physiological effects (see Table 4-2).

PHYSIOLOGICAL ROLES

Energy

The principal role of absorbed sugars is to provide a source of energy for body functions and activity and for heat to maintain body temperature. Glucose is the preferred source of energy for the brain and central nervous system, red blood cells, and lens of the eye. When carbohydrate intake is restricted, fat and protein stores may be used as an energy source. Although many organs can use fats for energy, glucose is the preferred fuel. Carbohydrate, whether it was originally from a sugar or a starch, provides 4 kcal/g. Because of incomplete absorption, sugar alcohols contribute varying amounts of kilocalories (see Table 4-1). Glycogen stores are a readily available source of glucose for the tissues.

Fat Storage

Sugars in the blood ensure replenishing of glycogen stores; however, excessive intake of energy from any source results

in converting glucose to fats in a process known as lipogenesis. When carbohydrates are eaten in excess of needs, lipogenesis results in increased fat stores.

Conversion to Other Carbohydrates

Monosaccharides are important constituents of many compounds that regulate metabolism. Examples include heparin, which prevents blood clotting; galactolipins, which are constituents of nervous tissue; and dermatan sulfate, which is present in tissues rich in collagen (especially the skin).

Conversion to Amino Acids

The liver can use part of the carbon framework from the sugar molecule and part of the protein molecule contributed by the breakdown of an amino acid to produce nonessential amino acids. These are physiologically essential, but are not required in the diet.

Normal Fat Metabolism

Oxidation of fats requires the presence of some carbohydrates. When carbohydrate intake is low, the body relies on energy from fat intake or stores. As detailed in Chapter 2, when fats are metabolized faster than the body can oxidize them, intermediate products, called ketone bodies, may accumulate. Ketones are normal products of lipid metabolism in the liver; muscles can use ketones for energy only if adequate amounts of glucose are available. An accumulation of ketones in the blood, or incompletely oxidized fatty products, results in ketosis.

Protein Sparers

Carbohydrates, by furnishing energy in the diet, are said to be protein-sparing. Energy is an essential physiological requirement. With insufficient carbohydrate intake, the body burns protein for fuel. If carbohydrate intake is adequate, protein can be used to build and repair tissue.

Intestinal Bacteria

Dietary fiber remains in the gastrointestinal tract longer than other nutrients. Undigestible fibers, such as lignin, cellulose, and hemicellulose, may be fermented by microflora in the large intestine. Fermentation produces gas and volatile fatty acids; cells lining the colon use these fatty acids for energy. Undigestible fiber functions as a prebiotic by encouraging growth of bacteria that synthesize some of the B-complex vitamins and vitamin K.

Gastrointestinal Motility

Dietary and certain functional fibers, particularly those that are poorly fermented, improve fecal bulk and laxation, ameliorate constipation, and perform various other functions (Table 4-2). Dietary fiber and functional fibers *accelerate* transit rate (the time it takes for waste products to move through the intestine) in individuals with a slow transit time (constipation). Viscous fiber *decreases* transit rate in individuals with a rapid transit time (diarrhea). The ability of fiber to bind water in the intestine and increase bulk from nondigestible substances decreases the length of time waste products are in the alimentary tract. An increased transit time lengthens the duration of tissue exposure to cancer-causing nitrogenous waste products. An added benefit of fiber is its stool-softening ability, which helps prevent constipation. Fiber in the colon increases stool bulk, exercising digestive tract muscles by increasing the radius of the colon and preventing the muscle from being chronically contracted. As muscle tone is maintained and colonic pressure declines, the gut is able to resist bulging out into pouches known as diverticula (Fig. 4-3).

Viscous fibers, also called soluble fiber, include pectins, gums, psyllium, mucilages, and algal polysaccharides. They influence the physiology of the upper gastrointestinal tract. Soluble fibers are physiologically important for their gel-forming ability, which results in increased viscosity of chyme and delays gastric emptying. Viscous fibers bind bile acids and decrease serum cholesterol levels. Viscous fibers also tend to improve glucose tolerance. Psyllium, added to many cereals and used as a laxative, is effective in reducing blood cholesterol levels.

Fiber-rich foods are not energy-dense and are retained longer in the stomach. They may cause one to feel full on a fewer number of kilocalories. Whether fiber plays a significant role in weight management has yet to be determined. Table 4-3 provides guidelines for assisting patients in increasing dietary fiber.

Other Nutrients

Carbohydrates are normally accompanied by other nutrients. Starchy foods are especially important for their contribution of protein, minerals, and B vitamins. Whole-grain products are superior because they contain fiber plus other

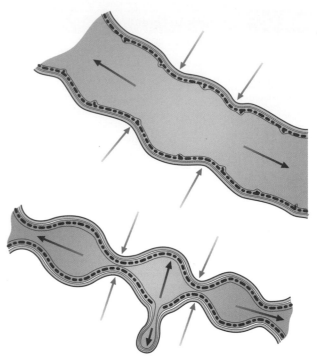

FIGURE 4-3 Mechanism by which low-fiber, low-bulk diets might generate diverticula. Where colon contents are bulk (*top*), muscular contractions exert pressure longitudinally. If lumen is smaller (*bottom*), contractions can produce occlusion and exert pressure against colon wall, which may produce a diverticular "blowout." (From Peckenpaugh NJ: *Nutrition essentials and diet therapy*, ed 11, St Louis, 2010, Saunders Elsevier.)

nutrients (see Table 1-2); enriched products should always be used in preference to products that are processed but not enriched.

 Dental Considerations

- Carbohydrate metabolism requires an adequate supply of B vitamins, phosphorus, and magnesium. Usually, adequate amounts of these nutrients accompany carbohydrate intake. However, this may not be true if refined sugars and breads are predominantly chosen.
- Ketosis can occur in patients with uncontrolled diabetes or in individuals who have inadequate carbohydrate intake, such as individuals who are ill or are following a high-protein, very-low-carbohydrate regimen because they are burning fat rather than carbohydrate. Among other concerns, ketosis creates a disturbance in the patient's acid-base balance. Question patients with acetone or fruity-smelling breath about their recent dietary intake.
- Increasing whole grains in the diet without increasing total energy intake may reduce risk of periodontal disease.[6]
- Concerns are not about consumption of sugars per se, but about overconsumption of sugar. Recommendations should focus on choosing nutrient-dense foods.
- Increasing whole grains in the diet may lead to improvements in blood pressure and gastrointestinal health, reduced body fat stores, and lower risk of cardiovascular disease, prediabetes, and type 2 diabetes.[7,8]

Nutritional Directions

- Carbohydrates alone do not cause obesity. Excessive caloric intake and inadequate energy output are the primary causes of obesity.
- Fiber tends to regulate the transit rate of foods in the gastrointestinal tract. The best source of dietary fiber to relieve constipation is bran, but it must be initiated slowly to avoid severe gas and bloating.
- Enthusiastic patients who eat excessive amounts of bran (50 to 60 g) gain no benefit from the surplus and expose themselves to unnecessary hazards, such as decreased mineral and vitamin absorption.
- Both fiber and whole grains have healthy benefits, but they are not interchangeable.

- Some vegetables and fruits (e.g., bananas, white potatoes, and apples) are high in pectins, which bind water. They are frequently used to control diarrhea but also can help relieve constipation by softening the stool.
- Even when an individual is trying to reduce caloric intake, consuming carbohydrates is important, especially vegetables, fruits, and whole-grain breads and cereals, to provide vital nutrients.
- Carbohydrates supply 4 kcal/g of energy and are a less-concentrated source of energy than fats (9 kcal/g).

Table 4-3	Guidelines for developing a high-fiber diet
Principles	**Guidelines**
Before recommending any changes, evaluate the patient's fiber and fluid intake. For patients ≤50 years old, the optimal level of dietary fiber is 38 g for men and 25 g for women; for patients ≥51 years old, the optimal level of dietary fiber is 30 g for men and 21 g for women	Fiber normalizes bowel movements to once or twice a day by either speeding or slowing the transit rate of food through the gastrointestinal tract. Food-preservation methods, such as cooking and freezing, only slightly decrease fiber content; however, grinding or pureeing foods may have pronounced effects on fiber action.
Rather than fiber supplements, foods that contain soluble and insoluble fibers are the best way to increase fiber	Include two to four servings daily of fruits, especially those with skins (e.g., figs, pears, apricots, nectarines, raisins, blueberries) and edible seeds (e.g., blackberries, raspberries, strawberries). Include three to five servings of vegetables daily, especially sweet potatoes, carrots, mushrooms, raw onions, pumpkin, spinach, turnip greens, kale, Brussels sprouts, parsnips, English peas, beets, okra, and broccoli. Vegetables (e.g., mushrooms, peppers, onions, tomatoes) can be added to meatloaf, spaghetti, chili, omelets, or scrambled eggs. Serve raw vegetables with low-fat dip as appetizers or snacks. (Take advantage of ready-to-use vegetables.) Add leafy greens, tomatoes, and sprouts to sandwiches. Include raw vegetables (e.g., zucchini, carrots, celery sticks) in brown-bag lunches. Choose fresh fruits and vegetables or plain popcorn instead of fried chips and cookies. Dietary fiber comes principally from whole-grain products; brown color is no guarantee of whole-grain content. Look for breads and cereals that list "whole grain" or "whole wheat" first in the ingredients list. Choose cereals with at least 2 g of fiber (5 g is ideal), but no more than 2 g of fat per serving. Experiment with brown rice, barley, whole-wheat pasta, and bulgur. Supplements made with concentrated or purified dietary fiber lack the nutritional balance provided by a varied diet that contains fruits, vegetables, whole-grain products, and legumes. Large amounts of purified fiber such as lignin and bran may result in important minerals, especially calcium, iron, and zinc, being bound by the fiber and excreted.
Fiber absorbs water in the intestines, so adequate fluids are important to keep the intestinal contents moving	Ensure intake of 10-12 cups of decaffeinated fluids a day to avoid problems such as fecal impactions.
Increase high-fiber foods gradually. Begin with 5- to 10-g increments to avoid adverse side effects. At least 6-8 weeks should be allowed for adaptation to prevent flatulence, abdominal cramping, and diarrhea/constipation	Substitute whole-wheat flour for one-quarter or one-half of the white flour in baked goods. Add bran, bran flakes, wheat germ, chopped nuts, seeds, or oatmeal to mixed meat dishes, casseroles, salads, cooked cereal, cookies, breads, muffins, and pancake batter. Use whole-grain crackers and unbuttered popcorn. Incorporate beans into soups, casseroles, nachos, or a salad. Use bran flakes for a crispy coating on meats or fish.
Increase intake of oat bran, beans, barley, and psyllium to help reduce cholesterol levels	Oat bran, rice bran, and corn bran are effective in reducing serum cholesterol. Use dried beans and peas as the main dish (in place of meat) at least once a week. Soluble dietary fiber is more effective in reducing blood cholesterol levels when the diet is also low in fat.

REQUIREMENTS

The Acceptable Macronutrient Distribution Range (AMDR) for carbohydrate is based on providing energy for the body, particularly brain cells. The brain is the only organ that requires glucose. The AMDR for digestible carbohydrate is 130 g per day for adults and children (see p. ii). Generally, men typically consume 200 to 330 g per day and women consume 180 to 230 g per day to meet energy requirements without exceeding acceptable levels of fat and protein. Research studies do not indicate a requirement for a specific amount of starch or sugar.

The AMDR for carbohydrate is limited to no less than 45% (to prevent excess fat intake) and no more than 65% (to ensure required nutrients from protein and fats that also provide essential micronutrients).[9] The American diet currently furnishes approximately 50% of the kilocalories from carbohydrates. The Dietary Reference Intakes (DRIs) compiled by the Institute of Medicine suggest a maximum intake of 25% or less of energy from added sugars.

The World Health Organization's (WHO) comprehensive report on nutrition recommends people limit their added sugar intake to 10% of their total kilocalories (e.g., 12 tsp of added sugars for 2200 kcal).[10] The WHO decision was based on economic, social, and political issues—not on scientific evidence—to prevent and control chronic health problems, especially obesity. The WHO-recommended level of 10% of total kilocalories is contradictory to the 2002 DRI recommendations (less than 25% of total kilocalories). For an individual consuming 2000 kcal per day, the maximum amount of added sugars, or 10% of total caloric intake, would be 11 tsp of added sugars (200 kcal).

The American diet contains an average of 15% of total kilocalories from added sugars.[11] As shown in Fig. 4-4, the average intake of caloric sweeteners was stable between 1985 and 1991, but increased from 1991 to 1999. Since 1999, there has been a sustained downward trend, resulting in an average of 379 kcal per day. Overall intake continues to exceed recommended limits.[12]

Adequate intake for total fiber intake is 14 g per 1000 kcal per day, or 38 g for men and 25 g for women daily. This amount is based on the amount needed to prevent CHD. Dietary fiber intake has remained relatively stable despite efforts to encourage consumers to increase intake, and a significant increase of whole-grain products on the market. More than 90% of adults and children fall short of meeting daily fiber recommendations, yet nearly 66% meet daily intake goals for total amount of refined grains.[13] Mean dietary fiber intake was 15.6 g per day for 1999-2000 and 15.9 g per day for 2007-2008.[14]

SOURCES

Carbohydrates are furnished by the following food groups: milk, grain, fruits, and vegetables. The only animal foods supplying significant quantities of carbohydrate are milk and milk products, which contain the disaccharide lactose. In cheese making, lactose is removed as a by-product. Consequently, most cheeses contain only trace amounts of lactose.

Other sugars are furnished from table sugar, syrups, jellies, jams, and honey. Sugars are incorporated into many popular foods (e.g., candy, beverages, cakes and desserts, chewing gum, and ice cream). Only about 25% of the sugar Americans consume is added to foods in homes, institutions, and restaurants. The remainder is added to foods during

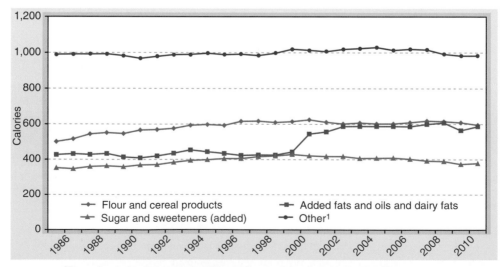

¹Sum of calories from: meat, eggs, and nuts; dairy; fruit; and vegetables

FIGURE 4-4 Average daily per capita calories from the U.S. food availability, by type of food product, adjusted for spoilage and other waste, 1985-2010. (From U.S. Department of Agriculture, Economic Research Service (ERS), *Food availability database and sugar and sweetener outlook*, January 2013.) http://www.ers.usda.gov/publications/sssm-sugar-and-sweeteners-outlook/sssm293.aspx

processing, e.g., canning; freezing; ingredients in breakfast cereals; condiments and salad dressings; soft drinks; cookies, crackers, and candies; flavored extracts and syrups; flour and bread products; and milk and dairy products.

Approximately 18% of caloric intake is from naturally-occurring sugars in fruits and vegetables. (This amount does not include sugar in milk.) Sugars, mainly glucose and fructose, are furnished by fruits and vegetables in varying amounts that depend on their maturity (ripe bananas contain more simple sugars than green bananas) and their water content (spinach contains less carbohydrate than potatoes).

The *Dietary Guidelines* address excessive sugar intake (Box 4-1). Because there is no physiological requirement for added sugars, *MyPlate* does not include a separate section for sugars; added sugars are included in the discretionary kilocalories. Eating sugar in moderation implies a proper balance among foods and nutrients, which should be the primary consideration in food selection. Eating lower amounts does not necessarily guarantee that a diet meets the *Dietary Guidelines*, nor does high sugar consumption mean a poorer quality diet.

Complex carbohydrates, or starches, are furnished by grain products (wheat, corn, rice, oats, rye, barley, buckwheat, and millet). Some vegetables, especially root and seed varieties (potatoes, sweet potatoes, beets, peas, and winter squashes), also contain considerable amounts of starch. Legumes, or dried beans and peas, are excellent sources of complex carbohydrates. Table 4-4 shows the complex carbohydrate and sugar content of the sample menu from Chapter 1, Fig. 1-2.

Dietary fiber, especially hemicellulose and cellulose, is furnished by whole-grain breads and cereals and legumes. Cellulose is found principally in the stems, roots, leaves, and seed coverings of plants; unpeeled fruits and leafy vegetables are good sources. Legumes are also a good source of dietary fiber (see Table 4-2). The pectin contributed by fruits and vegetables is an important source of viscous fiber. Small amounts of resistant starches occur naturally in underripe bananas, navy beans, lentils, barley, and whole-grain breads. A popular American snack food, popcorn (preferably without butter and salt), is also a whole-grain food. Table 4-4 lists the fiber content of foods of the sample menu from Chapter 1, Fig. 1-2.

The fiber in whole grains provides important contributions to health, but the fiber content of whole grains and products containing them varies widely. Consumers equate whole-grain label statements with claims about fiber content and choose products containing whole grains, expecting to increase fiber intake.[15] The fiber content of foods claiming "whole-grain" varies significantly and is very low (<3 g) in many cases. A product containing less than 3 g dietary fiber cannot be considered a "good" source of fiber. This consumer confusion is likely caused by unclear and inconsistent labeling for whole-grain–containing products, the need for a universally accepted definition of whole-grain foods, and lack of consumer education to encourage label reading.

BOX 4-1   Dietary Guidelines for Americans 2010 Recommendations Related to Carbohydrate Consumption*

Balance Calories to Manage Weight
- Prevent and/or reduce overweight and obesity through improved eating and physical activity behaviors.
- Control total calorie intake to manage body weight. For people who are overweight or obese, this will mean consuming fewer calories from foods and beverages.
- Maintain appropriate calorie balance during each stage of life—childhood, adolescence, adulthood, pregnancy and breastfeeding, and older age.

Foods and Food Components to Reduce
- Cut back on foods and drinks with added sugars or energy-containing sweeteners.
- Drink few or no regular sodas, sports drinks, and fruit drinks.
- Eat fewer grain-based or dairy-based desserts, other desserts, and candy, or eat smaller portions less frequently.
- Choose fewer servings of refined grains.

Foods and Nutrients to Increase
- Drink water, fat-free milk, 100% fruit juice, or unsweetened tea or coffee instead of sugar-sweetened drinks. Avoid fruit-flavored drinks.
- Eat fruit for dessert.
- Use the Nutrition Facts label to choose breakfast cereals and other packaged foods with less sugar and use the ingredients list to choose foods with little or no added sugars and to increase whole-grain intake.
- Eat a variety of vegetables, especially dark-green and red and orange vegetables, and beans and peas.
- Consume a sufficient amount of fruits and vegetables while staying within energy needs. Two cups of fruit and 2.5 cups of vegetables per day are recommended for a reference 2000 kcal intake, with higher or lower amounts depending on the kilocalorie level.
- Choose foods that provide more potassium, dietary fiber, calcium, and vitamin D, which are nutrients of concern in American diets. These foods include vegetables, fruits, whole grains, and milk and milk products.

*U.S. Department of Agriculture and U.S. Department of Health and Human Services: *Dietary guidelines for Americans, 2010*, ed 7, Washington, DC, December 2010, U.S. Government Printing Office.

Dental Considerations

- Assess total sugar intake and frequency, form, and time of day for carbohydrate intake. (See Chapter 18 for further discussion.)
- Encourage patients to increase fiber intake. Fiber helps reduce constipation, diverticulosis, and the risk of some colon cancers (see Table 4-3 for ideas to enhance fiber intake).
- Explain to the patient that a diet with adequate amounts of carbohydrate helps to maintain glycogen reserves, while a diet high in fat and low in carbohydrate results in poor glycogen reserves. Another point to emphasize is the need for glycogen stores in the heart, critical for continuous functioning of the heart muscle.
- Encourage patients to consume more whole-grain products and less refined sugar.

Table 4-4   Carbohydrate, dietary fiber, and added sugars content of the sample menu

Sample Menu	Carbohydrate (g)	Dietary Fiber (g)	Added Sugars (g)
Breakfast			
1 whole grain bagel	59	10	
2 tbsp light cream cheese spread	2		
1 tbsp seedless raisins	7		
12 oz skim milk	18		
12 oz black coffee			
Mid-Morning Snack			
1 medium orange	15	3	
12 oz water			
Lunch			
Sandwich with			
¼ c tuna			
1 egg	1		
1 tbsp light mayonnaise	2		4
1 tbsp pickle relish	4		6
¼ c thinly sliced cucumber	1		
2 slices tomato	2		
2 thin slices whole grain bread	20	6	4
¼ c cauliflowerettes	1	1	
8 baby carrots	8	2	
10 red pepper slices	2	1	
1 medium apple	19	3	
12 oz water			
Mid-Afternoon Snack			
1 oz dry roasted almonds (no salt)	5	3	
1 c seedless grapes	27	1	
8 oz herbal tea			
Dinner			
3 oz pot roast beef with			
¼ c gravy	2		
¼ c brown and wild rice blend	15	1	
1 c cooked kale	7	3	
¼ c tossed salad with lettuce, avocado, tomatoes, and carrots	7	4	
2 tbsp shredded low sodium Colby cheese			
2 tbsp vinaigrette salad dressing	3		9
1 medium wedge cantaloupe	6	1	
12 oz iced tea	1		
Evening Snack			
8 oz skim milk	12		
2 medium oatmeal cookies with raisins	18	1	21
TOTALS	264	40	44

From nutrient data SuperTracker. Accessed August 16, 2013: http://www.supertracker.usda.gov/default.aspx

Nutritional Directions

- A tablespoon of honey has more kilocalories than a tablespoon of sugar and only trace amounts of other nutrients. (Honey is not appropriate for children younger than 1 year old because of the risk of botulism.) Because of its retentive nature, honey is also more cariogenic than refined sugar.
- Food labels indicate the total amount of carbohydrate (starch, sugar, and fiber) in a serving. Because fiber is not absorbed, it does not contribute any kilocalories. A product with 25 g of carbohydrate may have only 80 kcal if at least 5 g of the carbohydrate is from fiber.
- Sugar may be identified as any of the following on food labels: sucrose, fructose, corn sweetener, cane sugar, evaporated cane juice, honey, molasses, high-fructose corn syrup, raw sugar, and maple syrup. Patients trying to reduce added sugars should avoid foods if one of these is the first ingredient listed.

HYPERSTATES AND HYPOSTATES

The role of carbohydrates in nutritional health and behavior continues to be misrepresented by the press and some professionals. Many stories have been published in the media linking sugar to practically every modern-day illness, including malnutrition, hypoglycemia, diabetes mellitus, blood lipid abnormalities, cardiovascular disease, hyperactivity, criminal behavior, obesity, malabsorption syndrome, allergies, gallstones, and cancer. The public's perception of sugar consumption continues to be at odds with scientific facts.

Normal physiological conditions and disease states affect carbohydrate metabolism, which is reflected in serum glucose levels. For individuals with diabetes, a blood glucose level that is greater than 130 mg/dL before meals or greater than 180 mg/dL 2 hours after meals indicates hyperglycemia; a blood glucose level less than 70 mg/dL indicates hypoglycemia.[16] Other factors concerning too much or too little carbohydrate are discussed subsequently.

Carbohydrate Excess

The preponderance of evidence based on scientific literature indicates sugar consumption at typical American levels does not directly contribute to any chronic health or behavioral problems, unless excessive sugar consumption results in energy imbalance and weight gain.[17,18] Excessive consumption of added sugars (greater than 25% of total energy) may result in an inadequate intake of foods containing necessary micronutrients. Intake of nutrients at most risk for inadequacy (vitamins E, A, and C, and magnesium) decrease as added sugars increase above 5% to 10% of total kilocalories. But the predominant issue is the low quality and overall high energy intake of all U.S. diets, regardless of sweetener content.[19] Weight gain that occurs with the amount of sugar intake is a result of excess caloric intake, not the physiological or metabolic consequences of sugar.[20] Americans need to cut back on their added sugar intake, but the average amount currently consumed is not above the level the IOM deems would result in an inadequate diet or an amount that would contribute to chronic diseases. Sugar increases palatability and may improve choices of certain foods otherwise disliked. Combining sugar with other nutritious foods, as in milk used for pudding, may increase the variety of foods consumed and enjoyed.

A principle concern in the *Dietary Guidelines* is consumption of adequate amounts of vitamins and minerals without consuming excess energy (see Box 4-1). Sweeteners contain no other nutrients (vitamins or minerals) and, when consumed as soft drinks and hard candies, provide nothing other than pleasure and energy. Consumers are drinking enormous amounts of kilocalories in liquid form. Frequently, soft drinks are substituted for milk.

Since 1977, soda has been the most popular beverage in the United States. Soft drinks and energy and sports drinks provide the most added sugars in the U.S. population.[21] On a good note, soft drink consumption fell from 51.5 gallons per capita in 2005 to 44.7 gallons per capita in 2010. Overall, consumption of soft drinks has decreased even among teenagers. In 2009-2010, youth ages 2-19 years consumed 155 kcal/day from sugar-sweetened beverages and adults consumed 151 kcal/day—a decrease from 1999-2000 of 68 kcal/day for youth and 45 kcal/day for adults.[22] Although federal regulations prohibit the sale of soft drinks to students during lunch in most high schools, vending machines may be accessible to students throughout the day.

Carbohydrate Deficiency

Frequently, carbohydrates are eliminated in an effort to lose weight. When carbohydrates are severely restricted, not only protein intake increases, but fat intake often increases. High-protein, low-carbohydrate diets do not necessarily lead to greater weight loss than traditional diets, and care must be taken to prevent elevated lipid levels that may accompany higher fat intake.[23,24] Extremely low-carbohydrate diets may lead to ketosis.

Consuming 47% to 64% energy from carbohydrates can result in a lower risk of becoming obese.[25] When complex carbohydrates are eliminated, an insufficient intake of B vitamins, iron, and fiber may occur. Vitamins and minerals are necessary for the body to use glucose, but these nutrients do not need to be present in the same foods. Only when sugar consumption interferes with or replaces a well-balanced intake does the diet become inadequate. When that occurs, sugar warrants the designation of "empty calorie," which indicates it is inadequate in vitamins, minerals, and trace elements. Fortification of foods has a positive effect on nutrient density of the diet. Nutrient density is the amount of nutrients of a food relative to the number of kilocalories provided.

Dental Caries

For many years, sucrose, the most frequently consumed form of sugar, has been considered the "arch villain" in dental caries formation. Sucrose and other carbohydrates have unusual biochemical properties that promote bacterial growth. Sucrose can lower the pH of plaque biofilm, hastening the dissolution of hydroxyapatite crystals of the enamel. Glucose, available from sucrose or any other carbohydrate food, can be used for energy by oral bacteria in plaque biofilm.

Many health professionals and consumers mistakenly believe that removing sucrose from the diet would largely eliminate dental caries. The American Dental Association (ADA) recognizes that carbohydrates provide the energy required for optimal nutrition. However, the American Academy of Pediatric Dentistry (AAPD) recommends fermentable carbohydrates that are consumed frequently or repeatedly (e.g., chewing gum, chewable tablets, lozenges, mints, and snack foods such as gummy bears) be replaced with products containing noncariogenic sweeteners, preferably xylitol.[26]

A fermentable carbohydrate that can reduce salivary pH to less than 5.5 is referred to as being cariogenic. The total amount of fermentable carbohydrate seems to be of less importance than the form in which it is eaten and the frequency of consumption. This may be related to variables influencing the length of time the carbohydrate is in contact with teeth and its potential for promoting growth of caries-forming, acid-producing bacteria. (See Chapter 18 for further discussion.)

Other monosaccharides and disaccharides, such as glucose, fructose, maltose, and lactose, are also readily metabolized by oral microorganisms, resulting in demineralization of tooth enamel. These sugars diffuse rapidly into plaque biofilm to become available for bacteria. In laboratory tests, the rate that fructose and glucose lowers plaque biofilm pH is similar to sucrose; they are considered as cariogenic as sucrose. Substituting glucose or fructose for sucrose would not be significantly effective in reducing caries rates. Lactose is less cariogenic than other sugars. The kind of sugar is not significant; the concentration or quantity of sugar in a foodstuff is not critical to its cariogenic potential.

Regular sodas and energy drinks contain fermentable carbohydrates and are highly acidic (Table 4-5). Despite differences in the carbohydrate content of carbonated beverages, fruit drinks, 100% fruit juice (approximately 10% carbohydrates), sport drinks (approximately 46% to 48% carbohydrates), energy drinks (approximately 9% to 10%

carbohydrates), flavored coffees and teas, and powdered drinks—all of these beverages seem to have similar cariogenic potential.

In addition to their sugar content, carbonated soda, fruit juices, and sport drinks are very acidic with pH ranges below 4.0. Dental erosion is the chemical removal of minerals from the tooth structure that occurs when an acidic environment causes enamel to dissolve gradually. This can occur with frequent exposure to liquids with a pH below 4.2. Citrus juices contain citric acid, which is especially damaging to tooth enamel; the citrate binds with calcium in saliva, reducing its potential to remineralize the tooth. Deleterious effects of 100% fruit juices can be minimized with calcium fortification.[27] Acidic, sugar-free products—regardless of whether naturally occurring or an additive—may increase the probability of dental erosion.[28] Research suggests the extent of enamel erosion caused by various beverages occurs in the following order (from greatest to least): energy drinks, sports drinks, regular soda, and diet soda.[29]

No definite relationship has been shown between total carbohydrate consumption and caries. Starches can cause acid production in plaque biofilm when consumed as part of a mixed diet containing fermentable carbohydrates. Some foods, such as potato chips or crackers, containing a high-carbohydrate, low-sugar content can contribute to the caries process when salivary amylase hydrolyzes complex carbohydrate to simple sugars. Starch molecules are large and cannot penetrate into plaque biofilm. Cooked and refined cereal grains are readily hydrolyzed by salivary amylases to produce maltose, which can lower pH and demineralize enamel. Some foods high in sugar are removed more quickly and do not lower the pH of plaque biofilm as much as starchy foods with less sugar. Starches, such as breads and pasta, are considered less cariogenic than sugars, but they tend to prolong the caries attack after it has been initiated (especially when sugar is added, as in sweet breads and cookies).

Some popular snack products contain sweeteners that are less cariogenic than sucrose. Sugar alcohols may decrease the risk of dental caries through any of the following mechanisms: (a) inhibiting the growth of S. mutans, (b) not promoting the synthesis of plaque biofilm, or (c) not lowering plaque biofilm pH. Studies evaluating evidence for an anticariogenic effect of sugar-free chewing gum concluded that sugar-free chewing gum has a caries-reducing effect, but more well-designed, randomized studies are recommended to confirm the findings.[30] The ADA has approved the use of their seal on sugarless gums by several gum manufacturers. The ADA recommends chewing gum after each meal for at least 20 minutes to reap the most benefits, if oral hygiene cannot be performed.

Sorbitol causes only a slight pH decrease in plaque biofilm. Bacteria in plaque biofilm are able to ferment sorbitol and mannitol, but only at a very slow rate over several weeks. After a period of adaptation, however, acid production increases.

Table 4-5	Destructive effects of beverages*	
Beverages	**Sugar (tsp)**	**pH†**
Mountain Dew	11	3.16
Pepsi Cola	9.8	2.49
Dr Pepper	9.5	2.92
Squirt	9.5	2.85
Coke Classic	9.3	2.53
Apple juice	9	3.42
Sprite	9	3.42
Gatorade Clear	5.5	2.4
Milk	3.5	6.4-6.8
Orange juice	2.5	3.30-4.19
Tomato Juice	<1	4.1
Water	0	7.0
Diet Dr Pepper	0	3.41
Diet Coke	0	3.39
Diet Mountain Dew	0	3.34
Fresca	0	3.2
Diet Pepsi Cola	0	3.06
Pepsi One	0	3.05
Lemon Juice	0	2.0-2.6

*Data from 21st Century Dental: *Drinks that eat teeth*. Accessed August 16, 2013: http://www.21stcenturydental.com/smith/pH_drinks.htm/
†Neutral pH = 7. Because the pH scale is logarithmic, one unit change in pH is associated with a 10-fold change in the acidity. For example, lemon juice has a pH of 2, whereas orange juice has a pH of 3.3. Lemon juice would therefore be more than 130 times as acidic as orange juice.

Xylitol is anticariogenic, exhibiting both passive and active anticaries effects, and directly inhibits the growth of *S. mutans*. Oral bacteria lack the enzymes to ferment xylitol; it does not lower plaque biofilm pH. An **anticariogenic** substance reduces the risk of caries by preventing bacteria from recognizing a cariogenic food. Some studies suggest that the anticariogenic effect of xylitol chewing gum may be enhanced by the chewing process.[31] Xylitol stimulates secretion of saliva, which contains a large number of bicarbonate ions to neutralize acid. One study concluded that a minimum of 5 to 6 g xylitol and three exposures per day are needed for clinical effect.[32]

Lactitol cannot be metabolized by bacteria in plaque biofilm and may provide a protective effect for teeth. However, it is only about one-third as sweet as sucrose. Saccharin inhibits tooth decay in rats. Aspartame does not support the growth of *S. mutans*, acid production, or plaque biofilm formation.

Obesity

A common misperception is that sugar is uniquely fattening. Because the taste of sugar is so pleasant, some rationalize that sugar becomes irresistible to the point of overconsumption or addiction. However, most individuals have a limit as to how sweet they like their foods and how much they can consume in a given period.

Four leading scientific and health organizations—the Food and Agriculture Organization, WHO, the Institute of Medicine, and the Academy of Nutrition and Dietetics—have all concluded that dietary sugars are not associated with causing illness or chronic diseases, including obesity. The evidence available to date continues to show no direct connection between total sugar intake and obesity.[36]

Some studies indicate an association between higher intake of whole grains (about three servings daily) with healthier body weights and fat stores. However, data from

---

🦷 Dental Considerations

- Scientific consensus[33] to date shows: (a) the link between sugar intake and obesity is inconsistent; (b) sugar intake alone does not cause diabetes; and (c) sugar intake is not an independent risk factor for CHD.
- Approximately 90% of commonly consumed snack foods contain fermentable carbohydrates (sugars or cooked starch or both).
- Snacks contribute significantly to the nutritional intake of young children and teenagers, who need larger amounts of energy for growth.
- Patients unable to tolerate adequate amounts at meals require snacks to promote healing and avoid loss of lean tissue.
- Although sucrose is a major factor in caries risk, provide factual information that does not overemphasize sugar's role in caries formation.
- Some foods, such as milk, yogurt, and aged cheese, actually protect the teeth by increasing oral pH and inhibiting acid production.
- If snacks are needed when oral hygiene cannot be performed, suggest low-fat milk products, aged cheese, or yogurt; or chew xylitol-containing gum.

- Complete and permanent elimination of sweets is unrealistic. The best advice is to (a) use sugar in moderation, (b) limit the frequency of sugar exposure, (c) consume sweets with a meal, and (d) brush the teeth after consuming sugar-containing products. If oral hygiene cannot be performed, chew xylitol, sorbitol, or xylitol-sorbitol chewing gum.
- Encourage patients to rinse their mouth with water after consuming acidic beverages rather than brushing their teeth, as this procedure may increase dental erosion.
- Assess patient consumption of acidic beverages. Patients with frequent consumption of acidic beverages, decreased salivary flow, prolonged holding habits, or mouth breathing could be at increased risk for dental erosion.[34]
- Excessive intake (more than 20 g per day) of sugar alcohol-containing gum and sweets may lead to unintended weight loss as a result of chronic diarrhea. One stick of sugar-free gum contains about 1.25 g sorbitol.
- Polyol-based, sugar-free products may cause dental erosion if they contain acidic flavoring.[35]

🥄 Nutritional Directions

- The association between eating and weight status is not the result of a single eating pattern but from a combination of food choices that are interrelated and cumulative in their effect.
- Educating patients to maintain healthy teeth can include recommending sweet-tasting foods without increasing risk of caries.
- The most important cause of dental caries is frequency of consuming fermentable carbohydrates that supply substrate to caries-producing oral bacteria.
- The potential for caries exists every time a carbohydrate is eaten because most foods promote acid formation if no procedures are taken to remove food debris or plaque biofilm, to buffer the acid produced, or to interfere with acid production.
- The amount of carbohydrate in a food is unrelated to its caries-forming potential; all carbohydrate foods are potentially cariogenic. Proteins and fats are **cariostatic**, or cannot be

metabolized by microorganisms in plaque biofilm, and are caries-inhibiting.
- Natural sugars, primarily fructose and glucose, in unprocessed foods, such as bananas and raisins, are potentially as cariogenic as sucrose.
- Brush the teeth before consuming acidic foods and rinse with water or chew sugarless gum after consuming acidic foods and beverages.
- Vegetables such as lettuce, celery, and broccoli contain a minimal amount of carbohydrate (5 g per serving), but do not cause acid production or demineralization of enamel in humans.
- Sugar alcohols are less likely to promote caries; xylitol seems to prevent caries formation.
- Highly acidic foods may prevent bacterial fermentation but cause enamel erosion.

Continued

Nutritional Directions—cont'd

- Replacing potentially cariogenic snacks with foods such as fresh fruits and vegetables; low-fat cottage cheese, cheese, and yogurt (flavored with nutmeg, cinnamon, or fresh fruit); peanuts; or low-fat popcorn can decrease caries and promote other health-conscious nutritional habits.
- Using a straw with beverages such as carbonated drinks or lemonade may reduce contact with teeth and may lessen risk of caries.
- Consumption of sodas should be limited to 8 oz or less daily with a meal.
- High-carbohydrate foods, especially complex unrefined carbohydrates, are high in fiber and other nutrients.

National Health and Nutritional Examination Surveys found no correlation between whole-grain intake and body mass index, but whole grains were related to positive nutrient profiles and chronic disease risk factors.[37] The *Dietary Guidelines* recommend a fiber-rich diet to help in the management of obesity as it provides bulk, which may help with satiety while reducing kilocalories consumed.

Excessive caloric intake leads to obesity, whether from carbohydrates, proteins, fats, or alcohol. Although excessive energy intake from sugar may lead to obesity, epidemiological studies and several individual studies show that obese patients actually consume less sugar than thin patients. Many sweet foods contain large amounts of fat. Too much carbohydrate is likely to be consumed when fat is severely restricted and overall food intake is not restricted to some degree.

Dental Considerations

- Scientific studies do not support the claim that sugars interfere with bioavailability of vitamins, minerals, or trace nutrients, or the notion that dietary imbalances are preferentially caused by increased sugar consumption. Do not assume that because a patient is obese, increased sugar intake is the culprit.

Nutritional Directions

- Encourage a well-balanced diet containing adequate nutrients with appropriate amounts of fruits, vegetables, and milk and dairy products.
- Several organs depend on glucose to function. A change to a minimal-carbohydrate, high-protein, high-fat diet may result in an inadequate intake of numerous nutrients and cognitive impairment.

NONNUTRITIVE SWEETENERS/ SUGAR SUBSTITUTES

The practice of flavoring foods without additional kilocalories is one of many approaches to the problems of excess energy intake and a sedentary lifestyle. Nonnutritive sweeteners, also called sugar sweeteners or artificial sweeteners, add sweetness but contain no or minimal carbohydrates (or energy) and do not raise blood sugars. Most are synthesized compounds from fruits, herbs, or sugar itself. The use of sugar substitutes also has beneficial ramifications for dental hygiene. The desire to decrease sugar consumption is being met through widespread and increasing use of numerous nonnutritive sweeteners. Consumption of low-calorie sweeteners is increasing faster than that of caloric sweeteners with a trend toward the purchase of more noncaloric sweetener-containing products.[38]

Nonnutritive sweeteners are used principally for their sweetening power, but they also make some foods more palatable. The large variety of sweeteners is desirable because each has certain advantages and limitations. Because each sweetener has different properties, the availability of various products helps satisfy various flavor and texture requirements in foods and beverages. Sweeteners may be combined because of their synergistic effect—that is, when combined, sweeteners yield a sweeter taste than that provided by each sweetener alone.

These sweeteners have the potential to reduce sugar and energy intakes, but Americans' BMIs have risen parallel to the rise in use of nonnutritive sweeteners. Although taste buds may be fooled by their sweetness, nonnutritive sweeteners do not produce a prolonged feeling of satiety. Concerns have been expressed that nonnutritive sweeteners may promote energy intake and contribute to obesity. Most of the possible mechanisms by which this occurs are not supported by available evidence.

Currently, data is insufficient to conclusively determine whether the use of sugar substitutes replacing caloric sweeteners reduces added sugars or carbohydrate intakes, or benefits appetite, energy balance, body weight, or other risk factors. Nevertheless, the American Heart Association concluded that nonnutritive sweeteners could be used in a structured diet to replace added sugars, thereby resulting in decreased total energy and weight loss/weight control, and promoting beneficial effects on related metabolic parameters.[39]

Whether use of these nonnutritive sweeteners decreases total caloric intake depends on other food choices. Making compensatory food choices, such as drinking a diet carbonated beverage to permit a piece of cheesecake, is ineffective in weight control, whereas replacing a high-calorie food with a low-calorie food, watching other food intake, and engaging in some form of exercise may be beneficial.

Many consumers question the safety of these products. All products on the market have been extensively researched and are safe for most people if consumed in moderation except for aspartame.[40] Aspartame is safe in moderate amounts for everyone except individuals who have phenylketonuria, a genetic disorder characterized by an inability to metabolize the amino acid phenylalanine. Table 4-6 summarizes information regarding sugar substitutes.

Table 4-6   Noncaloric sugar substitutes (nonnutritive sweeteners)*

	Acesulfame K	Aspartame	Neotame	Saccharin	Sucralose	Stevia (Rebaudioside A)	Monk Fruit (Lo han guo)
Description	200 times sweeter than sucrose	Made from 2 amino acids—phenylalanine and aspartic acid 200 times sweeter than sucrose	Derivative of 2 amino acids—aspartic acid and phenylalanine 7000-13,000 times sweeter than sucrose	300 times sweeter than sucrose	Sweetener made from sucrose; 600 times sweeter than sucrose	Derived from a South American plant called *Stevia rebaudina*; more than 300 times sweeter than sucrose	Grown in Asia 200 times sweeter than sugar
Assets	Leaves no aftertaste Excreted unchanged Excellent shelf life Works synergistically with other low-calorie sweeteners Stable to heat Does not promote tooth decay	No aftertaste Intensifies and extends flavors Does not promote tooth decay	Unique flavor-enhancing properties	Stable shelf life Synergistic effect with other low-calorie sweeteners Not metabolized Does not react with DNA	No aftertaste Very stable to heat Long shelf life Replaces sugar in equal amounts	Natural. steviol glycosides isolated and purified from stevia leaves Works synergistically with other sweeteners Readily soluble in water	Natural—crushed monk fruit is infused with hot water Used in China to treat colds, sore throat, and minor stomach and intestinal complaints
Limitations	None identified	Loses sweetness with lengthy heating or baking; not recommended for clients with phenylketonuria	None identified	Slight aftertaste	None identified	Exhibits a menthol-like or licorice aftertaste	
Safety	Tested in more than 90 studies JECFA† established an ADI‡ of 15 mg/kg of body weight	Most thoroughly studied additive available More than 500 studies over more than 3 decades confirm aspartame's safety§ ADI‡, 50 mg/kg body weight/day	More than 100 scientific studies show its safety	Over a century of safe human use More than 30 human studies indicate improbability of causing cancer in humans No association between saccharin and bladder cancer	More than 100 studies over a 20-year period show the safety of sucralose as a safe inert ingredient for all populations Does not promote tooth decay, cancer, genetic changes, birth defects	Stevia glycoside metabolized to stevia and excreted in urine; little to none absorbed JECFA† concluded no microbiological or nutritional safety concerns Used for decades in Japan and Paraguay and in 14 other countries. ADI‡—4 mg/kg body weight	Numerous safety studies in animals and humans show monk fruit is safe for its intended use in foods and beverages Heavily used in China and Japan
Status	Approved by FDA in July 1988 and reaffirmed its safety by broadening its approval in 2003	Approved for use by FDA in 1996; approved by regulatory bodies of more than 100 countries	Approved for use in Australia and New Zealand Approved by FDA in 2002	Warning label removed in 1977 Government, scientists, and industry agree that saccharin is safe Used in more than 100 countries	Approved by FDA in 1998 FDA approved it as a general purpose sweetener in 1999 Approved in more than 40 countries	Approved by FDA in 2008 as safe for people of all ages and populations as a general purpose sweetener in foods, excluding meat and poultry products	Approved for use by EFSA** in 2010 and European Commission in 2011 Approved for use as a sweetener and flavor enhancer by FDA in 2010

*Data from The Calorie Control Council. Accessed August 16, 2013: http://www.caloriecontrol.org/sweeteners-ande-lite/sugar-substitutes/. Calorie Control Council, 5775 Peachtree-Dunwoody Road, Ste 500-G, Atlanta, GA 30342.

†*JECFA,* Joint Expert Committee on Food Additives, a part of the World Health Organization.

‡*ADI,* acceptable daily intake.

§Magnuson BA, Burdock GA, Doull J, et al: Aspartame: a safety evaluation based on current use levels, regulations and toxicological and epidemiological studies. *Crit Rev Toxicol* 2007;37(8):629-727.

**European Food Safety Authority.

Dental Considerations

- Sugar substitutes can reduce energy content and decrease cariogenicity of a product. Used in moderation, nonnutritive sweeteners are beneficial for many people, especially patients with diabetes.
- Because aspartame contains phenylalanine, aspartame-containing products are labeled to warn patients with phenylketonuria to avoid their use.
- Use of sugar substitutes is especially advocated for between-meal snacks to decrease tooth exposure to sugar. For individuals who do not need to decrease energy intake, sugar alcohols may be recommended.
- Nonnutritive sweeteners are nonfermentable and do not promote caries formation; antimicrobial activity has not been observed. Saccharin and aspartame exhibit microbial inhibition and caries suppression.
- Dental professionals are often asked to provide advice regarding the importance of diet and the role of sugars and nonnutritive sweeteners in caries formation and weight control. A reduction of fermentable sugars and carbohydrates coupled with good oral hygiene practices will reduce incidence of dental decay.

Nutritional Directions

- Although nonnutritive sweeteners may not have cariogenic potential, bulking ingredients that allow them to pour and measure more like sugar (and other constituents of a product) may have cariogenic potential if they contain fermentable carbohydrates.
- Nonnutritive sweeteners do nothing to appease the appetite, but they do provide the pleasure of sweetness. They may enable patients to choose a wide variety of foods while managing their caloric or cariogenic intake.
- When deciding whether a young child should be given foods sweetened with a nonnutritive sweetener, consider the child's body weight, and limit the sweetener to below recommended levels (500 mg/day for saccharin, 50 mg/kg body weight for aspartame, 4 mg/kg body weight for stevia, and 15 mg/kg body weight for acesulfame-K). One packet of Sweet 'n Low (Cumberland Packing Corp) contains 40 mg of saccharin; one packet of Sweet One (Stadt Corp), contains 50 mg of acesulfame; and one packet of Equal (Nutrasweet Co.) contains 35 mg of aspartame. (Because there are no known side effects for sucralose, no maximum limits have been established for children.) Remember that children need energy for growth and development.
- Combinations of sweeteners can produce a sweet taste more similar to that of sugar than can a single high-intensity sweetener.
- During pregnancy, saccharin is not recommended because it is known to cross the placenta. Refer a pregnant patient to her obstetrician for counseling about use of any nonnutritive sweeteners.

HEALTH APPLICATION 4   High-Fructose Corn Syrup

In recent years, the lay press has drawn a lot of attention to numerous studies regarding high-fructose corn syrup (HFCS) and its association with the current obesity epidemic, diabetes mellitus, and other maladies. HFCS has been labeled "the devil's candy," "the crack of sweeteners," and "a sinister invention." Consumers are specifically concerned about HFCS; many of their changes in food choices are driven by efforts to consume foods they consider safe and healthy. In response to negative publicity and unfounded opinions about HFCS, consumers are purchasing fewer foods containing HFCS, so the food industry has reformulated many products to eliminate the sweetener.

HFCS was so named because it is made from corn; however, it is different from regular corn syrup, which is composed of glucose and glucose polymers. Some of the glucose molecules in corn are changed into fructose, making HFCS sweeter. Enzymatic processes involved in the production of HFCS are used to produce other foods and ingredients considered natural. The U.S. Food and Drug Administration (FDA) has stated that HFCS may be labeled as a natural ingredient. Whereas sucrose is 50% fructose and 50% glucose, HFCS contains between 42% and 55% fructose (and 45% to 58% glucose), not too different from sucrose, but significantly different from the original corn syrup product that is 100% glucose and no fructose. HFCS is comparable to sugar and honey in its sweetness and the way it is processed in the body. It was designed to be equal to sucrose in sweetness so they could be used interchangeably in foods and beverages.

HFCS is used principally in carbonated beverages and fruit preparations because of its stability in acidic products. After fructose and glucose (from sucrose, HFCS, or honey) are absorbed from the intestinal tract, each enters into its own metabolic pathway. In the bloodstream, the human body cannot distinguish these sweeteners from one another. The Academy of Nutrition and Dietetics developed an **Evidence Analysis Library,** a process in which an expert work group identifies practice-related questions, performs a systematic literature review, then develops and rates a conclusive statement for each question. For HFCS, they evaluated four short-term randomized controlled trials, two longitudinal studies, two cross-sectional studies, and five review articles to determine its physiologic effect compared to other nutritive sweeteners. "These studies consistently found little evidence that HFCS differs uniquely from sucrose and other nutritive sweeteners in metabolic effects (e.g., circulating glucose, insulin, postprandial triglycerides, leptin, and ghrelin), subjective effects (e.g., hunger, satiety, and energy intake at subsequent meals), and the adverse effect of weight gain."[41] Many studies dealing with HFCS were excluded from the evaluation because of limitations such as limited numbers of participants and duration, and research design flaws. The expert work group determined that, based on the research studies available, evidence of their conclusion was "fair," because of inconsistencies among the results from different studies or because of doubts about generalizability, bias, research design flaws, or adequacy of sample size. Fructose is clearly metabolized

HEALTH APPLICATION 4   High-Fructose Corn Syrup—cont'd

differently than glucose. Scientific studies indicate that large amounts of fructose consumed independent of glucose causes undesirable metabolic effects. But using typical conditions, HFCS and other caloric sweeteners do not appear to increase liver fat or contribute to insulin resistance.[42-44]

Some countries, such as Mexico, do not have the machinery available in the United States to manufacture HFCS. Cane sugar is still the sweetener in soft drinks in these areas, where cane sugar is inexpensive. But in the United States, the price for making and processing HFCS is less expensive than cane sugar. Many countries are seeing increasing rates of obesity and diabetes, even though little or no HFCS is present in their food supply. HFCS currently accounts for approximately 10% of sweeteners used around the world. The WHO states that worldwide obesity has more than doubled since 1980.[45]

Fructose intake provided 8.8% of total energy in 1977-1978 when most of the fructose was provided from fruits, vegetables, and honey.[46] HFCS intake increased between 1990 and 1999, then decreased significantly beginning in 2005; despite less consumption of HFCS, the prevalence of obesity has remained stable (Fig. 4-5). Overconsumption of either sweetener, or any calorie-containing food or beverage, along with fats and decreased physical activity, contribute to weight gain.

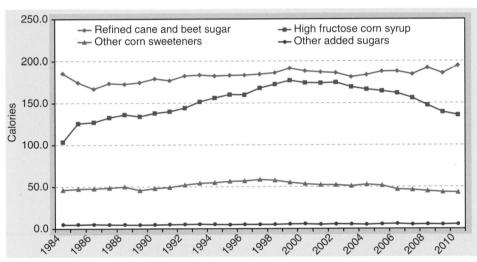

FIGURE 4-5 Added sugar and sweeteners: average daily per capita calories from the U.S. food availability, adjusted for spoilage and other waste (From U.S. Department of Agriculture, Economic Research Service (ERS), *Food availability database and sugar and sweetener outlook*, January 2013. http://www.ers.usda.gov/publications/sssm-sugar-and-sweeteners-outlook/sssm293.aspx)

Case Application for the Dental Hygienist

A healthy patient needs information on how to eat less refined sugar and more complex carbohydrates. He knows this regimen is encouraged, but does not know all the health reasons. Fiber intake is also important to him, but he is not knowledgeable about the types of food needed or the benefits.

Nutritional Assessment
- Willingness/motivation to learn
- Usual dietary habits; focus especially on carbohydrate
- Basic knowledge of carbohydrate and carbohydrate principles
- Usual food/nutrient intake
- Financial status, employment status, and where most of the food is consumed
- Support system—family, friends, coworkers
- Use of community resources
- Food shopping practices

Nutritional Diagnosis
Health-seeking behavior related to lack of knowledge concerning carbohydrate and carbohydrate principles for optimal nutrition.

Nutritional Goals
The patient will consume a high-fiber food and complex carbohydrate foods daily, and state three principles concerning carbohydrate.

Nutritional Implementation
Intervention: Explain that (a) the main function of carbohydrate is to provide energy for the body; (b) that excessive amounts of carbohydrate by themselves do not cause obesity, but excessive overall caloric intake increases body fat (and consequently weight); and (c) the role of carbohydrate in the dental caries process and enhancing plaque biofilm formation.
Rationale: Knowledge corrects misinformation.
Intervention: (a) Follow suggestions in Table 4-3. (b) Explain the importance of fiber. Recommend 30 to 38 g of fiber daily, and help the patient plan a diet that will provide this amount, incorporating his food preferences. Stress the importance of adequate fluid intake.
Rationale: These suggestions increase fiber in the diet. Fiber increases stool bulk, exercising digestive tract muscles and

Continued

Case Application for the Dental Hygienist—cont'd

preventing them from being chronically contracted. Muscle tone is maintained, colonic pressure is diminished, and the gut is able to resist bulging out into pouches. Additionally, fiber slows starch hydrolysis and delays glucose absorption.

Intervention: Explain sources of complex carbohydrates and fiber sources, and provide the patient with a list of these foods. Emphasize the importance of increasing fiber intake gradually and increasing noncariogenic, noncaloric fluid intake when increasing fiber.

Rationale: The patient's increased knowledge will encourage him to increase consumption of complex carbohydrate and fiber.

Intervention: (a) Recommend substituting non-nutritive sweeteners for sugar, especially at snack time. (b) Read a label with the patient to show the patient how to recognize sugars (they usually end in -*ose*). (c) Recommend substituting fresh fruit for juices to increase fiber. (d) Instruct him to limit products that contain complex carbohydrates and sugar, such as cookies and pastries.

Rationale: He wanted to reduce refined sugar intake, and these measures will help meet this personal goal.

Intervention: Refer him to an RDN and county extension agencies.

Rationale: These will provide expert knowledge and community resources for continued compliance.

Intervention: Review labeling: (a) "no sugar added" means sugar was not added, although the product may naturally contain sugar; (b) "sugar-free" means the product contains no added sucrose, but may have other sugars added, such as sorbitol; (c) a high-fiber food has been defined as containing 5 g or more per serving; (d) incorporate foods with 3 g or more of fiber per serving.

Rationale: Knowing the meaning of these terms facilitates making healthy food choices.

Evaluation

The patient consumes a bran muffin, beans, or other high-fiber foods daily and verbalizes that carbohydrates provide energy and fiber, carbohydrate has several roles in maintaining gut functioning, and most sugars end in -*ose*. Other indicators of success include reading a label correctly, modifying intake of refined sugars, and using the community resources.

STUDENT READINESS

1. Differentiate between the three classes of carbohydrates.
2. Identify sources of complex carbohydrates in the diet.
3. What are the main sources of fiber in the American diet? What are the main sources of starch?
4. List three of your favorite foods high in added sugar. What realistic modifications can you make to your diet with respect to these high-sugar foods?
5. Explain the functions of sugars and fiber in the diet in terms a patient can understand.
6. From cereal boxes at the local grocery store, identify some of the products that claim to be high in fiber: (a) evaluate the source of fiber on the ingredient label to determine if those are soluble or insoluble fibers, and (b) rank the cereals according to the amount of dietary fiber they contain. Which would you recommend?
7. Based on ready-to-eat cereals available at the grocery store, identify five that list a whole grain as the first ingredient.
8. Role play: To a patient consuming a very low-carbohydrate diet, discuss why this diet is neither healthy nor wise.
9. Role play: Advise a mother who has been told she should never give her infant anything that contains sugar because the infant will develop a sweet tooth?
10. What is the basis for WHO's recommendation of 10% or less of kilocalories from sugars? Why is the Institute of Medicine recommendation of 25% or less of energy intake different?
11. Match the carbohydrates on the left with the appropriate answer in the right column.

Dextrose	Cannot be used by the body
Glycogen	Milk
Fructose	Sweetest sugar
Lactose	Glucose
Cellulose	Storage form of carbohydrate in the body

CASE STUDY

A 22-year-old African American man presents with four carious lesions acquired since his last dental hygiene recare appointment. While questioning the patient, you learn that he frequently skips meals and relies heavily on snacks to get him through the day.

1. What further information about his dietary intake do you need?
2. Could the patient's snacking habits be related to his increase in dental caries?
3. Which types of foods should be suggested as snack foods and why?
4. What other precautions could the patient practice that might be helpful in preventing further caries problems?

References

1. Mann J, Cummings JH, Englyst HN, et al: FAO/WHO scientific update on carbohydrates in human nutrition: conclusions. *Eur J Clin Nutr* 61(Suppl 1):S132–S137, 2007.
2. Centers for Disease Control (CDC): Trends in intake of energy and macronutrients—United States, 1971–2000. *MMWR Morb Mortal Wkly Rep* 53(04):80–82, 2004.
3. U.S. Department of Agriculture and U.S. Department of Health and Human Services: *Dietary Guidelines for Americans 2010.* ed 7, Washington, DC, 2010, U.S. Government Printing Office.
4. Welsh JA, Sharma AJ, Grellinger L, et al: Consumption of added sugars is decreasing in the United States. *Am J Clin Nutr* 94(3):728–734, 2011.

5. Drewnowski A, Mennella JA, Johnson SL, et al: Sweetness and food preference. *J Nutr* 142(6):1142S–1148S, 2012.

6. Schwartz N, Kaye EK, Nunn ME, et al: High fiber foods reduce periodontal disease progression in men aged 65 and older: The Veterans Affairs normative aging study/dental longitudinal study. *J Am Geriatr Soc* 60(4):676–683, 2012.

7. Clemens R, Kranz S, Mobley AR, et al: Filling America's fiber intake gap: summary of a roundtable to probe realistic solutions with a focus on grain-based foods. *J Nutr* 42(7):S1390–S1401, 2012.

8. Kristensen M, Toubro S, Jensen MG, et al: Whole grain compared with refined wheat decreases the percentage of body fat following a 12-week, energy-restricted dietary intervention in postmenopausal women. *J Nutr* 142(4):710–716, 2012.

9. Institute of Medicine (IOM), National Academy of Sciences: *Dietary reference intakes for energy, carbohydrates, fiber, fat, protein, and amino acids (macronutrients)*. Washington, DC, 2002, National Academy Press.

10. Joint FAO/WHO Expert Consultation: *Diet, Nutrition, and the prevention of chronic diseases*. Geneva, Switzerland, 2003, World Health Organization. Accessed August 16, 2013: http://www.who.int/nutrition/topics/5_population_nutrient/en/index.html.

11. U.S. Department of Agriculture: *Sugar and Sweeteners Outlook, January 17, 2013. Electronic Outlook Report from the Economic Research Service (ERS), SSS-M-293*. Accessed August 16 2013: www.ers.usda.gov/media/984570/sssm293.pdf.

12. Welsh JA, Sharma AJ, Grellinger L, et al: Consumption of added sugars is decreasing in the United States. *Am J Clin Nutr* 94(3):728–734, 2011.

13. Clemens R, Kranz S, Mobley AR, et al: Filling America's fiber intake gap: summary of a roundtable to probe realistic solutions with a focus on grain-based foods. *J Nutr* 42(7):S1390–S1401, 2012.

14. King DE, Mainous AG 3rd, Lambourne CA: Trends in dietary fiber intake in the United States, 1999–2008. *J Acad Nutr Diet* 112(5):642–648, 2012.

15. Hornick B, Dolven C, Liska D: The fiber deficit, part II: consumer misperceptions about whole grains and fiber. *Nutr Today* 47(3):104–109, 2012.

16. American Diabetes Association: Standards of medical care in diabetes—2012. *Diabetes Care* 35(Suppl 1):S11–S63, 2012.

17. Schorin MD, Sollid, K, Edge MS, et al: The science of sugars, part 3: sugars and chronic disease risks. *Nutr Today* 47(5):252–261, 2012.

18. Haymond MW: *Fact and Fiction. Live Webinar: From Metabolism to Epidemiology: Understanding Dietary Sugars and Health, June 4, 2012.* Accessed August 15, 2013: http://beverageinstitute.org/us/webinar/from-metabolism-to-epidemiology/.

19. Marriott BP, Olsho L, Hadden L, et al: Intake of added sugars and selected nutrients in the United States, National Health and Nutrition Examination Survey (NHANES) 2003–2006. *Crit Rev Food Sci Nutr* 50(3):228–258, 2010.

20. Morenga LT, Mallard S, Mann J: Dietary sugars and body weight: systematic review and meta-analyses of randomised controlled trials and cohort studies. *BMJ* 346:e7492, 2012.

21. Crain Communications: *Bottoms up! A look at America's drinking habits. Advertising Age, published June 26, 2011.* Accessed August 16, 2013: http://adage.com/article/news/consumers-drink-soft-drinks-water-beer/228422/.

22. Kit BK, Fakhouri TH, Park S, et al: Trends in sugar-sweetened beverage consumption among youth and adults in the United States: 1999–2010. *Am J Clin Nutr* 98(1):180–188, 2013.

23. Hernandez TL, Sutherland JP, Wolfe P, et al: Lack of suppression of circulating free fatty acids and hypercholesterolemia during weight loss on a high-fat, low-carbohydrate diet. *Am J Clin Nutr* 91(3):578–585, 2010.

24. Smith SR: A look at the low carbohydrate diet. *N Engl J Med* 361(23):2285–2288, 2009.

25. Merchant AT, Vatanparast H, Barlas S, et al: Carbohydrate intake and overweight and obesity among healthy adults. *J Am Diet Assoc* 109(7):1165–1172, 2009.

26. American Dental Association: *Role of sugar-free foods and medications in maintaining good oral health, 2002.* Accessed August 16, 2013: http://www.ada.org/1874.asp/.

27. Ehlen LA, Marshall TA, Qian F, et al: Acidic beverages increase the risk of in vitro tooth erosion. *Nutr Res* 28(5):299–303, 2008.

28. Nadimi H, Wesamaa H, Janket SJ, et al: Are sugar-free confections really beneficial for dental health? *Br Dent J* 211(7):E15, 2011.

29. Owens BM, Kitchens M: The erosive potential of soft drinks on enamel surface substrate: an in vitro scanning electron microscopy investigation. *J Contemp Dent Pract* 8(7):11–20, 2007.

30. Mickenautsch S, Leal SC, Yengopal V, et al: Sugar-free chewing gum and dental caries—a systematic review. *J Appl Oral Sci* 15(2):83–88, 2007.

31. Council on Clinical Affairs: *Guideline on xylitol use in caries prevention.* Chicago, 2011, American Academy of Pediatric Dentistry (AAPD). Accessed October 4, 2013: http://www.guideline.gov/content.aspx?id=34770.

32. Milgrom P, Lyk A, Rothen M: Xylitol and its vehicles for public health needs. *Adv Dent Res* 21(1):44–47, 2009.

33. Schorin MD, Sollid K, Edge MS, et al: The science of sugars, part 4: sugars and other health issues. *Nutr Today* 47(6):275–280.41, 2012.

34. Ibid., Ehlen, 2008.

35. Ibid., Nadimi, 2011.

36. Position of the Academy of Nutrition and Dietetics: Use of nutritive and nonnutritive sweeteners. *J Acad Nutr Diet* 112(5):739–758, 2012.

37. Hur Y, Reicks M: Relationship between whole-grain intake, chronic disease risk indicators and weight status among adolescents in the National Health and Nutrition Examination Survey, 1999–2004. *J Acad Nutr Diet* 112(1):46–55, 2012.

38. Ng SW, Slining MM, Popkin BM: Use of caloric and noncaloric sweeteners in U.S. consumer packaged foods, 2005–2009. *J Acad Nutr Diet* 112(11):1828–1834, 2012.

39. Gardner C, Wylie-Rosett J, Gidding SS, et al: Nonnutritive sweeteners: current use and health perspectives. *Circulation* 126(4):509–519, 2012.

40. Ibid., Position of the Academy of Nutrition and Dietetics, 2012.

41. Ibid., Position of the Academy of Nutrition and Dietetics, 2012.

42. Schorin MD, Sollid K, Edge MS, et al: The science of sugars, part 2. Sugars and a healthful diet. *Nutr Today* 47(4):175–182, 2012.

43. Rippe JM, Angelopoulos TJ: Sucrose, high-fructose corn syrup, and fructose, their metabolism and potential health effects: what do we really know? *Adv Nutr* 4(2):236–245, 2013.

44. Bravo S, Lowndes J, Sinnett S, et al: Consumption of sucrose and high fructose corn syrup does not increase liver fat or ectopic fat deposition in muscles. *Appl Physiol Nutr Metab* 38(6):681–688, 2013.

45. World Health Organization: *Obesity and overweight fact sheet No. 311, May 2012.* Accessed August 16, 2013: Available at http://www.who.int/mediacentre/factsheets/fs311/en/index.html.

46. Bray GA, Nielsen JS, Popkin BM: Consumption of high-fructose corn syrup in beverages may play a role in the epidemic of obesity. *Am J Clin Nutr* 79(4):537–543, 2004.

ⓔ EVOLVE RESOURCES

Please visit http://evolve.elsevier.com/Stegeman/nutritional for additional practice and study support tools.

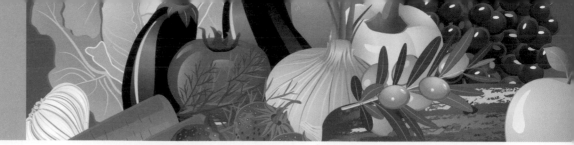

Chapter 5

Protein: The Cellular Foundation

Student Learning Outcomes

Upon completion of this chapter, the student will be able to complete the following student learning outcomes:

- List the possible fates of amino acids.
- Classify foods as sources of high-quality or lower-quality proteins.
- Explain how protein foods can be used to complement one another.
- Plan individualized menus to meet the recommended protein level for a diet containing animal foods, a vegetarian diet, and a vegan diet containing only plant proteins.

- Explain why various physiological states require different amounts of protein.
- Categorize the problems associated with protein deficiency or excess.
- Assess a patient's protein consumption in terms of deficiency or excess.
- Apply nutrition principles regarding food intake to prevent protein deficiency and protein excess into patient education.

Key Terms

Ad libitum
Bioavailability
Collagen
Complementary foods
Conditionally indispensable
Dipeptide
Erythema
Flexitarians
High-quality protein
Immune response
Immunocompromised
Immunoglobulins
Interstitial
Kwashiorkor
Lactovegetarian
Low-quality proteins

Marasmus
Necrosis
Necrotizing ulcerative gingivitis (NUG)
Nitrogen balance
Noma
Ovolactovegetarian
Ovovegetarian
Periodontium
Protein digestibility corrected amino acid (PDCAA) score
Protein-energy malnutrition (PEM)
Sarcopenia
Secretory immunoglobulin A (sIgA)
Thermogenesis
Vegan
Vegetarian

Test Your NQ

1. **T/F** A protein deficiency during childhood may lead to increased caries susceptibility related to alterations in tooth development and diminished salivary flow.
2. **T/F** Despite poor nutrition, malnourished children have a decreased rate of caries because they don't consume much sugar.
3. **T/F** Gelatin is a good source of high-quality protein.
4. **T/F** Older patients require less protein than younger adults.
5. **T/F** High protein intake strengthens the enamel of the tooth.

6. **T/F** An increase in protein intake without decreasing intake of other energy-containing nutrients may lead to an increase in fat stores rather than muscle.
7. **T/F** Amino acids are the building blocks of proteins.
8. **T/F** Marasmus is a protein-deficiency disorder.
9. **T/F** Protein requirements are based on the assumption that dispensable amino acids and kilocalories are provided in adequate amounts.
10. **T/F** Positive nitrogen balance occurs during periods of growth.

Until the middle of the 19th century, many scientists thought all life was composed of a single basic chemical: protein. Protein is present in every living cell, making up almost half of the dry weight of a cell. Second to water, protein is the most plentiful substance in the body. The United States is a nation of meat eaters, consuming more meat per capita than any other nation. Most Americans are unable or unwilling to plan a balanced meal without a meat entree. High-protein diets have been increasingly popular for weight reduction for many years, contributing to increased protein consumption. However, meat consumption has been declining for nearly a decade. Over the past few decades, beef consumption has trended downward as chicken's popularity has dramatically increased (Fig. 5-1). Consumers have numerous reasons for reducing their meat intake; the most frequently stated reasons are for health, economic (cost of meats has increased), and environmental concerns (a high meat diet is unsustainable). But the U.S. culture still values animal protein above other protein sources.

AMINO ACIDS

As described in detail in Chapter 2 and on the Evolve website, proteins are very large molecular structures containing the elements carbon, hydrogen, oxygen, and nitrogen, and sometimes sulfur and phosphorus. All the billions of proteins associated with life are made from combinations of 20 different amino acids. Amino acids can be compared to letters of the alphabet used in different sequences and combinations to make billions of words. An amino acid contains a basic, or amino, grouping ($-NH_2$) and an acidic, or carboxyl, grouping ($-COOH$). Figure 5-2 shows the general design of an amino acid.

The distinguishing feature of amino acids is the amine group, which is the body's source of nitrogen. The fundamental constituent of the protein molecule, called the side chain (R group), is the part of the structure that varies to form the many different amino acids found in humans.

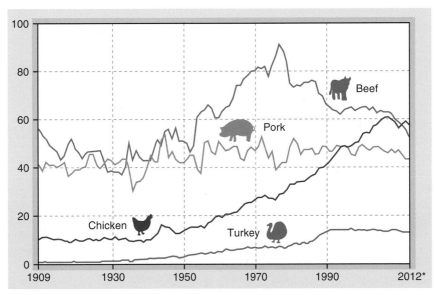

FIGURE 5-1 U.S. meat consumption per person, in pounds. Americans have been eating less beef and a lot more chicken. (From Earth Policy Institute. Wong, A/NPR: *A nation of meat of eaters: see how it all adds up.* June 27, 2012. Accessed August 17, 2013: http://www.npr.org/blogs/thesalt/2012/06/27/155527365/visualizing-a-nation-of-meat-eaters.)

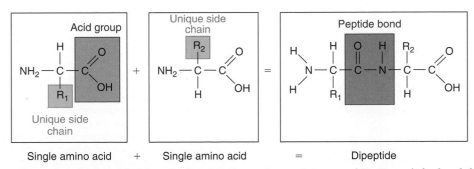

FIGURE 5-2 Structure of amino acids. (Modified from Mahan LK, Escott-Stump, S, Raymond JL: *Krause's food and the nutrition care process*, ed 13, St Louis, 2012, Saunders Elsevier.)

Amino acids combine with each other to make long chains. As shown in Figure 5-2, two amino acids together form a **dipeptide**. Several amino acids bound together form a polypeptide. Food and body proteins contain polypeptides. The number of amino acids in a protein varies greatly (from 100 to 300), but each protein has a specific number. The protein chain adopts a compact, folded, 3-dimensional structure (see Chapter 2, Fig. 2-9) that is essential to perform its basic function.

CLASSIFICATION

A prerequisite for life and health are the 20 amino acids, the building blocks of protein. These amino acids, listed in Table 5-1, can be classified as indispensable, dispensable, or conditionally indispensable. These classifications were previously known as essential, nonessential, and conditionally essential. Nine indispensable (essential) amino acids are required in the diet. Dispensable (nonessential) amino acids are essential for the body, but because they can be made from indispensable amino acids, they are not required in normal conditions. In certain nutritional or disease states, or stages of development, several dispensable amino acids become indispensable; these are classified as **conditionally indispensable.**

If any one of the indispensable amino acids is not available when a cell needs it for protein synthesis, the protein cannot be produced. The body is able to make adequate amounts of dispensable amino acids if a sufficient amount of protein is available to furnish the nitrogen needed and enough kilocalories are present to spare the catabolism (breakdown) of amino acids.

The amount of indispensable amino acids furnished by a food determines its ability to support growth, maintenance, and repair. A food with all the indispensible amino acids present is identified as a "complete" protein. When the nine indispensible amino acids are provided from a food in amounts adequate to maintain nitrogen balance and permit growth, the food is said to provide **high-quality protein**. **Nitrogen balance** refers to the balance of reactions in which protein substances are broken down or destroyed and rebuilt (Box 5-1). Healthy individuals excrete (in feces and urine, and from skin) the same amount of nitrogen as is consumed from their food. A patient with a burn or illness excretes more nitrogen than is ingested. In periods of growth, as in a child or pregnant woman, the body is in positive nitrogen balance (more protein is retained than is lost daily).

Complete protein foods have all the indispensible amino acids present in balanced amounts for human physiological requirements. If the quantity of one or more of the indispensible amino acids in a food is insufficient for optimal protein synthesis, the food is a source of low-quality protein. **Low-quality proteins**, if the only protein source consumed, support life but not normal growth. These include proteins found in legumes, nuts, and grains. The amino acid in short supply relative to need is referred to as the "limiting amino acid." High-quality proteins are well balanced in their indispensible amino acid content.

Table 5-1	Amino acids in the human diet	
Indispensable (Essential)	**Dispensable (Nonessential)***	**Conditionally Indispensable†**
Histidine**	Alanine	Arginine
Isoleucine	Aspartic acid	Cysteine
Leucine	Asparagine	Glutamine
Lysine	Glutamic acid	Glycine
Methionine	Serine	Proline
Phenylalanine		Tyrosine
Threonine		
Tryptophan		
Valine		

*Required in the diet when the body cannot produce enough to meet metabolic needs.

**Although histidine is considered indispensable, unlike the other eight indispensable amino acids, it does not fulfill the criteria of reducing protein deposition and inducing negative nitrogen balance promptly upon removal from the diet.

†Required in the diet when the body is unable to synthesize adequate amounts for metabolic functions for special pathophysiological conditions.

Data from Food and Nutrition Board, Institute of Medicine: *Dietary Reference Intakes for energy, carbohydrate, fiber, fat, fatty acids, cholesterol, protein, and amino acids (macronutrients)*. Washington, DC, 2002, National Academy Press.

BOX 5-1	Nitrogen Balance*

N balance: body protein constant
N intake = N excretion
Positive N balance: increase in body protein
N intake > N excretion
Negative N balance: decrease in body protein
N intake < N excretion

POSITIVE N BALANCE	**NEGATIVE N BALANCE**
Growth	Inadequate protein intake (e.g., fasting, gastrointestinal tract diseases)
Pregnancy or lactation	Inadequate energy intake
Recovery from illnesses, surgery, or trauma	Illnesses (e.g., fevers, infections, or wasting diseases)
Medications	Routine intake of glucocorticoids
Athletic training	Injury or immobilization
	Deficiency of indispensible amino acids
	Accelerated protein loss (e.g., albuminuria, protein-losing gastroenteropathy)
	Burns
	Increased secretion of thyroxine and glucocorticoids

*Because nitrogen is a unique component of protein metabolism, measurements of nitrogen and nitrogenous constituents in the blood and urine assess protein equilibrium in the body. Although "nitrogen balance" means that the output is equal to input, the amount of excreted nitrogen atoms is usually not the same as that ingested. For nitrogen equilibrium, not only must the diet contain the required amounts of protein, but also energy intake must be adequate to prevent protein being used for energy.

Table 5-2	Protein digestibility corrected amino acid score
Casein (milk protein)	1.00
Whey	1.00
Egg white	1.00
Beef protein	0.92
Soy	0.91
Whole wheat	0.40

Data from FAO/WHO Expert Consultation (1990) Protein Quality Evaluation. Food and Agricultural Organization of the United Nations, FAO Food and Nutrition Paper 51, Rome; European Dairy Association (1997) Nutritional Quality of Proteins. European Dairy Association, Brussels, Belgium; Renner, E. (1983) Milk and Dairy Products in Human Nutrition. W-Gmbh Volkswirtschaftlicher Verlag, München, pp. 90-130.

Protein digestibility corrected amino acid (PDCAA) score is the official method of evaluating protein quality for humans. Based on amino acid requirements of young children, it corrects for digestibility. After digestibility adjustments, proteins containing amino acids equal to or greater than requirements receive a PDCAA score of 1. Table 5-2 lists PDCAA scores for several proteins in foods. Proteins not containing indispensible amino acids in adequate amounts to support life have a low PDCAA score. Vegetable and some grain proteins are not digested as well as animal proteins, partly because the protein is encased in cell walls that make it less available to digestive enzymes. Vegetables and grains contain all the indispensible amino acids, but because one or more of these amino acids are present in a very low ratio, the protein they furnish has a low PDCAA score.

Dental Considerations

- Inquire about the patient's use of amino acid supplements because toxicity and amino acid imbalance syndromes may occur when an excess of one amino acid is ingested. For example, when large doses of tryptophan are taken, toxic metabolites build up, causing an unusual autoimmune disorder.

Nutritional Directions

- The PDCAA score indicates how well the body can digest and use a particular protein. The higher the number, the higher the protein quality because it contains all the indispensible amino acids in adequate amounts that are easily digested and absorbed.
- Protein from animals and fish (except for gelatin) are high-quality proteins, but are not essential to an adequate diet.

PHYSIOLOGICAL ROLES

Proteins are an essential part of a diet and perform many important physiological roles. However, protein is not the only important nutrient because others are essential for the body to fully use available protein. Proteins are the principal source of nitrogen for the body and are fundamental components of every human cell. Proteins are necessary for many

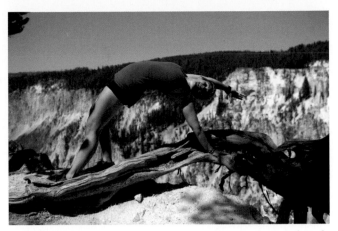

FIGURE 5-3 Protein is important to stimulate muscle growth and lean muscle mass, for physical strength and activity. (Reprinted with permission of D2 Studios, www.d2studios.net.)

physiological functions, which can be classified into the following seven categories:

1. *Generation of new body tissues.* Because protein is a constituent of all cells, it is necessary for growth. During periods of increased growth (infancy, childhood, adolescence, and pregnancy) and in periods of wound healing or recovery (illness, surgery, burns, or fever), the need for protein to build new tissues is increased. In some individuals, moderately high protein consumption may stimulate muscle protein growth, favoring retention of lean muscle mass, while improving metabolism (Fig. 5-3).[1]
2. *Repair of body tissues.* Body proteins are continuously being broken down, necessitating their replacement.
3. *Production of essential compounds.* Amino acids and proteins are constituents of regulatory enzymes, hormones, and other body secretions. The structural compound **collagen** is a protein substance in connective tissue that helps support body structures, such as skin, bones, teeth, and tendons. A low protein intake may affect all of these compounds.
4. *Regulation of fluid balance.* Protein dissolved in water forms a colloidal solution; in other words, it attracts water. Blood albumin (a protein) draws water from **interstitial** (space between tissue cells) fluid or cells to maintain blood volume. During protein deficiency, a decreased amount of protein in the blood causes a loss of osmotic balance, resulting in an accumulation of interstitial fluid (edema).
5. *Resistance to disease.* Antibodies, or **immunoglobulins**, the body's main protection from disease, are proteins. Low protein levels may negatively affect an individual's **immune response**, resulting in an inability to fight bacteria and other harmful organisms.
6. *Transport mechanisms.* Proteins enable insoluble fats to be transported through the blood.
7. *Energy.* When the nitrogen grouping is removed, the remaining carbon skeleton can be used for energy, furnishing 4 kcal/g. Although this is not one of its main functions, protein is used in this manner when (a) caloric

intake from carbohydrate and fat is inadequate, (b) protein intake exceeds requirements, and (c) indispensible amino acids are unavailable for synthesis of proteins.

REQUIREMENTS

Protein requirements for health are based on body size and rate of growth. The body requires more protein during growth periods or for maintenance and repair of a larger body mass. To a certain extent, the better the quality of protein (higher PDCAA score), the less quantity is required. Protein requirements are based on the assumption that indispensible amino acids and kilocalories are provided in adequate amounts.

The RDAs for protein vary proportionately for different ages and stages of life to adjust for growth rates. The IOM has determined that the daily minimum requirement of protein for adults is approximately 0.6 g/kg (see p. ii). Using 0.6 g/kg, a person weighing 150 lb (68.2 kg) would require 41 g of protein. Because RDAs provide a margin of safety, the IOM has established 0.8 g/kg daily as the RDA. With this standard, a patient weighing 150 lb (68.2 kg) requires 56 g protein. Table 5-3 lists the RDAs for protein for various stages of life. Ideally, protein needs are based on body weight, not energy intake. The average protein intake is approximately 100 g/day for men and 69 g/day for women.[2]

The *Dietary Guidelines* principally focus on maintaining a healthy body weight. Moderate evidence indicates that diets containing more than 35% of total kilocalories from protein are generally no more effective at controlling weight than 25% to 35% of total energy intake (see Table 5-3). Very few individuals consume protein amounts close to the highest acceptable macronutrient distribution range of 35% for their age/sex group. Box 5-2 provides guidelines related to protein intake to ensure adequate consumption of recommended nutrients. More and more Americans are becoming vegetarians (see *Health Application 5*). Vegetarians purposefully do not eat meat (beef, pork, poultry, seafood, other animal flesh, and sometimes by-products of animals). Protein consumption of many vegetarians is at the lower level, or below the 10% of kilocalories, recommended for Americans.

Some research indicates many adults may benefit from eating more than the minimum requirement. Many scientific studies indicate protein diets exceeding RDA (yet not the *Dietary Guidelines* maximum of 35% of kilocalories) could be beneficial in preventing sarcopenia and osteoporosis, maintaining mobility, and treating chronic diseases (e.g., type 2 diabetes and CHD).[3,4] Sarcopenia is the progressive loss of muscle mass and strength with aging, a condition many believe is normal for elderly individuals. Therefore, some researchers believe that overweight, obese, and older Americans may benefit by consuming 35% of their kilocalories from protein.

Conversely, the World Health Organization recommends 0.75 g protein per kilogram of lean body weight, which translates to 45 g protein daily for an average woman and 56 g for an average man. When any condition of health or disease causes a significant protein loss, an increased protein intake (greater than the RDA recommendation) prevents

Table 5-3	Protein recommendations			
		Recommended Dietary Allowances		
Life Stage/ Gender	Age (years)	Protein (g/kg)	Protein (g/d)	% Kilocalories
Infants	0-6 mo	1.52	9.1*	5-10
	7-12 mo	1.2	11	5-10
Children	1-3	1.05	13	5-10
	4-8	0.95	19	10-30
Males	9-13	0.95	34	10-30
	14-18	0.85	52	10-30
	19->70	0.80	56	10-35
Females	9-13	0.95	34	10-30
	14-18	0.85	46	10-30
	19->70	0.80	46	10-35
Pregnant	All ages	1.1	71 (+25 g/ day)	10-35
Lactating	All ages	1.3	71 (+25 g/ day)	10-35

Data from Institute of Medicine of the National Academies: *Dietary reference intakes for energy, carbohydrates, fiber, fat, protein, and amino acids.* Washington, DC, 2002, National Academy Press.
*Adequate intake, based on 0.8 g protein/kg body weight for reference body weight. For healthy, breastfed infants, the adequate intake is the mean intake.

BOX 5-2   2010 Dietary Guidelines Related to Protein

Foods to Reduce or Limit
- Reduce intake of kilocalories from solid fats.
  - Consume more nonfat or low-fat dairy products.
- Limit protein foods to 5.5-ounces a day (a deck of cards is about 3 ounces).

Foods to Increase
- Choose a variety of protein foods, which include seafood, lean meat and poultry, eggs, beans and peas, soy products, and unsalted nuts and seeds.
  - Eat more beans and peas, which are a natural source of fiber and protein.
  - Opt for lean meats, such as white meat of chicken without skin, loin and round cuts of beef and pork that are trimmed, flank or strip steak, and ground beef that's 90% lean or leaner.
  - Substitute beans for at least half of the meat, chicken, or pork in chili, burritos, pasta, or stir-fry dishes.
- Choose seafood in place of some meat and poultry.
  - Eat at least 8 ounces seafood a week (two 4-ounce or three 3-ounce servings).
  - Pregnant or breastfeeding women should eat 12 ounces seafood a week.
- Replace protein foods that are high in solid fats with proteins that are low in solid fats and kilocalories.
  - Replace high-fat meats with lean meats.

excessive loss of tissue and plasma proteins. Although these states increase protein requirements, RDAs have not been established for these conditions. Providing additional amounts through supplementation with high-quality proteins can help prevent protein malnutrition and shorten recovery periods. There is no compelling evidence for additional protein requirements for healthy adults undertaking resistance or endurance training, especially because Americans commonly ingest significantly more protein than is recommended.

Ordinarily, dietary protein is restricted only in some physiological disease states affecting the liver and kidney because these organs are heavily involved in protein metabolism and excretion of protein waste products. If the liver and kidney are diseased, excessive amounts of protein cannot be properly handled without further organ damage.

SOURCES

Foods with a high protein content are readily available in the United States. Table 5-4 lists the average protein content of some foods. Meat and milk food groups furnish most of the protein. Soy is a good source of protein and has other health benefits. Increased intake of cereal products also boosts protein intake. The protein content of items from the sample menu presented in Chapter 1, Fig. 1-2 is shown in Fig. 5-4.

Depending on sex, size, and activity level, *MyPlate* recommends 5.5 oz of cooked lean meat, poultry, or fish daily for adults. Protein foods, the purple portion of the plate, covers only one-fourth of the plate (see Fig. 1-3). About 3 Tbsp of chopped/ground meat, or the size of a small matchbox, equals 1 oz of meat; a small chicken drumstick or thigh is equivalent to 2 oz of meat; and a deck of cards or the size of your palm is approximately 3 oz. One-half cup of beans, or the amount that can fit in a cupped hand, or 1 Tbsp of peanut butter (size of a ping-pong ball) can be substituted for 1 oz of meat. Not to be overlooked, dairy is not optional, even though it is located above the plate where a glass would be placed. The *Dietary Guidelines* recommend 3 cups of fat-free or low-fat milk and dairy products daily for Americans 9 years of age and older, 2 to $2\frac{1}{2}$ cups for children 4 to 8 years, and 2 cups for children ages 2 to 3 years. Three cups of milk provide 24 g protein as well as other essential nutrients.

In most cases, digestibility and nutritional value are favorably affected by cooking procedures. Proper cooking sometimes facilitates digestion and use. Cooking makes egg albumin more readily digestible, and cooking soybeans increases amino acid bioavailability. Bioavailability indicates the amount of nutrient available to the body after absorption. Processing affects proteins in cereal by binding lysine (an amino acid), making it unusable by the body.

Table 5-4	Protein content of select foods	
Food	**Quantity**	**Protein (g)**
Pork chop, lean, cooked	2 oz	17
Beef, cooked, lean cuts	2 oz	17
Chicken, light meat, cooked	2 oz	16
Pinto beans, cooked	1 cup	15
Chicken, dark meat, cooked	2 oz	14
Cheddar cheese	2 oz	14
Nonfat dried skim milk powder	⅓ cup	14
Cottage cheese	½ cup	13
Cod fish, cooked	2 oz	13
Egg, hard boiled	2	13
American processed cheese	2 oz	10
Milk, whole, reduced fat, or low fat	1 cup	8-9
Peanut butter	2 Tbsp	8
Macaroni, cooked	1 cup	8
Thick milkshake	11 oz	7
Oatmeal, cooked	1 cup	6
Rice, brown, cooked	1 cup	5
Ice cream	1 cup	5
Rice, white, cooked	1 cup	4
Corn muffin, small	1	4
Enriched white bread	1 slice	2
Vegetables	½ cup	1-2
Fruits	½ cup	0.1-1

Data from U.S. Department of Agriculture, Agricultural Research Service. 2012. *USDA national nutrient database for standard reference, release 26.* Accessed October 1, 2013: http://ndb.nal.usda.gov/ndb/search/list.

Dental Considerations

- Most Americans consume almost twice as much protein as recommended in the RDAs.
- When assessment indicates a normal consumption of 1.5 g/kg or more above the RDA for protein, this is considered a high-protein diet. Further increases may not be beneficial and may contribute to increased fat stores and dehydration.
- An inadequate protein intake could affect any or all of the physiological functions of protein. If dietary intake seems inadequate, evaluate the patient's status in the areas described in "Physiological Roles" on p. 91.
- Assessing protein intake of patients with periodontal issues is especially important. Protein deficiencies may compromise the physiological systemic response to inflammation and infection, and periodontal problems may increase the protein requirement to promote healing in patients with inadequate or marginal protein intake.
- One rule of thumb is protein should provide 10% to 35% of caloric intake. If protein intake seems inappropriate, determine caloric or protein intake or both. The adequacy of intake can be established by using one of two methods. As an example, assuming consumption of 2200 kcal/day, the amount of protein based on total energy intake is calculated as follows:
  2200 kcal × 0.35 (maximum recommended % of total kcal from protein) = 770 kcal from proteins or less
  770 kcal ÷ 4 (kcal/g protein) = 193 g or less of protein
- The intake of 193 g protein is the highest level recommended. Because 35% is the upper limit, protein consumption above this level may jeopardize adequate intakes of nutrients available from other food sources.

Continued

Sample Menu		Ovolactovegetarian Menu	
Breakfast	Protein (g)	**Breakfast**	Protein (g)
1 c Frosted Mini Wheat cereal	5	1 c Complete wheat bran flakes cereal	4
12 oz skim milk	12	12 oz skim milk	12
12 oz black coffee	1	1/2 small banana	1
Mid-morning snack		**Mid-morning snack**	
1 small orange	1	1 small orange	1
12 oz water		12 oz water	
Lunch		**Lunch**	
Sandwich with		1 sandwich wrap, filled with	
3 oz tuna	22	vegetables and rice	16
1 medium boiled egg	6		6
1 tbsp light mayonnaise			
1 tbsp pickle relish			
1/4 c thinly sliced cucumber		1/4 c thinly sliced cucumber	
2 slices tomato		2 slices tomato	
2 thin slices whole grain bread	4		
1/4 c cauliflorets		1/4 c cauliflorets	
8 baby carrots	1	8 baby carrots	1
10 red pepper slices		10 red pepper slices	
1 medium apple		1 medium apple	
12 oz water		12 oz water	
Mid-afternoon snack		**Mid-afternoon snack**	
1 oz dry roasted almonds (no salt)	6	1 oz dry roasted almonds (no salt)	6
1 c seedless grapes	1	1 c seedless grapes	1
8 oz herbal tea		8 oz herbal tea	
Dinner		**Dinner**	
4 oz pot roast beef cooked with	36	1 c baked beans (vegetarian)	12
1/4 c mushrooms	2	1/2 c sauteed mushrooms	
1/2 c enriched white rice cooked with	2		
1/4 c low sodium vegetable juice (V8)	2	6 oz low sodium vegetable juice (V-8)	
1 c cooked kale	2	1 c cooked kale	2
2 c tossed salad with lettuce,	2	2 c tossed salad with lettuce, avocado,	
avocado, tomatoes, and carrots		tomatoes, and carrots	1
1 tbsp low sodium cheddar cheese	2	2 tbsp low sodium cheddar cheese	3
2 tbsp vinaigrette salad dressing		2 tbsp vinaigrette salad dressing	
1 medium wedge cantaloupe	1	1 medium wedge cantaloupe	1
12 oz iced tea		12 oz iced tea	
Evening snack		**Evening snack**	
12 oz skim milk	12	12 oz skim milk	12
1/2 whole wheat bagel with raisins	5	1/2 whole wheat bagel with raisins	5
and 1 tbsp fat free cream cheese	2	1 tbsp peanut butter	4
Totals	**126**		**81**

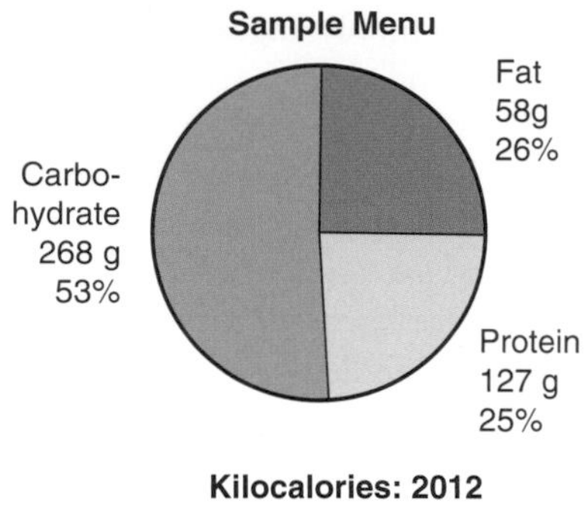

Sample Menu — Fat 58g 26%, Carbohydrate 268 g 53%, Protein 127 g 25%. Kilocalories: 2012

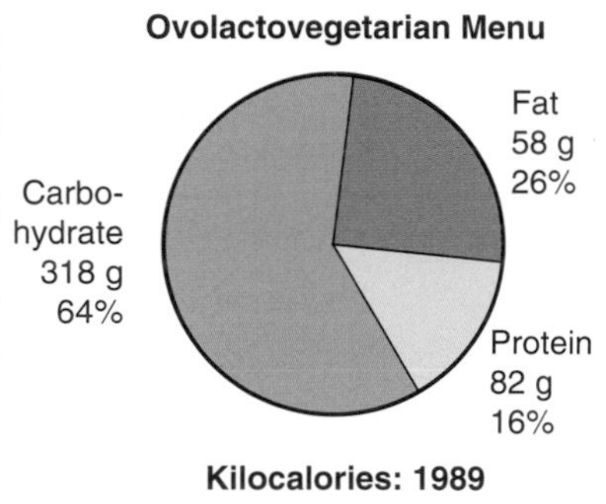

Ovolactovegetarian Menu — Fat 58 g 26%, Carbohydrate 318 g 64%, Protein 82 g 16%. Kilocalories: 1989

FIGURE 5-4 Protein content of sample menu and modifications for ovolactovegetarian diet. (USDA's Food and Nutrient Database for Dietary Studies, 5.0 [2012] was used to calculate nutrient values, using the SuperTracker.)

Dental Considerations—cont'd

- A second method of calculating percentage of protein intake based on actual protein intake: Protein intake of 55 g with kcal intake of 2200 kcal:

  55 (g protein) × 4 (kcal/g protein) = 220 kcal from protein

  220 (kcal from proteins) ÷ 2200 (total kcal intake) × 100(%) = 10% of total kcal from protein

  Because 10% is the lower limit, this patient's protein may be inadequate, and professional counseling may be warranted. Refer the patient to an RDN.

- Do not overemphasize animal sources of protein to patients on restricted incomes (e.g., elderly, homeless, and impoverished individuals). Too much emphasis on high-protein foods may result in inadequate amounts of other nutrients in the diet, especially when the food budget is low. Complementary sources of protein (described in *Health Application 5*), which are less expensive, can provide adequate protein.

- Evaluate food intake by gathering data from the patient in comparison with the recommended servings from *MyPlate* for the stage of growth, and Dietary Reference Intakes (DRIs) for kilocalorie and protein requirements (see p. ii).

Nutritional Directions

- Additional dietary protein is unnecessary for healthy adults participating in endurance or resistance exercise. Studies indicate that endurance athletes may need 1.2 to 1.4 g/kg per day and strength training athletes protein needs may need 1.2 to 1.7 g/kg protein per day.[5] The amount of protein needed by an athlete should be determined by a Board Certified Specialist in Sports Dietetics or an RDN specializing in sports nutrition.
- Protein requirements should be met by foods from several sources (including different animal protein foods) because of other nutrients that accompany the protein. For example, pork is an excellent source of thiamin, while red meats furnish a significant amount of iron. In contrast, too many egg yolks in the diet contribute excessive cholesterol.
- Animal sources of protein are generally the most expensive. When patients have limited resources, counsel them to (a) eat protein in adequate but not excessive amounts, (b) use a variety of proteins of lower quality (which are less expensive), and (c) purchase less expensive kinds of protein foods (see Chapter 16, Table 16-2).
- The color of the eggshell is not related to its nutritional value. The breed of the hen determines the color.
- Reinforce the lack of benefit and the possible danger of taking amino acid supplements if protein intake is adequate.

UNDERCONSUMPTION AND HEALTH-RELATED PROBLEMS

Although protein supplies in the United States are plentiful, and drastic protein deficiency is uncommon, several groups of individuals are susceptible to insufficient intakes: (a) elderly individuals, (b) individuals with low income, (c) strict vegetarians or vegans, (d) individuals with a lack of education or who are unwilling to shop wisely, and (e) patients who are chronically ill or hospitalized (e.g., patients with AIDS, anorexia nervosa, or cancer). The decision to intentionally restrict dietary protein to improve bone health is unwarranted. Recent epidemiological and meta-analysis studies suggest that dietary protein works synergistically with calcium to improve calcium retention and bone metabolism.[6]

Fewer than 10% of U.S. adults over 70 years of age get less than the recommended 0.8 g/kg body weight per day. Lower consumption of protein by older Americans may be related to cost, inability to prepare nutritious meals, depression, difficulty chewing, or concerns about the fat and cholesterol content of meats. Inadequate amounts of dietary protein contribute to sarcopenia. For the older population, a moderate increase in dietary protein intake (above the RDA of 0.8 g/kg) may be beneficial to bone health, while still falling within the safe and acceptable range for protein consumption.[7]

Certain physiological conditions and impaired digestion or absorption cause excessive protein losses and may precipitate **protein-energy malnutrition (PEM)**. Although PEM is uncommon in the United States, given the above-mentioned conditions, malnutrition is frequently unrecognized. PEM is usually accompanied by other nutritional deficiencies. Separating effects of different nutrient deficiencies by observing clinical symptoms is often difficult. PEM affects the whole body, including every component of the orofacial complex.

The occurrence of PEM during critical developmental stages, including prenatal and postnatal periods, may affect developing tissues or lead to irreversible changes in oral tissues. During tooth development, mild-to-moderate protein deficiency results in smaller molars, significantly delayed eruption, and retardation during development of the mandible. Smaller salivary glands result in diminished salivary flow; this saliva is different in its protein composition and amylase and aminopeptidase activity, compromising the immune function of saliva.

Poor nutrition results in delayed eruption and exfoliation of deciduous teeth. Although malnourished children have an increased rate of caries, the peak caries experience is delayed by approximately 2 years. The increased caries rate may simply be related to length of time a tooth is in the oral cavity; if the delay in exfoliation is greater than delay in eruption, the tooth is in the mouth a longer time, and it is exposed to caries-producing bacteria longer. Children with malnutrition (e.g., in developing countries and in many urban and rural areas in developed countries) have different dietary habits overall and oral environments that are not conducive to dental caries. However, the teeth in these populations are highly susceptible to dental caries. Increased caries susceptibility may be related to alterations in structure of tooth crowns and diminished salivary flow, or changes in saliva composition may be related to malnutrition issues.

Epithelium, connective tissue, and bone also may be poorly developed. An increase in acid solubility associated with chemical alterations of the exposed enamel surface may contribute to increased caries susceptibility.

The **periodontium** includes hard and soft tissues surrounding and supporting the teeth: gingiva, alveolar mucosa, cementum, periodontal ligaments, and alveolar bone. An insufficient intake of protein creates negative nitrogen balance, decreasing nitrogen reserves, blood protein levels, and resistance of the periodontium to infections. In addition, the ability of the periodontium to withstand the stress of injury or surgery is reduced, and recovery periods are longer. In malnourished children, **secretory immunoglobulin A (sIgA)** levels are depressed. sIgA is the predominant immunoglobulin, or antibody, in oral, nasal, intestinal, and other mucosal secretions. It provides the first line of defense in the oral cavity. Low sIgA levels in malnourished children probably play a role in their increased susceptibility to mucosal infections.

PEM may be a major reason for increased incidence of **noma** and **necrotizing ulcerative gingivitis (NUG)**, conditions that are strongly associated with depressed immune responses caused by nutritional deficiencies, stress, and infection (see Chapter 19, Fig. 19-4). Noma is a progressive **necrosis** (degeneration and cellular death) that usually manifests as a small ulcer on the gingiva that spreads to produce extensive destruction of lips, cheeks, and tissues covering the jaw with an accompanying foul odor. NUG is characterized by **erythema** (marginated redness of mucous membranes caused by inflammation) and necrosis of the interdental papillae. This painful gingivitis is generally accompanied by a metallic taste and foul oral odor. Cratered papillae often remain after treatment of the disease.

NUG sometimes occurs among college students who are under a great deal of psychological stress and have poor eating habits. It also can be observed in individuals who live in developed countries and are severely debilitated or **immunocompromised** (having an immune response weakened by a disease or pharmacological agent), or in children 2 to 6 years old who live in developing countries, are malnourished, and have recently experienced a stressful event, such as viral disease.

NUG can be precipitated by emotionally stressful situations that affect eating patterns, leading to acute deficiencies and depressed immune response to bacteria normally found in the oral cavity. Decreased host resistance to infection may permit gingival lesions to spread rapidly into adjacent tissues, producing extensive necrosis and destruction of orofacial tissues, whereas in a healthy individual, the lesion is limited to the gingiva alone. Wound healing is also delayed (see Chapter 19 for further discussion).

In other areas of the world, where quantities of high-quality protein and kilocalories are insufficient, PEM is commonly seen. **Kwashiorkor** develops when young children consume adequate kilocalories and inadequate high-quality protein (Fig. 5-5). It is almost exclusively seen in association with famine in the tropics. It usually appears after the child has been weaned from breast milk. **Marasmus** occurs in infants when both protein and kilocalories are deficient in the diet.

Kwashiorkor and marasmus are very serious health problems that have received much attention by the United Nations and the World Health Organization. Incaparina, a food powder made from corn, cottonseed, and sorghum with mineral and vitamin supplements; skim milk powder; and

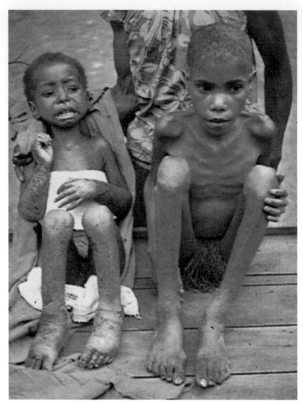

FIGURE 5-5 Kwashiorkor and marasmus in brothers. The younger brother, on the left, has kwashiorkor with generalized edema, skin changes, pale reddish yellow hair, and an unhappy expression. The older child, on the right, has marasmus, with generalized wasting, spindly arms and legs, and an apathetic expression. (From Peters W, Pasvol G, editors: *Tropical medicine and parasitology*, ed 5, London, 2006, Mosby.)

the addition of lysine to cereal products have been used to improve nutritional status in developing countries. However, most of these efforts to improve the nutritional status worldwide have not been well accepted for various reasons, and protein-energy problems in the world still exist.

Dental Considerations

- When assessing for marasmus or kwashiorkor, remember the main difference between the two conditions is the presence of some subcutaneous fat tissue in individuals with kwashiorkor and edema, especially in the abdomen, feet, and legs. Fat stores and edema are absent in marasmus. Assess the patient's financial status because poverty is a major cause of PEM and has been identified in rural and urban inner city areas in the United States. To assess for inadequate protein intake, look for frequent or extended periods of fasting, medications that cause anorexia, abnormal food intake, nausea and vomiting, and problems with hair (dull, dry, brittle, breaks easily), skin (flaky and dry), or fingernails (dry and cracked, spoon-shaped).
- Treatment of malnutrition requires referral to a healthcare provider or an RDN.

- Malnourished patients take longer to heal and regain strength and are at risk for frequent infections. Adequate infection control procedures are particularly important for these patients.
- The protein requirement of older adults is the same as that of young adults; however, older adults are frequently not motivated to eat because of low income level, transportation problems, depression and loneliness, edentulous status, and gustatory (taste and smell) changes. Decreased protein intake is common as a result of ill-fitting dentures or edentulousness. Closely assess protein intake of older patients.
- In the United States, noma-like lesions may occur in patients with cancer whose immune systems have been severely impaired by chemotherapy.

Nutritional Directions

- Suggest Meals-on-Wheels or community senior centers for older patients with an inadequate diet, and refer them to a social worker.
- Suggest protein supplementation of the diet by adding skim milk powder to milk, soups, or mashed potatoes (if the patient is not lactose intolerant) and by adding cheese to foods.

OVERCONSUMPTION AND HEALTH-RELATED PROBLEMS

An upper limit for safe levels of protein intake has not been determined. Most patients believe no upper limits for protein exist. Americans frequently eat 150% to 200% of the RDA for protein. Excessive protein intake can contribute to obesity because any energy-providing nutrient consumed in excess of physiological needs is converted to fat and stored.

For many years, general consensus in the medical community was that high protein intake had a negative impact on calcium and bone metabolism. Numerous studies have shown that a higher protein intake does not have an adverse effect on bone health except in a context of inadequate calcium supply.[8,9]

When protein intake is excessive, fluid imbalances may occur in all age groups, but especially in infants. Metabolism of 100 kcal of protein requires 350 g of water compared with 50 g of water for a similar amount of carbohydrates or fats. Water requirements are increased as well as the end products of protein metabolism in the bloodstream.

It is controversial whether popular high-protein diets are excessive in protein content. Usually a high-protein diet refers to 25% to 35% of kilocalories coming from protein foods. Regardless, this trend stimulated scientific research that has expanded the scientific knowledge base in this realm. Higher protein diets support weight control by enhancing loss of body fat with less muscle loss and improved control of blood glucose levels. Dietary protein may aid in weight loss by increasing satiation; increasing muscle mass, which burns more kilocalories; increasing thermogenesis (production of body heat); and decreasing energy efficiency. Protein intake generally increases satiety to a greater extent than carbohydrate or fat and may facilitate a reduction in ad libitum (as desired) energy consumption.

Obtaining adequate protein, or within the upper range of recommended amounts, is an important dietary concern, especially for weight loss or management, or for physical strength and activity. To maximize weight loss using a high-protein diet, the goal should be 120 g protein daily. Other macronutrients also need to be considered. If the principal source of protein is red meat and regular dairy products, intake of cholesterol and saturated fat content is high which raises the risk of CHD, including stroke. A study involving 29,000 postmenopausal women found participants who reported the highest protein intakes from red meat and dairy products had approximately a 40% higher risk of dying of CHD than those with the lowest intake of these foods.[10] Good choices of high protein, low fat foods include fish, skinless chicken, low fat dairy products, and lean beef and pork.

If carbohydrates are severely restricted by an individual eating primarily protein foods, high fiber foods are limited. High fiber plant foods help lower blood lipids. Restriction of plant-based carbohydrate foods limits nutrients that offer protection against cancer and other diseases and causes problems such as constipation and diverticulosis.

Although high protein intake is not associated with diminished kidney function in individuals with healthy kidneys, it appears that high protein diets may be harmful to the kidneys in individuals with preexisting metabolic renal dysfunction.[11,12] The American Diabetes Association recommends limiting protein intake to less than 20% of total kilocalories (100 g protein for a 2000-kcal diet).[13]

Dental Considerations

- Protein intake exceeding daily caloric requirements can result in additional fat stores and obesity.

Nutritional Directions

- Extremely high protein intake is especially undesirable in infants.
- Because proteins must be metabolized by the liver and filtered by the kidneys, excessive amounts (more than 200% of the RDA) result in additional work by or stress on these organs.

HEALTH APPLICATION **5**   Vegetarianism

Despite the fact that protein is not limited in the U.S. food supply, some people choose plant sources of protein for health reasons or because of philosophical, ecological, or religious convictions. Large numbers of vegetarian cookbooks and meatless "veggie" burgers and sausage-style products would lead one to believe vegetarianism is a growing consumer movement. The Vegetarian Resource Group indicates approximately 4% of the population are true vegetarians, or approximately 9 million Americans.[14] "Self-described" vegetarians are

not true vegetarians because they occasionally eat fish and poultry. These people are known as "semi-vegetarians" or flexitarians.

Technically, variations of vegetarian diets differ in the types of foods included. In a lactovegetarian diet, dairy products are consumed in addition to plant proteins (lacto- comes from the Latin word for milk, lactis). Meat, poultry, fish, and eggs are excluded. Milk and cheese products, which complement plant foods and enhance the amino acid content, are included.

Continued

HEALTH APPLICATION 5   Vegetarianism—cont'd

The ovolactovegetarian diet is supplemented with milk, cheese, and eggs (*ovo-* comes from the Latin word for egg, *ovum*). Only meat, poultry, and fish are excluded. If adequate quantities of eggs, milk, and milk products are consumed, all nutrients are likely to be provided in sufficient quantities. The ovovegetarian diet consists of protein foods from plants with the addition of eggs. Meat, poultry, fish, and dairy products are excluded. Strict supervision is unnecessary for these three groups. The vegan (or strict vegetarian) diet is the strictest type and contains only food from plants, including vegetables, fruits, and grains. No foods of animal origin are allowed (e.g., meat, milk, cheese, eggs, and butter).

Some groups, especially Seventh-Day Adventists, supplement protein intake with textured vegetable protein products. These meat substitutes are produced from vegetable proteins, usually soybeans. The protein in textured vegetable protein products is of good quality, but these products may have high sodium content.

Indispensible amino acids can be provided by plants, but larger amounts of these plant products must be consumed to match the protein obtained from animal sources. Indispensible amino acids present in low levels in grains are abundant in other plants, such as legumes. Beans are low in methionine and tryptophan, and corn is low in lysine and threonine. When eaten together, as in pinto beans and cornbread, they are said to be complementary foods, and less volume is required.

Protein from a single source is seldom consumed alone. Foods are usually combined without awareness that they are complementary to each other (e.g., beans are usually combined with rice, bread, or crackers [wheat], or tortillas or cornbread [corn]). When a combination of plant proteins is eaten throughout the day, the amino acids provided by each complement each other; that is, the deficiencies of one are offset by the adequacies of another. Additionally, small amounts of high-quality proteins can be combined with plant foods, as in macaroni and cheese or cereal and milk, to provide adequate amounts of indispensable amino acids. If caloric intake is adequate, protein requirements are met when a variety of protein-containing foods are eaten throughout the day. Foods providing complementary amino acids do not have to be consumed at the same time.

With some basic nutrition knowledge, vegetarian foods can be selected that are healthy and nutritionally balanced. The major difference is the protein source. The Vegetarian Food Pyramid (Fig. 5-6) and *My Vegan Plate* (Fig. 5-7) are designed specifically to address nutrient inadequacies and reduced mineral bioavailability of vegetarian and vegan diets. Figure 5-6 indicates the number of servings recommended for various caloric levels to meet recommended nutrient needs. Table 5-5 indicates changes in number of servings from the food groups to meet nutrient recommendations for various life stages. By using a variety of principally unrefined foods, and enough kilocalories to promote good health, protein quantity and other nutrients can be adequate for most individuals.

Vegetarian diets generally result in lower dietary intake of saturated fat and cholesterol, and high levels of dietary fiber, magnesium, potassium, vitamins C and E, and folate. Key nutrients that may fall short of the DRIs in the vegan diet and less often in the vegetarian diet include zinc, calcium, vitamins D and B_{12}, and long-chain n-3 fatty acids.[15-16]

Persons following a vegan diet must pay closer attention to food choices and will need supplementation or fortification of vitamins B_{12} and D, and possibly zinc and iodine. Vitamin B_{12} deficiency rates are especially high for pregnant women, adolescents, older adults, and those who have adhered to a vegetarian diet since birth.[17] Box 5-3 summarizes information that can be used in planning healthy and nutritionally balanced vegetarian diets that meet calcium and vitamins B_{12} and D requirements of adults. Commonly available fortified foods (e.g., fortified breakfast cereals and nondairy soymilks) are emphasized to ensure good sources of vitamins B_{12} and D, and calcium. Because of difficulties consuming adequate volumes of food to meet nutritional needs, the vegan diet is not recommended for infants, children, or pregnant/lactating women. Breastfed infants of two vegan mothers in the United States developed brain abnormalities as a result of vitamin B_{12} deficiency.[18] More information can be found at http://www.theveganrd.com/food-guide-for-vegans. During periods of rapid growth, vegans should be referred to an RDN.

Much can be said of the healthy aspects of vegetarian diets. Vegetarian diets can meet the DRIs as long as the variety and amounts of foods are adequate. That vegetarian diets and lifestyles seem to be conducive to good health is exemplified by vegetarians exhibiting better weight control, improved gastrointestinal function, fewer breast and colon cancers, better glucose control, a lower incidence of gallstones, lower blood pressure, a decreased rate of CHD, and greater longevity.[19-22] These advantages are not attributed solely to avoidance of meat products, but benefits from phytochemical-rich plant foods. For instance, beans, legumes, and whole-grain products help with blood glucose control; plant foods are associated with a lower risk of CHD. When working with a vegetarian patient, keep lines of communication open by respecting their decision, unless eating habits are potentially harmful. Patients who have an interest in pursuing a vegetarian diet should be encouraged to do so. All patients should be encouraged to have more meatless meals (see http://www.meatlessmonday.com/) and to consume more plant proteins.

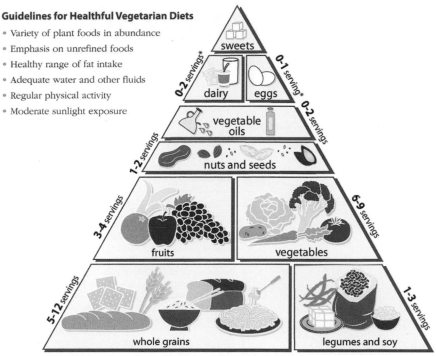

Guidelines for Healthful Vegetarian Diets

- Variety of plant foods in abundance
- Emphasis on unrefined foods
- Healthy range of fat intake
- Adequate water and other fluids
- Regular physical activity
- Moderate sunlight exposure

* A reliable source of vitamin B12 should be included if no dairy or eggs are consumed.

Other Lifestyle Recommendations **Daily Exercise** **Water**—eight, 8 oz. glasses per day **Sunlight**—10 minutes a day to activate vitamin D

Calories/day ▶	1600kcal/day	2000kcal/day	2500kcal/day	1600kcal/day	2000kcal/day	2500kcal/day
Food Groups	vegan servings/day			lacto-ovo servings/day		
Whole Grains	5	7	12	5	6	9
Legumes and Soy	3	3	3	3	3	3
Vegetables	6	8	9	6	8	9
Fruits	3	4	4	3	4	4
Nuts and Seeds	2	2	2	1	1	2
Vegetable Oils	1	2	2	1	2	2
Dairy Products	0	0	0	2	2	2
Eggs	0	0	0	1/2 egg	1/2 egg	1/2 egg
Sweets	Optional					

LOMA LINDA UNIVERSITY • SCHOOL OF PUBLIC HEALTH • DEPARTMENT OF NUTRITION
©2008 www.llu.edu/llu/sph/nutrition

FIGURE 5-6 The vegetarian food pyramid. (From Loma Linda University, School of Public Health. © 2008 Loma Linda University, School of Public Health, Department of Nutrition. Accessed August 17, 2013: http://www.vegetariannutrition.org/food-pyramid.pdf.)

Table 5-5 **Modifications to the vegetarian food pyramid (Fig. 5-6) for children, adolescents, and pregnant and lactating women**

	Food Group*		
Life Cycle	Vitamin B₁₂–rich Foods (servings)	Beans/Nuts/Seeds/Egg (servings)	Calcium-rich Foods (servings)
Child (4-8 years)	2	5	6
Adolescent (9-13 years)	2	6	10
Adolescent (14-18 years)	3	6	10
Pregnancy	4	7	8
Lactation	4	8	8

From Messina V, Melina V, Mangels AR: A new food guide for North American vegetarians. *J Am Diet Assoc* 2003;103(6):771-775.
*The number of servings in each group is the minimum amount needed. The minimum number of servings from other groups is not different from the vegetarian food guide (see Fig. 5-6). Additional foods can be chosen from any of the groups in the vegetarian food guide to meet energy needs.

Vegan MY ^ PLATE

Nutrition Tips:

*Choose mostly whole grains.
*Eat a variety of foods from each of the food groups.
*Adults age 70 and younger need 600 IU of vitamin D daily.
  Sources include fortified foods (such as some soymilks) or a vitamin D supplement.
*Sources of iodine include iodized salt (3/8 teaspoon daily) or
  an iodine supplement (150 micrograms).
*See www.vrg.org for recipes and more details.

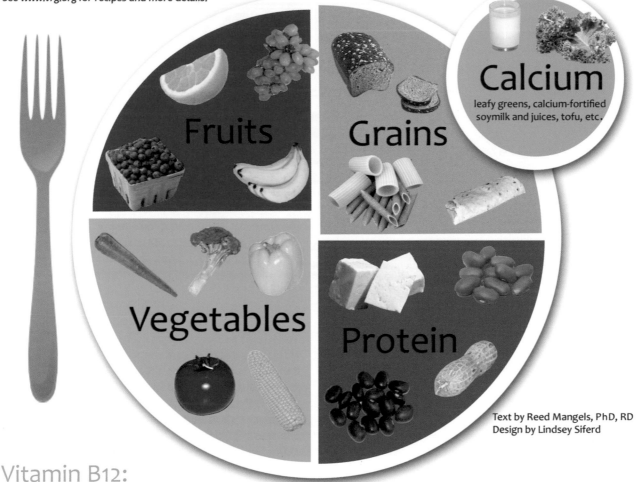

Calcium
leafy greens, calcium-fortified
soymilk and juices, tofu, etc.

Fruits

Grains

Vegetables

Protein

Text by Reed Mangels, PhD, RD
Design by Lindsey Siferd

Vitamin B12:

Vegans need a reliable source of vitamin B12. Eat daily a couple of servings of fortified foods
such as B12-fortified soymilk, breakfast cereal, meat analog, or Vegetarian Support Formula nutritional yeast.
Check the label for fortification. If fortified foods are not eaten daily,
you should take a vitamin B12 supplement (25 micrograms daily).

Note:

Like any food plan, this should only serve as a general guide for adults.
The plan can be modified according to your own personal needs. This is not personal
medical advice. Individuals with special health needs should consult a registered
dietitian or a medical doctor knowledgeable about vegan nutrition.

VRg. The Vegetarian
Resource Group P.O. Box 1463 Baltimore, MD 21203 www.vrg.org (410) 366-8343

FIGURE 5-7 My Vegan Plate. (From The Vegetarian Resource Group, P.O. Box 1463 Baltimore, MD 21203. Accessed August 17, 2013: http://www.vrg.org/nutshell/MyVeganPlate.pdf.)

**BOX
5-3**   **Tips for Planning Vegetarian Meals**

1. Choose a wide variety of foods.
2. The number of servings in each group is the minimum amounts needed. Choose more foods from any of the groups to meet energy needs.
3. A serving from the calcium-rich food group provides approximately 10% of adult daily requirements. Choose eight servings per day. These also count toward servings from the other food groups in the guide. For example, ½ cup (125 mL) of calcium-fortified fruit juice counts as a calcium-rich food and counts toward servings from the fruit group.
4. Include two servings every day of foods that supply omega-3 fats (see Chapter 6). Foods rich in omega-3 fats are found in the legumes/nuts group and in the fats group. A serving is 1 tsp of flaxseed oil, 3 tsp of canola or soybean oil, 1 Tbsp of ground flaxseed, or ¼ cup walnuts. For the best balance of fats in your diet, olive and canola oils should be chosen for cooking.
5. Nuts and seeds may be used in place of servings from the other choices in the fats group.

6. Be sure to get adequate vitamin D from daily sun exposure or through fortified foods or supplements. Cow's milk and some brands of soymilk and breakfast cereals are fortified with vitamin D.
7. Include at least three good food sources of vitamin B_{12} in your diet every day. These include 1 Tbsp of *Red Star* Vegetarian Support Formula nutritional yeast, 1 cup fortified soymilk, ½ cup cow's milk, ¾ cup yogurt, 1 large egg, 1 oz of fortified breakfast cereal, or ½ oz of fortified meat substitute. If these foods are not consumed regularly (at least three servings per day), take a daily vitamin B_{12} supplement of 5 to 10 µg or a weekly vitamin B_{12} supplement of 2000 µg.
8. If you include sweets or alcohol in your diet, consume these foods in moderation. Get most of your daily kilocalories from foods in the vegetarian food guide.

Adapted from Messina V, Melina V, Manges AR: A new food guide for North American vegetarians. *J Am Diet Assoc* 2003;103(6):771-775.

 Case Application for the Dental Hygienist

A single mother of two children comes to the clinic complaining about sensitivity to hot and cold foods and bleeding gums. She has recently lost her job, and child support payments are irregular. She is very concerned about the limited amount of protein foods she is able to purchase with her food stamps. Based on her diet diary, her caloric intake is 1800 kcal per day, and protein is approximately 50 g. Food intake is principally pastas, tortillas, chips, sweet pastries, and sodas.

Nutritional Assessment

- Willingness to learn
- Knowledge base of protein, carbohydrate, and fat principles for optimal nutrition
- Cultural beliefs
- Recent percentage of kilocalories from protein (11%)
- Types of protein intake and total nutrient intake
- Overall nutrient intake
- Carbonated beverage intake

Nutritional Diagnosis

Altered health maintenance and limited nutrition knowledge related to insufficient funds to purchase foods to provide adequate nutrients.

Nutritional Goals

The patient will verbalize three principles concerning protein as well as the benefits from other nutrients. The patient will consume foods providing complementary protein and incorporate some fruits and dairy products into her menus.

Nutritional Implementation

Intervention: Educate on: (a) the seven functions or roles of protein, (b) the difference between indispensable amino acids and

dispensable amino acids, (c) the difference between high-quality and lower quality protein, and (d) how to incorporate complementary protein into menus.
Rationale: Knowledge corrects inaccurate information.
Intervention: Discuss cheaper sources of protein (see Chapter 16, Table 16-2).
Rationale: Good sources of protein do not have to be high-priced meats.
Intervention: Encourage the use of milk and milk products.
Rationale: Dairy products are an excellent source of protein and provide other nutrients important to maintain health.
Intervention: Encourage incorporating fruits and vegetables into the menus.
Rationale: Protein is not the only nutrient needed to maintain good oral health. In addition, consumption of more fruits and vegetables models healthy eating to her children.
Intervention: Refer her to a social worker.
Rationale: The social worker will be knowledgeable about local and federal programs she is eligible for and can direct her to local food banks and other resources.

Evaluation

The patient should understand protein is important, but also realize it is possible to purchase cheaper sources of protein that provide all the indispensible amino acids. To determine this, have the patient repeat three of the principles she remembers from your teaching. The patient should also express her intention to use complementary proteins to provide adequate amounts of amino acids, which will provide other nutrients necessary for health, and purchase some dairy products, fruits, and vegetables each week.

STUDENT READINESS

1. Define bioavailability, kwashiorkor, sarcopenia, nitrogen balance, high-quality protein, and complementary proteins for a patient.
2. List and explain the functions of proteins.
3. Using your desirable body weight, how many grams of protein should you consume?
4. Given a patient weighing 180 lb who has a caloric intake of 2500 kcal, if the diet averages 15% protein, how many kilocalories are provided by protein? How many grams of protein is this? How does this compare with the RDA for this patient?
5. What would you tell a strict vegetarian (vegan) parent about feeding her infant?
6. What are the oral effects of too much protein in the diet? What are the oral effects of too little protein in the diet?
7. Explain the relationship between kilocalories and protein.
8. What are two methods of obtaining the indispensible amino acids from vegetarian foods? List two food combinations for each type of vegetarian diet that would provide adequate amounts of indispensible amino acids.
9. If a patient eats more protein than his or her body needs, what happens to the excess protein?
10. How do high protein diets help with weight loss or maintenance?
11. Using Tables 5-4 and Table 16-2, what suggestions would you offer to help a patient reduce the amount of money spent on food without compromising protein intake? Would this significantly affect intake of other nutrients?

References

1. Bray GA, Smith SR, de Jonge L, et al: Effect of dietary protein content on weight gain, energy expenditure, and body composition during overeating: a randomized controlled trial. *JAMA* 307(1):47–55, 2012.
2. Wright JD, Wang Y: *Trends in intake of energy and macronutrients in adults from 1999–2000 through 2007–2008.* NCHS Data Brief No. 49, November 2010. Accessed August 17, 2013: http://www.cdc.gov/nchs/data/databriefs/db49.htm.
3. Layman D: Dietary guidelines should reflect new understanding about adult protein needs. *Nutr Metab (Lond)* 6:12, 2009.
4. Protein Summit 2007: Exploring the impact of high-quality protein and optimal health. *Am J Clin Nutr* 87(Suppl):S1551–S1583, 2008.
5. Position of the American Dietetic Association, Dietitians of Canada, and the American College of Sports Medicine: Nutrition and athletic performance. *J Am Diet Assoc* 109(3):509–527, 2009.
6. Kerstetter JE, Kenny AM, Insogna KL: Dietary protein and skeletal health: a review of recent human research. *Curr Opin Lipidol* 22(1):16–20, 2011.
7. Surdykowski AK, Kenny AM, Insogna KL, et al: Optimizing bone health in older adults: the importance of dietary protein. *Aging Health* 6(3):345–357, 2010.
8. Calvez J, Poupin N, Chesneau C, et al: Protein intake, calcium balance and health consequences. *Eur J Clin Nutr* 66(3):281–295, 2012.
9. Beasley JM, Ichikawa LE, Ange BA, et al: Is protein intake associated with bone mineral density in young women? *Am J Clin Nutr* 91(5):1311–1316, 2010.
10. Kelemen LE, Kushi LH, Jacobs DR Jr, et al: Associations of dietary protein with disease and mortality in a prospective study of postmenopausal women. *Am J Epidemiol* 161(3):232–249, 2005.
11. Friedman AN, Ogden LG, Foster GD, et al: Comparative effects of low-carbohydrate high-protein versus low-fat diets on the kidney. *Clin J Am Soc Nephrol* 7(7):1103–1111, 2012.
12. Calvez J, Poupin N, Chesneau C, et al: Protein intake, calcium balance and health consequences. *Eur J Clin Nutr* 66(3):281–295, 2012.
13. American Diabetes Association: Standards of medical care in diabetes—2012. *Diabetes Care* 35(Suppl 1):S11–S63, 2012.
14. Stahler C: How often do Americans eat vegetarian meals? And how many adults in the U.S. are vegetarians? Posted on May 18, 2012. The Vegetarian Resource Group Blog. Accessed August 17, 2013: http://www.vrg.org/.
15. Marsh K, Zeuschner C, Saunders A: Health implications of a vegetarian diet: a review. *Am J Lifestyle Med* 6(3):250–267, 2012.
16. Position of the American Dietetic Association: Vegetarian Diets. *J Am Diet Assoc* 109(7):1266–1282, 2009.
17. Pawlak R, Parrott SJ, Raj S, et al: How prevalent is vitamin B_{12} deficiency among vegetarians? *Nutr Rev* 71(2):110–117, 2013.
18. Centers for Disease Control and Prevention (CDC): Neurologic impairment in children associated with maternal dietary deficiency of cobalamin, Georgia, 2001. *MMWR Morb Mortal Wkly Rep* 52(4):61–64, 2003.
19. Huang T, Yang B, Zheng J, et al: Cardiovascular disease mortality and cancer incidence in vegetarians: a meta-analysis and systematic review. *Ann Nutr Metab* 60(4):233–240, 2012.
20. Marsh K, Zeuschner C, Saunders A: Health implications of a vegetarian diet: a review. *Am J Lifestyle Med* 6(3):250–267, 2012.
21. Key TJ, Appleby PN, Spencer EA, et al: Cancer incidence in vegetarians. *Am J Clin Nutr* 89(5):1620S–1626S, 2009.
22. Orlich MJ, Singh PN, Sabaté J, et al: Vegetarian dietary patterns and mortality in Adventist Health Study 2. *JAMA Intern Med* 173(13):1230–1238, 2013.

ⓔ EVOLVE RESOURCES

Please visit http://evolve.elsevier.com/Stegeman/nutritional for additional practice and study support tools.

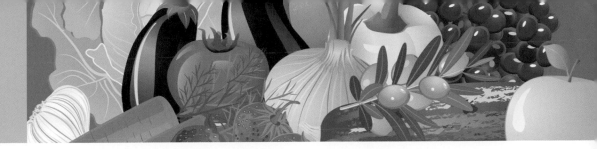

Chapter 6

Lipids: The Condensed Energy

Student Learning Outcomes

Upon completion of this chapter, the student will be able to achieve the following student learning outcomes:

- Describe how fatty acids affect the properties of fat.
- Explain the functions of fats in the body and how these affect oral health.
- Identify dietary sources for saturated, monounsaturated, polyunsaturated, omega-3 and *trans* fatty acids, and cholesterol.

- Calculate the recommended amount of dietary fat.
- Plan appropriate interventions when dietary modification of fat intake has been recommended to a patient.
- Select nutritional directions for various patient issues.

Key Terms

Adipose tissue
α-Linolenic acid
Atherosclerosis
Calorie-dense foods
Compound lipids
Docosahexaenoic acid (DHA)
Eicosapentaenoic acid (EPA)
Essential fatty acid (EFA)
Fatty acids (short-chain, medium-chain, long-chain)
Hyperlipidemia

Interesterified fats
Lipoproteins
Omega-3 fatty acids
Omega-6 fatty acids
Phospholipids
Plant sterols
Protein-sparing
Structural lipids
Trans fatty acid
Unsaturated fatty acid (UFA)

Test Your NQ

1. **T/F** No food containing more than 35% of its kilocalories from fat can be considered healthy.
2. **T/F** Fats containing vitamin E deteriorate and become rancid rapidly.
3. **T/F** A product containing more unsaturated fatty acids than saturated fatty acids is a healthier food choice than one containing a higher proportion of saturated fatty acids.
4. **T/F** Dietary fat intake should be less than 20% of total kilocalories.

5. **T/F** Bananas and avocados contain cholesterol.
6. **T/F** Oils are less fattening than solid fats.
7. **T/F** Fat intake has been linked more frequently to cancer than any other dietary factor.
8. **T/F** Nuts and cheeses are nutritious foods that should be recommended to all patients for snacks because they reduce the rate of caries.
9. **T/F** Fats contain 9 kcal/g.
10. **T/F** Omega-3 fatty acids are polyunsaturated fatty acids.

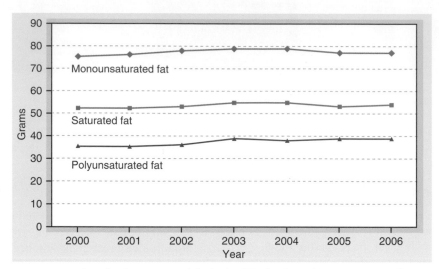

FIGURE 6-1 Saturated, monounsaturated, and polyunsaturated fat in the U.S. food supply, per capita per day, 2000-2006. (From Hiza HAB, Bente L: *Nutrient content of the U.S. food supply: developments between 2000 and 2006.* Home Economic Research Report No. 59. Washington DC, 2011, Center for Nutrition Policy and Promotion, U.S. Dept of Agriculture.)

Unsweetened coconut, mayonnaise, sour cream, blue cheese, salad dressing, almonds, pecans, olives, avocados, and sausages—what do all these foods have in common? More than 50% of the kilocalories in each of these foods come from fat, a vital nutrient in our diet.

Added fats and oils provide more kilocalories in the average American diet than any other food group. Examination of U.S. food supply trends indicates total fat intake, which remains at a high level, increased slightly since 2000. The trend reflects a very slight increase in fats provided by vegetable oils (Fig. 6-1).[1] Between 1977 and 2008, daily consumption of total fat declined from 39.7% to 33.4% of total caloric intake.[2] Consumers have become more aware of healthy food choices, but changes in eating patterns are difficult. Food manufacturers, producers, and grocers have responded to concerns by (a) trimming fat from meats, (b) providing leaner cuts of beef and pork, (c) replacing tropical oils and *trans* fats in processed foods, and (d) manufacturing foods containing less fat. In addition, some consumers have increased their consumption of fish and poultry and substituted lower fat milk for whole milk. The fat content of very lean beef and pork cuts currently compares favorably with a skinless chicken breast. Added fats and oils provide most of the kilocalories Americans consume (Fig. 6-2).

CLASSIFICATION

Fats in the diet should actually be called lipids. Lipids contain the same three elements as carbohydrates: carbon, hydrogen, and oxygen. Lipids contain less oxygen in proportion to hydrogen and carbon than carbohydrates. The structure and function of lipids are covered in detail in Chapter 2 and on the Evolve website. Because of their structure, they provide more energy per gram than either carbohydrates or proteins.

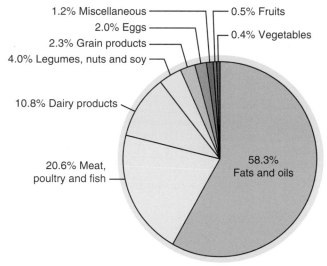

FIGURE 6-2 Added fats and oils provided more calories per day for the average American than all other food groups combined in 2006. (Data from Hiza HAB, Bende L: *Nutrient content of the U.S. food supply: developments between 2000 and 2006.* Home Economics Research Report No 59. Washington DC, 2011, Center for Nutrition Policy and Promotion, U.S. Dept of Agriculture.)

The two classes of water-insoluble substances are (a) simple lipids, or triglycerides, which occur in foods and in the body, and (b) **structural lipids**, which are produced by the body for specific functions. The structural component of lipids is **fatty acids**. Triglycerides with one or more of the fatty acids replaced with carbohydrate, phosphate, or nitrogenous compounds are called **compound lipids**. Dietary lipids used physiologically include triglycerides, fatty acids, phospholipids, and cholesterol. Lipoproteins are found solely in the body.

CHEMICAL STRUCTURE

Triglycerides are composed of fatty acids and glycerol, as shown:

Monoglycerides = glycerol + one fatty acid

Diglycerides = glycerol + two fatty acids

Triglycerides = glycerol + three fatty acids

A fatty acid is a chain of carbon atoms attached to hydrogen atoms with an acid grouping on one end. Glycerol is the alcohol portion of a triglyceride to which the fatty acids attach. Triglycerides are the most common fat present in animal or protein foods (Fig. 6-3). Monoglycerides and diglycerides are found in the small intestine and result from the breakdown of triglycerides during digestion. Free fatty acids, monoglycerides, and glycerol can cross cell membranes.

Each of the three fatty acids attached to the triglyceride can be different: they can be long, medium, or short, and saturated or unsaturated. Medium-chain and short-chain fatty acids are readily digested and absorbed, but most fats in foods (especially vegetable fats) contain predominantly long-chain fatty acids. Short-chain fatty acids contain less than six carbon atoms, medium-chain fatty acids contain 6 to 10 carbon atoms, and long-chain fatty acids contain 12 or more carbon atoms.

Saturated Fatty Acids

As discussed in Chapter 2, fatty acids are classified according to their degree of saturation. Saturation of a fatty acid depends on the number of hydrogen atoms attached to the carbon chain. Saturated fatty acids (SFAs) contain only single bonds, with each carbon atom having two hydrogen atoms attached to it (see Chapter 2, Fig. 2-15). Palmitic and stearic acids (see Chapter 2, Table 2-4), the two most prevalent SFAs, are structural components of tooth enamel and dentin.

Monounsaturated Fatty Acids

When adjacent carbon atoms are joined by a double bond because two hydrogen atoms are lacking, there is a gap between the hydrogen atoms in the chain; it is called an unsaturated fatty acid. Monounsaturated fatty acids (MUFAs) contain only one double bond (see Chapter 2, Fig. 2-12). The most abundant MUFA is oleic acid. Oleic acid is also a structural component of the tooth.

Trans Fatty Acids

Hydrogenation is a commercial process in which vegetable oil is converted to a solid margarine or shortening by adding hydrogen to the oil. This process results in naturally unsaturated vegetable oils being changed to a SFA by changing unsaturated bonds to saturated bonds. Hydrogenation can be controlled, so "tub" or "soft" margarine is "partially hydrogenated," or not completely saturated. The hydrogenation process not only increases the proportion of SFAs, but also changes the shape of the fatty acid. When the hydrogen atoms are rotated so that they are on opposite sides of the bond, in the *"trans"* position (see Chapter 2, Fig. 2-16), the fatty acid is called a *trans* fatty acid. Partial hydrogenation results in large numbers of fatty acids having this altered shape. Foods with *trans* fatty acids have a longer

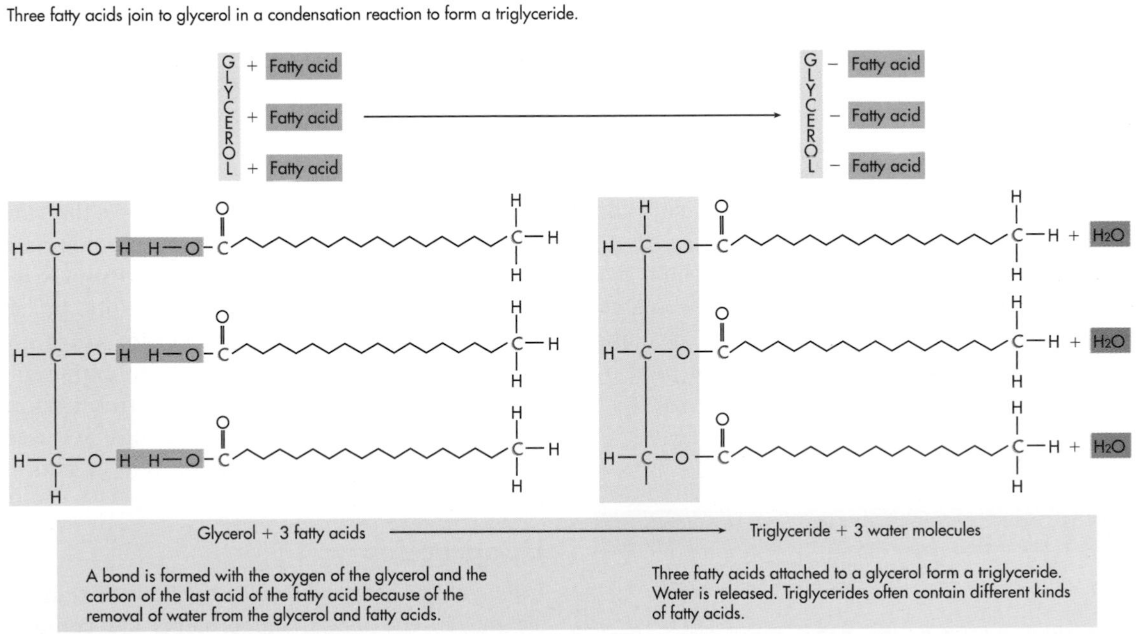

Three fatty acids join to glycerol in a condensation reaction to form a triglyceride.

Glycerol + 3 fatty acids ⟶ Triglyceride + 3 water molecules

A bond is formed with the oxygen of the glycerol and the carbon of the last acid of the fatty acid because of the removal of water from the glycerol and fatty acids.

Three fatty acids attached to a glycerol form a triglyceride. Water is released. Triglycerides often contain different kinds of fatty acids.

FIGURE 6-3 Formation and structure of a triglyceride. (Adapted from Grodner M, Roth SL, Walkingshaw BC: *Nutritional foundations and clinical applications*, ed 5. St Louis, 2012, Mosby Elsevier.)

shelf life, and flavors are stable. The most common *trans* fatty acid is elaidic acid, found in partially hydrogenated vegetable oils, such as tub margarines and cooking oils. A naturally-occurring *trans* fatty acid, vaccenic acid, with double bonds on adjacent carbons, is present in small amounts in milk and meat of ruminants (cows, sheep, and deer). Limited research suggests that these *trans* fats may possibly have health-enhancing potential.

Polyunsaturated Fatty Acids

When carbons in a fatty acid are connected by two or more double bonds, the fatty acid is polyunsaturated (see Chapter 2, Fig. 2-13). Linoleic acid and arachidonic acid are polyunsaturated fatty acids (PUFAs). These PUFAs are omega-6 fatty acids. Their first double bond is on the sixth carbon from the omega (terminal) end; they are also referred to as n-6 PUFAs.

Omega-3 fatty acids, or α-linolenic acids, make up another class of PUFAs. As shown in Chapter 2, Figure 2-13*A*, these fatty acids are unique in that the first double bond is located three carbon atoms from the omega end of the molecule; hence they are called omega-3s or *n-3*s. Omega-3 fatty acids include α-linolenic acid, which has 18 carbon atoms and two double bonds, and eicosapentaenoic acid (EPA), which has 20 carbon atoms and five double bonds.

CHARACTERISTICS OF FATTY ACIDS

The carbon chain length and degree of saturation determine various properties of fats, including their flavor and hardness, or melting point (the temperature at which a product becomes a liquid). Most SFAs are solid at room temperature; e.g., animal fats, being solid at room temperature, are predominantly saturated fats. Short-chain fatty acids (6 carbon atoms or less), MUFAs, and PUFAs that are liquid at room temperature are oils. Milk fat contains a large amount of short-chain SFAs.

Fats with a high proportion of unsaturated fatty acids may deteriorate or become rancid, resulting in unpleasant flavors and odors. Fats become rancid when subject to high temperatures and exposure to light, which cause oxidation and decomposition of fats. The decomposition results in peroxides that may be toxic in large amounts. Vitamin E, a fat-soluble vitamin, is an antioxidant and, to some degree, protects the oil to which it is added. However, in doing so, vitamin E is inactivated and cannot then be used by the body.

Dental Considerations

- Lipids are an integral part of many foods and are important physiologically.
- The primary form of fat in the body is triglyceride, not cholesterol.

Nutritional Directions

- Frying foods at low temperatures causes the food to absorb excessive amounts of fats, whereas frying at very high temperatures results in decomposition of some fats, which can be irritating to the intestine, causing gastrointestinal discomfort after meals containing fried foods.
- The relatively small amounts of *trans* fatty acids that occur naturally in meat and dairy products do not appear to be harmful.
- Butylated hydroxyanisole and butylated hydroxytoluene are antioxidants added to processed foods to retard or prevent spoilage.

COMPOUND LIPIDS

Phospholipids

Phospholipids contain phosphorus and a nitrogenous base in addition to fatty acids and glycerol. Detail on the biochemistry of phospholipids can be found online in Evolve. Fats from plant and animal foods contain phospholipids, but they are not required in the diet because the body produces adequate amounts of phospholipids. These substances cannot be absorbed intact; they are broken down into their chemical components before absorption. As a structural component of cell membranes, tooth enamel, and dentin, they are the second most prevalent form of fat in the body. As such, these substances are not used for energy, even in a state of severe starvation. Although the mechanism is not fully understood, phospholipids are involved in the initiation of calcification and mineralization in teeth and bones, and are present in higher amounts in the enamel matrix of teeth than in dentin.

Phospholipids are important in fat absorption and transport of fats in the blood. Phospholipids can mix with either fat-soluble or water-soluble ingredients and transport these products across membrane barriers.

Phospholipids include lecithin, cephalin, and sphingomyelins. Lecithin, the most widely distributed phospholipid, is present in all cells. Lecithin supplements have been marketed for reducing the risk of atherosclerosis (a complex disease of the arteries in which the interior lining of arteries becomes roughened and clogged with fatty deposits that hinder blood flow), for weight loss, and for other chronic health conditions. However, the value of lecithin in this role is questionable because lecithin is digested before its absorption. Cephalin is present in thromboplastin, which is necessary for blood clotting. Sphingomyelins are important constituents of brain tissue and the myelin sheath around nerve fibers. Phospholipids, especially lecithin, are used as additives in commercial products to prevent fat and water components from separating.

Lipoproteins

Lipoproteins are produced by the body to transport insoluble fats in the blood. Lipoproteins are compound lipids composed of triglycerides, phospholipids, and cholesterol combined with protein (see Chapter 2, Fig. 2-18). The liver

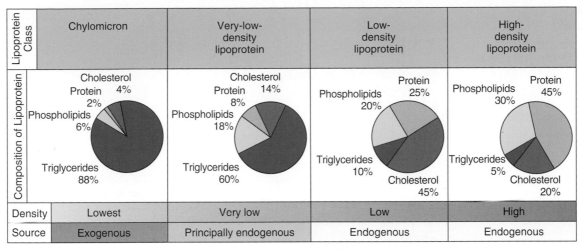

FIGURE 6-4 Characteristics of lipoproteins.

and intestinal mucosa produce lipoproteins. Four different types of lipoproteins are present in the blood: high-density lipoproteins (HDLs), low-density lipoproteins (LDLs), very-low-density lipoproteins (VLDLs), and chylomicrons.

The ratio of lipid to protein in lipoproteins varies widely; these variations affect their density. Density increases as lipids decrease and protein increases. Lipoproteins can be classified according to their density and composition, as shown in Figure 6-4. Phospholipids in lipoproteins are present in approximately the same proportions in all individuals.

HDLs, which have been thought to protect against development of CHD, contain greater amounts of protein and less lipid. LDL cholesterol typically constitutes 60% to 70% of the total blood cholesterol. It is considered the main agent in elevated serum cholesterol levels, or the "bad" cholesterol. Serum HDL, LDL, and VLDL are important predictors of heart disease, as discussed in *Health Application 6*.

CHOLESTEROL

Cholesterol is a fatlike, waxy substance classified as a sterol derivative with a complex ring structure (see Chapter 2, Fig. 2-17). More details on the structure and function of cholesterol are available online in the Evolve website. Because the body frequently produces more cholesterol than it absorbs, cholesterol intake is not essential. Cholesterol has important functions as a constituent of the brain, nervous tissue, and bile salts; a precursor of vitamin D and steroid hormones; and a structural component of cell membranes and teeth. Lipoproteins transport cholesterol in the blood.

PHYSIOLOGICAL ROLES

Energy

Dietary fats are a concentrated source of energy, furnishing 9 kcal/g. Foods high in fats are generally referred to as calorie-dense, a beneficial quality in some cases. **Calorie-dense foods** are high in fats (or fat and sugar) and low in

vitamins, minerals, and other nutrients. A characteristic of calorie-dense foods is that less volume of food is needed to furnish energy requirements. As an energy source, fats are also referred to as **protein-sparing** because they allow protein to be used for the important functions of building and repairing tissues.

Satiety Value

Dietary fats are important for their satiety value. Fats contribute to a feeling of fullness for a longer time than carbohydrates or protein because digestion of high-fat meals is slower than other energy-containing nutrients. This has given rise to such descriptions as "sticks to the ribs" in reference to rich, high-fat meals. The higher the fat content of a meal, the longer the food remains in the stomach. Nevertheless, approximately 95% of ingested fats are absorbed. Soft fats that are liquids at body temperature (e.g., margarine) are digested more quickly than hard fats (e.g., meat fats).

Palatability

Fats contribute to the palatability and flavor of foods. In cooking, they improve texture. A receptor on the tongue and a potential pathway for detection of a "fatty taste" has been identified, which may affect food preferences.[3,4] Preference for high-fat foods develops at an early age and persists through adulthood.

Complementary Relationships

Fat-soluble vitamins and linoleic acid are generally found in foods containing fat. The absorption of fat-soluble vitamins is facilitated by the presence of fats in the gastrointestinal tract.

Linoleic acid, an omega-6 fatty acid with 18 carbon atoms and two double bonds (see Chapter 2, Fig. 2-12), cannot be synthesized by the body and must be supplied from dietary sources. If linoleic acid is not furnished in the diet, signs of deficiency, including growth retardation, skin lesions, and reproductive failure, result. For this reason, linoleic acid is an **essential fatty acid (EFA)**.

Table 6-1	Common food sources and physiological actions of fatty acids	
Fatty Acid Classification	Common Food Sources	Physiological Action
Saturated Fatty Acid (SFA)		
	Coconut oil, butter fat, most fats and oils, cocoa butter, fully hydrogenated vegetable oils	Raises total, LDL and HDL cholesterol (except stearic acid)
Monounsaturated Fatty Acid (MUFA)		
Cis configuration	Some fish oils, beef fat, most fats and oils, nuts, seeds, avocados	Decreases total and LDL cholesterol when substituted for SFAs and decreases total cholesterol compared with dietary carbohydrate
Trans configuration	Partially hydrogenated vegetable oils	Raises total and LDL cholesterol similar to SFAs, decreases HDL more than saturated fatty acids, and raises total-to-HDL ratio more than SFAs
Trans configuration	Dairy fat, meat from ruminating animals (beef, lamb)	May have beneficial health effects, especially vaccenic acid; more research needed
Polyunsaturated Fatty Acid (PUFA)		
n-6 Fatty Acids		
Linoleic acid	Liquid vegetable oils, nuts, seeds	Decreases total and LDL cholesterol
Arachidonic acid	Meat, poultry, fish, eggs	Precursor for important biologically active substances; substrate for synthesis of a variety of proinflammatory compounds
n-3 Fatty Acids		
α-Linolenic acid	Flaxseed, canola oil, soybean oil, walnuts	Decreases cardiovascular risk
Eicosapentaenoic acid (EPA) Docosahexaenoic acid (DHA)	Fish oil, algae	Decreases risk of sudden death from cardiovascular conditions and has beneficial effects on nervous system development and health

Adapted from Kris-Etherton P, Innis S: Position of the American Dietetic Association and Dietitians of Canada: dietary fatty acids. *J Am Diet Assoc* 2007; 107(9): 1599-1611.

Arachidonic acid (18-carbon chain with four double bonds) and linolenic acid (18-carbon chain with three double bonds) are also considered EFAs, but healthy individuals can produce them from sufficient quantities of linoleic acid (see Chapter 2, Fig. 2-13). Linolenic acid can be converted rapidly into omega-3 fatty acids in the body. The conversion of linolenic acid to EPA and the conversion of linoleic acid to arachidonic acid are competitive because the processes use the same enzyme. Studies suggest that less than 10% of linolenic acid is converted to EPA. When intake of linoleic acid is substantially higher than intake of linolenic acid, less EPA is available. Linolenic acid may be a protective factor against CHD (Table 6-1).[5]

Omega-3 fatty acids are used to produce compounds regulating blood pressure, clotting, immune responses, gastrointestinal secretions, and cardiovascular functions; they also prevent heart arrhythmias and decrease triglyceride levels. Omega-3 fatty acids are essential for the development of brain and retinal tissues in fetal and neonatal development, and ongoing cognitive development in childhood. The presence of omega-3 fatty acids in the diet has been linked to reduction or amelioration of several chronic diseases, including CHD, atherosclerosis and atherosclerotic plaque, and mortality risk from CHD (Fig. 6-5),[6] rheumatoid arthritis, psoriasis, inflammatory and immune disorders, and serious eye problems such as macular degeneration (see Table 6-1). However, in numerous studies, supplementation

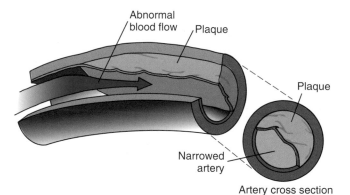

FIGURE 6-5 Atherosclerosis. An artery narrowed by the buildup of plaque. (From Workman ML, LaCharity L, Kruchko SL: *Understanding pharmacology*, 2011, St Louis, Saunders.)

has not been associated with either lower risk of all-cause mortality or major CHD outcomes.[7] Studies are exploring the relationship of omega-3 fatty acids with mental aging and Alzheimer disease.

Fat Storage

Adipose tissue, or body fat, has several roles: (a) it provides a concentrated energy source, (b) it protects internal organs, and (c) it maintains body temperature.

Energy

Excess dietary carbohydrates and protein are converted to fat and stored in adipose tissue. Fatty acids can be used as an energy source by all cells except red blood cells and central nervous system cells. People have been known to survive total starvation for 30 to 40 days with only water to drink.

Protection of Organs

Fatty tissue surrounds vital organs and provides a cushion, protecting them from traumatic injury and shock.

Insulation

The subcutaneous layer of fat functions as an insulator that preserves body heat and maintains body temperature. Excessive layers of fat can also deter heat loss during hot weather.

DIETARY FATS AND DENTAL HEALTH

Dietary fats are essential for oral health because they are incorporated into the tooth structure. There is some evidence from epidemiological and laboratory studies that fats may have a cariostatic effect. Individuals, whose diet may contain 80% fat from animal and seafood sources (e.g., Alaskan natives), have a very low incidence of dental caries, but this could possibly be a result of their low carbohydrate intake. Dietary fats probably have local rather than systemic influence because fats added to foods protect the teeth more than foods naturally high in fat. Precisely how fats reduce the caries rate is unknown; however, several hypotheses have been explored, as follows:

1. Some fatty acids, specifically oleic acid, are growth factors for lactic acid bacteria, whereas streptococcal organisms are inhibited by lauric acid (Lauricidin).
2. Long-chain fatty acids may reduce dissolution of hydroxyapatite by acids.
3. Oral food retention is reduced by fat intake.
4. Fats may lubricate the tooth surface and prevent penetration of acid to the enamel (i.e., the "greased" tooth is impervious to acid, protecting caries-susceptible areas).
5. Fats may produce a film on food particles and prevent partial digestion of food particles in the mouth.
6. Dietary fat delays gastric emptying, enhancing fluoride absorption, and increasing tissue fluoride concentration.

Bacterial inflammation and systemic immune response are believed to play a central role in the initiation and propagation of atherosclerosis. Periodontal diseases (including gingivitis and periodontitis) are oral conditions caused by bacteria (and poor oral hygiene) that are risk factors contributing to coronary artery disease. When bacteria are allowed to grow rampantly in the mouth, inflammation may occur throughout the body. Bacteria from dental plaque biofilm can cause blood clots when they escape into the bloodstream and could be involved in inflammation of the lining of blood vessels and atherosclerosis. This inflammation may serve as a base for development of arterial atherosclerotic plaques,

but—contrary to some concerns—omega-6 fatty acids do not seem to promote inflammation.[8] Research studies show that the inflammatory process can be attenuated by n-3 fatty acids.[9] Consumption of greater amounts of docosahexaenoic acid (DHA) and—to a lesser degree—EPA were associated with lower prevalence of periodontitis.[10]

Dental Considerations

- Although fat intake may have a positive effect on dental health, the medical history of the patient needs to be considered when providing nutrition education.
- Lipids as a source of energy provide 9 kcal/g, whereas carbohydrates and proteins provide 4 kcal/g.
- Fish consumption may have a favorable effect on blood platelets and other blood clotting mechanisms, reducing the risk of clot formation.
- The only proven benefit and suggested use of lecithin supplements is for individuals taking niacin to treat high cholesterol levels because niacin can deplete the body's stores of choline.
- Interview the patient to evaluate total fat intake. Everyone needs adequate amounts of fat to allow protein to perform its functions of building and repairing. If total energy intake is inadequate, healing is slower. Also, inadequate fat intake could lead to secondary deficiencies of fat-soluble vitamins.
- Foods such as nuts and certain cheeses (cheddar, Monterey Jack, Swiss) may protect teeth against acid attack, especially when consumed after fermentable carbohydrates. Even though they are generally considered nutritious foods, they have a relatively high fat content and may not be appropriate for all people.
- Because omega-3 fatty acids may be beneficial to health, determine the patient's frequency of fish consumption and supplement use. An increase in fish consumption is recommended for most patients, but some fish, especially mackerel and tuna, should be consumed in moderation because of their mercury content.
- Do not advocate indiscriminate use of omega-3 fatty acid supplements. Although fish oils are beneficial for many conditions, they may have a negative effect on blood glucose levels in patients with diabetes mellitus. If the patient is consuming omega-3 fatty acid supplements, inquire about the quantity. Intakes of more than 3 g should be supervised by a healthcare provider.
- Krill oil (a type of fish oil) contains omega-3 fatty acids, but is more expensive than other omega-3 supplements. Studies have not shown convincing evidence that health benefits of krill oil are superior to those of regular fish oil.
- If the patient is taking anticoagulants or aspirin, evaluate use of omega-3 fatty acids. These patients may be prone to bleeding problems or poor wound healing.
- Structural differences among the various *trans* fatty acids result in different health effects.

Nutritional Directions

- Although digestion of fried foods takes longer, the process is as complete as that of other foods in most individuals if food is fried at the proper temperature.
- Fats act as a lubricant in the intestines, decreasing constipation.
- Foods containing *trans* fats include stick margarine, vegetable shortening, peanut butter, commercially baked goods (cookies, crackers, biscuits, cake, and breads), potato chips, salad dressing,

Continued

Nutritional Directions—cont'd

and fast foods (french fries, doughnuts, and other fried foods). Products containing partially hydrogenated (or *trans*) fats should be limited because *trans* fats behave like saturated fat in the body.

- Patients should consult their healthcare provider or an RDN before taking an omega-3 fatty acid supplement. Foods containing omega-3 fatty acids should be included in the diet at least 2 times a week to enjoy good health and prevent many diseases.
- Educate patients on how to read labels of omega-3 fatty acid supplements. Supplements made from liver should be avoided because high levels of pesticides or heavy metals may be present.
- The potential relationship between periodontal disease and heart disease emphasizes important health reasons for good dental hygiene.
- Avoid choosing a product containing less *trans* fats but more saturated fat because both have undesirable effects on blood lipids.

DIETARY REQUIREMENTS

A certain amount of fat is needed to provide adequate amounts of fat-soluble vitamins and EFAs. The acceptable macronutrient distribution range for fat is estimated to be 20% to 35% of energy intake for adults (Table 6-2). The lower limit for fat intake was established to minimize the increase in blood triglyceride levels and decrease in HDL cholesterol levels that occur with higher intakes of carbohydrates. The upper limit of 35% kcal from fat was based on information indicating higher fat intake is associated with a greater intake of energy and SFA, which may be detrimental to health. Box 6-1 shows a method for calculating the IOM recommendation for dietary fat.

Between 2000 and 2008, Americans' fat consumption jumped 5%, reaching an average intake of 33% of the total caloric intake (Fig. 6-6).[11] The World Health Organization recommends a range of 15% to 30% of total kilocalories from fats.[12]

The Dietary Reference Intake also recommends that SFA and *trans* fatty acid intakes be as low as possible while consuming a diet providing an adequate intake of all essential nutrients. The *Dietary Guidelines* recommend less than 10% of kilocalories from saturated fats, replacing them with MUFAs and PUFAs and keeping *trans* fats as low as possible (see Table 6-2). Currently, approximately 11% of the kilocalories consumed by Americans are saturated.[13] Studies do not support substituting saturated fats with high carbohydrate (starchy) foods, but modifying the type of fat seems to protect against CHD better.[14,15]

Adequate intake established for linoleic acid is 0.6% of energy intake or 17 g/day for men and 12 g/day for women 19 to 50 years, and 14 g/day for men and 11 g/day for women older than 51 years (see p. ii). The *Dietary Guidelines* recommend a target of ≥250 mg per day for omega-3 fatty acids (EPA and DHA), but many specialists think that the target should be between 250 to 500 mg/day.[16] Currently daily intake is around 150 mg.[17]

SOURCES

Table 6-3 itemizes selected foods containing SFAs, MUFAs, and PUFAs. Foods contain a combination of fatty acids; each of the fatty acids attached to the glycerol may be different. For example, corn oil, with 57% PUFA, 29% MUFA, and 13.6% SFA, is considered a good source of PUFA. Of the food groups (excluding fats and oils), animal products contribute the largest proportion of fat, although their share has been declining. The most important sources of saturated fats are the meat and milk groups; cocoa butter and coconut and palm oils also are high in saturated fat. SFAs are found in animal fats, butter fat, coconut oil, cocoa butter, coffee creamers, and fully hydrogenated vegetable oils (see Tables 6-1 and 6-3). The

---

BOX 6-1	Calculating Total Daily Fat Recommendations for Specific Caloric Levels*

To calculate dietary fat:

1. Determine caloric level of the diet (see Dietary Reference Intake for Energy for Active Individuals, p. ii) (e.g., patient needs 2000 kcal).
2. Multiply the kilocalories by 0.35 to determine the number of kilocalories of fat the diet can contain (e.g., 2000 kcal × 0.35 [% of total kilocalories] = 700 kcal from fat).
3. Divide the answer by 9 to determine the grams of fat allowed daily (e.g., 700 kcal from fat ÷ 9 kcal/g of fat = 77.7 g of fat).

KILOCALORIE LEVEL	GRAMS OF FAT PER DAY
1200	<46
1500	<58
1800	<70
2000	<78
2200	<86
2400	<93

*Total fat intake limited to less than 35% of the total daily kilocalories.

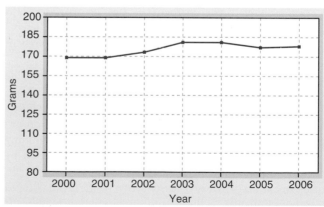

FIGURE 6-6 Total fat in the U.S. food supply, per capita per day, 2000-2006. (From Hiza HAB, Bente L: *Nutrient content of the U.S. food supply: developments between 2000 and 2006.* Home Economics Research Report No. 59. Washington DC, 2011, Center for Nutrition Policy and Promotion, U.S. Dept of Agriculture.)

Table 6-2	Fat recommendations for adults*				
Classification of Fat	Dietary Guidelines	IOM† Reference Dietary Allowance (RDA)/Adequate Intake‡ (AI)	IOM† Acceptable Macronutrient Distribution Range (AMDR)	American Heart Association§	American Diabetes Association¶	Canada's Food Guide**
Total fat	20% to 35% kcal	—	20% to 35% kcal	25% to 35% kcal	—	20% to 35% kcal
Saturated fatty acids (SFA)	<10% kcal	Minimize	Minimize	<7% kcal (stay away from tropical oils such as coconut oil, palm oil and palm kernel oils that are high in SFA)	<7% kcal	Limit butter, hard margarines, lard, and shortening
Trans fatty acids (TFA)	<1% kcal	Minimize¶¶	Minimize¶¶	>1% kcal	Minimize¶¶	Limit hard margarines, lard, and shortening
Omega-6 fatty acids (n-6 PUFA)		14 g/day for males; 11 g/day for females	5% to 10% kcal	Choose monounsaturated fatty acids (MUFA) or PUFA (vegetable oils, margarines with liquid vegetable oil as the first listed ingredient)		Use vegetable oils, such as canola, olive, and soybean
α-Linolenic acid		1.6 g/day for males; 1.1 g/day for females	0.6% to 1.2% kcal	No specific recommendation		
Omega-3 fatty acids (DHA and EPA)	2 servings fish/wk††			2 or more servings fish/wk	Nonfried fish 2-3 times/wk	Include foods rich in PUFA and plant oils (canola, walnut, flax)
Plant sterols				~2 g/day		

*Adults 19-70 years old.

†Institute of Medicine (IOM): *Dietary reference intakes for energy, carbohydrate, fiber, fat, fatty acids, cholesterol, protein, and amino acids*, Washington, DC, 2002, National Academies Press.

‡AI—observed median intake.

§American Heart Association: *Fats and oils*. Accessed August 19, 2013. Available at: http://www.heart.org/HEARTORG/GettingHealthy/FatsAndOils/Fats101/Fats-and-Oils-AHA-Recommendation_UCM_316375_Article.jsp.

¶Data from American Diabetes Association: Nutrition recommendations and interventions for diabetes. *Diabetes Care* 2008;31(Suppl 1):S61-S78; and Summary of revisions for the 2009 clinical practice recommendations. Diabetes Care 2009;32(Suppl 1):S3-S5.

¶¶Minimize while consuming a nutritionally adequate diet.

**Health Canada. *Eating well with Canada's food guide—a resource for educators and communicators, 2011.* Accessed August 19, 2013. Available at: http://www.hc-sc.gc.ca/fn-an/food-guide-aliment/educ-comm/index-eng.php

††Two servings of fish per week = 450-500 mg DHA and EPA.

| Table 6-3 | Fatty acids and cholesterol content of selected foods |

Food	Portion	Total Fat (g)	SFA (Saturated Fatty Acids) (g)	MUFA (Monounsaturated Fatty Acids) (g)	PUFA (Polyunsaturated Fatty Acids [Total]) (g)	Cholesterol (mg)
Milk and Milk Products						
Cheese, cheddar	1 oz	9.4	6.0	2.7	0.27	30
Cheese, Monterey	1 oz	8.5	5.3	2.5	0.25	25
Cottage cheese, 2%	4 oz	2.8	1.1	0.5	0.08	11
Cream cheese	1 oz	9.7	5.5	2.4	0.41	31
Ice cream, 10% fat	1 cup	14.5	8.9	3.9	0.60	58
Milk, 1%	1 cup	2.4	1.6	0.7	0.09	12
Milk, 2%	1 cup	4.7	2.9	1.4	0.17	20
Milk, whole, 3.7%	1 cup	8.9	5.6	2.6	0.33	34
Meats, Fish, and Eggs						
Beef, lean ground (85%/15%)	3 oz	113.2	5.0	5.7	0.41	76
Beef liver	3 oz	4.7	1.5	0.6	0.58	356
Chicken breast, skinless	3 oz	26.7	0.9	1.1	0.66	73
Chicken breast, with skin	3 oz	7.0	2.0	2.7	1.5	76
Chicken thigh, skinless	3 oz	7.4	2.1	3.0	1.5	122
Egg, large whole	1	5.3	1.6	2.0	0.71	186
Egg white	1	0.1	0	0	0	0
Pork chop, center loin, lean only	3 oz	8.5	3.0	3.9	0.54	69
Salmon, canned	3 oz	6.1	1.3	2.2	1.60	71
Salmon, Atlantic	3 oz	10.5	2.1	3.8	3.8	54
Shrimp	3 oz	1.4	0.4	0.3	0.5	179
Veal loin, lean only	3 oz	7.8	2.2	2.8	0.70	106
Fats and Oils						
Butter	1 tbsp	11.5	7.3	3	0.43	31
Cream, half-and-half	¼ cup	7.0	4.3	2	0.26	22
Margarine, corn oil soft	1 tbsp	8.4	1.7	2.7	3.7	0
Margarine, vegetable oil, stick	1 tbsp	8.3	1.4	2.8	3.46	0
Oil, canola	1 tbsp	14	1.0	8.9	3.9	0
Oil, corn	1 tbsp	13.6	1.8	3.8	7.4	0
Salad dressing, mayonnaise-type	1 tbsp	10.3	1.6	2.3	6.17	6
Shortening, partially hydrogenated soybean and cottonseed oil	1 tbsp	12.8	3.5	6.9	1.8	0

Data from U.S. Department of Agriculture: *USDA national nutrient database for standard reference, release 26.* Nutrient Data Laboratory Home Page. Accessed August 21, 2013: http://www.ars.usda.gov/ba/bhnrc/ndl

biggest food contributors of saturated fat consumed by Americans are regular cheese (9% of total saturated fat intake) and pizza, grain-based and dairy-based desserts, chicken and chicken dishes prepared with chicken (6% for each group).[18] Animal products and canola and olive oils supply approximately 50% of MUFAs. Oleic acid, the most prevalent MUFA, is present in most fats, oils, nuts, seeds, and avocados.

PUFAs from the n-6 series are derived from land plants, especially foods from the grain group, and additional fats and oils. Linoleic acid is the most prevalent PUFA in the food supply. Safflower, soybean, and corn oils provide the most linoleic acid; food sources are nuts and seeds. Almost 80% of all vegetable oil consumed in the United States is soybean oil.[19] It is also the principal source of omega-3 fatty acids in the U.S. diet. Conjugated linoleic acids are natural components of beef, lamb, and dairy products. Linolenic acid is present in plant products—flaxseed, canola, and soybean oils; soybeans; walnuts; flaxseed; and wheat germ.

Long-chain n-3 fatty acids (EPA and docosahexaenoic acid [DHA]), provided from seafood, include fatty fish such as mackerel, salmon, herring, and albacore tuna, and fish oils. Most shellfish contain very little omega-3s except oysters, which are considered a rich source. These foods are also low in saturated fat. The American Heart Association (AHA) guidelines recommend consumption of fish at least two times a week.

In 2003-2004, approximately 52% of the soybean oil used in the United States was partially hydrogenated; the food industry is working to produce a soybean oil that does not require hydrogenation and thus contains no *trans* fats.[20]

Trans fats are present in shortening; stick margarine; deep-fried fast foods such as french fries; and commercially baked pastries and desserts such as doughnuts, cookies, and crackers. Box 6-2 details how to limit the total amount of fat in the diet, focusing on reducing foods high in saturated and *trans* fats and choosing more foods containing unsaturated fats.

Only animal products contain cholesterol (see Table 6-3); it is not found in egg whites or plant foods (e.g., vegetable oils). It is highest in egg yolks, liver, and other organ meats.

BOX 6-2   Wise Choices of Dietary Fats

Purchasing and Planning

- Read nutrition labels on foods to determine the amount of fat and saturated fat in a serving. Low-fat is less than 3 g fat per serving.
- Choose fats and oils with 2 g or less saturated fat per tablespoon, such as tub margarines and vegetable oils (e.g., canola, corn, safflower, sunflower, and olive oil). Liquid vegetable oil should be listed as the first ingredient. Avoid saturated fats such as butter, lard, and palm and coconut oils.
- Avoid foods containing hydrogenated or partially hydrogenated fats because they contain *trans* fatty acids. Such foods include shortening, chips, doughnuts, cookies, snack crackers, cakes, fried foods, and some processed and convenience foods. Foods containing partially hydrogenated fats may have some redeeming factors if they contain canola or soybean oil that contain trace amounts of partially hydrogenated oil.
- Watch for reformulated products with zero *trans* fats.
- Substitute plain low-fat Greek style yogurt for mayonnaise or sour cream or purchase light sour cream (compare fat content on labels).
- Purchase fresh fruits, vegetables, and nuts for snacks rather than sugar-sweetened beverages, chips, pastries, and high kilocalorie pastries (e.g., muffins, doughnuts).
- Choose two or three servings of lean meat, skinless poultry, or fish, with a daily total of about 6 oz.
- Choose a vegetarian entree (e.g., dry beans and peas) at least once a week.
- Include fish (not fried) at least twice a week.
- Include a variety of fresh meats (not processed); producers breed animals to produce leaner beef and pork.
- Choose beef graded "select" because it contains fewer kilocalories as a result of less fat marbling. Fat content of meats also depends on the type of cut; leaner cuts include flank steak, sirloin or tenderloin, loin pork chops, and 85% or greater lean ground beef.
- Choose lean turkey or chicken sausage, or turkey bacon.
- Choose food made with whole grains.
- Use low-fat ground turkey or extra-lean ground beef in casseroles, spaghetti, and chili.
- Moderate the use of egg yolks (maximum of four egg yolks weekly) and organ meats (liver, brain, and kidney).
- Choose tuna packed in water, not in oil (compare fat content on labels).
- Select fat-free or low-fat milk and dairy products. Choose cheeses with 6 g or less of fat per ounce. (90% of the kilocalories in cream cheese are from fat.)

Food Preparation

- Use fats and oils (e.g., olive, canola, corn, sunflower, or cottonseed) sparingly in cooking (roast, bake, grill, or broil when possible). Baste meats with broth or stock.
- Use nonstick cookware and an aerosol cooking spray.
- Prepare and eat smaller portions.
- Use the paste method for making gravy or sauces: add flour or cornstarch to cold liquids slowly and blend well.
- Season with herbs, lemon juice, or stock rather than lard, bacon, ham, margarine, or fatty sauces.
- Remove skin from poultry and visible fat from beef and pork products.
- Skim fat from homemade soups or stews by chilling and removing the fat layer that rises to the top.
- A small amount of olive or canola oil in salads increases absorption of antioxidants and fat-soluble vitamins.
- Include olives and healthful fats, such as flaxseed oils, nuts, and avocados.
- Use good quality jam, preserves, or marmalade instead of butter or margarine.
- Rely on mustard, salad greens, shredded carrots, tomato slices, sweet peppers, and red onions to add moisture to sandwiches rather than fat-laden spreads.
- Top a baked potato with salsa and a dollop of fat-free Greek yogurt instead of butter or sour cream.
- Substitute two egg whites for one whole egg.
- Prepare broth-based chicken, vegetable, or bean-based soups rather than cream soups made with high-fat dairy products.
- Marinate leaner cuts of meat in lemon juice, flavored vinegars, or fruit juices.
- Sauté with olive oil instead of butter.
- Sprinkle slivered nuts, flaxseed, or sunflower seeds on salads instead of bacon bits.
- Choose a handful of nuts rather than chips or crackers.
- Place meat or poultry on a rack to allow the fat to drain.
- Steam, simmer, boil, broil, bake, grill, or microwave foods rather than frying them.
- Use smaller servings of oil-based or low-fat salad dressings.
- Use whole-grain flours to enhance the flavor of baked goods made with less fat.
- Choose nonhydrogenated peanut butter or other nut-butter spreads on celery, banana, or rice or popcorn cakes.
- Add avocado slices rather than cheese to a salad or sandwich.

Average cholesterol intake in the United States is slightly above the 300 mg recommended in the *Dietary Guidelines*. Average blood cholesterol values have declined since about 1960.

Food Choices

The percentage of fat by weight is widely used on food labels and advertising. Although this information is correct, it is misleading and confusing. The recommendation that fat intake should be limited to 35% refers to the percentage of fat based on total kilocalories of the product. As shown in Table 6-4, the percentage of fat in whole milk is 48% of the total kilocalories, not 3.25% as the label indicates.

The Nutrition Facts label on foods (see Fig. 1-7) indicates the grams and % Daily Value for fat, saturated fat, and *trans* fats in a serving of the product. All *trans* fats, including those from ruminant animals, are included on the Nutrition Facts Label; only conjugated linoleic acids are excluded. Before *trans* fats were added to the nutrition label, average consumption was 5.8 g, or 2.6% of kilocalories. Food manufacturers responded to labeling requirements by reducing *trans* fats in their products. Consumption of *trans* fatty acids decreased from about 4.6 g/person/day in the late 1990s to about 1.3 g/person/day in 2010, a reduction

of approximately 58% (Fig. 6-7).[21] This positive change should help lower the risk of CHD in adults.

Because a specific amount of *trans* fats has not been recommended, consumers find it difficult to interpret whether the product contains a high level or not. Even a motivated consumer may misinterpret a label indicating 4 g of *trans* fats as being acceptable. The AHA recommends less than 1% (2 g) of total kilocalories from *trans* fat daily, but zero intake of commercially produced *trans* fats is best. The Nutrition Facts label may indicate the product has no *trans* fats, but the ingredient label indicates "partially hydrogenated" oil. This is because the U.S. Food and Drug Administration allows the Nutrition Facts label to indicate the food has "zero" *trans* fats if the product contains less than 0.5 g per serving. A claim such as "zero" *trans* fat on the package is more helpful than the information on the Nutrition Facts label. Canadian regulations set the labeling threshold at 0.2 g per serving.

For most people, a decrease in red meat consumption is probably desirable, but complete elimination is questionable. In recent years, through improvements in breeding and feeding livestock, these products are lower in fat, saturated fat, kilocalories, and cholesterol. Important nutrients are present in beef, pork, and lamb; moderate consumption of

Table 6-4	Analysis of fat content of milk			
Type of Milk	Kilocalories (1 cup)	Total Fat (g)	Percentage of Fat by Weight	Percentage of Fat by Kilocalories
Whole milk (3.25%)	149	7.9	3.3	48
Low-fat milk (2%)	122	4.8	2	35
Low-fat milk (1%)	102	2.4	1	21
Skim milk	83	0.20	1	2

Data from U.S. Department of Agriculture: USDA *national nutrient database for standard reference, release 26*. Nutrient Data Laboratory Home Page. Accessed August 21, 2013. Available at: http://www.ars.usda.gov/ba/bhnrc/ndl

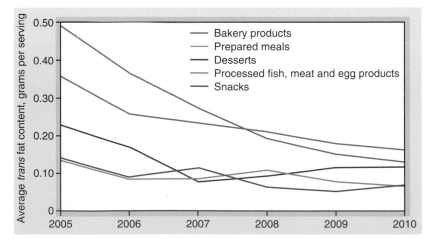

FIGURE 6-7 *Trans* fat levels in new products have dropped dramatically over the last 5 years. (From USDA, Economic Research Service calculations using Mintel Global New Products Database. From Rahkovsky I: *Trans* fats are less common in new food products. *Amber Waves,* Sept 20, 2012.)

these products is encouraged for everyone. Loin (sirloin, tenderloin, or center loin) and round cuts (top, bottom, eye, or tip) and lean or extra lean ground beef contain the least amount of fat. More important than the fat content of any product is its saturated and *trans* fatty acid content.

Dental Considerations

- Use Box 6-1 when assessing fat recommendations.
- Patients frequently consume more fat than they realize because of the "invisible" fats in dairy and meat products. Dental hygienists should interview patients to assess their intake of these foods.
- Foods having a higher fat content are more calorie-dense. For example, ¼ cup of peanuts and seven whole carrots have the same number of kilocalories (210 kcal). Carrots have only a trace of fat; peanuts contain 18 g of fat per ¼ cup. Knowledge of fat content of foods is necessary to assess for fat intake.
- Have patients read a Nutrition Facts label to determine whether the product is a good buy as well as a healthy choice with regard to fat.
- Encourage intake of fruits and vegetables, whole-grain foods, and low-fat dairy products, and discourage intake of fatty meats, fried foods, and processed foods that are low in fiber and high in saturated and *trans* fats.

Nutritional Directions

- Butter contains more saturated fats than most margarines; it also contains cholesterol, whereas soft margarines do not. However, butter does not contain *trans* fatty acids as do some margarines.
- An easy way to determine whether a food is low in fat is to hold up one finger for every 50 kcal in the food (based on the food label); if the total number of fingers you are holding is more than the total fat grams on the label, the item is low-fat; if the total number of fingers you are holding is less than the total fat grams, the item is high fat.
- Purchase processed foods that contain more PUFAs and MUFAs than SFAs. If the food label only lists the total fat, saturated fat, and *trans* fat content, subtract the total number of grams of saturated fat and *trans* fat from the total fat. For example, if the product contains 8 g of fat with 2 g of saturated fat and 1 g of *trans* fat, the 5 g of MUFAs and PUFAs is more than the 3 g from saturated and *trans* fats. This product is acceptable, but if there is another similar product that contains less than 3 g of saturated and *trans* fats, that product would be a wiser choice.
- Fully hydrogenated fats contain almost no *trans* fats but are very seldom found in foods.
- Tropical oils, including palm, palm kernel, and coconut oils, are saturated fats, and their consumption should be limited. In transitioning away from *trans* fats, it is important to avoid reverting to alternatives, such as palm or coconut oils, which are saturated fats and may increase the risk of CHD.
- Fruits, vegetables, and whole-grain foods should be used to replace high fat foods.
- A few fruits and vegetables contain a small amount of fat. Bananas contain a trace of fat (0.55 g or 0.5% fat by weight and 6% of the kilocalories); avocados contain 31 g of fat (15% by weight and 86% of the kilocalories). Both are good sources of several vitamins and minerals.

- Increasing intake of good dietary sources of omega-3 fatty acids is recommended over taking supplements.
- Teach patients to read labels and to understand that the percentage of fat should be determined based on the total kilocalories, not the weight, of the food. To determine fat content, use either of the following formulas:
  - Grams of fat × 9 = kilocalories provided by fat, or
  - Kilocalories of fat ÷ total kilocalories of the product × 100 = % fat content of the product.
- Fats and oils that are 100% fat are necessary to provide adequate PUFAs and fat-soluble vitamins; food items are averaged together to determine if an item exceeding 35% fat would cause the overall intake to exceed the maximum 35% desired fat level.
- Children younger than age 2 years grow rapidly; fat restriction is potentially unsafe for this age group because of uncertainties about the amounts of energy, cholesterol, and EFAs required for growth. After 2 years of age, the *Dietary Guidelines* are applicable.
- If vegetable oil is the first ingredient on the label, the *trans* fatty acid content will be lower than if the first ingredient listed is partially hydrogenated oil.

OVERCONSUMPTION AND HEALTH-RELATED PROBLEMS

Some conditions related to fat intake are observed in dental hygiene practice. The following conditions suggest alteration of the amount or type, or both, of dietary fat: obesity, diabetes mellitus, **hyperlipidemia** (elevated concentrations of any or all of the blood lipids, especially triglycerides and LDL cholesterol), fatty infiltration of the liver, and certain types of cancer.

Obesity

Excessive fat stores are a common disorder in the United States (as discussed in Chapter 1, *Health Application 1*). Although the cause is usually overconsumption of all energy nutrients, kilocalories from fat are so concentrated that relatively small quantities may rapidly increase caloric intake.

Blood Lipid Levels

Elevated blood lipids are related to diet and other risk factors. Hyperlipidemia is associated with CHD. Although many factors can affect blood lipid levels, the strongest dietary determinant of blood cholesterol is dietary saturated and *trans* fats. In contrast, stearic acid, found in beef and cocoa butter, has no detrimental effect on serum cholesterol. Total dietary fat content also affects serum lipid levels, but to a lesser extent than fatty acids. Reduction of total dietary fat content may help reduce saturated fat content. Based on results of metabolic and epidemiological studies, *trans* fatty acids act like SFAs by increasing the risk of CHD considerably (2.5- to 10-fold).

Because of unfavorable publicity about harmful effects of *trans* fatty acids and food labels disclosing how much is in a product, commercial food producers developed product alternatives to *trans* fats. Preserving the structural characteristics and palatability of these food products is not easy. In some cases, the hydrogenation process has been modified to reduce the amount of *trans* fatty acid to less than 10% of the oil content. A relatively new industrial process is used to produce customized fats, which are called interesterified fats, with properties suitable for commercial preparation. Highly saturated hard fats are blended with oils to produce fats with intermediate characteristics. Many of the *trans* fatty acid alternatives, especially those made from tropical fats containing SFA, may not have a desirable effect on blood lipids. Some zero *trans* fat margarines may have a higher amount of SFA than conventional margarines with *trans* fatty acid.[22] In short studies comparing the effects of *trans* fatty acid and interesterified fats, these new fats negatively affected blood lipids, but not as severely as *trans* fats.[23] Needless to say, more research is needed to determine the potential consequences of the products being used to replace *trans* fatty acids. Factors and dietary modifications influencing serum lipid levels are discussed in more detail in *Health Applications 6*.

Coconut oil recently has been touted as being "near miraculous," protecting against cancer and melting away excess body fat. These claims have not been supported by research. Coconut oil, containing 60% medium-chain triglycerides, is a solid at room temperature and does not deteriorate rapidly. Both virgin and conventional coconut oils contain the same saturated fats. More importantly, fatty acids in coconut oil are proven to increase total cholesterol and may decrease HDL levels.[24,25]

Cancer

One third of the more than 500,000 deaths caused by cancer in the United States each year can be attributed to diet and physical activity.[26] Research continues to examine whether the association between high-fat diets and various cancers is attributable to the total amount of fat, the particular type of fat, the kilocalories contributed by fat, or some other factor associated with high-fat foods. Increased body weight and weight gain are associated with higher risk of breast and ovarian cancer. MUFAs, omega-3 fatty acids, and other PUFAs have not been associated with increased risk of cancer. Different mechanisms may be involved in tumor development at different sites and stages of the cancer. Despite many uncertainties about a relationship between dietary fat and cancer risk, experts agree it is best to limit total fat intake by increasing the consumption of fish and lean meat, fruits, vegetables, and whole grain products, while decreasing high-fat meats and foods, especially those high in saturated fats.

Dental Considerations

- To distinguish obesity from edema, when the skin of an obese subject is palpated, it has a flabby consistency, in contrast to the mushy or spongy consistency found in edematous skin.
- Ask adult patients if they know their blood lipid levels. A high serum HDL level is considered desirable to prevent heart disease,

whereas elevated levels of cholesterol, triglycerides, LDL, and VLDL increase the risk of heart disease.
- Inquire about a family history of CHD and other risks associated with heart disease.
- Stay current on research differentiating health effects of commercially produced and naturally occurring *trans* fatty acids.
- Teach patients to read the Nutrition Facts label for saturated and *trans* fats to avoid substituting one unhealthy fat for another.

Nutritional Directions

- Linoleic acid should provide 10% of the total caloric intake. Serum cholesterol can be reduced by increasing intake of MUFAs and PUFAs (see Table 6-1).
- Reduce dietary cholesterol intake to less than 300 mg daily by limiting meats, whole milk and cheese, and eggs.
- "Low cholesterol" on a food label can be misleading. A cholesterol-free product, such as stick margarine, can still be high in saturated and *trans* fatty acids, which elevates blood cholesterol.
- Dietary saturated and *trans* fatty acids have a greater effect on serum cholesterol and LDL cholesterol than dietary cholesterol.
- The consumption of soluble fibers may decrease serum cholesterol.
- Wise food choices to prevent heart disease include unsaturated fats found in liquid vegetable oils, nuts, seeds, and omega-3 unsaturated fats from fatty fish such as salmon, sardines, and shellfish.
- Interesterified fat may be listed on food labels as fully hydrogenated oil.

UNDERCONSUMPTION AND HEALTH-RELATED PROBLEMS

Overconsumption of fat is a primary concern in healthcare, whereas underconsumption of fats is virtually nonexistent in the United States without medical or dietary intervention. However, clinical symptoms of fat deficiency may occur, especially in patients with malabsorption syndromes such as cystic fibrosis or patients in later stages of AIDS. EFA deficiency results in poor growth, dermatitis, reduced resistance to infection, and poor reproductive capacity.

When overall food intake, including fats, is poor, patients lose weight, depleting subcutaneous fat stores needed to maintain body temperature. Patients with anorexia nervosa are especially of concern (see Ch. 17).

Dental Considerations

- If a patient has a poor reserve of subcutaneous fat, monitor temperature closely. These patients are unable to regulate temperature as effectively as patients who have subcutaneous fat reserves.
- A patient with inadequate fat intake is thin, has dry skin and dull hair, and is sensitive to cold temperatures. If these signs and symptoms are noted, suggest examination by a healthcare provider.

- Although much is heard about the problems of fat consumption, fats have important physiological functions, and a certain amount must be provided in the diet.

FAT REPLACERS

As a result of health concerns regarding dietary fats, numerous foods are being manufactured containing less fat. Fat replacers may be helpful in reducing fat and energy consumption. Most of the formulations to replace fat are carbohydrate- and protein-based, but lipid-based materials are available. Each of these fat replacers possesses diverse sensory, functional, and physiological properties that affect their incorporation into various types of products (Table 6-5). Low-calorie salad dressing, low-fat yogurt, and imitation margarine are made by using modified starches and gums to reduce the oil or fat in the product.

By substituting fat replacers for fats, total fat intake can be reduced, and some weight loss may be achieved. However, an overall weight-loss program is still needed to effect weight loss. By consuming large portions of lower fat products, an individual can potentially negate the caloric and fat savings of the replacement foods. Fat substitutes seem to pose little risk to health, but data are sparse regarding possible benefits under conditions of normal consumer use.

Table 6-5 Fat replacers

Generic Name (Trade Name)	kcal/g	Appropriate Uses
Carbohydrate Based		
Cellulose	0	Dairy-type products, sauces, frozen desserts, salad dressings
Dextrins	4	Salad dressings, puddings, spreads, dairy-type products, frozen desserts
Fiber	0	Baked goods, meats, spreads, extruded products
Gums	0	Salad dressings, desserts, processed meats
Inulin	1-1.2	Yogurt, cheese, frozen desserts, baked goods, icings, fillings, whipped cream, dairy products, fiber supplements, processed meats
Maltodextrin	4	Baked goods, dairy products, salad dressings, spreads, sauces, frostings, fillings, processed meats, frozen desserts
Nu-Trim	4	Baked goods, milk, cheese, ice cream
Oatrim	1-4	Baked goods, fillings and frostings, frozen desserts, dairy beverages, cheese, salad dressings, processed meats, confections
Polydextrose	1	Baked goods, chewing gums, confections, salad dressings, frozen dairy desserts, gelatins, puddings
Polyols	1.6-3	Bulking agent
Starch and modified food starch	1-4	Processed meats, salad dressings, baked goods, fillings and frostings, sauces, condiments, frozen desserts, dairy products
Z-Trim	0	Baked goods, burgers, hot dogs, cheese, ice cream, yogurt
Protein-based		
Microparticulated protein (Simplesse)	1-2	Dairy products (e.g., ice cream, butter, sour cream, cheese, yogurt), salad dressings, margarine- and mayonnaise-type products, baked goods, coffee creamers, soups, sauces
Modified whey protein concentrate		Milk and dairy products (e.g., cheese, yogurt, sour cream, ice cream), baked goods, frostings, salad dressings, mayonnaise-type products
Fat Based		
Emulsifiers	9	Cake mixes, cookies, icings, vegetable dairy products
Esterified propoxylated glycerol (EPG)*		Formulated products, baking and frying
Olestra (Olean)	0	Salty snacks, crackers, fried products
Salatrim	5	Confections, baked goods, dairy products
Sorbestrin*	1.5	Fried foods, salad dressings, mayonnaise, baked goods

Data from Data from Calorie Control Council: *Glossary of fat replacers.* © 2012 Calorie Control Council. Accessed August 19, 2013. Available at: http://www.caloriecontrol.org
*May require FDA approval.

Dental Considerations

- Assess use of fat replacers.
- Evaluate overall dietary habits because a patient may think using fat replacers will make a desirable change in health without considering other aspects of the diet.
- If a patient exhibits symptoms such as gastrointestinal distress after consuming a product containing a fat substitute, recommend avoidance of that fat substitute.

Nutritional Directions

- Patients allergic to eggs or cow's milk could be at risk for an allergic reaction to Simplesse because it is made from egg white and milk protein.
- Intake of fat replacers needs to be balanced with variety and moderation in food choices to achieve an overall healthy, nutritious diet.

HEALTH APPLICATION 6 Hyperlipidemia

Despite years of research and copious studies, CHD is still a major concern in the United States, causing *Healthy People 2020* to establish 24 objectives for heart disease and stroke. Cardiovascular disorders include hypertension, CHD, stroke, congenital cardiovascular defects, and congestive heart failure. CHD prevalence in the United States has declined overall; mortality has declined because of improvements in treatment and a reduction in risk factors.[27] One of the *Healthy People 2020* objectives is to lower the death rate 20% from a baseline of 126.0 per 100,000 in 2007 to 100.8 per 100,000.[28] CHD accounts for approximately 36% of deaths (1 of every 2.8) in the United States. Heart disease remains the number one leading cause, and stroke is the number four leading cause of death in the United States.[29]

Hyperlipidemia, or increased plasma cholesterol and LDL levels, seems to be a major risk factor in CHD. The Committee who compiled the *Third Report of the Expert Panel (NCEP) on Detection, Evaluation, and Treatment of High Blood Cholesterol in Adults (ATP III)*[30] and the AHA routinely reevaluate guidelines and update recommendations for healthcare professionals to help prevent CHD. Continual scientific research provides more information allowing refinement of recommendations on detection and management of established risk factors, including evidence against the safety and efficacy of interventions previously considered promising. Most CHD is preventable through the adoption of healthy diet and lifestyles.

The AHA and National Cholesterol Education Program (NCEP) encourage a fasting lipoprotein profile (total cholesterol, LDL and HDL cholesterol, and triglycerides) for all adults older than age 20 years every 5 years along with an assessment for risk factors. LDL cholesterol levels less than 100 mg/dL throughout life are associated with a very low risk for CHD; LDL cholesterol greater than 100 mg/dL is the primary target of therapy. Reducing LDL cholesterol produces favorable outcomes for coronary lesions and reduces the likelihood of acute coronary syndromes. Table 6-6 shows levels that are considered desirable or optimal. Fortunately, the prevalence of elevated LDL levels decreased between 2001 and 2008, but this progress seems to have stalled in recent years.[31] This improvement may be attributed to changes in *trans* fatty acids in the food supply, use of statin medications, or overall dietary changes. More than 25% of adults ages 40 to 74 years continue to have high LDL levels.[32]

The National Institutes of Health, in a cooperative effort with the AHA, has summarized current strategies for implementing recommendations to reduce CHD in the "TLC Program," which is described in "Your Guide to Lowering Your Cholesterol with TLC: Therapeutic Lifestyle Changes."[33]

The programs provide guidelines for diet, physical activity, and weight management (Box 6-3). Maintaining a healthy diet and lifestyle offers the greatest potential of all known approaches for reducing the risk of CHD in the general public. For all individuals without CHD or CHD risk equivalents whose LDL cholesterol is less than 100 mg/dL, adoption of healthy life habits (including cigarette smoking cessation or abstinence, a healthy diet, weight control, and increased physical activity), is recommended, as well as routine medical checkups for blood pressure and cholesterol. These general recommendations also can be applied to patients with CHD or at risk for CHD. If the lipoprotein profile does not normalize after implementing these guidelines, drug treatment may be added.

With the implementation of therapeutic lifestyle changes, LDL cholesterol may decrease 20% to 30%. Other lifestyle changes shown in Box 6-4 also have a positive effect on preventing heart disease. Dietary recommendations are similar to those mentioned in Box 6-2. Natural food sources generally are recommended for nutrients rather than supplements. Other diets and lifestyle changes have also been successful in reducing CHD, namely the Dietary Approaches to Stop Hypertension (DASH) regime (see Chapter 12) and the Mediterranean diet, which promotes vegetables, monounsaturated fats, and nuts (see the Evolve website).[34,35]

Many other dietary factors have been proposed to help reduce the risk of CHD. Some of these are generally unproven or have uncertain effects on CHD. Although antioxidants seem to prevent CHD, antioxidant vitamin supplements or other supplements such as selenium[36] are not recommended to prevent CHD. Phytochemicals found in fruits and vegetables may be important in reducing the risk of atherosclerosis. Foods containing antioxidants from a variety of fruits and vegetables, whole grains, and vegetable oils, and spices like turmeric, garlic, and cinnamon, are recommended. Until more is known about the mode of action of these compounds, the most prudent practice to ensure optimum consumption of bioactive compounds by increasing intake of fruits and vegetables and replacing salt with spices.

Plant sterols are bioactive compounds found in all vegetable foods, which inhibit cholesterol absorption. Consumption of soy protein–rich foods, a source of plant sterols, may indirectly reduce CHD risk if they replace animal and dairy products that contain saturated fat and cholesterol. Small quantities of sterols are present in a variety of foods, including fruits, vegetables, nuts, seeds, cereals, and legumes. Plant sterols are absorbed at the same sites in the small intestine as cholesterol, and interfere with cholesterol absorption,

HEALTH APPLICATION 6   Hyperlipidemia—cont'd

resulting in a 5% to 17% reduction of LDL cholesterol.[37,38] An intake of approximately 2 to 3 g is needed to produce maximum effects. To sustain LDL cholesterol reductions from sterols, daily intake is necessary, as with medications. A plant sterol can be added into fat products and other foods to provide this beneficial product in a readily available source to increase dietary availability of sterols. In the United States, sterols are added to margarine spread, orange juice, and other products. A low-fat diet increases the effectiveness of these products.

The AHA recommends patients without CHD eat a variety of fish, preferably oily fish, at least twice a week. Individuals who already have CHD are advised to consume at least 1 g of EPA and DHA daily, preferably from oily fish, but the healthcare provider may recommend supplements.

Of all the dietary changes recommended, cholesterol intake probably has the least effect on plasma cholesterol concentrations in most individuals because of less endogenous cholesterol production in response to cholesterol absorption. Consuming an egg daily does not increase risk for CHD.[39] The AHA recommendations do not limit the number of eggs as long as total dietary cholesterol is limited to about 300 mg per day. One large egg contains 212 mg of cholesterol.

Most studies have found that reducing total dietary fat reduces serum cholesterol. Because fat consumption generally coincides with decreased saturated fat intake, changes in blood lipids may be related more to the type of fat consumed rather than total fat. However, a low-cholesterol, low-fat diet rarely reduces cholesterol more than 15%, and medications may be needed to reduce blood lipids further. A diet that limits fat to 35% of kilocalories with 5% to 10% from PUFAs and 10% from SFAs and *trans* fatty acids reduces total and LDL cholesterol concentrations in most patients with hyperlipidemia.[40] Lowering omega-6 PUFA intake any further would possibly increase the risk for CHD.[41] By replacing some SFAs with MUFAs and some PUFAs, and decreasing total fat, LDL is lowered without decreasing HDL concentrations. These changes result in a more palatable diet that is better received by Americans.

Because of Americans' high intake of sugar, which exceeds discretionary kilocalorie allowances, especially in the form of sugar-containing beverages, the AHA recommends reducing added sugar intake. A high intake of refined carbohydrates negatively affects lipid profile (decreases HDL, increases triglyceride and LDL). The AHA recommends a prudent upper limit of half of the discretionary kilocalorie allowance (no more than 100 kilocalories for women and 150 kilocalories for men).[42]

One of the most important facts for decreasing the risk of CHD is the types of foods chosen when lowering saturated fat intake. When a decrease in saturated fats is recommended, suggestions should be made regarding what types of foods/fats should be chosen to replace those kilocalories. Total dietary fat may not be a risk factor for CHD, but more likely, the types of fat eaten. Replacing saturated and *trans* fats with PUFA may benefit lipid profiles, but replacing them with refined carbohydrate foods increases risk factors.[43] Omega-6 PUFA intake should be increased, but not replace beneficial omega-3 PUFAs in an effort to reduce fat intake. Replacing SFA with MUFA may increase HDL levels, thereby improving lipoprotein profiles.[44] Previous recommendations to decrease fat intake have resulted in increased consumption of refined carbohydrates, which may actually have increased CHD risk. Overall dietary quality includes (a) carbohydrate quality (whole versus refined grains, and dietary fiber); (b) intake of specific individual fatty acids; (c) inclusion of a variety of healthful foods such as fruits, vegetables, nuts, fish, dairy products, and vegetable oils; (d) limited amounts of sugar-sweetened beverages and processed meats and foods; and (e) energy balance.[45] Recommendations will continue to change as research leads to knowledge about the effect of specific fatty acids on lipid profiles and CHD.

Table 6-6	Desirable/optimal blood lipid levels	
Lipid	**Desirable/Optimal Level (mg/dL)**	
Total cholesterol	<200	
LDL	<100	
HDL	>60	
Triglyceride	<150	

Data from National Cholesterol Education Program (NCEP): *Third report of the National Cholesterol Education Program (NCEP) on detection, evaluation, and treatment of high blood cholesterol in adults (Adult Treatment Panel III), final report.* Publication No. 02-5125. Bethesda, MD, 2002, National Institutes of Health, National Heart, Lung, and Blood Institute, and American Heart Association: *What your cholesterol means.* Accessed August 19, 2013. Available at: http://www.heart.org/HEARTORG/Conditions/Cholesterol/AboutCholesterol/What-Your-Cholesterol-Levels-Mean_UCM_305562_Article.jsp.

BOX 6-3   American Heart Association Healthy Diet Goals

For the first time, the American Heart Association has defined what it means to have ideal cardiovascular health, identifying seven health and behavior factors that impact health and quality of life. We know that even simple, small changes can make a big difference in living a better life. Known as "Life's Simple 7," these steps can help add years to your life:

- Do not smoke.
- Maintain a healthy weight.
- Engage in regular physical activity.
- Manage blood pressure.
- Eat a healthy diet.
- Take charge of cholesterol.
- Keep blood sugar, or glucose, at healthy levels.

From American Heart Association Nutrition Center: Healthy Diet Goals. © 2013 American Heart Association, Inc. Accessed October 5, 2013: http://www.heart.org/HEARTORG/GettingHealthy/NutritionCenter/HealthyDietGoals/Healthy-Diet-Goals_UCM_310436_SubHomePage.jsp.

<table>
<tr><td>

**BOX
6-4**

</td><td>

Practical Tips to Implement American Heart Association 2006 Lifestyle Recommendations

</td></tr>
</table>

- Know your caloric needs to achieve and maintain a healthy weight.
- Know the kilocalorie content of the foods and beverages you consume.
- Track your weight, physical activity, and kilocalorie intake.
- Prepare and eat smaller portions.

- Track and, when possible, decrease screen time (e.g., watching television, surfing the Internet, and playing computer games).
- Incorporate physical movement into habitual activities.
- Do not smoke or use tobacco products.
- If you consume alcohol, do so in moderation (equivalent of no more than 1 drink for women or 2 drinks for men per day).

Adapted from American Heart Association Nutrition Committee, Lichtenstein AH, Appel LJ, Brands M, et al: Diet and lifestyle recommendations revision 2006. A scientific statement from the American Heart Association Nutrition Committee. *Circulation* 2006;114(1):82-96.

Case Application for the Dental Hygienist

A 50-year-old patient complains to his dental hygienist that he has recently been having chest pain. He says a recent testing at his grocery store indicated his blood cholesterol level was elevated. A healthcare provider told him several years ago his cholesterol was slightly elevated and that he probably should lower his cholesterol intake. No formal diet education was ordered and no follow-up work has been done. His blood pressure is 145/90 mm Hg.

He continues to eat anything he wants. He realizes some foods are high in fat and should be avoided, but he is unable to identify these foods. When questioned about fat requirements and different types of fat, he says that he does not understand all of those big medical terms. He also indicates his parents ate what they wanted without all these problems and concerns.

Nutritional Assessment
- Readiness/willingness to learn
- Knowledge level concerning fat principles and how these relate to his diagnosis
- Total amount of fat intake
- Typical foods eaten
- Type of dietary habits: who purchases and prepares the food, where he lives, where most meals are eaten
- Blood pressure
- Serum lipids, if known
- Family medical history (parents still living, cause of death)

Nutritional Diagnosis
Altered health maintenance related to lack of knowledge of fat principles; diet and how it relates to the condition.

Nutritional Goals
The patient will adhere to a low-fat, low-cholesterol diet; list foods high and low in fat; and state how disease may improve or deteriorate with diet.

Nutritional Implementation
Intervention: Emphasize the importance of having a thorough examination annually by a healthcare provider and a confirmation of laboratory work with a complete fasting lipid profile.
Rationale: Dietary changes and lifestyle changes are probably indicated; however, the best individuals to diagnose and prescribe treatment are a healthcare provider and RDN.
Intervention: Explain how diet and lifestyle affect his condition: (a) saturated and *trans* fats increase the rate of fatty deposits in the arteries; (b) high cholesterol intake also adversely affects this

process; (c) physiological roles of fat (see p. 108); (d) smoking increases the risk of heart disease; and (e) maintaining a body mass index (BMI) within normal range decreases risk.
Rationale: Knowledge increases compliance.
Intervention: Explain the difference between PUFAs and SFAs: (a) use actual Nutrition Facts labels; (b) provide a list of foods high and low in these two types of fat; (c) keep fat intake to less than 35% of total kilocalories; less than 10% of caloric intake from SFAs and *trans* fatty acids, up to 20% from MUFAs, and up to 10% from PUFAs.
Rationale: If the patient knows the difference between the two types of fat, he can make informed choices to help reduce the likelihood of heart disease.
Intervention: Explain the difference between the types of lipids and cholesterol: (a) provide a list of foods high and low in cholesterol; (b) limit daily cholesterol intake to 300 mg or less; (c) explain that "cholesterol-free" does not mean "fat-free."
Rationale: Reducing serum cholesterol levels may help slow the effects of heart disease.
Intervention: Inquire at each recare appointment if the patient has had a blood lipid profile check recently (HDL, greater than 35 mg/dL for men; LDL, less than 100 mg/dL). Use these as motivators to stay on a healthy diet.
Rationale: These values can provide concrete evidence for motivation and compliance.
Intervention: Monitor blood pressure values at each recare appointment. Inform the patient that hypertension is another risk factor for heart disease. Refer to the healthcare provider for elevated values.
Rationale: If the patient is aware of his blood pressure and the harmful effects of blood pressure elevation, he will make attempts to lower it.
Intervention: Teach the patient how to read nutrition labels (use an actual food label for teaching); use a margarine brand that lists the first ingredient as liquid oil. Explain the different claims on labels, such as "fat-free," "low-fat," and "reduced-fat." (See Box 1-3.)
Rationale: Labels can be confusing. Accurate information can promote healthy food choices, and reduce the incidence of heart disease.
Intervention: Suggest the patient decrease the amount of dietary fat and saturated fats: advise him to (a) eat smaller servings of meat; (b) trim visible fat from meats; (c) consume more skinless poultry and fatty fish; (d) avoid fried foods; and (e) use less salad

Case Application for the Dental Hygienist—cont'd

dressing, change the type of fat (use olive oil), or reduce the amount of fat in the salad dressing (fat-free or low-fat).

Rationale: These are all ways to decrease fat intake, thereby decreasing the progression of atherosclerosis. The use of more fish increases intake of omega-3 fatty acids.

Evaluation

If the patient lists foods higher and lower in fat and makes better choices to consume a low-fat, low-cholesterol diet, dental hygiene

care was effective. In addition, dental hygiene care was successful if the patient can identify the healthiest low-fat, low-cholesterol choices from three food labels; state how fat and cholesterol can lead to further deterioration of his disease; and verbalize that fat speeds up the accumulation of fatty deposits. Other factors to evaluate include whether (a) blood lipid levels improve, (b) blood pressure is within normal values, and (c) the patient has begun a smoking cessation program.

STUDENT READINESS

1. Describe the following terms: lipoproteins, hyperlipidemia, structural lipids, and EFA.
2. A patient wants to know which foods to consume to (a) increase PUFAs, (b) increase MUFAs, and (c) decrease SFAs. Name three sources of each.
3. In observing physical properties of fats, how could you estimate the polyunsaturated and saturated fat content of a food?
4. What unsaturated fatty acid is essential in the diet? What are the functions of unsaturated fatty acids in the body?
5. Compare the Nutrition Facts labels of three brands of stick margarine, three brands of tub margarine, two brands of diet margarine, and two brands of spray margarine. How do they differ in their polyunsaturated-to-saturated fat ratio? List the first ingredient of each.
6. Describe the functions of fat in the diet.
7. Evaluate one day of your intake for types of foods consumed and amounts of cholesterol, *trans* fatty acid, and saturated fat. If that day represented your average cholesterol and saturated fat intake over an extended period, determine whether the cholesterol or saturated fat content of intake should be reduced. List some simple, realistic suggestions for decreasing their intake.
8. Describe the role of cholesterol in the body.
9. Calculate the caloric value of the following items:
   2 slices bacon (8 g of fat, 4 g of protein)
   1 tbsp margarine (12 g of fat)
   1 tbsp whipped margarine (8 g of fat)
   1 tbsp mayonnaise (6 g of fat)
   1 tbsp lard (13 g of fat)
10. A patient asks if it is possible to lose or gain 1 lb of body fat every day. What would you say?
11. Calculate the grams of fat a patient could consume on (1) a 1500-kcal diet and (2) a 2000-kcal diet to meet the *Dietary Guidelines.*
12. List five points you think a patient should know about fats in general.

References

1. Hiza HAB, Bende L: *Nutrient content of the U.S. food supply: developments between 2000 and 2006.* Home Economics Research Report No 59. Washington DC, Center for Nutrition Policy and Promotion, U.S. Dept of Agriculture, 2011. Accessed August 19, 2013: http://www.cnpp.usda.gov/Publications/FoodSupply/Final_FoodSupplyReport_2006.pdf.
2. Biing-Hwan L, Guthrie J: *Nutrition quality of food prepared at home and away from home, 1077–2008.* Economic Research Service, Economic Information Bulletin Number 105, 2012. Accessed August 20, 2013: http://www.ers.usda.gov/publications/eib-economic-information-bulletin/eib105.aspx
3. Tucker RM, Mattes RD: *Are free fatty acids effective taste stimuli in humans?* Presented at the symposium "The Taste for Fat: New Discoveries on the Role of Fat in Sensory Perception, Metabolism, Sensory Pleasure and Beyond" held at the Institute of Food Technologists 2011 Annual Meeting, New Orleans, LA, June 12, 2011.
4. Gaillard D, Laugerette F, Darcel N, et al: The gustatory pathway is involved in CD36-mediated orosensory perception of long-chain fatty acids in the mouse. *FASEB J* 22(5):1458–1468, 2008.
5. Pan A, Chen M, Chowdhury R, et al: α-Linolenic acid and risk of cardiovascular disease: a systematic review and meta-analysis. *Am J Clin Nutr* 96(6):1262–1273, 2012.
6. Mozaffarian D, Lemaitre RN, King IB, et al: Plasma phospholipid long-chain ω—3 fatty acids and total and cause-specific mortality in older adults: a cohort study. *Ann Intern Med* 158(7):515–525, 2013.
7. Rizos EC, Ntzani EE, Bika E, et al: Association between omega-3 fatty acid supplementation and risk of major cardiovascular disease events: a systematic review and meta-analysis. *JAMA* 308(10):1024–1033, 2012.
8. Johnson GH, Fritsche K: Effect of dietary linoleic acid on markers of inflammation in healthy persons: a systematic review of randomized controlled trials. *J Acad Nutr Diet* 112(7):1029–1041, 2012.
9. Kay EK: n-3 Fatty acid intake and periodontal disease. *J Am Diet Assoc* 110(11):1650–1652, 2010.
10. Naqvi AZ, Buettner C, Phillips RS, et al: n-3 Fatty acids and periodontitis in US adults. *J Am Diet Assoc* 110(11):1669–1675, 2010.
11. Wright JD, Wang CY: *Trends in intake of energy and macronutrients in adults from 1999–2000 through 2007–2008.* NCHS Data Brief No. 49, Washington, DC, 2010, U.S. Department of Health and Human Services.
12. Reddy KS, Katan MB: Diet, nutrition and the prevention of hypertension and cardiovascular diseases. *Pub Health Nutr* 7(1A Supp l001):167–186, 2004.
13. Ibid., Wright.
14. Hooper L, Summerbell CD, Thompson R, et al: Reduced or modified dietary fat for preventing cardiovascular disease. *Cochrane Database Syst Rev* 5:CD002137, 2012.
15. Baum SJ, Kris-Etherton PM, Willett WC, et al: Fatty acids in cardiovascular health and disease: a comprehensive update. *J Clin Lipidol* 6(3):216–234, 2012.
16. International Food Information Council: *EPA and DHA: Time to establish a dietary reference intake level? Food Insight 2009 Aug.* Accessed August 18, 2013. Available at: http://www.

foodinsight.org/Newsletter/Detail.aspx?topic=EPA_and_DHA_T.

17. International Food Information Council: *Food insight interviews Dr. Bill Harris on omega-3 and omega-6 fatty acids.* Accessed August 18, 2013. Available at: http://www.foodinsight.org/Newsletter/Detail.aspx?topic=Food_Insight_.

18. U.S. Department of Agriculture (USDA) and U.S. Department of Health and Human Services: *Dietary guidelines for Americans 2010*, ed 7, Washington DC, 2010, U.S. Government Printing Office.

19. Soy Connection: *Soybean oil overview.* Accessed August 18, 2013. Available at: http://www.soyconnection.com.

20. Soy Connection: *Trans fat fact sheet.* Accessed August 18, 2013. Available at: http://www.soyconnection.com.

21. Doell D, Folmer D, Lee H, et al: Updated estimate of *trans* fat intake by the US population. *Food Addit Contam Part A Chem Anal Control Expo Risk Assess* 29(6):861–874, 2012.

22. Stender S, Astrup A, Dyerberg J: What went in when *trans* went out? *N Engl J Med* 361(3):314–316, 2009.

23. Hayes KC, Pronczuk A: Replacing *trans* fat: the argument for palm oil with a cautionary note on interesterification. *J Am Coll Nutr* 29(3 Suppl):S253–S284, 2010.

24. Cunningham E: Is there science to support claims for coconut oil? *J Am Diet Assoc* 111(5):786, 2011.

25. Siri-Tarino PW, Sun Q, Hu FB, et al: Meta-analysis of prospective cohort studies evaluating the association of saturated fat with cardiovascular disease. *Am J Clin Nutr* 91(1):535–546, 2010.

26. American Cancer Society: *Diet and physical activity: what's the cancer connection?* Accessed August 18, 2013: http://www.cancer.org/Cancer/CancerCauses/DietandPhysicalActivity/diet-and-physical-activity.

27. Centers for Disease Control and Prevention: Prevalence of coronary heart disease—United States, 2006–2010. *MMWR Morb Mortal Wkly Rep* 60(40):1377–1381, 2011.

28. Centers for Disease Control and Prevention: *Healthy People 2020 Topics and Objectives. Heart Disease and Stroke.* Accessed August 18, 2013. Available at: http://healthypeople.gov/2020/topicsobjectives2020/overview.aspx?topicid=21.

29. Murphy SL, Jiaquan X, Kochanek KD: Deaths: preliminary data for 2010. *Natl Vital Stat Rep* 60(4):1–68, 2012. Accessed August 20, 2013: http://www.cdc.gov/nchs/data/nvsr/nvsr60/nvsr60_04.pdf

30. National Cholesterol Education Program: *Third report of the National Cholesterol Education Program (NCEP) expert panel on detection, evaluation, and treatment of high blood cholesterol in adults.* NIH Publication No. 02-5215. Bethesda, MD, 2002, National Institutes of Health. Accessed August 18, 2013: www.nhlbi.nih.gov/guidelines/cholesterol/atp3full.pdf.

31. Kaufman HW, Blatt AJ, Huang X, et al: Blood cholesterol trends 2001-2011 in the United States: analysis of 105 million patient records. *PLoS ONE* 8(5):e63416, 2013.

32. Kuklina EV, Carroll MD, Shaw KM, et al: *Trends in high LDL cholesterol, cholesterol-lowering medication use, and dietary saturated-fat intake: United States, 1976–2010.* NCHS Data Brief Number 117. Hyattsville, MD, 2013, National Center for Health Statistics. Accessed August 20, 2013: http://www.cdc.gov/nchs/data/databriefs/db117.htm

33. U.S. Department of Health and Human Services, National Institutes of Health: *Your guide to lowering your cholesterol with TLC.* NIH Publication No 06-5235, 2010.

34. Salehi-Abargouei A, Maghsoudi Z, Shirani F, et al: Effects of dietary approaches to stop hypertension (DASH)-style diet on fatal or nonfatal cardiovascular diseases—incidence: a systematic review and meta-analysis on observational prospective studies. *Nutrition* 29(4):611–618, 2013.

35. Estruch R, Ros E, Salas-Salvadó J, et al: Primary prevention of cardiovascular disease with a Mediterranean diet. *N Engl J Med* 368(14):1279–1290, 2013.

36. Rees K, Hartley L, Day C, et al: Selenium supplements for the prevention of cardiovascular disease. *Cochrane Database Syst Rev* 1:CD009671, 2013.

37. Bruckert E, Rosenbaum D: Lowering LDL-cholesterol through diet: potential role in the statin era. *Curr Opin Lipidol* 22(1):43–48, 2011.

38. Gylling H, Hallikainen M, Nissinen MJ, et al: The effect of a very high daily plant stanol ester intake on serum lipids, carotenoids, and fat-soluble vitamins. *Clin Nutr* 29(1):112–118, 2010.

39. Rong Y, Chen L, Zhu T, et al: Egg consumption and risk of coronary heart disease and stroke: dose-response meta-analysis of prospective cohort studies. *BMJ* 346:e8539, 2013.

40. Harris WS, Mozaffarian D, Rimm E, et al: Omega-6 fatty acids and risk for cardiovascular disease: a science advisory from the American Heart Association Nutrition Subcommittee of the Council on Nutrition, Physical Activity, and Metabolism; Council on Cardiovascular Nursing; and Council on Epidemiology and Prevention. *Circulation* 119(6):902–907, 2009.

41. Bruckert E, Rosenbaum D: Lowering LDL-cholesterol through diet: potential role in the statin era. *Curr Opin Lipidol* 22(1):43–48, 2011.

42. Johnson RK, Appel LJ, Brands M, et al: Dietary sugars intake and cardiovascular health. *Circulation* 120(11):1011–1020, 2009.

43. Siri-Tarino RW, Sun Q, Hu FB, et al: Saturated fat, carbohydrate, and cardiovascular disease. *Am J Clin Nutr* 91(3):502–509, 2010.

44. Jenkins DJ, Chiavaroli L, Wong JM, et al: Adding monounsaturated fatty acids to a dietary portfolio of cholesterol-lowering foods in hypercholesterolemia. *CMAJ* 182(18):1961–1967, 2010.

45. Mozaffarian D: The great fat debate: taking the focus off of saturated fat. *J Am Diet Assoc* 111(5):665–666, 2011.

ⓔ EVOLVE RESOURCES

Please visit http://evolve.elsevier.com/Stegeman/nutritional for additional practice and study support tools.

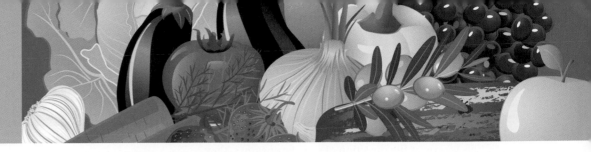

Chapter 7

Use of the Energy Nutrients: Metabolism and Balance

Student Learning Outcomes

Upon completion of this chapter, the student will be able to achieve the following student learning outcomes:

- Calculate energy needs according to the patient's weight and activities.
- Explain physiological sources of energy.
- Identify factors affecting the basal metabolic rate.
- Assess factors affecting energy balance.

- Summarize the effects of inadequate energy intake.
- Explain the principles for and importance of regulating energy balance to a patient.
- Individualize dental hygiene considerations to patients regarding energy metabolism.
- Relate nutritional directions to meet patients' needs regarding energy metabolism.

Key Terms

Adenosine triphosphate (ATP)
Anabolism
Appetite
Basal energy expenditure
Basal metabolic rate (BMR)
Calorimeter
Catabolism
Coenzyme
Cofactor
Gluconeogenesis
Glycemic effect
Glycogenesis
High-energy phosphate compounds
Hormones
Hunger

Indirect calorimetry
Insulin
Ketoacidosis
Ketonuria
Ketosis
Kilocalorie (kcal)
Lipogenesis
Lipolysis
Metabolism
Normoglycemic
Oxidation
Pedometer
Postabsorptive state
Renal failure
Thermic effect

☉ Test Your NQ

1. **T/F** Insulin is a hormone that decreases blood glucose levels.
2. **T/F** Even during sleep, the body requires energy.
3. **T/F** BMR stands for blood malnutrition reaction.
4. **T/F** A malnourished patient would have a low BMR.
5. **T/F** The hypothalamus controls hunger and satiety.
6. **T/F** Hunger is the same as appetite.
7. **T/F** Fats are a good source of quick energy.
8. **T/F** The kidneys play an important role in maintaining nutrient balance within the body.
9. **T/F** Ketoacidosis can occur as a result of strict carbohydrate restriction.
10. **T/F** Vitamins are a source of energy.

After foods are chewed and digested, the macronutrients (carbohydrate, protein, fat, and alcohol) supplying physiological energy for the body are converted to glucose, fatty acids, and amino acids. These basic nutrient units are delivered to cells where, at the direction of specific enzymes, they can be used.

Recall from earlier chapters that no single nutrient can be isolated from the others because nutrients are concurrently distributed in foods and share many points of interaction in digestion, absorption, and metabolism. Metabolism encompasses the continuous processes whereby living organisms and cells convert nutrients into energy, body structure, and waste.

METABOLISM

In metabolic activity, the two major chemical reactions are catabolism and anabolism. Catabolism is splitting complex substances into simpler substances; anabolism is using absorbed nutrients to build or synthesize more complex compounds (see Chapter 2 or online at Evolve for more detail). Anabolism and catabolism are continuous reactions in the body. Cells in the epithelial lining of the oral and gastrointestinal mucosa are replaced approximately every 3 to 7 days. Despite this rapid turnover, the rate of catabolism is usually equal to that of anabolism in a healthy adult. During certain stages of life, such as growth periods or pregnancy, more anabolism is occurring than catabolism. Conversely, when illness or stress occurs, excessive catabolism is evident.

Other phases of metabolism include delivery of nutrients to the cells where they are needed, and delivery of wastes to sites where they can be excreted. After absorption of the macronutrients, glucose, fatty acids, and amino acids can be used to yield energy via a common pathway within the mitochondria of cells (Fig. 7-1). The catabolic end products of carbohydrates, proteins, and fats are carbon dioxide, water, and energy. Nitrogen is an additional end product of protein.

The Krebs cycle (also called citric acid cycle or tricarboxylic acid [TCA] cycle) converts glucose, fatty acids, and amino acids to a usable form of energy, requiring many enzymes. Additional information on the TCA cycle can be found in Chapter 2 and online at Evolve. For activation of some enzymes, vitamins or minerals or both must be available. An enzyme needing vitamins for activation is called a coenzyme. Thiamin, riboflavin, and niacin are B vitamins essential as coenzymes in the TCA cycle. An enzyme may also require a cofactor. A cofactor functions in the same way as coenzymes, but the molecule required is a mineral or electrolyte.

Anabolic processes require energy. Examples of anabolism are the building of new muscle tissue or bone and the secretion of cellular products such as hormones. Hormones are "messengers" produced by a group of cells that stimulate or retard the functions of other cells. Hormones principally control different metabolic functions that affect secretions and growth. Anabolism involves the use of

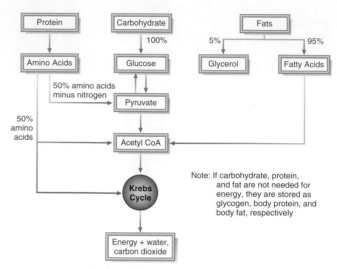

FIGURE 7-1 Metabolic pathways. (From Peckenpaugh NJ: *Nutrition essentials and diet therapy*, ed 11, St Louis, 2010, Saunders.)

glucose, amino acids, fatty acids, and glycerol to build various substances that make up the body itself and the other substances necessary for the body to function. All nutrients are intertwined in this process. For instance, dispensible amino acids are ordinarily used to build proteins, but glucose can be the basis for anabolism of amino acids and fatty acids.

ROLE OF THE LIVER

The liver plays a major regulatory role by controlling the kinds and quantities of nutrients in the bloodstream. All monosaccharides are converted to glucose in the liver to provide an energy supply for the cells. Glycogen, a polysaccharide, also can be broken down to glucose and released into the circulating blood as needed. Other end products of digestion may be oxidized to provide energy; converted to glucose, protein, fat, or other substances; or released to circulate at prescribed levels in the blood for use by cells throughout the body.

ROLE OF THE KIDNEYS

Kidneys perform the important metabolic task of removing waste products from the blood, and along with the liver, control the levels of many nutrients in the blood. Metabolic end products from cells, unnecessary substances absorbed from the gastrointestinal tract, potentially harmful compounds that have been detoxified by the liver, and drugs are removed from the blood by the kidneys.

Kidneys accomplish this task by a process of filtration and reabsorption. Glucose, amino acids, vitamins, water, and various minerals are reabsorbed or excreted by the kidneys, depending on the body's need. Excess nitrogen from protein catabolism also is excreted by the kidneys. Kidneys help maintain nutrient balance within the body. Other routes of excretion of waste products are through the bowel; the skin, which excretes water and electrolytes; and the lungs, which remove carbon dioxide and water.

Dental Considerations

- The goal of nutrition in a dental setting is to promote anabolism for growth or healing.
- Uncontrolled blood glucose levels may cause numerous complications, such as poor wound healing and increased risk of infection for patients with diabetes.
- The kidneys' ability to reabsorb nutrients may be altered by certain medications, especially diuretics, or a kidney disorder. Function also depends on fluid balance.

Nutritional Directions

- The liver is a vital organ for metabolism of food and drugs.
- The kidneys help the body dispose of waste products and drugs. Adequate fluid intake (9 to 11 cups per day) facilitates this process.
- If the kidneys are not working properly, drugs and nutrients may be retained or lost. Both are undesirable.

CARBOHYDRATE METABOLISM

Monosaccharides are transported through the portal vein to the liver for **glycogenesis**, a process in which sugars, including fructose, galactose, sorbitol, and xylitol, may be stored as glycogen. Glucose is the circulating sugar in the blood; it is the major energy supply for cells. The level of circulating glucose is closely monitored by the liver and is constantly maintained at a **normoglycemic** level (normal blood glucose range), between 70 and 100 mg/dL. **Insulin** is a hormone that lowers blood glucose levels. Blood glucose levels peak at 140 mg/dL 30 to 60 minutes after a meal and return to normal within 3 hours in individuals with normal secretion and use of insulin. This consistent blood glucose level is significant, indicating the necessity of a certain amount of glucose in the blood for normal functioning of body tissues (Fig. 7-2). Hyperglycemia (elevated blood glucose) and hypoglycemia (decreased blood glucose) are very serious conditions that could be fatal; the precipitating cause for either should be identified. Many patients with diabetes who take insulin or an antidiabetic medication that can cause hypoglycemia, or both, may exhibit symptoms related to hypoglycemia, particularly if they have not eaten within a 4- to 5-hour time span. These patients need to be treated with a carbohydrate source before continuing treatment (see *Health Application 7*).

Individuals with diabetes often respond differently to different carbohydrate sources. It is important for patients with diabetes to closely manage and monitor their glycemic levels. The blood glucose response to different foods and different combinations of food cannot be accurately

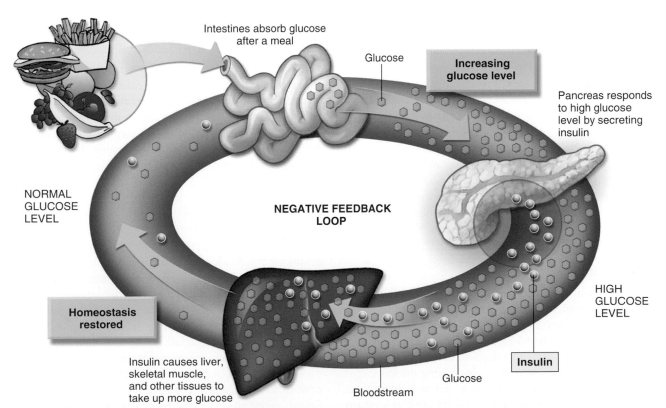

FIGURE 7-2 Role of insulin. Insulin operates in a negative feedback loop that prevents blood glucose concentration from increasing too far above the normal (or setpoint) level. Insulin promotes uptake of glucose by all cells of the body, enabling them to catabolize or store it, or both. The liver and skeletal muscles are especially well adapted for storage of glucose as glycogen. Excess glucose is removed from the bloodstream. If the glucose level falls below the setpoint level, hormones such as glucagon promote the release of glucose from storage into the bloodstream. (From Thibodeau GA, Patton KT: *Anatomy and physiology*, ed 7, St Louis, 2010, Mosby Elsevier.)

predicted from the amount of simple sugars or complex carbohydrates ingested.[1] White bread, potatoes, and white rice have a glycemic effect similar to sucrose. **Glycemic effect** is the rate at which glucose increases in the bloodstream after a particular food is eaten.

A complex hormonal system maintains a constant blood glucose level. Insulin is the primary hormone that lowers blood glucose levels. When hyperglycemia occurs, insulin is secreted to decrease blood glucose levels. Conversely, hypoglycemia elicits the secretion of several hormones (thyroid hormone, epinephrine, glucagon, and growth hormone) to increase blood glucose levels. The liver can elevate blood glucose levels by converting amino acids from protein, and glycerol from fats to glucose. The process of synthesizing glucose from noncarbohydrate sources is known as **gluconeogenesis** (see Chapter 2 or online at Evolve for additional details).

Dietary carbohydrates ensure optimal glycogen stores and are digested faster than other energy nutrients. The liver can degrade glycogen to glucose. The amount of energy available from glycogen stores is generally less than a day's energy expenditure, or approximately 1200 to 1800 kcal. Red blood cells, and cells in the heart, brain, and renal medulla prefer glucose as their energy source.

PROTEIN METABOLISM

Amino acids are transported through the portal vein into the liver. The liver is an "aminostat," monitoring the intake and breakdown of most of the amino acids. Individual amino acids are released by the liver to enter the general circulation at specific levels, so each amino acid is available as needed to synthesize each individual protein. Amino acids transported in the blood are rapidly removed for use by cells. If individual amino acids increase above a specific level in the blood, they are removed and oxidized for energy.

Protein metabolism is in a constant dynamic state, with catabolism and anabolism occurring continuously to replace worn-out proteins in cells. Even during anabolic periods such as growth, muscle catabolism is elevated as each cell remodels itself. Anabolic and catabolic processes are controlled by the liver and hormones. Insulin, thyroxine, and growth hormone stimulate protein synthesis.

Anabolism

A small reservoir of amino acids, which is called the *amino acid metabolic pool,* is available for anabolism and to maintain the dynamic state of equilibrium. This metabolic pool, containing approximately 70 g of amino acids, is less than most Americans consume in a day and could hardly be classified as a large storage of protein. Increasing muscle size is considered an increase in body mass, not protein storage. High-protein diets are neither safe nor effective as a means to increase muscle mass without physical activity or exercise to promote muscle development. To maintain a satisfactory protein status, a daily supply of essential amino acids obtained from the diet is necessary.

Anabolism depends on the presence of all essential amino acids simultaneously. It is not a stepwise process in which the synthesis of a protein can be started at one point, but completed when the needed amino acid appears later.

Protein synthesis is also affected by caloric intake. If caloric intake is inadequate, tissue proteins are used for energy, resulting in increased nitrogen excretion. This process requires the B vitamin pyridoxine.

Catabolism

Amino acids are catabolized principally in the liver, but metabolism also occurs to some extent in kidney and muscle. Removal of the nitrogen grouping from amino acids, a process requiring the B vitamins pyridoxine and riboflavin, yields carbon skeletons and ammonia. The carbon skeletons can be (a) used to make nonessential amino acids, (b) used to produce energy via the TCA cycle, or (c) converted to fats and stored as fatty tissue. Not all ingested protein is used to build muscle.

When amino acids are not needed for protein anabolism, and energy is not needed, they are converted to fat and stored in the body. If caloric intake is inadequate, proteins are used for energy rather than to build or repair lean body mass or produce essential protein-based compounds.

Urea is the major waste product of protein catabolism. Ammonia is a toxic substance the liver converts to urea to be excreted by the kidneys. The levels of urea and ammonia vary directly with dietary protein levels.

LIPID METABOLISM

Hormones involved in carbohydrate metabolism also control fat metabolism. Insulin increases fat synthesis, whereas thyroxine, epinephrine, growth hormone, and glucocorticoids increase fat mobilization. The liver is the principal regulator of fat metabolism and lipoprotein synthesis. Fatty acids can be hydrolyzed or modified by shortening, lengthening, or adding double bonds before their release from the liver into the circulation. The liver produces cholesterol, removes it from the blood, and uses it to make bile acid.

Metabolism of chylomicrons in the liver results in triglycerides being transported to the tissues for energy or other uses or carried to adipose tissue to be stored. Serum triglycerides are the result of not only absorption from foods, but also the conversion of carbohydrates and proteins into fats. Triglycerides can be synthesized in the intestinal mucosa, adipose tissue, and liver. Fats are synthesized in the process of **lipogenesis** and broken down during **lipolysis** (the splitting or decomposition of fat). These continual processes are in equilibrium when energy needs are balanced.

The process of hydrolyzing triglycerides into two-carbon entities to enter the Krebs cycle for energy production is known as **oxidation**. A discussion of oxidation can be found in Chapter 2 and online at Evolve. During oxidation, 1 lb of fat results in the release of 3500 kcal for energy—more than most individuals use in a 24-hour period. When excessive amounts of fats are oxidized for energy, the liver is overwhelmed, and acidic metabolic products, or ketones, are formed. Ketones are not oxidized in the liver, but are carried to the skeletal and cardiac muscles, where, under normal circumstances, they are rapidly metabolized.

If the glucose supply is reduced, the capacity of the tissues to use ketone bodies may be exceeded. Accumulation of ketone bodies in the body is known as ketosis. Ketosis may lead to ketoacidosis (acidic condition due to accumulation of large quantities of ketone bodies in the blood). The signs and symptoms of ketoacidosis include nausea, vomiting, and stomach pain. Ketoacidosis can be a dangerous condition for several reasons. Bases must neutralize these strong acids (ketones) to maintain acid-base balance in the blood. Ketones are excreted in the urine, a condition known as ketonuria, along with sodium. If adequate amounts of base are not available, acidosis may result. In addition to the loss of sodium ions, large amounts of water are lost, which can lead to dehydration (or rapid weight loss for an individual reducing caloric intake). When blood glucose levels remain low for several days, brain and nerve cells adapt to use ketones for some of their fuel requirements.

Carbohydrates play a predominant role in heavy exercise when the muscle's oxygen supply is limited, but triglycerides provide about half the energy with continued exercise. Although fats can be stored as adipose tissue in virtually inexhaustible amounts, their slower rate of metabolism makes them a less efficient source of quick energy. The amount of energy available is highly variable in individuals, but usually at least 160,000 kcal is available from body fat stores.

ALCOHOL METABOLISM

Although alcohol is considered a drug, the kilocalories it provides can be used by the body for energy, providing approximately 7 kcal/g. When consumed in excessive amounts, alcohol is a toxin. Caloric content of alcoholic beverages can be calculated by using the equations in Box 7-1. Alcoholic beverages contain negligible nutrients.

Alcohol is metabolized primarily by the liver. Alcohol provides an alternative fuel that is oxidized instead of fat; this

---

BOX 7-1	Calculation of Energy Value of Alcoholic Beverages

The equation for determining energy (caloric) value of liquors is as follows:

Ounces of beverage × proof × 0.8 kcal/proof/1 oz

Example: 1.5 oz × 86 proof × 0.8 kcal/proof/1 oz = 103.2 kcal

The equation for determining energy (caloric) value of beer and wines is as follows:

Ounces of beverage × % of alcohol × 1.6

Example: 12 oz × 5% × 1.6 = 96 kcal

From Gastineau CF: Nutrition note: alcohol and calories. *Mayo Clin Proc* 1976; 51(2):88.

---

may result in accumulation of lipids in the liver. Not much is known about safe amounts of alcohol consumption without risk of liver damage.

A well-balanced diet accompanied by habitual consumption of alcoholic beverages in excess of energy needs can be a risk factor for weight gain. However, excessive amounts of alcohol in a person who is an alcoholic tend to result in poor appetite for food and may lead to weight loss and malnutrition. In addition to causing liver damage, alcohol can interfere with the transport, activation, catabolism, and storage of almost every nutrient. Alcohol has a marked effect on blood pressure and risk of hypertension.[2]

The *Dietary Guidelines* advise moderation in alcohol consumption: one drink a day for women and no more than two drinks a day for men. (An alcoholic beverage is defined as 12 oz of regular beer, 5 oz of wine, or 1.5 oz of 80-proof distilled spirits.) For middle-aged and older adults, one to two drinks daily results in the lowest mortality rate.[3] This is perhaps a result of the protective effects of moderate alcohol consumption on CHD. Alcohol consumption seems to provide little, if any, health benefit for younger individuals. Alcoholic beverages should be avoided by women who may become pregnant, are pregnant or breastfeeding.

METABOLIC INTERRELATIONSHIPS

The body is an overwhelmingly complex system. Whether excessive food intake is in the form of protein, carbohydrate, fat, or alcohol, most excess energy intake is stored as adipose tissue (Fig. 7-3). (Glycogen is another storage form of energy; however, the amount of glycogen stored in the body is limited.)

Protein from the metabolic pool of amino acids and in lean muscle mass is generally not considered a good source of energy, but it can be used for energy if caloric intake is below caloric expenditure. Fat is a good source of energy, but carbohydrate is the preferred fuel. However, the body cannot metabolize excessive quantities of fat without some side effects—ketoacidosis, hyperlipidemia, and accumulation of fat in the liver.

Carbohydrates can be used in forming nonessential amino acids. Proteins contribute to synthesis of some lipids (e.g., lipoproteins). Although lipids do not contribute significantly to the synthesis of amino acids, glycerol from triglycerides can be used for synthesis of carbohydrates. Fatty acids and some amino acids can be converted to glucose.

Catabolism of all classes of foodstuffs involves oxidation through the TCA cycle to produce energy. The quantity of kilocalories in the diet from carbohydrate or lipids influences protein metabolism. In some situations, one nutrient can be substituted for another because of their interrelationship. For example, a decrease in carbohydrate intake increases lipolysis; protein excess can be used for energy. Because the body can easily adapt to shifts in either carbohydrate or fat as the main source of energy, and in view of substantial body fat stores, large variations in macronutrient intake (energy sources) and energy expenditure are well tolerated.

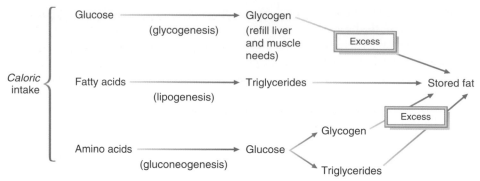

FIGURE 7-3 Metabolic pathways of excess energy. (From Nix S: *Williams' basic nutrition and diet therapy*, ed 13, St Louis, 2009, Mosby Elsevier.)

In addition to energy-providing nutrients, vitamins and minerals are essential for digestion, absorption, and metabolism of carbohydrate, protein, and fat. Although vitamins and minerals are not required in the large quantities that macronutrients are, their presence is just as important. When a deficiency occurs, reactions do not proceed normally. For example, although protein may be consumed alone (as in liquid protein supplements), many other nutrients, including vitamins and minerals, must be present for the protein to be used by cells. Each nutrient has its specific function; all the nutrients must be present simultaneously for optimal benefits.

A detailed discussion of metabolic interrelationships is beyond the scope of this text. These interrelationships are important, and for optimal use of nutrients, food sources of all the nutrients should be consumed. The easiest way to obtain optimal nutrition is to include a variety of foods from all the food groups.

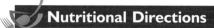

Dental Considerations

- Glycogen stores are depleted with a carbohydrate-poor diet even when high levels of fat and protein are eaten. A patient who ingests a carbohydrate-poor diet has decreased energy reserves and is prone to prolonged healing periods and fatigue.
- Blood glucose concentrations are increased only slightly when fructose, sorbitol, or xylitol is given because these sugars are absorbed more slowly; less insulin is required for their metabolism. Caution with portion size is still a consideration for individuals with diabetes.
- Patients with compromised liver or renal function may postpone progression of their condition by avoiding excessive amounts of protein.
- Ketoacidosis does not result from the rapid breakdown of adipose tissue alone; severe curtailment of carbohydrate intake must occur simultaneously. Ensure patients consume an adequate amount of carbohydrate.
- Ketoacidosis frequently occurs in patients with uncontrolled diabetes mellitus (see *Health Application 7*) or who are fasting (as a result of illness or weight reduction) because the body is burning fat rather than carbohydrate. Question patients with fruity-smelling breath about recent food and fluid intake, weight loss, and conditions such as diabetes mellitus.

- High ketone levels may be associated with starvation or high-protein, low-carbohydrate, low-calorie diets. These result in decreased appetite and occasionally nausea, which can worsen the condition.
- Symptoms of hypoglycemia include weakness or light-headedness; confusion; pale color; sweating; and rapid, shallow breathing; or the patient may have no symptoms, yet have low blood glucose levels.

Nutritional Directions

- A diet high in protein without limiting total energy intake may convert excess protein to fat stores.
- Increasing protein intake does not necessarily (or may not) increase muscle tissue, and may lead to dehydration.
- High-protein, low-carbohydrate diets have been promoted as an effective way of excreting kilocalories by creating a state of ketoacidosis to lose weight. The amount of kilocalories lost may be insignificant when considering the risk involved.

METABOLIC ENERGY

Without energy from chemical reactions, people could not bat an eye, wiggle a toe, or think a thought. Energy is required for all physiological functions. Energy from food is converted into forms the body can use: electrical for the brain and nerves, mechanical for muscles, thermal for body heat, and chemical for synthesis of new compounds.

The potential energy value of foods and energy exchanges within the body are expressed in terms of the kilocalorie. A kilocalorie (kcal) is the amount of heat required to increase the temperature of 1 kg of water 1°C. A kilocalorie is 1000 times larger than the small calorie. Although kilocalorie is the proper term, it is commonly used interchangeably with calorie or Calorie (abbreviated Cal).

Carbohydrate, fat, protein, and even alcohol provide energy for humans. (Vitamins and minerals are not energy sources, but are necessary for energy-producing reactions.) Physiological energy values commonly used are 4 kcal/g carbohydrate, 9 kcal/g fat, 4 kcal/g protein, and 7 kcal/g alcohol.

Measurement of Potential Energy

The amount of energy, or kilocalories, available in a food may be precisely calculated by placing a weighed amount of food inside a device used to measure kilocalories, called a calorimeter. As a food is burned, an increase in water temperature indicates the heat given off or potential (free) energy of that food.

Energy Production

The metabolism of basic nutrients results in production of cellular energy, which is stored as adenosine triphosphate (ATP). ATP is an instant source of cellular energy for mechanical work, transport of nutrients and waste products, and synthesis of chemical compounds generated from the Krebs cycle. ATP units, also called high-energy phosphate compounds, are the currency, or "money," the body uses for energy. Because ATP can be metabolized without oxygen, the reaction is classified as anaerobic. The body must always have a supply of ATP, and several systems ensure a constant supply in the body. More detailed discussion of ATP can be found in Chapter 2 and online at Evolve.

Increasing kilocaloric intake from carbohydrates and fats would not produce optimal energy without adequate protein intake. Energy use is remarkably sensitive to the quantity and the quality of dietary protein.

BASAL METABOLIC RATE

Even during sleep, the body requires energy for the basic minimum tasks of respiration and circulation, and for many intricate activities within each cell. Basal metabolic rate (BMR) indicates the energy required for involuntary physiological functions to maintain life, including respiration, circulation, and maintenance of muscle tone and body temperature. The BMR is lowest while lying down, awake, rested, and relaxed in a comfortable environment, not having eaten for 12 to 15 hours. The BMR can be measured in a clinical setting using indirect calorimetry, which indirectly measures the rate of oxygen used while the person is resting (see Fig. 7-4). Because digestion and absorption require energy, the BMR is the amount of energy required when the body is in a postabsorptive state (digestion and absorption are minimal).

Factors Affecting the Basal Metabolic Rate

Various factors can increase or decrease the BMR, which determines energy needs.

Sleep

Metabolic rate is lowest after a few hours of sleep because muscles are more relaxed. Approximately 10% less energy is needed for the BMR during this relaxed state.

Age

From birth through age 2 years, growth results in the highest BMR, which then decreases until the puberty growth spurt,

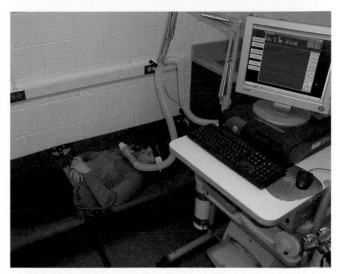

FIGURE 7-4 Measuring basal metabolic rate. (From Nix S: *Williams' basic nutrition and diet therapy*, ed 13, St Louis, 2009, Mosby Elsevier.)

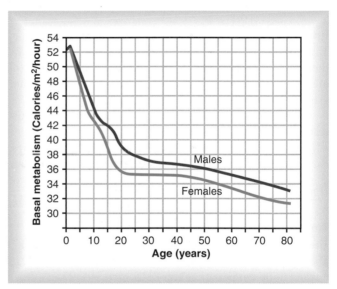

FIGURE 7-5 Normal basal metabolic rates at different ages for each sex. (From Guyton AC, Hall JE: *Textbook of medical physiology*, ed 12, St Louis, 2011, Elsevier.)

and is followed by a gradual decline for the rest of the life cycle (Fig. 7-5).

Pregnancy and Lactation

During the last trimester of pregnancy, the BMR increases approximately 15% to 30%. The amount of energy necessary to produce milk for lactation can increase the BMR 40%.

Surface Area

The more body surface area, the greater the BMR. Because of greater surface area, a tall, thin person requires more energy than a short one of similar weight.

State of Health

Illnesses and diseases may increase or decrease the BMR. Patients recovering from a wasting illness require extra energy to build new tissue. Additionally, the activity level may be influenced by such conditions as lack of sleep, exhaustion, tenseness, fatigue, or depression.

Body Composition and Gender

In adults, lean body mass is the best single predictor of the BMR. Because cells in muscles and glands are more active than cells in bone and fat, body composition influences the BMR. The amount of lean body tissue versus fat tissue in adults is a distinguishing factor; normally, women have more fat tissue and use fewer kilocalories. Differences in the BMR may be primarily related to typical variations in body composition, rather than directly related to gender.

Muscle tone is an important factor in metabolism; the state of tension or relaxation also has an effect. An athlete who has better muscle tone than a sedentary individual of similar size and shape requires more kilocalories.

Endocrine Glands: Chemical Messengers

Thyroxine, the iodine-containing hormone secreted by the thyroid gland, has a greater influence on the rate of metabolic processes than secretions from any other gland.

Adrenal glands affect metabolism to a lesser degree. Stimulations by fright, excitement, or even joy can cause a temporary increase in the BMR by releasing catecholamines, particularly epinephrine. The pituitary gland accounts for about a 15% to 20% increase in the BMR during growth of children and adolescents.

Temperature

The BMR can be affected by body temperature or climate. The BMR is slightly higher in cooler climates to maintain normal body temperature. The BMR increases when a fever is present.

Fasting and Starvation

Individuals who are undernourished or fasting for long periods have a lower than normal BMR. This is a result of decreased muscle mass and an adaptive body process to conserve energy. Numerous studies indicate the body responds to dieting the way it does to famine, by decreasing the BMR.

TOTAL ENERGY REQUIREMENTS

Basal energy expenditure includes kilocalories necessary to maintain BMR, plus additional kilocalories needed for thermic effect, voluntary activities, and any increased needs from catabolic processes (e.g., disease states or fever) or anabolic processes (e.g., growth or pregnancy) for a 24-hour period. The thermic effect of food refers to increased energy expenditure resulting from the consumption of food or the number of kilocalories needed for digestion.

BMR can be estimated using several methods based on a patient's age, gender, and body size. For most individuals, the BMR accounts for 65% to 70% of the body's total energy requirement. Calculations determining a patient's BMR are inexact, but many general guidelines have been formulated. One quick guideline for adults is as follows:

$$10 \times \text{ideal weight (lb)} = \text{kilocalories needed for BMR daily}$$

Food digestion requires energy. The thermic effect of a mixed diet is estimated to be approximately 10% of the energy required for BMR. Many times this factor is omitted in calculations determining total energy expenditure.

Voluntary Work and Play

The most variable factor affecting total energy needs is muscle activity, which is influenced by the physical activity level (Table 7-1). Mental activity uses almost no extra energy (approximately 3 to 4 kcal per hour). Activity level normally accounts for 20% to 30% of the daily energy requirement.

The *Dietary Guidelines* and *MyPlate* guidelines address the need for regular physical activity. Along with these sources, the Physical Activities Guidelines from the U.S. Department of Health and Human Services recommends 2.5 hours per week of moderate intensity activities for substantial health benefits.[4] The exercise or activity should be one the individual enjoys to enhance the likelihood of consistent participation. Inactive individuals may need to gradually increase the duration and intensity of the exercise.

Estimated Energy Requirements

The estimated energy requirements established by the Institute of Medicine indicate the daily kilocalorie intake needed to maintain energy balance in healthy individuals of a specific age, gender, weight, height, and level of physical activity (see p. ii). These levels are recommended to sustain body weights in the desired range for good health (BMI 18.5 to 25 kg/m^2), while maintaining a lifestyle with adequate levels of physical activity. A recommended dietary allowance was not established because energy intakes greater than the estimated energy requirement could result in weight gain. Weight gain resulting in a BMI greater than 25 kg/m^2 is associated with an increased risk of early mortality. Numerous studies substantiate a morbidity risk of type 2 diabetes, hypertension, CHD, stroke, gallbladder disease, osteoarthritis, and some types of cancer for BMIs greater than 25 kg/m^2. The IOM suggests that at the end of adolescence, BMI should be around 22 kg/m^2 to allow for a moderate weight gain in midlife without exceeding the 25 kg/m^2 threshold.[5]

Dental Considerations

- Encourage intake of adequate amounts of the macronutrients and energy to spare protein for growth or healing, as needed. If energy is insufficient, healing is prolonged.
- Low-carbohydrate diets are not as effective in supporting high activity levels as a high intake of complex carbohydrates. For athletic patients, advise increased intake of complex carbohydrates.
- For healthy men, the BMR usually ranges from about 1580 to 1870 kcal daily, whereas approximately 1150 to 1440 kcal is needed for women. If energy intake is inadequate, physical status may deteriorate. A referral to a healthcare provider or RDN is needed to improve nutrient intake.
- Increased thyroxine activity (hyperthyroidism) may double the BMR and can cause vitamin deficiencies because the quantity of many enzymes is increased. Unless physical activity is above average, the BMR represents the largest proportion of a patient's energy requirement. Determination of the BMR can be used to evaluate adequacy of caloric intake.

Nutritional Directions

- The BMR may be elevated or depressed. A high BMR requires more kilocalories; fewer kilocalories are needed for a low BMR.
- Because the BMR decreases about 2% every 10 years after age 25 years, many patients gain weight because previous eating habits are maintained without increasing activity.
- A naturally higher BMR is a reason why children and pregnant women do not feel as cold as adults under the same weather conditions. Do not overdress children based on an adult's perception.

ENERGY BALANCE

The proper energy balance for stable weight is maintained when caloric intake equals the amount of energy needed for body processes and physical activities (Fig. 7-6). Energy balance is maintained when the kilocalorie intake equals the amount of energy needed for body processes and physical activities. This statement sounds simple, but very few Americans are able to maintain energy balance at an appropriate body weight. Many factors help create this unbalanced equation; because it is a complex system, there are no easy answers. An alarming and increasing number of Americans are overweight; energy consumption increased by more than 168 kcal per day for men and approximately 335 kcal for women between 1971 and 2000.[6] Caloric consumption, estimated to be 1877 kcal/day for women and 2618 kcal/day for men, is significantly above the government recommendation of 1600 kcal/day for women and 2200 kcal/day for men. Dental hygienists need to be aware of the complexities of maintaining energy balance to be more understanding of patients who have problems managing their weight.

Many healthy patients are able to control energy intake to balance energy output with little effort; their **appetite**, or desire to eat, controls food intake to balance energy

Table 7-1	Energy expenditure during various activities		
Activity (1 hour)	130 lb	155 lb	180 lb
Aerobics, general	384	457	531
Aerobics, low impact	295	352	409
Carpentry, general	207	246	286
Cleaning, dusting	148	176	204
Construction, exterior, remodeling	325	387	449
Cycling, 14 to 15.9 mph, vigorous bicycling	590	704	817
Cycling, <10 mph, leisure bicycling	236	281	327
Diving, springboard or platform	177	211	245
Downhill snow skiing, moderate	354	422	490
Downhill snow skiing, racing	472	563	654
Electrical work, plumbing	207	246	286
Fishing, general	177	211	245
Football or baseball, playing catch	148	176	204
Football, competitive	531	633	735
Football, touch, flag, general	472	563	654
Frisbee playing, general	177	211	245
Golf, walking and carrying clubs	266	317	368
Handball	708	844	981
Health club exercise	325	387	449
Hiking, cross country	354	422	490
Horseback riding	236	281	327
Housework, light	148	176	204
Judo, karate, jujitsu, martial arts	590	704	817
Marching, rapidly, military	384	457	531
Mowing lawn, walk, power mower	325	387	449
Painting	266	317	368
Polo	472	563	654
Pushing stroller, walking with children	148	176	204
Racquetball, playing	413	493	572
Raking lawn	254	303	351
Rowing machine, light	207	246	286
Rowing machine, vigorous	502	598	695
Running, 5 mph (12-minute mile)	472	563	654
Running 6 mph (9-minute mile)	590	704	817
Running, 7 mph (8.5-minute mile)	679	809	940
Walking 2.0 mph	177	211	245
Walking 3.0 mph, moderate	195	232	270
Walking 4.0 mph, very brisk	295	352	409

Adapted from NutriStrategy Software. Kilocalories are calculated based on research data from *Medicine and Science in Sports and Exercise*, The Official Journal of the American College of Sports Medicine. Copyright © 2010 by NutriStrategy. Accessed August 18, 2013. Available at: http://www.nutristrategy.com/activitylist4.htm

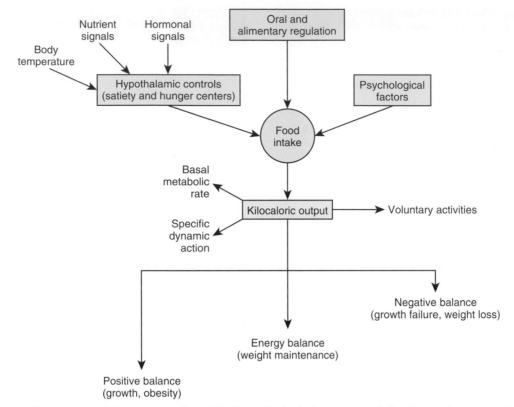

FIGURE 7-6 Factors affecting energy balance. (From Davis JR, Sherer K: *Applied nutrition and diet therapy for nurses*, ed 2, Philadelphia, 1994, Saunders.)

expenditure. Hunger, or the physiological drive to eat, is regulated by a complex network of factors (see Fig. 7-6). Appetite is frequently used in the same sense as hunger, but it usually implies desire for specific types of food and is related to the pleasurable sensation of eating.

Hunger and appetite greatly affect weight balance. When more kilocalories are consumed than the body needs, the excess is stored as fat, resulting in weight gain. One pound of body fat is equivalent to 3500 kcal. Overweight patients have a very difficult time losing extra pounds and maintaining their energy balance to keep off unwanted pounds. Weight control can be approached by either decreasing the number of kilocalories consumed or increasing physical activities. A combination of both is most effective (Box 7-2).

Intake is generally regarded as the key to weight regulation. The weight of most patients tends to remain stable for long periods with only a 1- to 5-lb gain or loss of adipose tissue over a year. Even small daily deviations from balance can result in gradual yet significant fluctuations in fat stores. For instance, an additional 100 kcal daily would result in a 10-lb weight gain over one year and a 100-lb gain over 10 years.

Physiological Factors

The hypothalamus, located in the middle of the brain, is especially important in controlling hunger. A satiety center and a hunger (or feeding) center are present within the hypothalamus.

BOX 7-2	**Equation for Weight Loss**

The total energy expenditure for a sedentary individual 67 inches tall who weighs 191 lb (BMI = 30) is 2235 kcal.

For 1 lb weight loss per week, decrease caloric intake by 500 kcal/day:

2235 − 500 = 1735 kcal/day

The result of a 500-kcal deficit in 1 week:

500 × 7 = 3500 kcal

A kilocalorie reduction combined with exercise to lose 2 lb/week can be accomplished by increasing caloric expenditure by 500 kcal/day.

Cycling at a rate of 15 mph or running at a rate of 10 minutes/mile for 45 minutes = 525 kcal:

525 × 7 = 3675 kcal

This would result in a weight loss of 2 lb/week or 8 lb/month.

Stimulation of the hunger center causes insatiable hunger; damage to this area results in no desire for food. Stimulation of the satiety center results in complete satiety. If the satiety center of the hypothalamus is destroyed, the appetite becomes voracious, resulting in obesity. The feeding center stimulates the drive to eat, whereas the satiety center inhibits the feeding center.

Usually the body discerns food characteristics such as sweetness and viscosity to gauge intake. The body may use this information to determine how much food is needed to meet its caloric requirements. Many researchers have hypothesized that nonnutritive sweeteners may confuse the body's ability to discern that the taste and feel of food in the mouth is providing caloric intake. It is possible that, by substituting noncaloric sweetened foods and beverages for natural sweeteners, the body learns it can no longer use the taste sense to gauge energy intake, resulting in increased caloric intake.[7,8] More research is needed to determine the effect low-calorie products have on the appetite.[9]

Several mechanisms affect the amount eaten at a particular meal. Distention of the stomach results in inhibitory signals that suppress the feeding center, reducing the desire to eat. Cholecystokinin in response to fat in the duodenum has a strong direct effect on the feeding center, causing the person to cease eating. Food in the stomach and duodenum causes the secretion of glucagon and insulin, both of which suppress the feeding center.

The hypothalamus is also responsive to body temperature. Cold temperatures lead to increased food intake, resulting in a higher metabolic rate and more fat stores for insulation.

The relationship between exercise and food intake is unclear. Exercise has been reported to increase, decrease, or have no effect on appetite. These findings cannot be explained, but may be related to the timing or duration of the exercise, individual metabolic differences, or some unknown reason. Generally, acute exercise decreases food intake after the activity, but regular exercise promotes increased energy intake.

Nutrient and hormonal signals affect the brain and liver to stimulate satiety and feeding centers in the brain (Table 7-2). Numerous studies have shown physiological control of energy intake is unreliable. Energy balance must be adjusted through some other mechanism.

Psychological Factors

Appetite is affected by the fact that eating is rewarding or pleasurable and makes us feel good. The eating behavior of obese individuals is thought to be influenced more by external cues, including time, taste, smell, and sight of food, than it is in individuals of normal weight. Greater weight usually means the individual is responding to feelings and emotions rather than actual hunger. Boredom and stress are factors that frequently affect eating habits of obese individuals.

Energy Expenditure

Contrary to popular opinion, obese women have a similar or higher metabolic rate than thinner women. The effect of this is less weight gain for a given increase in caloric intake. Genetics may also play a role in the BMR. Some families have low metabolic rates, but not all individuals with a low BMR are obese.

Exercise tolerance of obese individuals is less than normal, but any activity uses more kilocalories because of the amount of additional mass that has to be moved. Not all inactive patients are obese, so activity level does not seem to be a principal determinant in development of obesity. Because of differences in body composition (percentage of muscle and fat), the BMR affects energy expenditure for various activities. Weight loss resulting from a specific energy deficit is invariably smaller than expected. Conversely, overconsumption fails to produce weight gains anticipated. Adjustments in energy expenditure seem to be adaptive.

Because food is abundant in the United States, and most Americans enjoy eating, increased physical activity is needed to balance energy intake. Walking is a physical activity that has been emphasized because it is inexpensive and convenient, and most individuals are physically able to walk, even if they initially need to walk at a slow rate. Numerous studies have shown that using a pedometer (a small meter worn at the waist that monitors the number of steps a person takes) results in a significant increase in the number of steps per week.[10-12] Usually the goal is 10,000 steps a day, but individuals are encouraged to start at a comfortable pace and distance, and gradually increase intensity and distance.

INADEQUATE ENERGY INTAKE

A deficiency in energy intake may result in a depressed rate of growth in children and weight loss in adults. Intentional weight loss may be helpful or harmful, depending on the methods used for losing weight. Decreased fat stores are normally the goal, but loss of muscle may be an undesirable side effect (Fig. 7-7).

Inadequate energy intake may result in malnutrition and become a serious problem in the face of a physiologically stressful situation. Inadequate intake may be intentional, as in the case of anorexia nervosa (discussed in Chapter 17), a psychological disorder in which undernourishment is not perceived by the individual. Inadequate intake causes a vicious downward spiral in which metabolic imbalances decrease hunger and may become life-threatening without proper treatment.

Table 7-2	Stimuli affecting food intake	
	Food Intake	
Signal	**Increased**	**Decreased**
Food odors	Pleasant	Repulsive
Taste	Desirable	Offensive
Climate (temperature)	Cold	Hot
Gastrointestinal	Hunger pains	Distention Cholecystokinin Glucagon
Glucose level	Low	High
Lipoprotein	High	Low
Nutrient stores	Decreased	Increased

From Davis JR, Sherer K: *Applied nutrition and diet therapy for nurses*, ed 2, Philadelphia, 1994, Saunders.

Dental Considerations

- Observe emotional factors. Depression and stress as well as other emotional factors result in overeating and decreased activity in some patients. Referral to a healthcare provider may be indicated.
- A positive energy balance is desirable during periods of growth; a proportionately larger amount of energy is needed by pregnant and lactating women, and by children.
- When nutrient stores decrease, the feeding center of the hypothalamus becomes active, and the patient becomes hungry; when nutrient stores are abundant, the patient feels satiated and loses the desire to eat. If the hypothalamus is injured in any way (as in a head injury or stroke), hunger and satiety may be altered.
- If kilocalories are underestimated, the body must use stored energy (fat and protein), putting the patient at risk for malnutrition. If excessive kilocalories are consumed, the body converts excess kilocalories to fat.
- A patient with a BMI between 18.5 kg/m² and 25 kg/m² has approximately 13 to 44 lb of body fat, which could provide 50,000 to 200,000 kcal.
- It is out of the scope-of-practice for the dental hygienist to counsel patients on weight loss. Refer patients to an RDN.

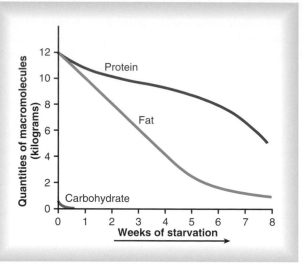

FIGURE 7-7 Effects of starvation on the body. Three major macromolecules serve as primary energy sources: carbohydrates, fats, and proteins. During starvation, the carbohydrate stores (glycogen) are rapidly depleted. However, stored lipids can mobilize and provide much of a person's energy needs for several weeks. Eventually, lipid stores run low, and the body starts using proteins as a major source of energy, causing the breakdown of muscle and other protein-rich tissues. Muscle damage during starvation usually leads to death. (From Guyton AC, Hall JE: *Textbook of medical physiology*, ed 12, St Louis, 2011, Elsevier.)

Nutritional Directions

- Exercise may enhance the BMR by increasing the amount of lean body mass, which uses more energy than fat.
- To gain 1 lb of fat, a patient must consume 3500 kcal more than are used.
- To lose 1 lb of weight, energy intake must be 3500 kcal less than the number of kilocalories used.
- A decrease from prior activity level or additional caloric intake may result in weight gain.

- Large variations from energy balance are well tolerated, but may be reflected in gains or losses of fat.
- Although quitting smoking is linked to an increased risk of weight gain, encourage patients who smoke to enroll in a smoking cessation program along with a weight-loss program. Remind the patient that the benefits of not smoking outweigh the potential risk factors of weight gain associated with quitting smoking (see *Health Application 19* in Chapter 19).

HEALTH APPLICATION **7** Diabetes Mellitus

Diabetes mellitus is a heterogeneous group of metabolic abnormalities in which carbohydrates, proteins, fats, and insulin are ineffectively metabolized, leading to disturbances in fluid and electrolyte balances (Fig. 7-8). It is a chronic, lifelong disease. Diabetes mellitus is specifically related to hormonal pancreatic secretions, but involves the entire endocrine system.

Diabetes mellitus is presently one of the most common disorders, with rates increasing at an alarming pace, especially in children and adolescents. African Americans, Hispanic Americans, and Native Americans have the highest incidence of diabetes mellitus of all cultural population groups. In addition to metabolic complications secondary to diabetes mellitus, life expectancy is approximately 70% to 80% that of the

general population. The Centers for Disease Control and Prevention estimates more than 18.8 million individuals in the United States have diabetes mellitus, 79 million have prediabetes, and an additional 7 million have diabetes but are not aware of it.[13] Type 2 diabetes mellitus can be prevented or delayed by changes in lifestyles of high-risk individuals. Exercise improves the body's sensitivity to insulin and helps the body metabolize glucose better, preventing development of diabetes in individuals who are at high risk.

The two most prevalent types of diabetes mellitus are characterized by different metabolic defects and can appear to be very different conditions (Table 7-3). Type 1 diabetes mellitus, which affects 5% to 10% of individuals with the disease, is distinguished by little or no endogenous insulin production.

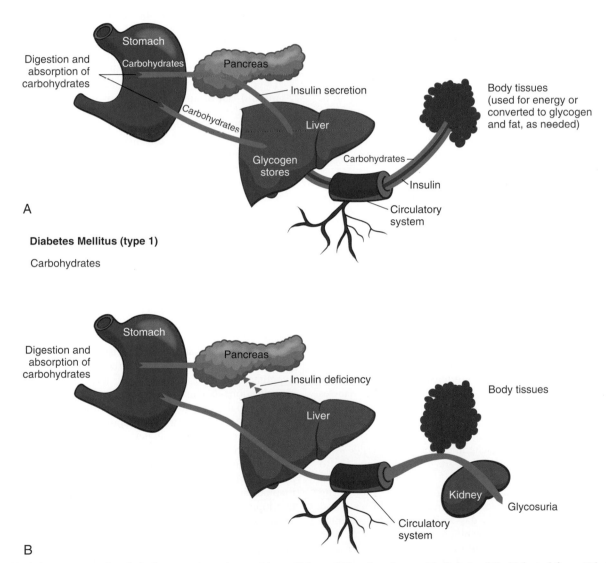

FIGURE 7-8 Comparison of carbohydrate use in patients without diabetes (**A**) and patients with diabetes (**B**). (Adapted from *What Is diabetes?* Indianapolis, 1973, Eli Lilly & Co.)

HEALTH APPLICATION **7**   Diabetes Mellitus—cont'd

This condition most commonly manifests in young people but can occur at any age. (Type 1 diabetes mellitus was formerly known as juvenile or insulin-dependent diabetes; the name was changed because adults also develop type 1 diabetes.) Onset is sudden with all the clinical symptoms associated with this condition. Patients are prone to ketosis and must receive exogenous insulin for life.

Approximately 90% to 95% of Americans with diabetes have type 2 diabetes mellitus, which results from insulin resistance, usually with a relative insulin deficiency. Family history, age, history of gestational diabetes, obesity (BMI greater than 27 kg/m^2), and sedentary lifestyle are risk factors associated with diabetes. For obese patients, increased fat stores cause some degree of insulin resistance. In many cases, insulin is secreted in adequate or higher-than-normal amounts, but glucose uptake by body cells (except for the brain) is decreased.

Abnormalities in insulin levels precipitate clinical manifestations. Insulin deficiency or defects in insulin action or both result in hyperglycemia, the main manifestation of type 2 diabetes mellitus. Symptoms of hyperglycemia include thirst, frequent urination, hunger, blurry vision, fatigue, frequent infections, and dry, itchy skin; or the patient can be asymptomatic.

Treatment should be implemented as soon as possible after diagnosis to prevent complications of metabolic alterations secondary to diabetes mellitus. Elevated blood glucose levels can damage almost every major organ of the body. Early, tight control of diabetes can postpone and minimize many of these severe complications. Chronic complications develop slowly over long periods as body tissues are adversely exposed to hyperglycemia and hypoglycemia. Hyperglycemia in type 2 diabetes mellitus causes macrovascular and microvascular disease (involving large and small vessels) and can damage almost every major organ of the body. Patients with uncontrolled diabetes experience slow wound healing, frequent abscesses, periodontal disease, a predisposition to bacterial infections, a compromised immune system, skin irritations, pruritus (itching), numbness and tingling of the extremities, and visual disturbances. The American Diabetes Association defines uncontrolled blood glucose levels as three consecutive readings of 200 mg/dL or greater.[14] Because of the increased risks of hyperglycemia on the oral cavity, the patient may need to be rescheduled for dental visits when the patient's blood glucose levels are in a safe range (70 to 200 mg/dL).

Obtaining a blood glucose level using a glucose monitoring system (a personal meter used to monitor capillary blood glucose levels) provides a day-to-day, minute-to-minute reading. It is a "snapshot" of the blood glucose level at the time it is taken. This is valuable information to obtain before a dental procedure because blood glucose levels can vary throughout the day. It is measured in milligrams per deciliter (mg/dL) or millimoles per liter (mmol/L).

Another valuable reading is the glycosylated hemoglobin (A_{1C}) assay, a widely accepted and reliable measure of a blood glucose level over the past 3 months. It provides a guide for long-term planning and possible adjustments to diabetes treatment. However, hemoglobin A_{1C} does not show the ups and downs in a given day, just an average level over 3 months. This reading helps evaluate metabolic control and determines whether the target range is maintained.[15]

Hyperlipidemia and hypertension are common risks for individuals with diabetes, and are often treated more aggressively than for individuals without diabetes. For example, a patient with diabetes who has a blood pressure of 130/80 mm Hg or greater begins treatment for hypertension, whereas someone without diabetes receives the same treatment when blood pressure readings are 140/90 mm Hg or greater.[14] Changes in capillary membranes result in renal complications (leading to renal failure, the inability of kidneys to excrete toxic waste materials), obstruction of circulation in the extremities (leading to gangrene), and progressive blood vessel damage in the retina of the eye (leading to blindness). Neuropathy, or deterioration of nervous tissue, also is frequently seen in patients with diabetes mellitus. Abnormalities of the gastrointestinal tract causing nausea, early satiety, and frequent vomiting interfere with food intake and absorption.

Hypoglycemia, or low blood glucose levels (less than 70 mg/dL) can occur when a patient is taking insulin or an antidiabetic medication whose side effect is hypoglycemia. Symptoms include rapid heartbeat, hunger, shakiness, blurry vision, sweating, fatigue, dizziness, and irritability. However, the patient may be unaware of their symptoms, so as a precautionary measure, obtain blood glucose readings before treatment to prevent a medical emergency. A patient whose blood glucose level is less than 70 mg/dL should be treated with 10 to 15 g of a carbohydrate source, such as 3 glucose tablets, 1 tube of glucose gel, 8 hard candies (disk), 4 oz of regular soda, or 4 oz of fruit juice. Wait 15 minutes and retest. If the blood glucose level is still less than 70 mg/dL or symptoms remain, repeat. When the blood glucose level is greater than 70 mg/dL, continue with treatment, and offer a meal or snack within 30 minutes. If the patient is experiencing severe hypoglycemia (e.g., he or she is uncooperative, unable to take fluids, or unconscious), administer glucagon to bring the blood glucose value into an appropriate range. Call the community emergency medical services for assistance.

Medical nutrition therapy is the cornerstone for preventing hyperglycemia and hypoglycemia and decreasing chronic complications. No single dietary plan can be appropriate for all individuals with different personalities and lifestyles. The objective of a meal plan is to empower patients to maintain good control of their diabetes or to promote near-normal blood glucose, lipid, and blood pressure levels. Additionally, food choices should promote overall health by providing optimal nutrition and allowing physical activity; achieving or maintaining an ideal body weight; and preventing or delaying development or progression of periodontal disease, and cardiovascular, renal, retinal, neurological, and other complications associated with diabetes, insofar as these are related to metabolic control. The meal plan should be flexible to allow personal and cultural preferences and lifestyles, while respecting the individual's wishes and willingness to make changes.

Beginning in 2002, each of the American Diabetes Association's nutritional recommendations was assigned a grade (*A*, *B*, *C*, or *E*) based on the weight of the scientific evidence that supports it. An *A* rating means supportive evidence is based on multiple, well-conducted studies; *B* is an intermediate rating, signifying some supporting evidence is available; *C* means supporting evidence is limited; *E* means the recommendation is based on expert consensus. These are reviewed annually, and grades are reevaluated based on new research.

HEALTH APPLICATION 7   Diabetes Mellitus—cont'd

Table 7-4 lists some of the more than 51 nutrition recommendations.

The American Diabetes Association, the Academy of Nutrition and Dietetics, and the U.S. Public Health Service compiled the exchange system to allow meal plan flexibility in addition to reasonable constancy of carbohydrate, protein, fat, and energy intake. These exchange lists divide foods into six groups; within each group, all food items are approximately equal in carbohydrate, protein, and fat content. Serving sizes vary so that foods in each list are calorically equivalent. Foods within any group can be traded, or exchanged, with other foods in the same group. Use of the exchange system is not essential, but it is a good tool for teaching macronutrient content of foods, is easy for patients to follow, and can be adapted easily to meet individual needs.

Because of increased awareness of nutrient metabolism in diabetes, the "diabetes meal plan" has been liberalized in favor of modifying the patient's usual eating habits to be more consistent with the *Dietary Guidelines* and *MyPlate*. When kilocalorie content is controlled, all foods containing carbohydrate, protein, fat, and alcohol are limited because these sources of energy are potential sources of glucose.

Carbohydrate counting focuses on total carbohydrate consumption. Because carbohydrate is the major factor in blood glucose fluctuations, the given amount of carbohydrate affects insulin requirements more than the protein and fat content. Carbohydrate counting provides greater precision in estimating carbohydrate intake than the diabetic food exchange lists.

For individuals with a healthy weight and normal lipid profile, the American Diabetes Association recommends the same guidelines as advocated by the National Cholesterol Education Program, discussed in Chapter 6. Because many patients with diabetes have undesirable lipid levels, a moderate increase in monounsaturated fat with a moderate intake of carbohydrate is recommended.

Table 7-3	Comparison of type 1 and type 2 diabetes mellitus	
	type 1	**type 2**
Prevalence	Approximately 5% to 10% of cases	90% to 95% of cases (1 in 5 adults >65 years old)
Age at onset	Most frequently during childhood or puberty, but may occur at later ages	Frequently >40 years, but occurring more frequently in overweight children and adolescents
Precipitating cause	Genetic, autoimmune destruction of the pancreatic cells that produce insulin	Obesity and inactivity
Type of onset	Sudden, but may develop slowly in adults	Usually gradual; may go undetected for years
Family history of diabetes	Frequently positive	Usually positive
Nutritional status at time of onset	Normal weight with recent weight loss, but occasionally obese	Usually overweight (BMI >25) with increased percentage of body fat predominantly in the abdominal region
Symptoms	Polydipsia, polyphagia, ketoacidosis, weight loss	Glycosuria without ketonuria; absent or mild polyuria and polydipsia
Blood glucose stability	Fluctuates widely in response to changes in insulin, diet, exercise, infection, and stress	Fluctuations less marked
Control of diabetes	Difficult	Easy, especially if diet is followed
Ketosis	Frequent	Seldom
Plasma insulin	Negligible or absent	May be low (not absent) or high, with insulin resistance
Vascular complications and degenerative changes	Occurs after diabetes is present for approximately 5 years	Increased risk of macrovascular and microvascular complications
Medical nutrition therapy	Required	May eliminate need for hypoglycemic agents or insulin or both
Medication	Insulin required for all	Usually can be controlled with hypoglycemic agents; insulin may be necessary for some

Table 7-4	American Diabetes Association nutritional recommendations

A to C, E Rating*	Recommendation
Diabetes Prevention	
A	Among individuals at high risk for developing type 2 diabetes, structured programs that emphasize lifestyle changes, including moderate weight loss (7% body weight) and regular physical activity (150 min/wk), with dietary strategies, including reduced calories and reduced intake of dietary fat, can reduce risk for developing diabetes and are recommended.
B	Individuals at high risk for type 2 diabetes should be encouraged to achieve the U.S. Department of Agriculture (USDA) recommendation for dietary fiber (14 g fiber/1000 kcal) and foods containing whole grains (one-half of grain intake).
Carbohydrates	
A	Monitoring carbohydrate, whether by carbohydrate counting, exchanges, or experience-based estimation, remains a key strategy in achieving glycemia control.
A	Sucrose-containing foods can be substituted for other carbohydrates in a meal plan or, if added to a meal plan, covered with insulin or other glucose-lowering medications. Care should be taken to avoid excess energy intake.
A	Sugar alcohols and nonnutritive sweeteners are safe when consumed within daily intake levels established by U.S. Food and Drug Administration (FDA).
B	A dietary pattern that includes carbohydrate from fruits, vegetables, whole grains, legumes, and low-fat milk is encouraged for good health.
B	The use of glycemic index and load may provide modest additional benefit over that observed when total carbohydrate is considered alone.
B	As for the general population, patients with diabetes are encouraged to consume a variety of fiber-containing foods. Evidence is lacking to recommend a higher fiber intake for patients with diabetes than for the population as a whole.
Proteins	
A	For patients with type 2 diabetes, ingested protein can increase insulin response without increasing plasma glucose concentrations. Protein should not be used to treat acute hypoglycemia or prevent nighttime hypoglycemia.
E	For patients with diabetes and normal renal function, there is insufficient evidence to suggest that usual protein intake (15% to 20% of energy) should be modified.
E	High-protein diets are not recommended as a method for weight loss at this time. Long-term effects of protein intake >20% of calories on diabetes management and its complications are unknown. Although such diets may produce short-term weight loss and improved glycemia, it has not been established that these benefits are maintained long-term, and long-term effects on kidney function for patients with diabetes are unknown.
Fats	
A	Limit saturated fat to <7% of total calories.
B	Two or more servings of fish per week (with the exception of commercially fried fish filets) provide n-3 polyunsaturated fatty acids and are recommended.
B	Intake of *trans* fat should be minimized.
E	In patients with diabetes, limit dietary cholesterol to <200 mg per day.
Energy Balance, Overweight, and Obesity	
A	In overweight and obese insulin-resistant patients, modest weight loss has been shown to improve insulin resistance. Weight loss is recommended for all such individuals who have or are at risk for diabetes.
A	For weight loss, either low-carbohydrate or low-fat, calorie-restricted diets may be effective in the short-term (up to 1 year).
B	Physical activity and behavior modification are important components of weight loss programs and are most helpful in maintenance of weight loss.
B	Bariatric surgery may be considered for some patients with type 2 diabetes and BMI ≥35 kg/m^2 and can result in marked improvements in glycemia. Long-term benefits and risks of bariatric surgery in patients with prediabetes or diabetes continues to be studied.
Micronutrients	
A	There is no clear evidence of benefit from vitamin or mineral supplementation in patients with diabetes (compared with the general population) who do not have underlying deficiencies.
A	Routine supplementation with antioxidants, such as vitamins E and C and carotene, is not advised because of lack of evidence of efficacy, and concern related to long-term safety.
E	Benefit from chromium supplementation in individuals with diabetes or obesity has not been shown; chromium supplementation cannot be recommended.

Table 7-4	American Diabetes Association nutritional recommendations—cont'd
A to C, E Rating*	**Recommendation**
Alcohol	
B	In individuals with diabetes, moderate alcohol consumption (when ingested alone) has no acute effect on glucose and insulin concentrations, but carbohydrate coingested with alcohol (as in a mixed drink) may increase blood glucose.
E	If adults with diabetes choose to use alcohol, daily intake should be limited to a moderate amount (≤1 drink per day for women and ≤2 drinks per day for men).
E	To reduce risk of nocturnal hypoglycemia in individuals using insulin or insulin secretogogues, alcohol should be consumed with food.

Data from American Diabetes Association: Nutrition recommendations and interventions for diabetes. *Diabetes Care* 2008;31(Suppl 1):S61-S78; and American Diabetes Association: Summary of revisions for the 2009 clinical practice recommendation. *Diabetes Care* 2009;32 (Suppl 1):S3-S5.
*ABC rating—evidence based on research criteria: *A*, strong supporting evidence; *B*, some supporting evidence; *C*, limited supporting evidence; *E*, based on expert consensus.

Case Application for the Dental Hygienist

On a routine recare appointment, Ronnie, who is 10 years old, reports that he was diagnosed with type 2 diabetes about a year ago. He appears to be about 100 lb overweight. After talking with him, you learn that he does not want to be labeled as "different" from his friends, so he eats when and what they do. Typically, they eat cheeseburgers, pizza, french fries, shakes, and regular sodas throughout the day. He says he does not have time to eat breakfast. He does not floss his teeth, has numerous caries, and has bleeding on probing.

Nutritional Assessment
- Observe height, weight, BMI, and age
- Knowledge of diabetes guidelines
- Motivation level
- Food/nutrient intake
- Eating habits
- Support from family and friends
- Activity level

Nutritional Diagnosis
Altered nutrition: Body requirements less than kilocalorie intake in relation to energy expenditure.

Nutritional Goals
The patient will have gradual weight loss until a BMI for age is below the 85th percentile.

Nutritional Implementation
Intervention: Provide Ronnie and his parents with the name of an RDN who can provide necessary nutritional counseling.
Rationale: Well-balanced food choices that naturally contain a large amount of vitamins and minerals, rather than high-calorie foods, are needed to maintain his health and promote growth. The RDN's knowledge of nutrition and expertise in counseling is recommended to provide adequate nutrients safely and effectively without affecting his linear growth.
Intervention: Explain that some of his food choices are not good for his overall physical or oral health.
Rationale: Consuming too many carbohydrates at meals and snacks affects his blood glucose level and increases the risk of caries.

Intervention: Explain that carbohydrates, proteins, and fats all provide kilocalories, but fats are the most concentrated source of energy.
Rationale: To maintain his weight while still growing, wise food choices are advisable. Foods high in fat and sugar will not help him in his attempts to look handsome and may worsen his diabetes status.
Intervention: Stress the importance of consuming complex carbohydrate and fiber, and reducing intake of fat and kilocalories.
Rationale: Complex carbohydrate and fiber intake is effective in helping maintain a lower caloric intake without excessive hunger. Fat reduction enhances weight maintenance because a lower fat intake may help reduce energy intake and decrease risk of developing heart disease.
Intervention: Discuss the benefits of eating at routine times.
Rationale: This is important for control of his diabetes and may allow him time to brush his teeth after eating, reducing his risk of caries.
Intervention: Discuss the importance of a plan incorporating diet, exercise, and behavior modification.
Rationale: This combination of therapies has proven more effective for long-term weight control.
Intervention: Explain that good oral hygiene is very important for patients with diabetes because of an exaggerated response to plaque bacteria.
Rationale: Knowledge may help increase compliance.
Intervention: Suggest becoming involved in some sports, or increasing his activity level by walking to friends' homes, or participating in some recreational activity such as skating.
Rationale: Weight and diabetes control is improved when energy expenditure is increased along with decreased caloric intake. Additionally, physical activity helps increase muscle mass and improves strength.

Evaluation
The patient consulted with the RDN and did not gain any weight before the next recall visit. Also, no new caries developed.

STUDENT READINESS

1. Define the terms energy, thermogenic effect, basal metabolism, and basal energy expenditure.
2. Calculate your total caloric needs for 1 day (BMR plus estimated voluntary energy expenditures plus thermogenic effect).
3. Assuming height and weight are the same, is the BMR higher or lower in:

   A man or a woman?

   An athlete or a sedentary person?

   A 40-year-old or a 20-year-old?

   A woman who is not pregnant or a woman who is pregnant?
4. How many kilocalories of protein, fat, and carbohydrate are in 1 cup of homogenized milk that contains 8.5 g of protein, 8.5 g of fat, and 12 g of carbohydrate?
5. A boxer achieved a dramatic weight loss of about 18 kg (39.6 lb) in approximately 60 days. A strict diet, heavy exercise, thyroid supplements, and a diuretic drug produced significant weight loss. His defeat in a boxing match shocked some of his fans. What happened to his physical condition? Explain.

CASE STUDY

Jay G. is a 16-year-old high school athlete on the football and baseball teams. He recently developed three dental caries. His classmates have encouraged him to eat a high-protein, low-carbohydrate diet. His mother is concerned about this and talks to her best friend, who is a dental hygienist.

1. What points do you think the dental hygienist should mention to this mother?
2. For increased energy expenditure, what should be the primary source of nutrients?
3. Would decreasing dietary carbohydrate content have a positive effect on the rate of dental caries?
4. What is the effect of a high protein intake?
5. On a high-protein, low-carbohydrate diet (approximately 120 g of protein, 80 g of carbohydrate, 2800 kcal), where would most of his energy requirements come from? Is this good or bad?
6. Which vitamins are important in the production of energy?
7. Is the diet varied? Does the diet provide recommended amounts of fruits, vegetables, grains, and other nutrients?

References

1. Franz MJ, Powers MA, Leontos C, et al: The evidence for medical nutrition therapy for type 1 and type 2 diabetes in adults. *J Am Diet Ass* 110(12):1852–1888, 2010.
2. Chen L, Smith G, Harbord RM, et al: Alcohol intake and blood pressure: a systematic review implementing a Mendelian randomization approach. *PLoS Med* 5(3):e52, 2008.
3. King DE, Mainous AG, 3rd, Geesey ME: Adopting moderate alcohol consumption in middle age: subsequent cardiovascular events. *Am J Med* 121(3):201–206, 2008.
4. U.S. Department of Health and Human Services: *2008 Physical activity guidelines for Americans.* Available at: http://www.health.gov/paguidelines/guidelines/default.aspx. Accessed August 18, 2013.
5. Institute of Medicine (IOM), National Academy of Sciences: *Dietary reference intakes for energy, carbohydrates, fiber, fat, protein and amino acids (macronutrients),* Washington, DC, 2002, National Academy Press.
6. Centers for Disease Control and Prevention (CDC): Trends in intake of energy and macronutrients—United States, 1971-2000. *MMWR Morb Mortal Wkly Rep* 53(4):80–82, 2004.
7. Brown RJ, de Banate MA, Rother KI: Artificial sweeteners: a systematic review of metabolic effects in youth. *Int J Ped Obes* 5(4):305–312, 2010.
8. Renwick AG, Molinary SV: Sweet-taste receptors, low-energy sweeteners, glucose absorption and insulin release. *Br J Nutr* 104(10):1415–1420, 2010.
9. Academy of Nutrition and Dietetics: Position of the Academy of Nutrition and Dietetics: Use of nutritive and nonnutritive sweeteners. *JAND* 112:739–758, 2012.
10. Belanger-Gravel A, Godin G, Bilodeau A, et al: The effect of implementation intentions on physical activity among obese older adults: a randomized control study. *Psychol Health* 28(2):217–233, 2013.
11. Huberty J, Beets M, Beighle A: Effects of a policy-level intervention on children's pedometer-determined physical activity: preliminary findings from Movin' Afterschool. *J Public Health Manag Pract* 2013 [Epub ahead of print]. Accessed August 19, 2013: http://www.ncbi.nlm.nih.gov/pubmed/23676476.
12. Eather N, Morgan PJ, Lubans DR: Social support from teachers mediates physical activity behavior change in children participating in the Fit-4-Fun intervention. *Int J Behav Nutr Phys Act* 2013. Accessed August 19, 2013; http://www.ncbi.nlm.nih.gov/pubmed/23676476.
13. Centers for Disease Control and Prevention: *National Diabetes Fact Sheet: General information and national estimates on diabetes in the United States, 2011.* Atlanta, GA, 2011, U.S. Department of Health and Human Services.
14. American Diabetes Association: Standards of medical care in diabetes—2012. *Diabetes Care* 35(Suppl 1):S11–S63, 2012.
15. Nathan DM, Kuenen J, Borg R, et al: Translating the A1C assay into estimated average glucose values. *Diabetes Care* 31(8):1473–1478, 2008.

ⓔ EVOLVE RESOURCES

Please visit http://evolve.elsevier.com/Stegeman/nutritional for additional practice and study support tools.

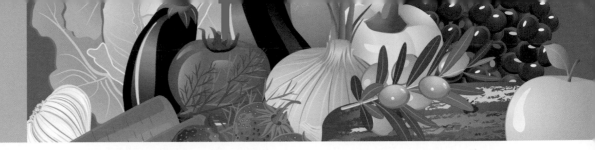

Chapter 8

Vitamins Required for Calcified Structures

Student Learning Outcomes

Upon completion of this chapter, the student will be able to achieve the following student learning outcomes:

- List the fat-soluble vitamins.
- Compare the characteristics of water-soluble vitamins with those of fat-soluble vitamins.
- Identify functions, deficiencies, surpluses, and toxicities, and oral symptoms for vitamins A, D, E, K, and C.

- Select food sources for vitamins A, D, E, K, and C.
- Individualize dental hygiene considerations for patients regarding vitamins A, D, E, K, and C.
- Relate nutritional directions to meet patients' needs regarding vitamins A, D, E, K, and C.

Key Terms

Alopecia
Ameloblasts
Anticoagulant
Antioxidants
Calcitonin
Collagen
Diplopia
Enamel hypoplasia
Epiphyses
Fibroblasts
Follicular hyperkeratosis
Hematopoiesis
Hormone
Hypercarotenemia
Hypervitaminosis A
Leukoplakia
Lysosomes
Meta-analysis
Night blindness

Odontoblasts
Osteoblasts
Osteocalcin
Osteoclasts
Osteodentin
Osteomalacia
Petechiae
Prostaglandins
Prothrombin
Phytochemicals
Retinoic acid
Rhodopsin
Scorbutic
Secondary deficiency
Tocopherols
Tocotrienols
Vitamins
Xeroderma
Xerophthalmia

Test Your NQ

1. **T/F** Fat-soluble vitamins are stored in the body.
2. **T/F** Vitamins do not provide energy.
3. **T/F** Vitamin E is found in vegetable oils and green leafy vegetables.
4. **T/F** Fat-soluble vitamins include A, D, E, and K.
5. **T/F** Animal foods are the principal dietary source of beta-carotene.
6. **T/F** Xerophthalmia occurs with a deficiency of vitamin A.
7. **T/F** The liver and kidney help convert vitamin D to its active form.
8. **T/F** An excess of vitamin D causes rickets.
9. **T/F** Vitamin K is essential for regulation of blood calcium and phosphorus levels.
10. **T/F** Vitamin C is needed for wound healing.

OVERVIEW OF VITAMINS

Nutrients never work single-handedly, but in partnership with each other. Vitamins are catalysts for all metabolic reactions using proteins, fats, and carbohydrates for energy, growth, and cell maintenance. Because only small amounts of these chemical substances obtained from food facilitate millions of processes, they may be regarded as "miracle workers."

Eating fats, carbohydrates, and proteins without enough vitamins means the energy from these nutrients cannot be used. The opposite is also true. Vitamins do not provide energy, and they cannot be used without an adequate supply of fats, carbohydrates, proteins, and minerals. Most vitamins come in several forms; each form may perform a different task. Vitamins are easily destroyed by the heat, oxidation, and chemical processes used in their extraction. In this text, water-soluble vitamins, fat-soluble vitamins, and minerals are presented based on their function in calcified structures (teeth and periodontium) or their role in oral soft tissues (oral mucous membranes and salivary glands) to familiarize you with nutrients that might be involved when oral changes are observed. Most dental hygiene students are well aware of the role of several minerals in calcified structures in the oral cavity, but vitamins presented in this chapter are also important for healthy teeth and the periodontium (Box 8-1).

Most nutrients have various functions; some are involved in both calcified and soft oral tissues. Oral physiological roles for these nutrients are presented in appropriate chapters, but information such as requirements and food sources is found only when the vitamin is first discussed. Fat-soluble and water-soluble vitamins differ in many ways, but a basic understanding of their fundamental similarities can facilitate learning.

Requirements

Although vitamins are vital to life, they are required in minute amounts. Vitamins are similar to hormones because of their potent effects, but they must come from an outside source because they either cannot be produced by the body or cannot be produced in adequate amounts to meet physiological needs. Each vitamin is essential, although the amount needed may vary from 2.4 µg per day for vitamin B_{12} to 550 mg per day for choline.

Although the DRIs list the amounts of vitamins for different ages and sexes, many factors (e.g., smoking; use of alcohol, caffeine, or drugs; and stress) modify an individual's requirements. Periods of rapid growth, pregnancy or lactation, fever, and recovery from accidents, disease, surgery, and burns are all considered stressful. Requirements for most vitamins, especially water-soluble vitamins, are increased during periods of stress because of elevated metabolic activity (Box 8-2).

Deficiencies

If adequate amounts of the nutrient are unavailable to sustain biochemical functions, a nutritional deficiency occurs. A nutritional deficiency as a result of decreased intake is called a primary deficiency. A vitamin deficiency caused by inadequate absorption or use, increased requirements, excretion, or destruction is called a secondary deficiency. Nutrients are codependent; a deficiency of one may cause deficiency symptoms of another.

Although specific vitamin deficiency syndromes are rare in the United States, several groups are at risk (see Box 8-2). Vitamin levels in the blood are often unmeasurable, so a nutritional deficiency may be identified on the basis of clinical signs and symptoms and their response to vitamin supplementation. However, one of the peculiarities of

---

BOX 8-1	Vitamins Required for Calcified Structures

Fat-Soluble Vitamins
Vitamin A
Vitamin D
Vitamin E
Vitamin K

Water-Soluble Vitamins
Vitamin C

BOX 8-2	Groups at Potential Risk of Nutritional Deficiencies

- Older adults
- Impoverished, low-income
- Vegans
- Chronic disease states
- Alcoholics
- Inadequate intake
- Smokers
- Excessive caffeine use
- Polypharmacy
- Physiological stress
- Periods of rapid growth
  - Pregnancy
  - Lactation
  - Infants, children, adolescents
- Medical conditions causing
  - Inadequate absorption
  - Inadequate use
  - Excessive excretion
  - Destruction
- Physical stress
  - Surgery
  - Accidents
  - Disease
  - Burns
  - Fever

vitamins is that the symptoms of a deficiency frequently resemble the symptoms caused by an overdose, making definitive diagnosis difficult.

Characteristics of Fat-Soluble Vitamins

Although the four fat-soluble vitamins (A, D, E, and K) differ in function, use, and sources, they have several similar characteristics: (a) they are soluble in fat or fat solvents; (b) they are fairly stable to heat, as in cooking; (c) they are organic substances (contain carbon); (d) they do not contain nitrogen; (e) they are absorbed in the intestine along with fats and lipids in foods; and (f) they require bile for absorption.

Fat-soluble vitamins are different from water-soluble vitamins mainly because larger amounts can be stored in the body. Vitamins A and D are stored for long periods, so minor shortages may not be identified until drastic depletion has occurred. For example, vitamin A can be stored in the liver to meet basic needs for at least 1 year. Observable signs and symptoms of a dietary deficiency are often not identified until they are in an advanced state. Dietary deficiencies occur when foods consumed do not provide necessary amounts of a nutrient.

Because several forms of each of the fat-soluble vitamins can be used by the body, vitamins A, D, and E were previously measured by their biological activity based on the growth of animals. International units (IU) reflect this biological activity in animal studies and do not always represent absorption rates in humans. Because of this, the retinol activity equivalents (RAE) standard was created for vitamin A. The RDAs for vitamins A and E were determined based on the biological effectiveness of each form because the different forms of these vitamins have varying activity levels. After measurement of all active forms of the vitamins, the quantity is converted to micrograms or milligrams and totaled to indicate the amount of vitamin in that food. RAE reflect vitamin A activity of foods. Although previous food tables listed IUs, more accurate weight measurements in micrograms or milligrams are now used.

Characteristics of Water-Soluble Vitamins

B-complex vitamins and vitamin C are water-soluble and are organic substances. In contrast to vitamin C and fat-soluble vitamins, B-complex vitamins contain nitrogen. Water-soluble vitamins have vital roles as coenzymes, which are necessary for almost every cellular reaction in the body. Vitamin C is discussed in this chapter with the fat-soluble vitamins because of its vital role as a structural component of teeth; it is also important in oral soft tissues. B-complex vitamins are discussed in Chapter 11.

Most water-soluble vitamins are readily absorbed in the jejunum. High concentrations of these vitamins result in decreased absorption efficiency. The body stores very small amounts of each of these vitamins; few water-soluble vitamins produce toxic symptoms. Because of their limited storage, daily intake is important.

Dental Considerations

- Assessment is crucial to determine requirements for vitamins. Assess for the following: smoking, alcohol use, excessive caffeine use, medications, physiological stress, or surgery. If any of the aforementioned is present, vitamin requirements in the diet may need to be altered.
- Dietary and physical assessments are more diagnostic for vitamin deficiencies than laboratory values. A combination of the three assessments provides the greatest amount of information on an individual's nutrition status.
- Evaluate nutrient intake of groups at high risk for developing nutritional deficiencies; older adults, impoverished/low-income patients, and patients with chronic diseases should be questioned. If indicated, refer the patient to an RDN.

Nutritional Directions

- No vitamin contains kilocalories, but some vitamins, especially the B-complex vitamins, are essential to the production of energy.
- The use of mineral oil as a laxative can interfere with absorption of fat-soluble vitamins.

VITAMIN A (RETINOL, CAROTENE)

Retinol is the dietary source of vitamin A from animal sources, and beta-carotene is the principal carotenoid present in plant pigments. Retinoic acid is the most biologically active form of vitamin A.

Physiological Roles

Vitamin A has many hormone-like roles in the body. It is also required for normal bone growth and development, and facilitating the transcription of DNA into RNA.

Vision

Retinol is converted to retinal in the eye. Retinal combines with opsin, a protein in the eye, to form the visual pigment, rhodopsin. Night blindness may result from inadequate vitamin A to permit rhodopsin production. This condition takes years to develop in adults, but occurs much sooner in children because they have fewer body stores.

Growth

Vitamin A is necessary for growth of soft tissues and bones. In skeletal tissue, vitamin A is necessary for resorption of old bone and synthesis of new bone. Retinoic acid, produced by the body from retinal, is the form of vitamin A involved in the development of teeth, especially in the formation of ameloblasts (in enamel) and odontoblasts (in dentin) along with growth of bone. Vitamin A deficiency during preeruptive stages of tooth development leads to enamel hypoplasia and defective dentin formation. Vitamin A also is involved with normal teeth spacing and promotes osteoblast function of the alveolar bone.

Cancer

Vitamin A and carotene have consistently been associated with cancer prevention because of their importance to the development and integrity of cells. The antioxidant role of vitamin A is discussed in *Health Application 8.* Antioxidants prevent cell membrane damage by free radicals that are produced by cells and tissues using free oxygen. Unchecked by an antioxidant, free radicals can damage the structure and impair the function of cell membranes. Research is inconclusive in regard to use of beta-carotene to prevent cancer. Studies suggest vitamin A, retinoids, and beta-carotene may resolve oral leukoplakia, but relapse is common. Leukoplakia (see Figs. 17-10 and 17-13) is a white plaque that forms on oral mucous membranes that cannot be wiped away. It has the potential to become cancerous. Despite the potential to resolve leukoplakia, evidence does not indicate that any of these nutrients prevent malignant transformation.[1] Whether beta-carotene or some other components in fruits and vegetables can help to resolve leukoplakia has not been determined. Supplementation is not advised other than increasing consumption of fruits and vegetables because some studies show an increased risk of lung cancer among smokers using beta-carotene supplements.[2,3] Based on clinical studies, the American Cancer Society does not support vitamin A supplementation for cancer prevention.[3]

Requirements

As shown in Table 8-1, the RDA for vitamin A is 900 µg RAE for men and 700 µg RAE for women (1 RAE = 1 µg = 12 µg beta-carotene = 3.3 IU). The tolerable upper intake level (UL) is 3000 µg RAE per day. The need for vitamin A is increased during periods of rapid growth, when gastrointestinal problems affect its absorption or conversion (e.g., cystic fibrosis, celiac disease, Crohn's disease, or chronic diarrhea), and in hepatic diseases that limit vitamin A storage or conversion of beta-carotene to its active form. Although no UL has been established for beta-carotene, the IOM does not advise supplements for healthy people.[4]

Average intake in the United States meets the RDA, and because vitamin A can be stored in the liver, most adults have sufficient quantities to maintain health. Inadequate intake occurs in lower socioeconomic groups as a consequence of inadequate vegetable and fruit intake.

Sources

Vitamin A, as preformed retinol, is found in organ meats, such as liver. It is also found in milk, cheese, butter, eggs, cod liver oil, and fortified foods (e.g., breakfast cereals). Sometimes retinol is added to skim milk and margarine. Beta carotene or provitamin A is also present in yellow, orange, and green leafy vegetables (e.g., spinach, turnip greens, broccoli) (Table 8-2). Although not as well absorbed as from animal sources and

Table 8-1	Institute of Medicine recommendations for vitamin A					
	EAR (µg/day)*		RDA (µg/day)†			
Life Stage	Male	Female	Male	Female	AI (µ/day)‡	UL (µg/day)§‖
0-6 months					400	600
7-12 months					500	600
1-3 years	210	210	300	300		600
4-8 years	275	275	400	400		900
9-13 years	445	420	600	600		1700
14-18 years	630	485	900	700		2800
>18 years	625	500	900	700		3000
Pregnancy						
14-18 years		530		750		2800
19-50 years		550		770		3000
Lactation						
14-18 years		885		1200		2800
19-50 years		900		1300		3000

Data from Institute of Medicine (IOM), Food and Nutrition Board: *Dietary reference intakes for vitamin C, vitamin K, arsenic, boron, chromium, copper, iodine, iron, manganese, molybdenum, nickel, silicon, vanadium, and zinc,* Washington, DC, 2000, National Academy Press.

*EAR (estimated average requirement)—the intake that meets the estimated nutrient needs of half of the individuals in a group.

†RDA (recommended dietary allowance)—the intake that meets the nutrient needs of almost all (97% to 98%) individuals in a group.

‡AI (adequate intake)—the observed average or experimentally set intake by a defined population or subgroup that seems to sustain a defined nutritional status, such as growth rate, normal circulating nutrient values, or other functional indicators of health. An AI is used if insufficient scientific evidence is available to derive an EAR. For healthy human milk–fed infants, the AI is the mean intake. *The AI is not equivalent to a RDA.*

§UL (tolerable upper intake level)—the highest level of daily nutrient intake that is likely to pose no risk of adverse health effects to almost all individuals in the general population. As intake increases above the UL, the risk of adverse effects increases. Unless specified otherwise, the UL represents total nutrient intake from food, water, and supplements.

‖Preformed vitamin A.

Table 8-2	Food sources of Vitamin A	
Food	**Portion**	**Vitamin A (μg RAE)**
Beef liver, cooked	1 slice	6425
Cod liver oil	1 tbsp	4080
Chicken liver, cooked	1 liver	1752
Sweet potato, baked	1 large	1730
Butternut squash, baked	½ cup	572
Raw carrots, chopped	½ cup	534
Spinach, cooked	½ cup	472
Collard greens, cooked	½ cup	386
Skim milk, fortified	1 cup	338
Turnip greens, cooked	½ cup	274
Cantaloupe	1 cup	270
Special K	1 cup	225
Mustard greens, cooked	½ cup	221
Romaine lettuce, shredded	1 cup	205
Dandelion greens, cooked	½ cup	180
Spinach, raw	1 cup	141
Apricots, dried	½ cup	117
Margarine	1 tbsp	116
Butter	1 tbsp	97
Whole egg	1	80
Cheddar cheese	1 oz	75
Broccoli, cooked	½ cup	60
Apricot, raw	1	34

Data from U.S. Department of Agriculture, Agricultural Research Service. 2013. *USDA national nutrient database for standard reference, Release 26.* Accessed August 30, 2013. Available at: http://www.ars.usda.gov/nutrientdata

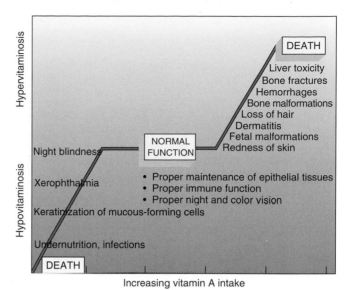

FIGURE 8-1 Vitamin A intake. This chart shows how changing the amount of vitamin A in the diet can lead to hypovitaminosis A or hypervitaminosis A. In extreme, either condition can lead to death. (From Patton KT, Thibodeau GA: *Anatomy and physiology,* ed 8, St Louis, 2013, Mosby Elsevier.)

fortified foods, beta-carotene is still a valuable source of this vitamin. Beta carotene is deep red in pure form and derives its name from carrots, from which it was first isolated. Chlorophyll disguises carotenoids in green vegetables. Most yellow, orange, and dark green fruits and vegetables are high in carotene or vitamin A content. The deeper the color, the more vitamin A activity is present in a fruit or vegetable.

Absorption and Excretion

Absorption is optimal when body stores are depleted, and when adequate amounts of other interrelated nutrients are present. The presence of vitamin E and the hormone thyroxine also enhances the use of vitamin A.

The liver stores approximately 90% of vitamin A, while smaller quantities are stored in the kidneys, lungs, and adipose tissue. Adequate serum proteins are necessary to mobilize vitamin A from the liver. Vitamin A is not readily excreted by the body, but a small amount is lost in urine.

Hyper States and Hypo States

Extreme levels of vitamin A (high or low) can cause serious problems, even resulting in death (Fig. 8-1).

Toxicity

When present in high concentrations, unbound vitamin A causes damage to cell membranes, especially in red blood cells and lysosomes (small bodies occurring in many types of cells). Large amounts of vitamin A supplements can exceed the storage capacity of the liver. If this occurs, free vitamin A enters the bloodstream and exerts toxic effects on cell membranes. High levels of vitamin A in the body are referred to as hypervitaminosis A.

Maternal consumption of vitamin A supplements before conception and during the first trimester of pregnancy has been associated with fetal birth defects (see Table 13-3 for effects of vitamin A toxicity during pregnancy). Toxicity is evident in infants by bulging of the fontanelle as a result of increased cerebrospinal fluid pressure. Other clinical symptoms include headache; nausea and vomiting; diplopia (double vision); lethargy and irritability; and alopecia (hair loss); dryness of the mucous membranes; reddened gingiva (Fig. 8-2); thinning of the epithelium; cracking and bleeding lips; and increased activity of osteoclasts (cells associated with bone resorption), which leads to decalcification, desquamation of oral mucosa, bone growth retardation, softening of the skull, and liver abnormalities.

Excess vitamin A (primarily in the form of retinol) may have a negative impact on bone health.[5] How this change in bone mineral density may affect alveolar bone is unknown.

Toxicity from excessive intake of vitamin A food sources is possible, but most cases are a result of too much supplementation. Beta-carotene is much less toxic than vitamin A. The body converts only the amount of carotenoids it needs into vitamin A. Although beta-carotenes are not toxic, overconsumption may result in hypercarotenemia, yellow pigmentation of the skin occurring first on the palms of the hands and soles of the feet, which is caused by carotene storage in fatty tissue (Fig. 8-3). This condition subsides when ingestion of beta-carotene is diminished.

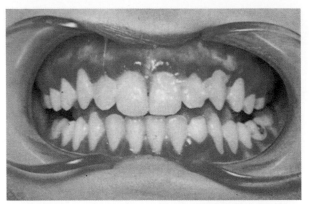

FIGURE 8-2 Hypervitaminosis A. Bright red marginal discoloration of the gingiva shown here is characteristic. (Courtesy of Dr. M.D. Muenter. From McLaren DS: *A colour atlas and text of diet-related disorders,* ed 2, London, 1992, Mosby–Year Book.)

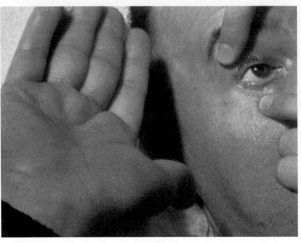

FIGURE 8-3 Hypercarotenosis. The face, eye, and palm of the hand. The sclerae remain clear, distinguishing the condition from jaundice. (Courtesy of Dr. I.A. Abrahamson, Sr. From McLaren DS: *A colour atlas and text of diet-related disorders,* ed 2, London, 1992, Mosby–Year Book.)

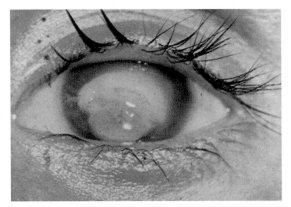

FIGURE 8-4 Xerophthalmia. (From McLaren DS: *A colour atlas and text of diet-related disorders,* ed 2, London, 1992, Mosby–Year Book.)

Deficiency

Inadequate dietary intake is the primary reason for vitamin A deficiency, found most commonly in children younger than 5 years of age. It also may result from chronic fat malabsorption. Vitamin A deficiency is rarely seen in the United States, but it is a major nutritional problem in developing countries. Mild vitamin A deficiency may contribute to a depressed immune response.

Inadequate vitamin A intake results in degeneration of epithelial cells in the eye and cessation of tear secretion. Lids are swollen and sticky with pus, and eyes are sensitive to light in xerophthalmia, sometimes resulting in permanent blindness. The first symptom of xerophthalmia is night blindness, followed by the occurrence of xerotic spots on the conjunctiva, called Bitot's spots. These eye ulcerations may spread and result in blindness if left untreated (Fig. 8-4).

Degeneration of epithelial cells results in an inability to produce mucus. This occurs not only in epithelial cells, but also in the intestines and lungs. Xeroderma can progress until the whole body is covered with dry, flaky, scaly skin that is similar to dandruff. It is followed by follicular hyperkeratosis, in which the skin is thickened, dry, and wrinkled (Fig. 8-5). Keratinization may also affect the oral mucosa and

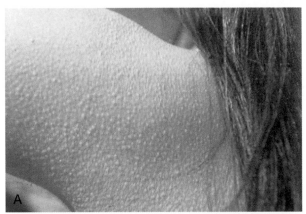

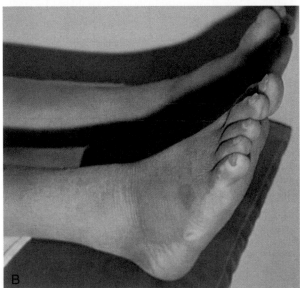

FIGURE 8-5 A, Follicular hyperkeratosis caused by vitamin A deficiency. **B,** Hyperkeratosis. The skin over parts of the body is thickened, dry, and wrinkled, associated with vitamin A deficiency. (From McLaren DS: *A colour atlas and text of diet-related disorders,* ed 2, London, 1992, Mosby–Year Book.)

the respiratory and gastrointestinal tracts. In these areas, degeneration of epithelial cells results in increased risk of infection, and delayed or impaired wound healing.

Severe vitamin A deficiency may result in enamel hypoplasia and defective dentin formation in developing teeth. Enamel hypoplasia involves defects in the enamel matrix and incomplete calcification of the enamel and dentin. Odontoblasts lose their ability to arrange themselves in normal parallel linear formation, resulting in degeneration and atrophy of ameloblasts. The normal deposition of dentin is altered.

Dental Considerations

- Vitamin A or beta-carotene supplements are not recommended for most healthy adults.
- Assess for signs of vitamin A deficiencies (loss of night vision, keratomalacia, corneal ulceration, or Bitot spots), especially in young and older patients. When in doubt, refer to a healthcare provider or RDN.
- In contrast to vitamin A, beta-carotene is not toxic, but large amounts can cause a temporary change in skin color. Hypercarotenemia may be distinguished from jaundice because the sclera retains its normal white color.
- Jaundice or any disorder affecting fat absorption also affects fat-soluble vitamin absorption, making these patients prone to vitamin A deficiency.
- Drugs such as orlistat (Xenical, Alli) used for weight loss and food components such as olestra negatively affect fat and fat-soluble vitamin absorption, especially the absorption of vitamin A and beta-carotene. Patients taking orlistat should follow a low-fat diet and take a multivitamin 2 hours before or after taking the drug.
- An alcoholic or alcoholic-cirrhotic patient may be deficient in vitamin A because of the effects of ethanol and impaired liver function.
- Vitamin A toxicity can be masked, especially when protein-energy malnutrition is present.
- Excessive intake of either vitamin E or C may decrease absorption of vitamin A. Do not encourage use of vitamin E and vitamin C supplements or vitamin E–rich or vitamin C–rich foods if the patient is at risk of vitamin A deficiency.

Nutritional Directions

- Vitamin A from animal or fortified foods is used better by the body than beta-carotene.
- Vegans need to consume a minimum of five servings of dark green, yellow, and orange fruits and vegetables daily to receive the recommended amount of vitamin A.
- Fortified foods and vitamin supplements should be used judiciously; severe, life-threatening liver damage or increased risk of hip fractures can result from chronic use in excess of the RDA.
- Discourage patients from taking more than the RDA in over-the-counter vitamin preparations unless specifically advised to do so by a healthcare provider or RDN.
- Recommend storing vitamins in a cool, dark place to prevent deterioration.
- Women of childbearing age need to limit intake of preformed vitamin A (retinol, retinyl, and retinoyl acetate) found in liver, fortified foods (breakfast cereals), and dietary supplements, to about 100% of the daily value because of the increased risk of neural defects during the first trimester of pregnancy.

VITAMIN D (CALCIFEROL)

Although vitamin D has been called a vitamin, it is more appropriately classified as a hormone (a compound secreted by one type of cell that acts to control the function of another type of cell). Skin cells are able to make vitamin D when the precursor 7-dehydrocholesterol, present in the skin, is exposed to ultraviolet (UV) light or sunshine. Vitamin D from food, ergocalciferol (vitamin D_2) or cholecalciferol (vitamin D_3), is biologically inert. Further processing occurs in the liver with conversion of vitamin D_2 or vitamin D_3 into 25-hydroxycholecalciferol (calcidiol), and a final change to the active form of 1,25-dihydroxycholecalciferol (calciferol) primarily by the kidney (Fig. 8-6).

Until recently, vitamin D was viewed primarily as a protective agent against bone disease, such as rickets. Research has shown, however, that vitamin D receptors are present in approximately 36 different types of cells, and the hormone is involved in the maintenance of more than 200 human genes.[6,7] Reports from many nations have highlighted a variety of vitamin D insufficiency and deficiency diseases. More research is needed to learn about the impact of vitamin D on different stages of the life cycle and in racial and ethnic groups.[8]

Physiological Roles

Vitamin D is intricately related to calcium and phosphorus, each being required for optimal use of the other. Vitamin D helps the body absorb and regulate calcium. The primary role of vitamin D is mineralization of bones and teeth, and regulation of blood calcium and phosphorus levels. It functions with the parathyroid and thyroid (calcitonin) hormones to regulate intestinal absorption of calcium and phosphorus, enhance renal calcium and phosphorus reabsorption, and regulate skeletal calcium and phosphorus reserves.

Vitamin D may also be involved in the functioning of cells involved in hematopoiesis (formation of red blood cells), the skin, cardiovascular function, and immune responses. Its regulatory role helps keep serum calcium in the appropriate range to maintain cardiac and neuromuscular function. Calciferol (1,25-dihydroxycholecalciferol) interacts with osteoblasts (cells that help produce collagen, and build and reform new bone) to increase the withdrawal of osteocalcin (calcium-binding noncollagen protein in bone) and other bone-building compounds, or interacts with parathyroid hormone to mobilize calcium stores from the skeleton when calcium is needed.

Requirements

The vitamin D requirement is difficult to determine and there are varying recommendations. When sufficient sunlight is available, people may not require an exogenous dietary source of vitamin D. Because many North Americans have limited exposure to sunlight, however, and because many factors can interfere with UV light–dependent synthesis of vitamin D in the skin, vitamin D is considered

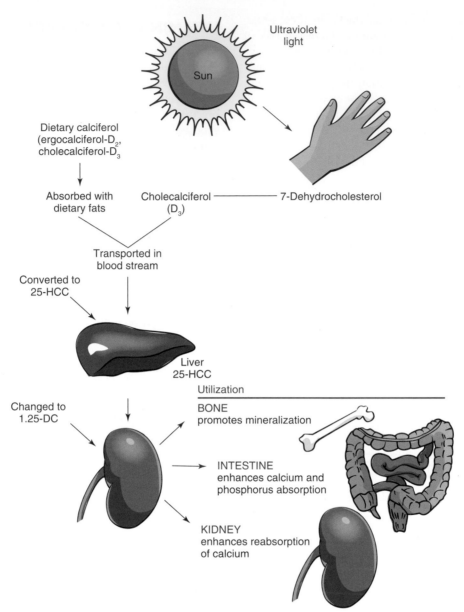

FIGURE 8-6 Vitamin D metabolism. (Adapted from Davis JR, Sherer K: *Applied nutrition and diet therapy for nurses*, ed 2, Philadelphia, 1994, Saunders Elsevier.)

an essential dietary nutrient. Vitamin D is measured in micrograms (mcg or µg) or IU. One microgram is equivalent to 40 IU.

The IOM determined that an adequate intake of vitamin D for ages 1 to 70 years old is 15 µg (600 IU); the recommended amount increases to 20 µg (800 IU) after age 70 (Table 8-3). The International Osteoporosis Foundation recommends 20 to 25 µg (800 to 1000 IU) for older adults.[9] The National Osteoporosis Foundation urges adults older than age 50 years to get at least 800 to 1000 IU of vitamin D to prevent fractures; they recommend supplementation to get adequate amounts because of difficulty obtaining it from food sources, especially for individuals diagnosed with osteoporosis.[10] Any supplements needed should be in the form of vitamin D_3 because it is more potent than D_2.[11] The U.S. Preventive Services Task Force found inconclusive

evidence to support supplementation of vitamin D_3 and does not recommend daily vitamin D_3 supplements unless a deficiency exists (determined by laboratory data) or the patient is diagnosed with osteopenia or osteoporosis (determined by radiograph).[12]

ULs for various life stages also were established for vitamin D. The estimated average requirement intake to prevent rickets is 10 µg or 400 IU. The American Academy of Pediatrics has recommended 10 µg (400 IU) of vitamin D for infants. Therefore, supplementation is needed for infants who are breastfed or consuming less than 1 L/day of formula. This practice should begin within the first few days following birth.[13]

Some medical researchers have expressed strong doubts in scientific journals about the adequacy of the current dietary reference intake for vitamin D. One reason the IOM

Table 8-3	**Institute of medicine recommendations for Vitamin D**		
Life Stage*	EAR µg/day (IU)†	RDA µg/day (IU)‡||	UL µg/day (IU)¶
0-6 months	10 µg/day (400 IU)	10 (400)‡	25 (1000)
7-12 months	10 (400)	10 (400)‡	37.5 (1500)
1-3 years	10 (400)	15 (600)	62.5 (2500)
4-8 years	10 (400)	15 (600)	75 (3000)
9-13 years	10 (400)	15 (600)	100 (4000)
14-18 years	10 (400)	15 (600)	100 (4000)
19-30 years	10 (400)	15 (600)	100 (4000)
31-50 years	10 (400)	15 (600)	100 (4000)
51-70 years	10 (400)	15 (600)	100 (4000)
>70 years	10 (400)	20 (800)	100 (4000)
Pregnant and Lactating			
19-50 years	10 (400)	15 (600)	100 (4000)

Data from Institute of Medicine (IOM), Food and Nutrition Board: *Dietary reference intakes for calcium and vitamin D*, Washington, DC, 2011, National Academy Press.
*All groups except pregnancy and lactation are males and females.
†EAR (estimated average requirement)—the intake that meets the estimated nutrient needs of half of the individuals in a group.
‡RDA (recommended dietary allowance)—the intake that meets the nutrient needs of almost all (97% to 98%) individuals in a group.
||As cholecalciferol: 1 µg cholecalciferol = 40 IU vitamin D.
¶UL (tolerable upper intake level)—the highest level of daily nutrient intake that is likely to pose no risk of adverse health effects to almost all individuals in the general population. As intake increases above the UL, the risk of adverse effects increases. Unless specified otherwise, the UL represents total nutrient intake from food, water, and supplements.

is hesitant to recommend further increases in intake is because of potential toxicity from vitamin D. More research is needed to validate the health benefits and appropriate level of vitamin D. Because U.S. residents comprise different ethnicities and locations and sensitivities, a "one-size-fits-all" recommendation may not be appropriate.

American and Canadian diets do not provide sufficient vitamin D.[8] A study involving healthy children and adolescents indicates low prevalence of vitamin D blood concentrations are related to low intake, race, and season of the year.[8]

Sources

Sunlight

The body's ability to produce adequate amounts of vitamin D from sunlight is the reason the sun has been considered a source of health. UV radiation is the principal cause of sunburn and cellular damage that leads to skin cancer. UV radiation penetrates uncovered skin and converts a precursor of vitamin D to previtamin D_3, which becomes the active form of vitamin D_3, or calcitriol. Most people experience an increase in vitamin D levels during the summer months because changes in the angulation of the sun occur throughout the year. During summer months, 10 minutes a day without sunblock on hands and face can replete the body's supply.

Many people in the northern hemisphere (above a line approximately between the northern border of California and Boston), especially older adults and darker-skinned individuals, may lack sufficient exposure to UV radiation, especially mid-October through mid-March. Cloud cover, fog, haze, shade, and pollution can reduce the UV energy needed for vitamin D. UV radiation does not penetrate glass. Sunscreens with a sun protection factor of 15 or more block both UVA and UVB rays,[14] interfering with the formation of vitamin D_3. Dermatologists continue to advise sunscreen and clothing protection for anyone in the sun more than 20 minutes. Although sunscreen inhibits vitamin D production, its use and moderation in sun exposure are important to protect against skin cancer. By age 70 years, the skin generally produces vitamin D at only half the level it did at age 20 years.

Food

Although adequate quantities of vitamin D may be derived from exposure to sunlight, additional food sources are necessary in most cases. Naturally-occurring vitamin D content in foods is limited and variable; food tables do not normally list vitamin D content. This information has been added to the National Nutrient Database for Standard Reference (available at http://www.nal.usda.gov/fnic/foodcomp/search/).

Natural sources include oily fish such as salmon, mackerel, sardines, and tuna, as well as cod liver oil and fish oils (Table 8-4). A diet composed of the best (unfortified) food sources of vitamin D may supply only 2.5 µg (1000 IU) daily.

Because vitamin D deficiencies are prevalent in the United States, the U.S. Food and Drug Administration allows vitamin D fortification of orange juice and other foods; this provides a good alternative source for people who do not drink milk. Other foods, such as margarine, infant formulas and cereals, prepared breakfast cereals, chocolate beverage mixes, and yogurt, also may be fortified with vitamin D (see Table 8-4).

Foods are not legally required to be fortified, but approximately 98% of the milk in the United States is fortified to provide 10 µg (400 IU) of cholecalciferol per quart. Vitamin D fortification of milk enhances absorption and utilization of the calcium and phosphorus inherent in milk and vice versa. Children especially benefit from vitamin D fortification of milk for bone growth. Vitamin D from fortified regular and low-fat cheeses is absorbed and metabolized well by the body.[15] Because fortification is optional, it cannot be taken for granted.

Nutrition labels can be used to assess daily intake of vitamin D; this information plus the amount of exposure to sunlight must be considered to ensure adequate amounts of vitamin D. Vitamin D is in multivitamins, prenatal vitamins, calcium–vitamin D combinations, and individual vitamin D supplements. Most multivitamins provide 400 IU per dose.

Table 8-4	Food sources of vitamin D	
Food	**Portion**	**Vitamin D (IU)**
Cod liver oil	1 tbsp	1360
Salmon, cooked	3 oz	447
Sardines, canned in oil, drained	3 oz	164
Tuna fish, canned in water, drained	3 oz	154
Orange juice, fortified with vitamin D	1 cup	137
Milk (skim, 1%, or 2%), fortified with vitamin D	1 cup	116
Chocolate milk, lowfat, fortified with vitamin D	1 cup	108
Raisin Bran	1 cup	91
Yogurt, nonfat, fortified with vitamin D	6 oz	88
American cheese, fortified with vitamin D	1 oz	85
Margarine, fortified	1 tbsp	60
Egg	1 large	44
Beef liver, cooked	1 slice	33

Data from U.S. Department of Agriculture, Agricultural Research Service. 2013. *USDA national nutrient database for standard reference, Release 26.* Accessed August 31, 2013. Available at: http://www.ars.usda.gov/nutrientdata

Traditionally, supplement manufacturers have used vitamin D_2 (ergocalciferol), but this form is less effective than vitamin D_3 at increasing calcidiol levels in the blood.

Absorption

As with other nutrients, optimal absorption occurs when all closely interrelated nutrients (particularly calcium and phosphorus) are present in sufficient quantities. Conversely, diets high in fiber can result in less vitamin D absorption.

Hyper States and Hypo States

Toxicity

Vitamin D has the potential to become toxic at high levels. The risk for harm increases as the intake level exceeds the UL.[15] For example, uncontrolled use of vitamin D supplements by older patients with osteoporosis led to occult vitamin D intoxication, resulting in diminished bone mass.[16]

When synthetic vitamin D supplements are taken orally in large amounts for 6 weeks, toxicity signs may occur. Nausea, vomiting, poor appetite, weight loss, constipation, dizziness, and weakness are signs of vitamin D toxicity. Vitamin D toxicity can also increase blood levels of calcium, causing mental changes, confusion, and heart rhythm abnormalities.[17] Amounts above 10,000 IUs/day may result in kidney and tissue damage.[15] Calciferol poisoning can result in enhanced bone resorption, leading to deposition of calcium and phosphate in soft tissues and irreversible kidney and cardiovascular damage.[17] Unless symptoms are detected

and the source of vitamin D is removed immediately, permanent damage results.

The most common reason for vitamin D toxicity is prolonged intake of excessive supplements or cod liver oil; otherwise, toxicity through diet is unlikely. Toxicity from excessive vitamin D intake may occur when a concentrated calciferol preparation is mistakenly given. An infant given a commercial formula and a vitamin supplement can easily ingest vitamin D well above the adequate intake level.

Deficiency

Vitamin D research indicates it may potentially protect against a wide variety of diseases.[18] In adults, vitamin D deficiency has been linked in research studies to conditions as diverse as asthma, cancer, CHD, hypertension, diabetes mellitus, depression, some infectious diseases, autoimmune disorders, and schizophrenia.[19] Many vitamin D researchers believe that by diligently shielding ourselves from sunlight, many benefits of this vitamin may be missed.[20,21] Also, the melanin that makes skin dark effectively filters out UVB, so dark-skinned individuals are much more likely than fair-skinned individuals to have low levels of vitamin D.

Vitamin D deficiency affects skeletal structure in children and adults. Signs of deficiency are commonly found in children because of increased requirements, decreased stores, decreased exposure to the sun, or use of sunscreens. In elderly patients, deficiencies are created by consuming inadequate diets with little exposure to the sun, reduced skin thickness, inability of the kidney to convert vitamin D to its active form, or inadequate absorption of vitamin D from the gastrointestinal tract. Plasma vitamin D is significantly lower in older patients than among the younger population; it is consistently higher for older men than women. A healthcare provider may recommend vitamin D and calcium supplements to older patients to prevent osteoporosis. When supplementation is recommended, care must be used to prevent toxic overdoses. Vitamin D deficiency is associated with muscle weakness, causing older individuals to tire easily and experience difficulty climbing stairs and rising from a chair. This muscle weakness frequently results in falls.

Rickets. Laboratory values indicating serum calcium or phosphorus above or below normal values, the failure of bones to grow properly in length, and x-ray films showing abnormal epiphyses (the terminal end or growth points of bones) indicate deficiencies (Fig. 8-7). Because vitamin D is intricately related to calcium and phosphorus functions, a change in any of these three nutrients affects the others.

The name rickets came from the word *wrikken,* meaning "to bend or twist." Rickets, caused by vitamin D deficiency, usually occurs in children 1 to 3 years old and is characterized by weak bones and skeletal deformities. Rachitic deformities such as bowlegs or knock-knees develop (Fig. 8-8A). The epiphyses of bones do not develop normally in children, so bones are twisted and warped. Other bone changes include a row of beadlike protuberances (rachitic rosary) on each

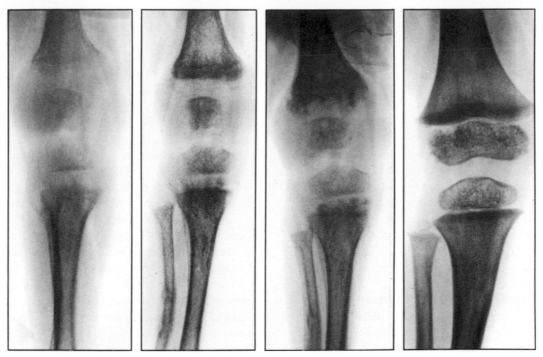

FIGURE 8-7 Active rickets of the knees. The metaphyses of the bones are concave and irregular, and the zone of uncalcified osteoid is enlarged. These x-rays show the progressive changes over 10 months, during which healing took place in this case. (Courtesy of Prof. A. Prader. From *A colour atlas and text of diet-related disorders,* ed 2, London, 1992, Mosby–Year Book.)

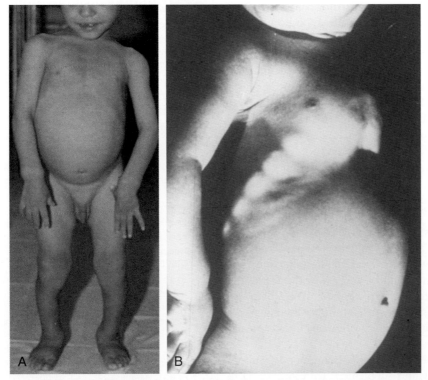

FIGURE 8-8 A, Bowlegs in rickets. The typical lateral curvature indicates that the weakened bones have bent after the second year as a result of standing. **B,** Rachitic rosary in a young infant. (**A,** From McLaren DS: *A colour atlas and text of diet-related disorders,* ed 2, London, 1992, Mosby–Year Book. **B,** From Kliegman RM, Stanton BMD, St. Geme J, Schor NF: *Nelson textbook of pediatrics*, ed 19, Philadelphia, 2011, Saunders Elsevier.)

side of the narrow, distorted chest (pigeon breast) at the juncture of the ribs and costal cartilage (Fig. 8-8*B*). A narrow pelvis, making future childbearing difficult in women, is also observed.

Rickets develops during a time of extremely rapid growth when children have had only a brief period to acquire vitamin D stores. Adequate intake of vitamin D during pregnancy and lactation is important because vitamin D is passed from the mother to the infant before birth and in breast milk. However, adequate vitamin D cannot be met solely by breastfeeding. Rickets is being diagnosed in the United States more frequently because of rising numbers of breastfed infants, lack of sun exposure, or use of sunscreens.[20,21]

The alveolar bone is affected similar to other bones in the body when rickets occurs. The trabeculae of the alveolar bone also weaken. Delayed dentition and small molars are observed in infants and children who are vitamin D deficient.

Enamel Hypoplasia and Dental Decay. A landmark study conducted in 1973 reported the possibility of increased risk of enamel hypoplasia in children of mothers experiencing vitamin D deficiency during pregnancy.[22] In addition, a few patients with evidence of rickets develop enamel hypoplasia as a result of a lack of vitamin D. Whether these teeth are more susceptible to dental caries is uncertain. The enamel does not seem to be weakened, but the rougher surface may facilitate adherence of dental biofilm and food residue. Finally, the research findings regarding an association between vitamin D status and dental decay indicate a possible association.[23,24]

Periodontitis. A deficiency in vitamin D could influence periodontal status. Studies suggest an association of adequate vitamin D intake with an overall healthier periodontium with less inflammation and a decreased risk of tooth loss.[25,26] Vitamin D inadequacy may also impact wound healing, causing negative treatment outcomes following periodontal surgery.[25-27]

Osteomalacia. Vitamin D deficiency in adults is called osteomalacia; it is also intricately related to calcium intake. Osteomalacia is characterized by decreased bone mineralization or softening of the bones, which may lead to deformities of the limbs, spine, thorax, and pelvis. The main symptoms are skeletal pain and muscle weakness, resulting in kyphosis, or an uneven gait. Oral manifestations include loss of the lamina dura around the roots of the teeth. The condition is more prevalent in women of childbearing age with calcium depletion because of multiple pregnancies or inadequate intake or in women who have little exposure to sun.

A healthcare provider or RDN may recommend a vitamin D supplement or a calcium supplement with vitamin D to maximize absorption of calcium, especially women who are at high risk for osteoporosis because of small frame size. Medication may also be prescribed to prevent further deterioration of bone mineral density.

Osteoporosis. Osteoporosis was previously thought of as a calcium deficiency, but research indicates that vitamin D levels are as important as calcium intake. As discussed previously, vitamin D deficiency interferes with mineralization of the skeleton, reducing bone density and increasing risk of bone fractures. Osteoporosis is a disease characterized by fragile bones and is associated with an increased incidence of bone fractures, especially the hip. Osteoporosis is discussed further in *Health Application 8.*

Cancer and Cardiovascular Risks. Laboratory, animal, and epidemiologic evidence suggests vitamin D may be protective against some cancers. Numerous studies indicate that higher vitamin levels in blood are associated with reduced prostate, colon and colorectal cancers, and breast cancer.[28,29] In animal studies, tumor growth has been reduced by giving vitamin D. The relationship of vitamin D and cancer is uncertain; evidence is based on limited data, and more studies are needed to determine optimal levels and intakes of vitamin D to reduce cancer risk.

Vitamin D may also be important for heart health. Evidence suggests that vitamin D may be related to a reduced risk of CHD. Individuals with lower blood levels of vitamin D had an increased risk of CHD. More research is needed to determine just how vitamin D affects these conditions and how much vitamin D is needed to promote CHD.[7,30]

Dental Considerations

- Assess for vitamin D toxicity and deficiency, especially in young children, pregnant and lactating women, and older adults.
- Vitamin D supplements should be given only in prescribed amounts based on laboratory values because patients vary widely in their susceptibility to vitamin D toxicity. Do not recommend patients buy vitamin D supplements. Refer them to a healthcare provider or RDN.
- If supplemental doses of vitamin D are used, cloudiness or a red color of the urine may indicate toxicity and should be brought to the healthcare provider's attention.
- Conditions leading to vitamin D deficiency include any abnormalities that (a) interfere with intestinal absorption (e.g., diarrhea, steatorrhea, celiac disease, Crohn's disease, and cystic fibrosis), and (b) abnormalities in calcium balance and bone metabolism caused by disease states such as renal failure. Evaluate the patient's health status for risk of vitamin D deficiency.
- Patients with minimal or no exposure to sunlight should be monitored for adequate vitamin D intake or supplementation or both to maintain adequate vitamin D stores. Question the patient regarding living environment or hobbies to determine exposure to sunlight.
- Determine the use of sunscreens. Consistent use of sunscreens may contribute to vitamin D deficiency in some patients. Sunscreens with a sun protection factor of 8 or greater block the UV rays from the sun necessary to produce vitamin D.
- Anticonvulsant drugs, such as phenytoin and phenobarbital, inactivate vitamin D, directly affecting skeletal and intestinal metabolism to cause osteomalacia. If a patient is taking these drugs over a long period, vitamin D supplements and some daily sun exposure may be beneficial.
- Low skeletal bone mass may also be associated with periodontal bone loss and tooth loss.

Nutritional Directions

- The bright sunlight between 11 AM and 2 PM offers maximum conversion. For light-skinned individuals, 10 to 20 minutes of daily sun exposure results in adequate conversion.
- Toxicity may result from excess intake of cod liver oil or from taking excessive vitamin D supplements.
- Older individuals, especially individuals living in a long-term care facility, are at high risk for vitamin D deficiency.
- Read the label on vitamin supplements; select brands that contain vitamin D$_3$ or cholecalciferol. Ergocalciferol is less effective.
- Provide meal or snack ideas to include fortified cereal with fortified low-fat milk; raw vegetables with a fortified yogurt dip; or topping a salad with salmon.
- Encourage patients to consume adequate amounts of fruits and vegetables, to exercise, not to smoke, and to drink alcohol only in moderation for overall health.

VITAMIN E (TOCOPHEROL)

Eight different compounds are collectively called vitamin E: four **tocopherols** and four **tocotrienols**. Biological activity of each form varies; α-tocopherol is the most active form and is used more efficiently by the body.

Physiological Roles

Vitamin E is the most important fat-soluble antioxidant. Vitamin E protects the integrity of normal cell membranes and effectively prevents hemolysis of red blood cells. It also protects vitamins A and C, beta-carotene, and unsaturated fatty acids from oxidation. Vitamin E supplementation improves the immune response in healthy older adults; this effect may be mediated by increases in **prostaglandins**, which enhance growth of white blood cells. These functions promote resistance of the periodontium to inflammation. In larger amounts, vitamin E is an **anticoagulant**, or blood thinner. The role of vitamin E as an antioxidant is discussed further in *Health Application 8*.

Requirements

The dietary reference intakes for vitamin E (adequate intake, RDA, and UL) are based solely on the α-tocopherol form because humans are unable to convert and use other forms. The RDA for vitamin E is 15 mg of α-tocopherol for healthy individuals 14 years old and older except for lactating women (Table 8-5). One milligram of α-tocopherol is the same as 1.5 IU. High intakes of polyunsaturated fatty acids increase the vitamin E requirement. Most polyunsaturated oils contain vitamin E, but chemical reactions may have rendered the antioxidant ineffective. If an individual's systemic stores are low, the vitamin E requirement is increased.

The daily UL is 1000 mg of α-tocopherol (1500 IU of natural vitamin E is equivalent to 1000 IU of synthetic vitamin E). The UL was established because of the adverse health effect of bleeding problems. Supplemental amounts in excess of the RDA should not be recommended.

Table 8-5	Institute of Medicine recommendations for α-tocopherol*			
Life Stage	EAR (mg/day)†	RDA (mg/day)‡	AI (mg/day)§	UL (mg/day)‖
0-6 months			4	ND¶
7-12 months			6	ND¶
1-3 years	5	6		200
4-8 years	6	7		300
9-13 years	9	11		600
14-18 years	12	15		800
19-70 years	12	15		1000
>70 years	12	15		1000
Pregnancy				
≤18 years	12	15		800
19-50 years	12	15		1000
Lactation				
≤18 years	16	19		800
19-50 years	16	19		1000

Data from Institute of Medicine (IOM), Food and Nutrition Board: *Dietary reference intakes for vitamin C, vitamin E, selenium, and carotenoids,* Washington, DC, 2000, National Academy Press.
*α-Tocopherol includes the only form of α-tocopherol that occurs naturally in foods, and some of the forms that occur in fortified foods and supplements, but not all forms because some that are used in fortified foods and supplements have not been shown to meet human requirements.
†EAR (estimated average requirement)—the intake that meets the estimated nutrient needs of half of the individuals in a group.
‡RDA (recommended dietary allowance)—the intake that meets the nutrient needs of almost all (97% to 98%) individuals in a group.
§AI (adequate intake)—the observed average or experimentally set intake by a defined population or subgroup that seems to sustain a defined nutritional status, such as growth rate, normal circulating nutrient values, or other functional indicators of health. An AI is used if insufficient scientific evidence is available to derive an EAR. For healthy human milk–fed infants, the AI is the mean intake. *The AI is not equivalent to an RDA.*
‖Institute of Medicine (IOM), Food and Nutrition Board: *Dietary reference intakes for vitamin A, vitamin K, Arsenic, boron, chromium, copper, iodine, iron, manganese, molybdenum, nickel, silicon, vanadium, and zinc.* Washington, DC, 2000, National Academy Press.
¶ND, Not determinable because of lack of data of adverse effects in this age group and concern about lack of ability to handle excess amounts. Source of intake should be from food and formula so as to prevent high levels of intake.

Sources

Vitamin E is available from vegetable oils and margarine made from them; whole-grain or fortified cereals; wheat germ; nuts; green leafy vegetables; and some fruits. Meats, fish, and animal fats contain very little vitamin E. Table 8-6 lists the amounts of vitamin E in some foods. Because vitamin E is widely distributed in foods, dietary deficiencies seldom occur if a well-balanced, varied diet is consumed.

Although the recommended levels are now designated in mg, food labels list the vitamin E content of the food or supplement in IUs because the daily value is measured in IUs. The daily value for vitamin E is 30 IU (or 20 mg of α-tocopherol). Dietary supplements label vitamin E as "dl" α-tocopherol, which means the vitamin E is a synthetic form, in contrast to "d" α-tocopherol, which means it is natural.

Table 8-6	Food sources of vitamin E	
Food	**Portion**	**Vitamin E (mg)**
Wheat germ oil	1 tbsp	20.3
Total cereal	1 cup	18.0
Almonds	1 oz	7.4
Special K cereal	1 cup	4.7
Hazelnuts	1 oz	4.3
Tomato sauce, canned	1 cup	3.5
Peanut butter	2 tbsp	2.9
Corn oil	1 tbsp	2.0
Spinach, cooked	½ cup	1.9
Sweet potato, baked	1 large	1.3
Soybean oil	1 tbsp	1.1
Peach, fresh	1 medium	1.1
Safflower oil	1 tbsp	1.0
Tomato juice, canned	1 cup	0.8
Margarine	1 tbsp	0.6
Pecans	1 oz	0.4
Raisin Bran cereal	1 cup	0.4
Apple, raw	1 medium	0.3
Apricot, raw	1	0.3
Walnuts	1 oz	0.2
Lima beans, cooked	½ cup	0.1

Data from U.S. Department of Agriculture, Agricultural Research Service. 2013. *USDA national nutrient database for standard reference, Release 26.* Accessed August 31, 2013. Available at: http://www.ars.usda.gov/nutrientdata

Dental Considerations

- Vitamin E may help the immune system function better, so assess intake of vitamin E in immunocompromised patients.
- Vitamin E supplementation is not recommended, but may be of special concern for patients with vitamin K deficiency or with known coagulation defects, or for patients receiving anticoagulation therapy, which interferes with vitamin K activity, because it can increase risk for hemorrhaging.
- In contrast to other vitamins, naturally occurring α-tocopherol from foods is twice as potent as the synthetic form, making it a more desirable choice than synthetic supplements.

Nutritional Directions

- When oils are reused in frying, heavy losses of vitamin E occur.
- An increase in fruits and vegetables provides more low-fat sources of vitamin E.
- Because of widespread publicity of scientific studies linking vitamin E to decreased risk of heart disease, diabetes, cancer, Alzheimer disease, and cognitive decline, many patients may choose to use supplements. Advise patients to limit vitamin E supplements to the RDA unless they are instructed otherwise by their healthcare provider.
- Adverse effects of excessive amounts of vitamin E are associated with vitamin E supplements only; food sources of vitamin E are not associated with adverse reactions.
- If vitamin E supplements are recommended by a healthcare provider or RDN, they should be consumed with a meal containing fat to assist with absorption.[32]
- Vitamin E supplements cannot replace other proven and effective ways to reduce disease risks—not smoking, getting regular exercise, maintaining a healthy weight, and eating a well-balanced, healthy diet.

Absorption and Excretion

Absorption of vitamin E is inefficient, ranging from 20% to 80% in healthy individuals. Efficiency of absorption depends on the body's ability to absorb fat and seems to decline as the amount of dietary vitamin E increases.

Hyper States and Hypo States

Scientific studies suggest that this antioxidant may reduce the risk of CHD, some types of cancer, cataracts, age-related macular degeneration, Parkinson and Alzheimer disease. However, evidence is inconclusive that vitamin E reduces the risk of CHD and other chronic diseases. Vitamin E supplements do not seem to reverse any disease, including cancer.[31]

Higher doses of vitamin E may disturb the balance of beneficial, naturally-occurring antioxidants. Individuals who benefit from vitamin E supplementation are premature infants; infants, children, or adults who cannot absorb fats and oils because of diseases in the gastrointestinal tract; individuals with sickle cell anemia; smokers; and individuals consuming an extremely low-fat diet. Low vitamin E levels in the blood are associated with subsequent decline in physical function, but normal levels of vitamin E can be maintained by consuming vitamin E–rich foods.[32]

VITAMIN K

Three forms of vitamin K, a fat-soluble vitamin, have been identified, all belonging to a group of chemical compounds known as quinones. The naturally occurring vitamins are K_1 (phylloquinone), which occurs in green plants, and K_2 (menaquinone), which is formed by *Escherichia coli* bacteria in the large intestine and is found in animal tissues. The fat-soluble synthetic compound menadione (vitamin K_3) is two to three times as potent as the natural vitamin.

Physiological Roles

Vitamin K–dependent proteins have been identified in bone, kidney, and other tissues. These proteins bind calcium and may be involved in bone crystalline formation. Vitamin K functions as a catalyst in synthesis of blood-clotting factors, primarily in maintaining **prothrombin** levels, which is the first stage in forming a clot. A low prothrombin level results in impaired blood coagulation.

Requirements

The RDA is 120 μg for men and 90 μg for women. No UL for vitamin K has been established (Table 8-7).

Table 8-7	Institute of Medicine recommendations for vitamin K	

	AI*	
Life Stage	Male (µg/day)	Female (µg/day)
0-6 months	2	2
7-12 months	2.5	2.5
1-3 years	30	30
4-8 years	55	55
9-13 years	60	60
14-18 years	75	75
>18 years	120	90
Pregnancy		
≤18 years		75
19-50 years		90
Lactation		
≤18 years		75
19-50 years		90

Data from Institute of Medicine (IOM), Food and Nutrition Board: *Dietary reference intakes for vitamin A, vitamin K, arsenic, boron, chromium, copper, iodine, iron, manganese, molybdenum, nickel, silicon, vanadium, and zinc,* Washington, DC, 2000, National Academy Press.
*AI (adequate intake)—the observed average or experimentally set intake by a defined population or subgroup that seems to sustain a defined nutritional status, such as growth rate, normal circulating nutrient values, or other functional indicators of health. An AI is used if insufficient scientific evidence is available to derive an estimated average requirement. For healthy human milk–fed infants, the AI is the mean intake. *The AI is not equivalent to an RDA.*

Table 8-8	Food sources of vitamin K	

Food	Portion	Vitamin K (µg)
Kale, cooked	½ cup	531
Spinach, cooked	½ cup	444
Broccoli, cooked	½ cup	110
Brussels sprouts, cooked	½ cup	109
Green leaf lettuce	1 cup	46
Asparagus, cooked	½ cup	28
Cabbage, raw	½ cup	27
Peas, cooked	½ cup	21
Lima beans, cooked	½ cup	5
Ground beef, cooked	3 oz	2
Yogurt, nonfat	6 oz	2

Data from U.S. Department of Agriculture, Agricultural Research Service. 2013. *USDA national nutrient database for standard reference, Release 26.* Accessed August 31, 2013. Available at: http://www.ars.usda.gov/nutrientdata

Sources

Although limited amounts of vitamin K are stored in the body, a shortage of vitamin K is unlikely because it is derived from food and microflora in the gut. Green leafy vegetables are high in vitamin K, but meats and dairy products also provide significant amounts (Table 8-8).

Bacterial flora in the jejunum and ileum synthesize vitamin K and provide about half of the body's requirement. However, synthesis of vitamin K by intestinal bacteria does not provide adequate amounts of the vitamin; therefore, a restriction of dietary vitamin K can alter clotting factors.

Absorption and Excretion

Vitamin K absorption decreases with high levels of vitamin E supplementation. Some vitamin K is stored in the liver, and some becomes a component of lipoproteins. Ordinarily, 30% to 40% of the amount absorbed is excreted via bile into the feces as water-soluble metabolites, with approximately 15% excreted in the urine.

Hyper States and Hypo States

No toxicity symptoms have been documented from oral intake of vitamin K. Synthetic menadione has caused toxic effects, however.

Primary vitamin K deficiency is uncommon, but disease or drug therapy may cause deficiencies. Any condition of the biliary tract affecting the flow of bile prevents vitamin K absorption. Vitamin K deficiency is common in celiac disease and sprue, which affect absorption in the small intestine, and other diarrheal diseases (e.g., ulcerative colitis) as a result of malabsorption. In vitamin K deficiency or in patients taking anticoagulants, blood-clotting time is delayed, increasing the risk of bleeding problems.

Impairment of vitamin K function in bones of postmenopausal women may be a factor in the effects of declining estrogen production. Typical vitamin K intake may be inadequate to support bone health in postmenopausal years.[33] Low dietary intake of vitamin K has been linked to reduced bone mass density in women, increasing the risk of hip fractures. However, high-dose supplementation with high levels of vitamin K did not stop age-related bone loss.[34]

Newborns may develop hemorrhagic disease secondary to vitamin K deficiency because the gut is sterile during the first few days after birth. Newborns are usually given a single dose of vitamin K intramuscularly immediately after birth to prevent hemorrhage.

Dental Considerations

- Excessive amounts of vitamin A or E, or both have a detrimental effect on vitamin K absorption.
- Mineral oil interferes with absorption of vitamin K and should not be consumed close to a meal.
- Vitamin K should never be confused with the symbol "K," which is used to designate potassium or kosher foods. If information is confusing or unclear, double-check with a healthcare provider or RDN.
- Vitamin K may be used prophylactically before any oral surgery to prevent prolonged bleeding in patients who have a condition that inhibits clotting.
- Frequently, blood-thinning agents may be discontinued for several days before any oral surgery to prevent excessive bleeding, or the patient may be hospitalized for a few days.
- Cholestyramine prescribed for hyperlipidemia binds with bile salts. The presence of bile is required for vitamin K absorption. Patients taking cholestyramine are at risk of vitamin K deficiency,

Continued

Dental Considerations—cont'd

so assess for bleeding problems, such as petechiae (pinpoint, flat red spots) or ecchymosis (bruising).
- Antibiotic therapy inhibits vitamin K–producing intestinal microflora and seems to be a factor in the origin of vitamin K deficiency, especially with impaired hepatic or renal function.
- Patients receiving oral anticoagulants (usually warfarin) to prevent blood clots from forming may develop serious hemorrhaging problems. They should keep vitamin K intake consistent and should not consume vitamin K supplements.

Nutritional Directions

- A lack of vitamin K may lead to bleeding problems.
- Vitamin K is stable to heat; cooking does not affect the vitamin K content of foods.

VITAMIN C (ASCORBIC ACID)

Physiological Roles

As a coenzyme, vitamin C has numerous metabolic roles. It is important in the production of collagen (the primary structural protein in connective tissue, cartilage, and bone), which plays a vital role in wound healing. During the development of connective tissue, bones, and teeth, vitamin C is important in the formation of fibroblasts (collagen-forming cells), osteoblasts, and odontoblasts. Vitamin C strengthens tissues and promotes capillary integrity. Vitamin C facilitates development of red blood cells by enhancing iron absorption and use. It also aids the body in utilizing folate and vitamin B_{12}. It has a coenzymatic function in the metabolism of amino acids and biosynthesis of bile acids, thyroxine, epinephrine, and steroid hormones. Vitamin C can also affect immune responses because of its high concentration in white blood cells.

Vitamin C functions as an antioxidant in numerous physiologic reactions. In its role as an antioxidant, it protects cells and tissues against damage caused by free radicals, toxic chemicals, and pollutants. More details on the role of vitamin C as an antioxidant are found in *Health Application 8*.

Requirements

The RDA is established at 90 mg daily for men and 75 mg daily for women, increasing during pregnancy and lactation (Table 8-9). The requirement for vitamin C is increased under many situations in which it is directly involved (e.g., stress, healing, and infections). It is detrimentally affected by many drugs (e.g., tobacco, alcohol, oral contraceptives, and aspirin), which increase requirements, and is usually the first nutrient to be depleted. Smokers may benefit from an additional intake of 35 mg per day because they are more likely to experience biological processes that damage cells and deplete vitamin C. The UL is 2000 mg per day.

Table 8-9	Institute of Medicine recommendations for vitamin C						
	EAR (mg/day)*		RDA (mg/day)†		AI (mg/day)‡		UL (mg/day)§
Life Stage	Male	Female	Male	Female	Male	Female	
0-6 months					40	50	ND‖
7-12 months					50	50	ND‖
1-3 years	13	13	15	15			400
4-8 years	22	22	25	25			650
9-13 years	39	39	45	45			1200
14-18 years	63	56	75	65			1800
19-70 years	75	60	90	75			2000
>70 years	75	60	90	75			2000
Pregnancy							
≤18 years		66		80			1800
19-50 years		70		85			2000
Lactation							
≤18 years		96		115			1800
19-50 years		100		120			2000

Data from Institute of Medicine (IOM), Food and Nutrition Board: *Dietary reference intakes for vitamin C, vitamin E, selenium, and carotenoids,* Washington, DC, 2000, National Academy Press.

*EAR (estimated average requirement)—the intake that meets the estimated nutrient needs of half of the individuals in a group.

†RDA (recommended dietary allowance)—the intake that meets the nutrient needs of almost all (97% to 98%) individuals in a group.

‡AI (adequate intake)—the observed average or experimentally set intake by a defined population or subgroup that seems to sustain a defined nutritional status, such as growth rate, normal circulating nutrient values, or other functional indicators of health. An AI is used if insufficient scientific evidence is available to derive an EAR. For healthy human milk–fed infants, the AI is the mean intake. *The AI is not equivalent to an RDA.*

§UL (tolerable upper intake level)—the highest level of daily nutrient intake that is likely to pose no risk of adverse health effects to almost all individuals in the general population. As intake increases above the UL, the risk of adverse effects increases. Unless specified otherwise, UL represents total nutrient intake from food, water, and supplements.

‖Not determinable because of lack of data of adverse effects in this age group and concern about lack of ability to handle excess amounts. Source of intake should be from food and formula so as to prevent high levels of intake.

Table 8-10	Food sources of Vitamin C	
Food	**Portion**	**Vitamin C (mg)**
Papaya	1 large	476
Red sweet pepper, raw	1 medium	152
Guava	1	126
Orange juice	1 cup	124
Strawberries	1 cup	98
Grapefruit	1 medium	88
Orange	1	83
Pineapple	1 cup	79
Kiwi	1	64
Cantaloupe	1 cup	59
Mango	1	59
Broccoli, cooked	½ cup	51
Strawberries	½ cup	49
Brussels sprouts, cooked	½ cup	48
Tomato juice	1 cup	45
Sweet potato, baked	1 large	35
Cauliflower, cooked	½ cup	28
Turnip greens, cooked	½ cup	20
Tomato	1 medium	17
Tomato sauce, canned	1 cup	17
Cabbage, raw	½ cup	16
Potato, baked	1 large	14

Data from U.S. Department of Agriculture, Agricultural Research Service. 2013. *USDA national nutrient database for standard reference, Release 26.* Accessed August 31, 2013. Available at: http://www.ars.usda.gov/nutrientdata

Sources

The RDA can usually be met by choosing one serving daily of foods known as an excellent source of vitamin C (e.g., citrus fruits and juices, cantaloupe, green and red peppers, broccoli, kiwi, strawberries, and mango). Good sources include peaches, cabbage, potatoes, sweet potatoes, and tomatoes; at least two servings of these sources a day may be required to meet the RDA (Table 8-10).

Hyper States and Hypo States

Intakes exceeding the UL of 2000 mg may result in stomach upset and diarrhea, and interfere with vitamin B_{12} absorption.

Healthcare professionals in the United States generally consider vitamin C deficiency, or scurvy, to be a disease of historical significance only. Many Americans exceed the RDAs for vitamin C. However, smokers have an elevated risk of vitamin C deficiency.

Scurvy, caused by vitamin C deficiency, can occur in 20 days. It is characterized by spontaneous gingival hemorrhaging, perifollicular petechiae (Fig. 8-9), follicular hyperkeratosis, diarrhea, fatigue, depression, and cessation of bone growth.

Inadequate amounts of vitamin C during tooth development may cause changes in ameloblasts and odontoblasts, resulting in **scorbutic** changes in the teeth or changes similar to those caused by scurvy. Atrophy of ameloblasts and

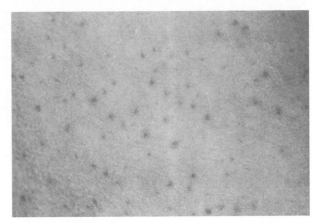

FIGURE 8-9 Perifollicular petechiae. Minimal bleeding into the hair follicles is often one of the earliest clinical manifestations of vitamin C deficiency. (Courtesy of Dr. H.H. Sandstead. From McLaren DS: *A colour atlas and text of diet-related disorders,* ed 2, London, 1992, Mosby–Year Book.)

odontoblasts leads to a decrease in their orderly polar arrangement in a vitamin C–deficient environment. Any new dentin deposits forming at this time are similar to **osteodentin** (dentin that resembles bone); the pulp also atrophies and is hyperemetic. Dentin deposits completely cease in severe vitamin C deficiency, with hypercalcification of predentin. Dentinal tubules also lack their normal parallel arrangement. In scorbutic adults, the dentin reabsorbs and is porotic.

Gingivitis, caused by ascorbic acid deficiency, also affects the periodontium, resulting in tooth mobility. This effect is probably related to weakened collagen secondary to vitamin C deficiency, which results in resorption of the alveolar bone (Fig. 8-10).

Apparently the simple image of antioxidants as valiant warriors protecting the body from rampaging free radicals

Dental Considerations

- Older patients (especially those who live alone or who avoid acidic foods to control gastroesophageal reflux), patients undergoing peritoneal dialysis or hemodialysis, smokers, and drug abusers are at greatest risk to become scorbutic. Assess for deficiency: periodontal disease, deep red to purple gingiva, hyperplasia, bleeding on probing, reported nosebleeds, melena (stools containing blood), vomiting, and petechiae (especially lower legs and back).
- Adequate vitamin C intake can slow the progression of a common cold. There is no clear evidence that amounts above the RDA of vitamin C will reduce the frequency or severity of a cold.
- Vitamin C chewable tablets, syrup, or cough drops are associated with enamel erosion and dentin hypersensitivity.
- Steroids, antibiotics, and salicylates can increase excretion of vitamin C.
- Deficient vitamin C intake (5 mg or less per day) increases the propensity of the gingiva to become inflamed or bleed on probing, but serum levels and gingiva return to normal with an intake of 65 mg per day.[35]
- Evaluate the vitamin C intake because low levels may affect the severity of periodontal disease.[36]

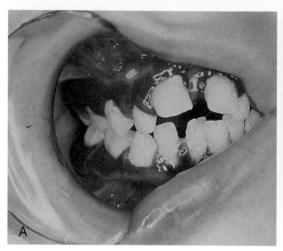
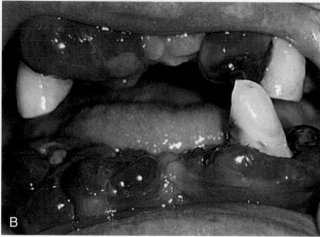

FIGURE 8-10 A, Ascorbic acid deficiency. The gingiva is blue-red and grossly swollen. The earliest changes involve the interdental papillae, which swell and tend to bleed easily. **B,** Effects on the periodontium result in tooth mobility. (From Swartz MH: *Textbook of physical diagnosis: history and examination*, ed 7, St Louis, 2014, Saunders Elsevier.)

Nutritional Directions

- Vitamin C requirements are readily available from small amounts of food. One orange contains 98 mg of vitamin C, which is enough vitamin C for healthy nonsmoking adults.
- Patients who smoke need an additional 35 mg of vitamin C daily; a man who smokes should consume 125 mg instead of 90 mg of vitamin C each day. (Refer patients who smoke to smoking cessation program as discussed in Chapter 19, *Health Application 19*.)
- Deficiency symptoms may develop within 20 to 40 days after dietary elimination of vitamin C.

- Storage is important to prevent oxidation of vitamin C. To retain more vitamin C, fruit juices should be kept in an airtight container that is appropriate for the amount stored. For example, 2 cups of juice in a pint container with an airtight lid protects the vitamin C content better than 1 pint of juice in a gallon container.
- Ascorbic acid is another name for vitamin C.
- Megadoses of vitamin C (2000 mg or greater per day) can interfere with vitamin B_{12} and copper use.

HEALTH APPLICATION 8   Antioxidants

Free radicals are highly unstable and reactive molecular fragments. They contain one or more unpaired electrons, which try to gain electrons to become more stable. During this process, the free radicals oxidize (damage) body cells. UV radiation from the sun, air pollution, ozone, and smoking are just a few conditions that can generate free radicals in the body. Antioxidants donate electrons to the free radicals to make them stable. This protects the body cells from damage. The antioxidant is oxidized and destroyed. In some situations, an antioxidant can regain or regenerate an electron to allow it to function.

Although antioxidants have some properties in common, each one has unique properties. Methods of measuring antioxidants and the effects of each antioxidant are being tested.[37] According to one comparative analysis, the best sources of antioxidants are beans (specifically small red, kidney, pinto, and black beans), fruits (particularly blueberries, cranberries, blackberries, prunes, raspberries, strawberries, apples, cherries, and plums), pecans, and potatoes.[38]

Much has been learned about the functions of vitamins C and E, beta-carotene, and other phytochemicals (biologically active substances found in plants), and the minerals selenium, zinc, copper, and manganese in their roles as antioxidants. Numerous studies have suggested that antioxidants may be important in preventing CHD, cancer, age-related eye disease,

and other chronic conditions associated with aging. Ascorbic acid is one of the strongest antioxidants and radical scavengers, serving as a primary defense against free radicals in the blood. However, the connections between vitamin C and these processes have yet to be established. Research has proven vitamin C and other antioxidants in amounts greater than the RDA are desirable. This is especially true if increased levels are achieved by improving food choices.

Increased serum antioxidant concentrations are associated with a reduced risk of periodontitis. Research studies with antioxidants have indicated conflicting conclusions in regard to reduction of CHD and prevention of cancers. A meta-analysis (systematic method that uses statistical analysis to integrate the data from numerous independent studies) published in the *Journal of the American Medical Association* analyzed research studies involving beta-carotene, selenium, and vitamins A, C, and E supplementation.[39] The consensus was that supplements of beta-carotene, vitamin A, and vitamin E significantly increased mortality by 7%, 16%, and 4%, respectively. Vitamin C and selenium had no significant effect on mortality. A systematic review and meta-analysis found no evidence to support antioxidant supplementation prevents mortality in healthy people or patients with CHD.[40] Neither vitamin E nor vitamin C supplementation reduced the risk of major CHD.[41,42]

is too simplistic. The American Heart Association does not recommend antioxidant supplements, waiting for more convincing data.[42] Because of the lay press publicity surrounding the potential health benefits, many Americans are taking some form of antioxidant supplement to prevent chronic diseases.

High intake levels of some antioxidants are well tolerated by most individuals, but several known factors must be considered before recommending supplements. Toxic effects occur with vitamin A; organ damage and deaths have been reported. Vitamin E supplements can antagonize vitamin K activity and enhance the effect of anticoagulant drugs. Adverse effects of vitamin C include diarrhea, increased risk of kidney stones, and decreased absorption of vitamin B_{12}. Although vitamin C increases iron absorption, large amounts decrease availability of vitamin B_{12} and copper. Erosion and hypersensitivity of tooth enamel are unique adverse effects of chewable vitamin C tablets. Simultaneous intake of carotenoids with α-tocopherol may inhibit the absorption of vitamin E. Possibly unexplored interactions may occur between large amounts of antioxidants and other nutrients. If a patient chooses to take vitamin C supplements, there is no benefit in taking more expensive ones, such as products containing bioflavonoids, over simple ascorbic acid.

Antioxidants may counteract the effects of cell damage produced by metabolic reactions and environmental factors such as pollution, smoking, and toxic chemicals in the diet.

However, the health toll of a smoking habit is not corrected by simply eating right or taking vitamins (see Chapter 19, *Health Application 19*). Recommendations for supplemental amounts of these nutrients should be reserved for claims that have been well substantiated by clinical trials that prove cause and effect and explore related side effects. Patients should also be cautioned about taking megadoses of vitamins and minerals because side effects, nutrient-nutrient interactions, and drug-nutrient interactions can occur. Individuals who are seriously ill with cancer, CHD, or other conditions should talk with their healthcare provider about everything they put into their bodies, including vitamins, supplements, or herbs.

The *Dietary Guidelines* emphasize consumption of a varied diet to help prevent several chronic diseases. Dietary patterns high in fruits and vegetables are associated with a lower risk of disease. Advice to patients should be to eat a healthy diet that includes many fruits and vegetables, especially those that are high in vitamins C and E, and beta-carotene. A pill cannot provide what is available from a healthful diet—so the bottom line is to "eat your fruits and veggies." Antioxidant supplements cannot be expected to undo a lifetime of unhealthy living. Adequate intake ideally should be in the form of improving dietary selections rather than supplements because as-yet unidentified components present in food may be beneficial and protective. Beyond diet, decreased exposure to free radicals and increased physical activity are essential.

Case Application for the Dental Hygienist

A healthy patient asks your advice about taking vitamin C supplements to prevent periodontal disease. She is unsure what foods to eat or what to look for if an excess or deficiency develops.

Nutritional Assessment
- Income
- Living arrangements, cooking and storage facilities
- Dietary assessment
- Tobacco and other drug use
- Knowledge level about vitamin C
- Beliefs about water-soluble vitamins
- Knowledge level about periodontal disease
- Physical status, especially any bleeding problems
- Use of over-the-counter or healthcare provider–prescribed supplements or medications
- Emotional state

Nutritional Diagnosis
Health-seeking behavior related to inadequate/insufficient knowledge about vitamin C and periodontal disease.

Nutritional Goals
The patient will consume foods high in vitamin C and state beliefs/information about vitamin C and periodontal disease.

Nutritional Implementation
Intervention: Teach the following about vitamin C: (a) functions, (b) requirements, and (c) sources. Teach the following about periodontal disease: (a) causes and (b) preventive factors.

Rationale: This provides the patient with a sound knowledge base about vitamin C and periodontal disease.

Intervention: Explain hyper- and hypo-vitamin C states.

Rationale: Large amounts of vitamin C decrease absorption of vitamin B_{12} and cause diarrhea, gastrointestinal distress, and kidney stones. Because vitamin C helps maintain capillary integrity, a vitamin C deficiency results in bleeding problems. Encourage food sources rather than supplements for increasing vitamin C.

Intervention: Provide oral hygiene instruction.

Rationale: The primary cause of periodontal disease is plaque biofilm. Providing education to effectively remove the plaque biofilm is essential. A vitamin deficiency does not cause periodontal disease, but it could exacerbate existing periodontal issues.

Evaluation
The patient should consume citrus fruits, strawberries, cantaloupes, and mangos. Additionally, the patient states that supplements are unnecessary for vitamin C, and large doses may interfere with absorption of other nutrients. She further states that if she does develop any bleeding problems, she will seek help. Lastly, the patient should verbalize information concerning excesses and deficiencies of vitamin C.

STUDENT READINESS

1. How do water-soluble vitamins differ from fat-soluble vitamins? What do these differences mean as you choose foods for your own menu? What do these differences mean as you teach patients about nutrition?

2. Which fat-soluble vitamins are toxic? What are the symptoms of toxicity?

3. A patient asks why so many foods are now fortified with vitamin D. How would you respond?

4. Plan a one-day menu that meets the RDA for vitamin E.

5. Keep a record of your food intake for one day. Use a table of nutrient values of foods (http://www.ars.usda.gov/main/main.htm) or a nutrient analysis program (https://www.supertracker.usda.gov/default.aspx) or Nutritrac (a link on the Evolve website) to determine your vitamin A intake. Was intake adequate? What are some wiser food choices to improve nutrients that were below the RDA?

6. Prepare a menu for one day that provides adequate amounts of vitamins A and D. Eliminate all sources of milk products and canned fish. What does this do to vitamin D intake? Now remove various types of egg products, green leafy vegetables, and dark yellow vegetables, and see the effect on the vitamin A content of the meal plan.

7. Justify the rationale of vitamin D supplementation of milk products in the United States. What age groups benefit most from vitamin D supplementation in milk?

8. What is the role of antioxidants in cancer prevention? What foods are advocated to prevent this condition?

9. Name the deficiency and toxicity conditions associated with vitamins A, D, K, and C.

10. Name five foods other than oranges that are good sources of vitamin C.

11. In a small group, discuss the pros and cons of the controversial issue of mandatory food labeling on nutrition supplements.

References

1. Connolly RM, Nguyen KN, Sukumar S: Molecular pathways: current role and future directions of the retinoic acid pathway in cancer prevention and treatment. *Clin Cancer Res* 19:1651–1659, 2013.

2. Mondul AM, Sampson JN, Moore SC, et al: Metabolomic profile of response to supplementation with ß-carotene in the alpha-tocopherol, beta-carotene cancer prevention study. *Am J Clin Nutr* 98(2):488–493, 2013.

3. American Cancer Society: *Vitamin A and beta-carotene.* Last revision: May 4, 2012. Accessed August 31, 2013 Available at: www.cancer.org/Treatment/TreatmentsandSideEffects/ComplementaryandAlternativeMedicine/HerbsVitaminsandMinerals/vitamin-a-and-beta-carotene.

4. Institute of Medicine (IOM), Food and Nutrition Board: *Dietary reference intakes for vitamin A, vitamin K, arsenic, boron, chromium, copper, iodine, iron, molybdenum, nickel, silicon, vanadium, and zinc,* Washington, DC, 2001, National Academy Press.

5. Mata-Granados JM, Cuenca-Acevedo JR, Luque de Castro MD, et al: Vitamin D insufficiency together with high serum levels of vitamin A increases the risk for osteoporosis in postmenopausal women. *Arch Osteoporos* 8:124, 2013.

6. Wacker M, Holick MF: Vitamin D-effects on skeletal and extraskeletal health and the need for supplementation. *Nutrients* 5:111–148, 2013.

7. Prentice RL, Pettinger MB, Jackson RD, et al: Health risks and benefits from calcium and vitamin D supplementation: Women's Health Initiative clinical trial and cohort study. *Osteoporos Int* 24(2):567–580, 2013.

8. Au LE, Rogers GT, Harris SS, et al: Associations of vitamin D intake with 25-hydroxyvitamin D in overweight and racially/ethnically diverse US children. *J Acad Nutr Diet* http://dx.doi.org/10.1016/j.jand.2013.05.025, [Epub ahead of print], 2013.

9. Dawson-Hughes B, Mithal A, Bonjour JP, et al: IOF position statement: vitamin D recommendations for older adults. *Osteoporos Int* 21:1151–1154, 2010.

10. National Osteoporosis Foundation: *NOF responds to the U.S. Preventive Services Task Force recommendations on calcium and vitamin D.* February 26, 2013. Accessed August 31, 2013. Available at http://www.nof.org/news/903.

11. Heaney RP, Recker RR, Grote J, et al: Vitamin D_3 is more potent than vitamin D_2 in humans. *J Clin Endocrinol Metab* 96(3):E447–E452, 2011.

12. U.S. Preventive Services Task Force: *U.S. Preventive Services Task Force issues final recommendation on vitamin D and calcium supplements to prevent fractures.* Accessed August 31, 2013. Available at: http://www.uspreventiveservicestaskforce.org/bulletins/vitdbulletin.pdf.

13. Perrine CG, Sharma AJ, Jefferds ED, et al: Adherence to vitamin D recommendations among US infants. *Pediatrics* 125(4):627–632, 2010.

14. Narayanan DL, Saladi RN, Fox, JL: Ultraviolet radiation and skin cancer. *Int J Dermatol* 49:978–986, 2010.

15. Wagner D, Sidhom G, Whiting SJ, et al: The bioavailability of vitamin D from fortified cheese and supplements is equivalent in adults. *J Nutr* 138:1365–1371, 2008.

16. Harvard Women's Health Watch: *The sunshine D-lemma.* (serial online). Accessed August 31, 2013. Available at: http://www.health.harvard.edu/press_releases/vitamin-d-has-the-potential-to-ward-off-a-number-of-serious-diseases.htm.

17. Institute of Medicine (IOM), Food and Nutrition Board: *Dietary Reference Intakes: calcium and vitamin D,* Washington, DC, 2011, National Academy Press.

18. Gallagher JC: Vitamin D and aging. *Endocrinol Metab Cl N Am* 42(2):319–332, 2013.

19. Office of Dietary Supplements, National Institutes of Health: *Dietary supplement fact sheet: Vitamin D.* Accessed August 31, 2013. Available at: http://ods.od.nih.gov/factsheets/VitaminD-HealthProfessional/.

20. Paxton GA, Teale GR, Nowson CA, et al: Vitamin D and health in pregnancy, infants, children and adolescents in Australia and New Zealand: a position statement. *Med J Aust* 198(3):1–8, 2013.

21. Wall CR, Grant CC, Jones I: Vitamin D status of exclusively breastfed infants aged 2-3 months. *Arch Dis Child* 98:176–179, 2013.

22. Purvis RJ, Barrie WJ, MacKay GS, et al: Enamel hypoplasia of the teeth associated with neonatal tetany: A manifestation of maternal vitamin D deficiency. *Lancet* 2:811–814, 1973.

23. Hujoel PP: Vitamin D and dental caries in controlled clinical trials: systematic review and meta-analysis. *Nut Rev* 71(2):88–97, 2013.

24. Grant WB: A review of the role of solar ultraviolet-B irradiance and vitamin D in reducing risk of dental caries. *Dermatoendocrinol* 3:193–198, 2011.

25. Garcia N, Miley D, Dixon DA: Vitamin D and periodontal disease. *Handbook of vitamin D in human health* 4:242–253, 2013.

26. Jimenez M, Giovannucci E, Kaye EK, et al: Predicted vitamin D status and incidence of tooth loss and periodontitis. *Public Health Nutr* 7:1–9 (Epub ahead of print. Accessed Sepember 2, 2013. Available: CJO2013. doi:10.1017/S1368980013000177, 2013.

27. Bashutski JD, Eber RM, Kinney JS, et al: The impact of vitamin D status on periodontal surgery outcomes. *J Dent Res* 90(8): 1007–1012, 2011.

28. Anderson LN, Cotterchio M, Vieth R, et al: Vitamin D and calcium intakes and breast cancer risk in pre- and postmenopausal women. *Am J Clin Nutr* 91:1699–1707, 2010.

29. Jenab M, Bueno-de-Mesquita HB, Ferrari P, et al: Association between pre-diagnostic circulating vitamin D concentration and risk of colorectal cancer in European populations: a nested case-control study. *BMJ* 340:b5500, 2010.

30. Lutsey PI, Michos ED: Vitamin D, calcium, and atherosclerotic risk: evidence from serum levels and supplementation studies. *Curr Atheroscler Rep* 15:293, 2013.

31. Russnes KM, Wilson KM, Epstein MM, et al: Total antioxidant intake in relation to prostate cancer incidence in the health professionals follow up study. *Int J Cancer* 201.; Accessed September 2, 2013. Available on doi:10.1002/ijc.28438.

32. Borel P, Preveraud D, Desmarchelier C: Bioavailability of vitamin E in humans: an update. *Nutr Rev* 71(6):319–331, 2013.

33. Lukacs J: Differential associations for menopause and age in measures of vitamin K, osteocalcin and bone density: a cross sectional exploratory study in healthy volunteers. *Menopause* 13(5):799–808, 2006.

34. Cheung AM, Tile L, Lee Y, et al: Vitamin K supplementation in postmenopausal women with osteopenia (ECKO Trial): a randomized controlled trial. *PLoS Med* 5(10):e196, 2008.

35. Jacob RA, Omaye ST, Skala JH, et al: Experimental vitamin C depletion and supplementation in young men: nutrient interactions and dental health effects. *Ann N Y Acad Sci* 498: 333 346, 1987.

36. Amaliya, Timmerman MF, Abbas F, et al: Java project on periodontal diseases: the relationship between vitamin C and the severity of periodontitis. *J Clin Periodontol* 34(4):299–304, 2007.

37. D'Aiuto F, Nibali L, Parkar M, et al: Oxidative stress, systemic inflammation, and severe periodontitis. *J Dent Res* 89(11):1241–1246, 2010.

38. Milan C, ČíŽová H, Denev P, et al: Different methods for control and comparison of the antioxidant properties of vegetables. *Food Control* 21:518–523, 2010.

39. Bjelakovic G, Nikolova D, Gluud LL, et al: Mortality in randomized trials of antioxidant supplements for primary and secondary prevention: systematic review and meta-analysis. *JAMA* 297(8):842–857, 2007.

40. Myung SK, Woong J, Cho B, et al: Efficacy of vitamin and antioxidant supplements in prevention of cardiovascular disease: systematic review and meta-analysis of randomized controlled trials. *Br Med J* 346:f10, 2013.

41. Sesso HD, Buring JE, Christen WG, et al: Vitamins E and C in the prevention of cardiovascular disease in men. *JAMA* 300(18): 2123–2133, 2008.

42. American Heart Association Scientific Position: *Vitamin and mineral supplements.* Accessed September 1, 2013. Available at: http://www.heart.org/HEARTORG/GettingHealthy/Nutrition Center/Vitamin-and-Mineral-Supplements_UCM_306033 _Article.jsp.

ⓔ EVOLVE RESOURCES

Please visit http://evolve.elsevier.com/Stegeman/nutritional for additional practice and study support tools.

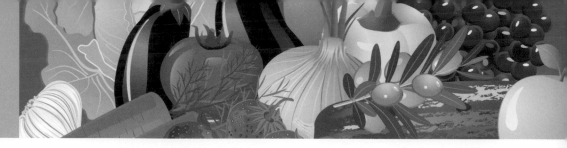

Chapter 9

Minerals Essential for Calcified Structures

Student Learning Outcomes

Upon completion of this chapter, the student will be able to achieve the following objectives:

- List the minerals found in collagen, bones, and teeth, and describe their main physiological roles and sources.
- Describe causes and symptoms of mineral excesses or deficits.
- Discuss the role of water fluoridation in the prevention of dental caries.

- Describe advantages and disadvantages of mineral supplementation.
- Individualize dental hygiene considerations to patients regarding calcium, phosphorus, magnesium, and fluoride.
- Utilize nutritional directions to provide patient education regarding calcium, phosphorus, magnesium, and fluoride.

Key Terms

Amorphous
Apatite
Bioavailability
Compressional forces
Fluorapatite
Fluorosis
Hydroxyapatite
Hypercalcemia
Hypercalciuria
Hypocalcemia

Mineralization
Osteoclasts
Osteoids
Osteoporosis
Periodontal disease
Phytochemicals
Remodeling
Rickets
Tensional forces
Tetany

Test Your NQ

1. **T/F** Meats are good sources of phosphorus.
2. **T/F** The only nutrients essential for strong healthy bones are calcium and phosphorus.
3. **T/F** Tooth exfoliation may be an oral sign of osteoporosis.
4. **T/F** Systemic fluoride causes changes in tooth morphology that increase caries resistance.
5. **T/F** To obtain adequate calcium, a teenager needs to drink 2 cups of milk a day.

6. **T/F** Water fluoridation is economically inefficient because very little of the water is actually consumed.
7. **T/F** All women should take calcium supplements to prevent osteoporosis.
8. **T/F** Calcium absorption is increased when a sugar is present.
9. **T/F** Caffeine intake may decrease calcium loss.
10. **T/F** All bottled waters contain fluoride.

BONE MINERALIZATION AND GROWTH

Calcified structures in the body, which include bones and teeth, are composed of a matrix of organic and inorganic substances. Dentin, cementum, and bone originate with a protein matrix, or collagen deposition. Collagen is present throughout the periodontium as the primary connective tissue fiber in the gingiva and major organic constituent of alveolar bone. Collagen is continuously being remodeled (resorption and reformation of bone) throughout growth and development. Defective collagen synthesis affects formation of bones and teeth.

The organic matrix of bone is 90% to 95% collagen fibers, which are secreted by osteoblasts. Collagen formation requires the presence of a variety of substances, including protein; vitamin C; and the minerals iron, copper, and zinc. When collagen is formed, apatite, a calcium phosphate complex, automatically crystallizes adjacent to the collagen fibers.

In bones that have not undergone calcification, osteoids are formed rapidly. Most develop into the finished product, hydroxyapatite crystals (inorganic component of bones and teeth).

Immediately after collagen formation, mineralization begins. Mineralization is the deposition of inorganic elements (minerals) on an organic matrix (mainly composed of protein in combination with some polysaccharides and lipids). In addition to calcium and phosphorus, numerous other minerals, especially magnesium, sodium, potassium, and carbonate ions, are incorporated into the mineral matrix.

Adequate nutritional components are necessary during collagen formation and mineral deposition phases to prevent structural imperfections. The crystalline mineral matrix provides great compressional strength similar to marble. The combination of collagen and crystalline mineral matrix forms a material resembling reinforced concrete.

The skeleton is constantly growing, changing, and remodeling itself. Approximately 0.4% to 10% of total bone calcium remains in a shapeless or amorphous form. This calcium is a reserve source that can be rapidly used when serum calcium levels decrease. Osteoblasts deposit fresh calcium salts where new stresses have developed, and where osteoclasts (connected with absorption of bone) are removing calcium deposits. Bone absorption by osteoclasts is controlled by parathyroid hormone (PTH). The rate of osteoblast and osteoclast activity is normally in equilibrium, except during periods of growth. In older adults, bone resorption may exceed mineralization, causing osteoporosis.

This dynamic state accommodates changing demands of the body. Bone strength is adjusted in proportion to the degree of stress on the bone. Continual physical stress stimulates calcification and osteoblastic deposition of bone.

FORMATION OF TEETH

Teeth are composed of three calcified tissues: enamel, dentin, and cementum. Enamel and dentin are principally composed of hydroxyapatite crystals similar to those in bone. Approximately 20% of dentin, cementum, and bone is organic material, principally collagen; only 1% of the enamel is organic material. Dentin lacks the osteoblasts and osteoclasts found in bone; enamel and dentin do not contain blood vessels or nerves. As with bone, the mineral crystallization structure makes teeth extremely resistant to compressional forces; collagen fibers make teeth tough and resistant to tensional forces. Actions in which pressure attempts to diminish a structure's volume are referred to as compressional forces; tensional forces are actions in which pressure stretches or strains the structure.

After a tooth erupts, no more enamel is formed, but mineral exchanges occur slowly in response to the oral environment. Changes in mineral composition of enamel occur by exchange of minerals in saliva, rather than from the pulp cavity. Minerals, such as fluoride, sodium, zinc, and strontium, can replace calcium ions. Carbonate can be substituted for phosphate; carbonate and fluoride can be substituted for hydroxyl ions. These changes may alter the solubility of apatite. Despite the changes that occur in enamel composition, enamel maintains most of its original mineral components throughout life.

The crystalline structure of enamel is one of the most insoluble and resistant proteins known. This special protein matrix, in combination with a crystalline structure of inorganic salts, makes enamel harder than dentin. It is comparable in hardness to quartz. Enamel is more resistant to acids, enzymes, and other corrosive agents than dentin.

Dentin, the main tissue of teeth, contains the same constituents as bone, but its structure is more dense. Its principal component is hydroxyapatite crystals embedded in a strong meshwork of collagen fibers. Odontoblasts line the inner surface of dentin and provide nourishment for the dentin.

Cementum, which covers the dentin in the root area, is another bonelike substance, but because it contains fewer minerals, it is softer than bone. It contains many collagen fibers originating in the alveolar bone. Compressional forces cause the cementum to become thicker and stronger. Cementum exhibits characteristics more typical of bone than enamel and dentin. Minerals are absorbed and deposited at rates similar to that of alveolar bone.

Development of normal, healthy teeth is affected by metabolic factors, such as PTH secretion, and the availability of calcium, phosphate, vitamin D, protein, and many other nutrients. If these factors are deficient, calcification of teeth may be defective and abnormal throughout life.

INTRODUCTION TO MINERALS

Minerals are inorganic elements with many physiological functions. Numerous inorganic elements in the body account for only about 4% of total body weight, or 6 lb for a 150-lb person. Minerals are subdivided into those required in larger amounts (major minerals) and those required in smaller amounts (micronutrients, also called trace elements)

Major Minerals (greater than 100 mg/day)
Calcium (Ca)*
Phosphorus (P)*
Sodium (Na)
Potassium (K)
Magnesium (Mg)*
Chlorine (Cl)
Sulfur (S)

Trace Elements (less than 100 mg/day)
Iron (Fe)*
Copper (Cu)*
Zinc (Zn)*
Manganese (Mn)*
Iodine (I)*
Molybdenum (Mo)*
Fluorine (F)*
Selenium (Se)*
Chromium (Cr)
Cobalt (Co)

Ultratrace Elements (No Recommended Dietary Allowances)
Boron (B)*
Arsenic (As)
Nickel (Ni)*
Silicon (Si)
Tin (Sn)
Vanadium (V)*
Cadmium (Cd)
Lead (Pb)
Bromide (Br)
Lithium (Li)
Aluminum (Al)

Data from Institute of Medicine, Food and Nutrition Board: *Dietary reference intakes for calcium and vitamin D*, Washington, DC, 2011, National Academy Press; Institute of Medicine, Food and Nutrition Board: *Dietary reference intakes for water, potassium, sodium, chloride, and sulfate*, Washington, DC, 2005, National Academy Press; Institute of Medicine, Food and Nutrition Board: *Dietary reference intakes for calcium, phosphorus, magnesium, vitamin D, and fluoride*, Washington, DC, 1997, National Academy Press; Institute of Medicine, Food and Nutrition Board: *Dietary reference intakes for vitamin A, vitamin K, arsenic, boron, chromium, copper, iodine, iron, manganese, molybdenum, nickel, silicon, vanadium, and zinc*. Washington, DC, 2001, National Academy Press.
*Tolerable upper intake levels have been established.

(Box 9-1). Despite the smaller amounts required, trace elements are just as important as major minerals.

CALCIUM
Physiological Roles

At least 99% of the body's calcium is found in the skeleton and teeth. Calcium is indispensable for skeletal function, which requires adequate dietary calcium to achieve full accretion of bone mass prescribed by genetic potential. Calcium (and phosphorus) in the bone, but not in the enamel of teeth, functions as a "savings account" for maintaining serum calcium levels. Only 1% of the body's calcium is found in blood, but as such, it controls body functions such as blood clotting, transmission of nerve impulses, muscle contraction and relaxation, membrane permeability, and activation of certain enzymes. Research indicates that calcium intake is important not only for bone health, but also for reducing the risk of many other disorders, from hypertension to obesity to colon cancer.

Saliva is supersaturated with calcium; saliva is a source of calcium to mineralize an immature or demineralized enamel surface and reduce susceptibility to caries. Calcium and phosphate in saliva provide a buffering action to inhibit caries formation. This buffer prevents dissolution of minerals in the enamel by plaque biofilm.

Requirements

The IOM has established an RDA and an estimated average requirement for calcium. The RDA is 1000 mg per day for ages 19 to 50 years. During growth periods, primarily from 9 to 18 years of age, the requirement is higher because peak bone mass appears to be related to calcium intake during periods of bone mineralization (Table 9-1). Approximately 85% to 90% of adult bone mass is acquired by age 18 years in girls and age 20 years in boys.[1] Typically, calcium intake of teens between ages 13 to 19 years falls below the RDA for calcium. On the other hand, adequate intake of calcium is observed in those ages 20 to 59 years.[2] Women may continue to increase bone growth and density through their 20s, but never achieve the bone mass levels observed in most men. From age 30 years until menopause, women tend to maintain bone mass; however, bone mass loss accelerates after menopause. The IOM recommends dietary intake of 1200 mg/day for females over 50 years of age.

Women are less likely than men to exceed their RDA. The estimated mean calcium intake for women over age 60 years during the 2009-2010 *National Health and Nutrition Examination Survey* (NHANES) was 842 mg per day compared with 966 mg/day for men in the same age category. Fortunately, when women in this age group include a calcium supplement, intake is boosted to 1266 mg/day, within their target range and surpassing the males' intake of 1153 mg/day.[2]

Americans usually consume less than two servings of dairy products per day.[3] Inadequate calcium intake can be attributed to (a) uninformed choices, or not selecting adequate sources of calcium on a daily basis; (b) the mistaken beliefs that adults do not need milk, or that milk contributes too many kilocalories to the diet; (c) economic hardships, plus a lack of knowledge regarding inexpensive sources of calcium-rich foods; (d) lactose intolerance or allergies to dairy products; (e) access to and consumption of soda; and (f) dislike of calcium-rich foods.

Generally, inadequate calcium intake affects bone mass more than tooth structure. Inadequate calcium and vitamin D intake during tooth formation and maturation may result in hypomineralization of developing teeth. After tooth formation, dietary calcium does not affect caries rate.

Table 9-1	Adequate intake for calcium			
Life Stage Group	**EAR* (mg/day)**	**RDA† (mg/day)**	**AI‡ (mg/day)**	**UL§ (g/day)**
Infants (birth–6 months)			200	1.0
Infants (6-12 months)			260	1.5
Children (1-3 years)	500	700		2.5
Children (4-8 years)	800	1000		2.5
Adolescents (9-13 years)	1100	1300		3.0
Adolescents (14-18 years)	1100	1300		3.0
Adults (19-30 years)	800	1000		2.5
Adults (31-50 years)	800	1000		2.5
Adults (51-70 years)				
Males	800	1000		2.0
Females	1000	1200		2.0
>70 years	1000	1200		2.0
Pregnancy and lactation	Same as for their age group			

Data from Institute of Medicine, Food and Nutrition Board: *Dietary reference intakes for calcium and vitamin D*, Washington, DC, 2011, National Academy Press.
*EAR (estimated average requirement)—the intake that meets the estimated nutrient needs of half of the individuals in a group.
†RDA (recommended dietary allowance)—the intake that meets the nutrient needs of almost all (97% to 98%) individuals in a group.
‡AI (adequate intake)—the observed average or experimentally set intake by a defined population or subgroup that seems to sustain a defined nutritional status, such as growth rate, normal circulating nutrient values, or other functional indicators of health. An AI is used if insufficient scientific evidence is available to derive an EAR. For healthy human milk–fed infants, the AI is the mean intake. The AI is not equivalent to an RDA.
§Tolerable upper intake level (UL)—the highest level of daily nutrient intake that is likely to pose no risk of adverse health effects to almost all individuals in the general population. As intake increases above the UL, the risk of adverse effects increases. Unless specified otherwise, the UL represents total nutrient intake from food, water, and supplements.

Calcium Balance

Despite wide variations in calcium intake, serum calcium is relatively constant because each cell has a vital need for calcium. If the serum calcium level declines, bones are used as calcium reserves. When calcium withdrawal from bones exceeds deposits, calcium imbalance occurs. Decreased bone density caused by insufficient calcium is a slow process.

Calcium-to-Phosphorus Ratio

Serum levels of calcium and phosphorus are inversely related; this relationship is called the serum calcium-to-phosphorus ratio. If the calcium level increases, phosphorus levels decrease, and vice versa. This relationship acts as a protective mechanism to prevent high combined concentrations, which can lead to calcification of soft tissue and stone formation.

Sufficient phosphorus intake is necessary to decrease calcium loss. The ideal dietary calcium-to-phosphorus ratio for adults of 1:1 is required for mineralization of bone. Excessive intake of phosphorus compared with calcium reduces serum calcium concentration.

Stimulation of PTH results in the possible loss of bone mass. This ratio does not warrant as close attention under normal conditions as in disorders such as renal disease, when dangerously high levels of phosphorus and calcium may cause calcification in soft tissues.

Numerous studies have investigated the relationship of calcium-to-phosphorus ratios and alveolar bone resorption of edentulous patients. Calcium requirements are increased when dietary phosphate is high, which is typical of the American diet; a relationship may exist between calcium intake and edentulous ridge resorption.

Absorption and Excretion

Calcium balance, achieved when intake equals excretion, does not solely depend on adequate calcium intake. Several hormones, including PTH, estrogen, glucocorticoids, and thyroid hormone, help to regulate calcium absorption. Under normal conditions, less than one-third of the calcium consumed is absorbed. Maximum calcium absorption occurs when it is consumed in small amounts and ingested several times throughout the day. In other words, individuals should consume 30% of the daily value or 300 mg/serving three or four times a day.

Absorption occurs in the small intestine and is affected by many factors, as shown in Figure 9-1. Calcium absorption from various dairy products is similar, whereas calcium present in many dark green leafy vegetables is not readily absorbed. During periods of increased need, especially during growth, pregnancy, and lactation, calcium absorption increases. Calcium absorption decreases with age, probably because of decreased gastric acidity. The rate of absorption is lowest in postmenopausal women because of diminished estrogen levels.

Although several plant foods contain large amounts of calcium, absorption is poor. Oxalates (oxalic acid) in vegetables and phytates (phytic acid) from wheat bran bind with calcium in these foods to reduce absorption, but they do not interfere with calcium absorption from other foods. Dark leafy green vegetables (e.g., kale, turnip greens) contain minimal amounts of oxalic acid, and calcium from these vegetables is readily absorbed. Excessive dietary fiber (more than 35 g/day) also interferes with calcium absorption.

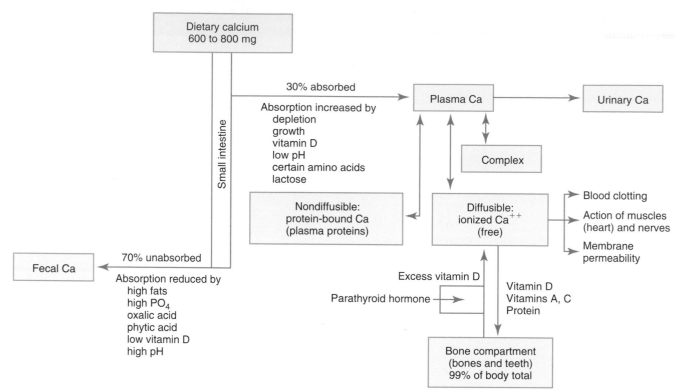

FIGURE 9-1 Calcium absorption and use. (Adapted from Schlenker ED, Roth SL: *Williams' essentials of nutrition and diet therapy*, ed 10, St Louis, 2011, Elsevier.)

High-protein intakes, typical in the United States, have a high phosphorus content. Phosphorus increases uptake of calcium by bone. The usual intake of protein and phosphorus does not cause calcium loss when intake is adequate, whereas a diet low in protein and phosphorus may have adverse effects on calcium balance with inadequate calcium intake. Generally, weight loss causes bone mineral loss. Higher protein diets have been criticized for potential harmful effects on bone because they increase urinary calcium.

PTH works concurrently with vitamin D to prevent calcium from being excreted and stimulates calcium release from bone when serum levels of calcium are low. Increasing synthesis of vitamin D by PTH also results in increased calcium absorption.

Sources

Milk and other dairy products supply the greatest amount of available calcium (Table 9-2). Not only are they preferred sources of calcium because of their high calcium content, but lactose and other nutrients in dairy products enhance calcium absorption. Milk also provides other essential nutrients. Box 9-2 lists portion sizes for various foods that provide approximately 300 mg of calcium.

Since 1999, food manufacturers have been fortifying products such as fruit juices, fruit-flavored drinks, breakfast cereals, and breads with calcium. Numerous calcium-fortified foods introduced to the market have been well received. Food products containing natural or fortified calcium must use certain terminology on packaging, shown in Table 9-3.

> **BOX 9-2   Calcium Equivalents**
>
> The following foods contain approximately 300 mg of calcium:*
> 1 cup milk
> 1 cup soymilk, calcium fortified
> 1½ oz cheddar cheese
> 1½ oz mozzarella cheese
> 1½ slices swiss cheese
> 1 cup yogurt
> 1 slice processed cheese
> 2 cups ice cream
> 1 cup orange juice, calcium fortified
> 1½ cup dark green leafy vegetables†
> 1¼ cup soybeans, cooked
> 1 can (3.75 oz) sardines
> 1 serving cheese pizza

Data from U.S. Department of Agriculture, Agricultural Research Service. 2012. *USDA national nutrient database for standard reference, release 25.* Nutrient Data Laboratory Home Page, Accessed August 20, 2012: http://www.ars.usda.gov/ba/bhnrc/ndl
*The RDA for calcium is 1000 mg for individuals 19 to 50 years old.
†Calcium from vegetable sources is not easily absorbed by the intestine and is not as effective in fulfilling calcium requirements.

Approximately 43% of the U.S. population purchase supplements containing calcium.[4] The U.S. Preventive Services Task Force found inconclusive evidence to support the use of a calcium supplement.[5] Further, excessive calcium intake may increase the risk of CVD.[6,7] Calcium supplements combined with vitamin D may result in small but

Table 9-2	Calcium and phosphorus content of selected foods		
Food	Portion	Calcium (mg)	Phosphorus (mg)
Romano cheese	3 oz	905	646
Swiss cheese	3 oz	673	482
Cheddar cheese	3 oz	613	435
Orange juice, calcium fortified	1 cup	500	117
Yogurt, nonfat plain	1 cup	488	385
Milk (1%, skim)	1 cup	299	247
Soy milk, calcium fortified	1 cup	299	104
American cheese	3 oz	296	182
Buttermilk, low-fat	1 cup	284	218
Salmon, canned	3 oz	212	301
Oats, instant, fortified	1 cup	187	180
Cottage cheese, low-fat (1%)	1 cup	138	303
Spinach, cooked	½ cup	122	50
Fruit-flavored drink, fortified	1 cup	101	0
Turnip greens, cooked	½ cup	99	21
Shrimp, cooked	3 oz	77	260
White beans, cooked	½ cup	65	151
Okra, cooked	½ cup	62	26
Kale, cooked	½ cup	47	18
Broccoli, cooked	½ cup	31	52
Parsnips, cooked	½ cup	29	54
Rutabaga, cooked, mashed	½ cup	22	49
Mixed nuts	1 oz	20	123
Bologna	3 oz	19	56
Ground beef (85% lean)	3 oz	15	168
Cola	12 oz	7	37

Data from U.S. Department of Agriculture, Agricultural Research Service. 2012. *USDA national nutrient database for standard reference, release 26.* Nutrient Data Laboratory Home Page. Accessed August 20, 2013: http://www.ars.usda.gov/ba/bhnrc/ndl

Table 9-3	Food labeling for calcium
Daily Value (DV) of Calcium in a Food	FDA-Authorized Labeling Terms
10% DV of calcium	Calcium enriched Calcium fortified More calcium
10% to 19% DV of calcium	Contains calcium Provides calcium Good source of calcium
≥20% DV of calcium	High in calcium Rich in calcium Excellent source of calcium

significant reductions in bone loss and are effective in reducing falls and fractures.[8] This strong trend toward the use of calcium supplements is especially evident among older adults. Benefits may be less than expected, partly because of limited bioavailability of supplemental calcium. Bioavailability refers to the amount of a nutrient available physiologically and is based on its absorption rate.

A calcium supplement contains elemental calcium along with other substances, such as carbonate or citrate. The amount of elemental calcium varies among supplements.

For example, calcium carbonate is 40% calcium by weight, whereas calcium citrate is 21% calcium. Some calcium supplements are better absorbed when taken with food, absorption being dependent on the availability of gastric acids. Others may be better absorbed when taken on an empty stomach. Calcium-citrate-malate, calcium lactate, calcium gluconate, and calcium sulfate are other forms of calcium in supplements or fortified foods.

Hyper States and Hypo States

Clinical conditions are associated with excesses and deficiencies of calcium. Hypercalcemia (too much calcium) and hypocalcemia (too little calcium) are critical metabolic conditions that can lead to loss of consciousness, fatal respiratory failure, or cardiac arrest. These problems are seldom caused directly by calcium intake; however, loss of bone density can be related to intake.

Hypercalcemia

Hypercalcemia, or excessive levels of calcium in the blood, is rarely the result of dietary intake. Hypercalcemia can result in renal insufficiency, kidney stones or hypercalciuria (high levels of calcium in the urine). Idiopathic hypercalcemia is observed occasionally in infants 5 to 8 months old, sometimes with genetic causes. Overdoses of cholecalciferol or excessive amounts of vitamin D preparations can also cause hypercalcemia. Treatment involves providing a low-calcium diet with no vitamin D. Hyperparathyroidism, certain types of bone disease, vitamin D poisoning, sarcoidosis, cancer, and prolonged excessive intake of milk may cause adult hypercalcemia.

Hypocalcemia

Hypocalcemia, or deficient levels of serum calcium, results in tetany, a neuromuscular disorder of uncontrollable cramps and tremors involving the muscles of the face, hands, feet, and eventually the heart. Depressed serum calcium levels may be caused by hypoparathyroidism, some bone diseases, certain kidney diseases, and low serum protein levels.

Excessive Calcium Intake

Excessively high calcium intake may cause dizziness, flushing, nausea or vomiting, constipation, kidney stone formation, irregular heartbeat, tingling sensations, xerostomia, fatigue, and high blood pressure. It also may inhibit iron and zinc absorption.

Inadequate Calcium Intake

Rickets, discussed in Chapter 8 in connection with vitamin D deficiency, results in porous, soft bones. Rickets develops during childhood as a result of inadequate amounts of calcium being deposited in the bone. Calcium intake may be adequate, but absorption is poor because of inadequate vitamin D.

Osteoporosis is an age-related disorder characterized by decreased bone mass, causing bones to be more susceptible to fracture. Numerous factors, including decreased estrogen, inadequate calcium or vitamin D intake, and lack of weight-bearing activity are implicated. The relationship of calcium intake to bone density indicates a protective effect

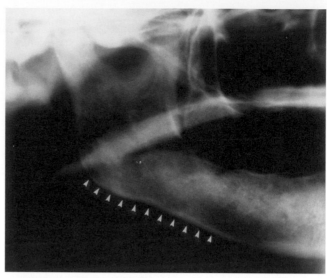

FIGURE 9-2 Radiographic appearance of osteoporosis affecting bone of the maxillofacial complex. This portion of a panoramic radiograph depicts thinning of the gonial and interior cortices of an edentulous mandible (*arrows*). A slight increase in the general size of marrow spaces is also apparent. (Courtesy of B.W. Benson, DDS, MS, Associate Professor, Department of Diagnostic Sciences, The Texas A&M University System, Baylor College of Dentistry, Dallas, TX.)

in women reporting high lifetime calcium intake, but not in women who increased intake after menopause. Building bone during the formative years is the best insurance against osteoporosis.

An oral sign of osteoporosis is loss of calcium in the alveolar bone, contributing to tooth exfoliation (Fig. 9-2). The condition usually goes undetected, however, until pain or spontaneous fracture occurs. Osteoporosis is discussed further in *Health Application 9*. Periodontal disease, or the breakdown of healthy periodontal tissue, can be exacerbated by calcium deficiency.[9]

Dental Considerations

- Physical inactivity results in bone depletion. In young individuals, recovery of calcium deposits is usually rapid, but older adults may never regain bone density.
- Consumption of calcium in the amounts recommended in the Dietary Reference Intakes (DRIs) is appropriate for fracture healing and should not exceed the tolerable upper intake level (UL).
- Patients with achlorhydria (the absence of hydrochloric acid in the stomach) may not absorb calcium supplements on an empty stomach and should take them with meals.
- Hyperparathyroidism induces bone disease. Alveolar bone is especially at risk, exhibiting extensive bone resorption.
- Patients who have had bariatric surgery for obesity are at risk of decreased bone mineral density.[10]
- Interventions for limiting or preventing further bone loss include encouraging exercise and foods rich in vitamin D and calcium.
- Patients who use excessive alcohol or caffeine, or smoke cigarettes, are at risk of calcium loss.

- Suggest alternatives for increasing calcium intake for patients with lactose intolerance (see Chapter 2, *Health Application 2*).
- Calcium supplements may interact with certain medications, including glucocorticoids, cellulose sodium phosphate (Calcibind), etidronate (Didronel), phenytoin (Dilantin), bisphosphonates, and tetracycline. Supplements should be taken 1 to 3 hours before or after the medication.
- Aluminum and magnesium-containing antacids and corticosteroids increase urinary excretion of calcium.
- Mineral oil and some laxatives can decrease calcium absorption.
- Poor patient compliance may be expected if several tablets are necessary, the supplement is too expensive, or gastrointestinal problems (e.g., gas, bloating, diarrhea) occur. More than 500 mg of calcium per tablet may cause constipation.

Nutritional Directions

- Adequate daily calcium, phosphorus, and vitamin D intake is important to support bone formation and maintenance. Consume the level recommended for each.
- Calcium supplement absorption can be enhanced by taking it with some form of sugar; lactose, dextrose, and sucrose enhance its absorption.
- Evaluate calcium supplements for their solubility, which affects absorption. For calcium to be absorbed from a supplement, the tablet must first dissolve. To measure how well a calcium tablet dissolves in the body, drop a tablet in a solution of $4\frac{1}{2}$ oz water and $1\frac{1}{2}$ oz vinegar to produce an environment similar to that of the stomach. Stir occasionally. At least two-thirds of a high-quality tablet dissolves within 30 minutes.
- Compare the amount of elemental calcium provided (actual amount of calcium in the supplement) and cost per tablet. Refer patients who are appropriate candidates for calcium supplementation to a healthcare provider or RDN.
- Decreased calcium intake in women results in lower levels of estrogen production, which can be harmful to the bones. Estrogen enhances calcium absorption and enables more efficient use of calcium.
- Moderate alcohol intake enhances bone density mass as a result of less bone remodeling, but excessive amounts increase the risk of bone loss later in life.

- Weight-bearing exercise has a positive effect on calcium deposition in bone during childhood and adolescence. Weight-bearing exercise and resistance training prevent, and in some cases reverse, bone loss in adults.
- When daily calcium intake appears to be low, encourage increased consumption of dairy products. If the patient has an aversion to milk, powdered milk can be added to many items, or other high-calcium foods can be used.
- Green leafy sources of calcium that are low in oxalic acid include kale, turnip greens, rutabaga, and okra. Oxalates inhibit the absorption of calcium. This is particularly helpful information for vegans or those not consuming dairy products.
- Do not take calcium supplements within 1 to 2 hours of eating large amounts of fiber, especially foods containing large amounts of phytates and oxalates.
- After menopause, calcium and vitamin D supplements slow bone loss and reduce fractures when coupled with an approved osteoporosis-related therapy, such as estrogen replacement therapy or a bisphosphonate or both. If an adverse reaction to the osteoporosis medication is reported, encourage the patient to check with the healthcare provider before discontinuing it.

PHOSPHORUS

Physiological Roles

Phosphorus is the second most abundant mineral in the body, with approximately 85% in the skeleton and teeth. Its presence in all body cells is necessary for almost every aspect of metabolism, including (a) transfer and release of energy stored as adenosine triphosphate; (b) composition of phospholipids, DNA, and RNA; and (c) metabolism of fats, carbohydrates, and proteins. Phosphorus also helps regulate the acid–base balance in the body.

Requirements

The RDA of phosphorus for adults older than 18 years of age is 700 mg. The ideal calcium-to-phosphorus ratio is 1:1. Because phosphorus is more readily available than calcium in the U.S. food supply, intake is generally 1.5 times higher than calcium. Although harmful effects from excessive amounts of phosphorus have not been reported, the IOM established a tolerable upper intake level to reflect normal serum levels (Table 9-4).

Absorption and Excretion

Approximately 60% to 70% of dietary phosphorus is absorbed in the jejunum. Its absorption can be inhibited by the same dietary factors affecting calcium absorption: phytate, excessive fat, iron, aluminum, and calcium intake. The kidneys excrete excessive amounts of phosphorus to maintain optimal body levels.

Sources

Phosphorus is abundant in foods, which is the reason deficiencies have not been observed. A diet adequate in calcium and protein contains enough phosphorus because all three minerals are present in the same foods (see Table 9-2). In addition to milk products, meats are a good source of phosphorus. Dietary restriction of phosphorus is extremely difficult because of its wide use as a food additive in baked goods, cheese, processed meats, and soft drinks. The daily reference values on a Nutrition Facts label are 1000 mg and can be multiplied by the daily value to determine the phosphorus content.

Hyper States and Hypo States

Both excesses and inadequacies of phosphorus can lead to medical complications, including impaired bone health. Hyperphosphatemia (serum level greater than 2.6 mg/dL) may occur in cases of hypoparathyroidism or renal insufficiency. Excessive amounts of phosphorus bind with calcium, resulting in tetany and convulsions.

Hypophosphatemia may occur with long-term ingestion of aluminum hydroxide antacids, which bind phosphorus, interfering with absorption, or it may occur in certain stress conditions in which the calcium-to-phosphorus balance is disturbed. Intestinal conditions, such as sprue and celiac disease, can result in phosphorus malabsorption and thus deficiencies. The principal clinical symptom of hypophosphatemia is muscle weakness. Even small phosphorus

Table 9-4	Institute of Medicine recommendations for phosphorus			
Life Stage*	EAR (mg/day)†	RDA (mg/day)‡	AI (mg/day)§	UL (g/day)‖
Birth–6 months	—	—	100	ND¶
7-12 months	—	—	275	ND¶
1-3 years	380	460	—	3
4-8 years	405	500	—	3
9-18 years	1055	1250	—	4
19-70 years	580	700	—	4
>70 years	580	700	—	3
Pregnancy				
≤18 years	1055	1250	—	3.5
19-50 years	580	700	—	3.5
Lactation				
≤18 years	1055	1250	—	4
19-50 years	580	700	—	4

Data from Institute of Medicine (IOM), Food and Nutrition Board: *Dietary reference intakes for calcium, phosphorus, magnesium, vitamin D, and fluoride*, Washington, DC, 1997, National Academy Press.
*All groups except Pregnancy and Lactation are males and females.
†EAR (estimated average requirement)—the intake that meets the estimated nutrient needs of 50% of the individuals in a group.
‡RDA (recommended dietary allowance)—the intake that meets the nutrient needs of almost all (97% to 98%) individuals in a group.
§AI (adequate intake)—for healthy infants fed human milk, AI is the estimated mean intake.
‖UL (tolerable upper intake level)—the UL is the highest level of daily nutrient intake that is likely to pose no risk of adverse health effects to almost all individuals in the general population. As intake increases above the UL, the risk of adverse effects increases. Unless specified otherwise, the UL represents total nutrient intake from food, water, and supplements.
¶ND—not determinable because of lack of data of adverse effects in this age group and concern with regard to lack of ability to handle excess amounts. Source of intake should be from food only to prevent high levels of intake.

depletions may cause increased calcium excretion, resulting in a negative calcium balance and bone loss.

During tooth development, a phosphorus deficiency can result in incomplete calcification of teeth, failure of dentin formation, and increased susceptibility to caries.

Dental Considerations

- A phosphorus deficiency is more likely to develop or occur in alcoholics; older adults with inadequate dietary intake; patients with disordered eating, inappropriate weight loss, and long-term diarrhea; and patients taking aluminum-containing antacids or diuretics. Assess the phosphorus status and document any signs or symptoms of a deficiency for these patients. A referral to the healthcare provider or RDN may be needed.
- Low phosphate intake may lead to an increased rate of caries formation, but additional or supplemental phosphate may not be helpful in preventing dental caries.

Nutritional Directions

- Phosphorus is abundant in foods, and a deficiency is unlikely. Educate patients that the goal is to maintain an equal calcium-to-phosphorus ratio. For example, an excessive consumption of soft drinks (more than 24 to 36 oz/day) in place of milk can interrupt the calcium-to-phosphorus balance.
- Adequate intake of phosphorus from dairy products may be a factor in lower blood pressure.[11]
- Hyperphosphatemia can be a risk factor for cardiovascular disease[11]

MAGNESIUM

Physiological Roles

Bones contain almost two-thirds of the body's magnesium. It is the third most prevalent mineral in teeth, with dentin containing about two times more than enamel. Magnesium has an important function in maintaining calcium homeostasis and preventing skeletal abnormalities. Magnesium is involved in more than 300 enzymatic reactions, including energy metabolism, insulin activity, and glucose use. Magnesium is vital to the structural integrity of muscles, especially the heart muscle, and nerves. Its role in enzymes is fundamental to energy (adenosine triphosphate) production. It is also crucial in controlling blood pressure and preventing stroke.[12]

Requirements

The RDA for magnesium ranges from 240 mg/day for 9-year-old children to 420 mg/day for men (Table 9-5). Although it is impossible to get too much magnesium from food alone, excessive amounts can be obtained from supplements. The tolerable upper intake level is provided for patients using supplements and other nonfood sources of magnesium.

Sources

Whole-grain products, nuts and beans are some of the best sources of magnesium (Table 9-6). Magnesium (Mg) is part of the chlorophyll molecule (Fig. 9-3); therefore, green leafy vegetables are also good sources. In addition, bananas and chocolate are sources of magnesium. Although whole grains

Table 9-5	Institute of Medicine recommendations for magnesium						
	EAR (mg/day)†		RDA (mg/day)‡		AI (mg/day)§		
Life Stage*	Male	Female	Male	Female	Male	Female	UL (mg/day)‖
Birth–6 months	—	—	—	—	30	30	ND¶
7-12 months	—	—	—	—	75	75	ND¶
1-3 years	65	65	80	80			65
4-8 years	110	110	130	130			110
9-13 years	200	200	240	240			350
14-18 years	340	300	410	360			350
19-30 years	330	255	400	310			350
>30 years	350	265	420	320			350
Pregnancy							
≤18 years		335		400			350
19-30 years		290		350			350
31-50 years		300		360			350
Lactation							
≤18 years		300		360			350
19-30 years		255		310			350
31-50 years		265		320			350

Data from Institute of Medicine (IOM), Food and Nutrition Board: *Dietary reference intakes for calcium, phosphorus, magnesium, vitamin D, and fluoride,* Washington, DC, 1997, National Academy Press.
*All groups except Pregnancy and Lactation are males and females.
†EAR (estimated average requirement)—the intake that meets the estimated nutrient needs of 50% of the individuals in a group.
‡RDA (recommended dietary allowance)—the intake that meets the nutrient needs of almost all (97% to 98%) individuals in a group.
§AI (adequate intake)—for healthy infants fed human milk, AI is the estimated mean intake.
‖UL (tolerable upper intake level)—the UL is the highest level of daily nutrient intake that is likely to pose no risk of adverse health effects to almost all individuals in the general population. As intake increases above the UL, the risk of adverse effects increases. Unless specified otherwise, the UL represents total nutrient intake from food, water, and supplements.
¶ND—not determinable because of lack of data of adverse effects in this age group and concern with regard to lack of ability to handle excess amounts. Source of intake should be from food only to prevent high levels of intake.

Table 9-6	Magnesium content of selected foods	
Food	Portion	Magnesium (mg)
Sesame seeds	1 oz	101
Spinach, cooked	½ cup	78
Cashew nuts	1 oz	74
Lima beans, cooked	½ cup	63
Peanut butter	2 tbsp	49
Navy beans, cooked	½ cup	48
Brown rice, cooked	½ cup	42
Potato, baked	1 medium	37
Sunflower seeds	1 oz	37
Split peas, cooked	½ cup	35
Dark chocolate	2.6 oz bar	23
Beets, cooked	½ cup	20
Bread, multigrain	1 slice	20
Yellow corn, cooked	½ cup	19
Broccoli, cooked	½ cup	16
Kale, cooked	½ cup	12
Mustard greens, cooked	½ cup	9

Data from U.S. Department of Agriculture, Agricultural Research Service. 2012. *USDA national nutrient database for standard reference, release 26.* Nutrient Data Laboratory Home Page. Accessed August 20, 2013: http://www.ars.usda/gov/ba/bhnrc/ndl

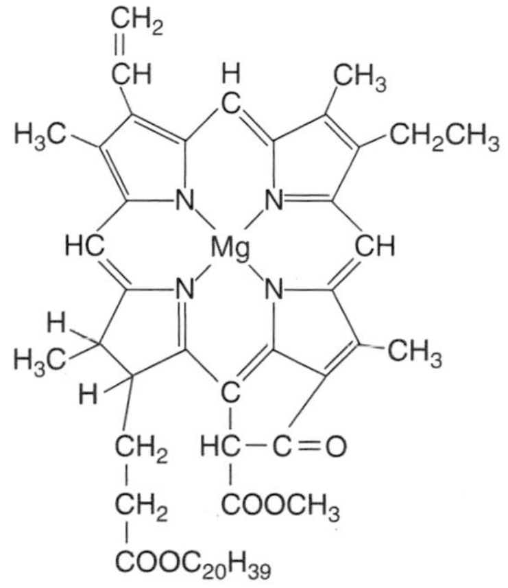

FIGURE 9-3 Structure of chlorophyll. All chlorophyll molecules are essentially alike; they differ only in details of the side chains. Magnesium is basic to all chlorophyll molecules.

are good sources of magnesium, enrichment of refined grain products does not replace magnesium lost during processing. Nonfood sources of magnesium include laxatives and antacids.

Hyper States and Hypo States

Because kidneys regulate plasma magnesium levels, toxicity has been associated with kidney failure. There is no evidence of harmful effects related to overconsumption of magnesium from food sources. A high dose of magnesium acts like a laxative (e.g., milk of magnesia).

In certain diseases or under stressful conditions, deficiencies may occur. Magnesium in bone is not available to replace serum magnesium deficits. A deficiency may result from numerous disease states, including gastrointestinal abnormalities with diarrhea, renal disease, general malnutrition, alcoholism, and medications interfering with magnesium conservation. Magnesium deficiency symptoms include neuromuscular dysfunction, personality changes, disorientation, muscle spasms, seizures, tremors, anorexia, nausea, apathy, and cardiac arrhythmias.

Dietary deficiencies may affect teeth and their supporting structures. Changes in ameloblasts and odontoblasts result in hypoplasia of the enamel and dentin during development. Alveolar bone formation may be reduced, along with a widening of the periodontal ligament space and gingival hyperplasia.

Dental Hygiene Considerations

- Decreased food intake, impaired magnesium absorption, and the use of certain diuretics may contribute to hypomagnesemia, or a below-normal blood serum concentration of magnesium. Encourage a well-balanced diet with liberal intake of foods high in magnesium.

Nutritional Directions

- Diets high in unrefined grains and vegetables provide more magnesium than diets that include a lot of refined foods, meats, and milk products.
- Magnesium plays a major role in blood pressure regulation; magnesium from foods is more effective than from supplements.[12]

FLUORIDE

Physiological Roles

In a strict nutritional sense, fluoride is not a nutrient essential for health. Fluoride present in low concentrations in soft tissues does not have any known metabolic function. However, because of its benefits to dental and bone health, fluoride is considered a desirable element for humans. Saliva contains varying amounts of fluoride; the amount of fluoride ingested has little effect on salivary levels.

Fluoride is advantageous to dental health because of its systemic effects before tooth eruption and topical effects after tooth eruption (Fig. 9-4). The caries-preventing properties of systemic and topical fluoride are cumulative.

Fluoride ions can replace hydroxyl ions in the hydroxyapatite crystal lattice. This fluoridated hydroxyapatite, or **fluorapatite**, is less soluble and makes the tooth more resistant to acid demineralization. Additionally, it enhances remineralization when the tooth is subject to the caries process

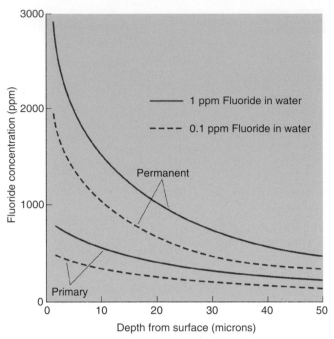

FIGURE 9-4 Concentration gradients of fluoride in outer enamel from permanent and deciduous teeth, from areas with 1 part per million (ppm) and 0.1 ppm of fluoride in the drinking water. (From Gron P: Inorganic chemical and structural aspects of oral mineralized tissues. In Shaw JH, editors: *Textbook of oral biology*, Philadelphia, 1978, Saunders, pp 484-507.)

(Fig. 9-5, *A*). Calcium and phosphate are present in saliva and plaque at higher concentrations than fluoride. When small pits develop in the enamel, fluoride is believed to promote deposition of calcium phosphate to remineralize the enamel surface.

Primary teeth benefit from the presence of fluoride during tooth development beginning at 6 months of age. Fluoride is present in the inner part of the enamel and dentin at lower concentrations; this occurs mainly during the amelogenesis/odontogenesis stage. Enhanced concentration in the surface enamel occurs during the maturation stage of tooth development. Fluoride can be readily incorporated into the apatite crystal from topically-available fluoride during the maturation stage, but this reversible process is superficial, rather than fluoride being distributed throughout the enamel thickness, as shown in Figure 9-5, *B*.

The presence of fluoride in saliva also interferes with the demineralization process, resulting in a less cariogenic environment. Topically-available fluoride reduces dental caries by inhibiting demineralization, promoting remineralization, and interfering with formation and function of acidogenic bacteria. Higher concentrations of fluoride inhibit *Streptococcus mutans*, *Streptococcus sobrinus*, and *Lactobacillus* in plaque biofilm, and accelerate remineralization during early stages of enamel caries development.

Maximum protection of fluoride against caries occurs during the first 6 to 10 years of life, but adults and children continue to benefit from the presence of fluoride. Systemic fluoride uptake by calcified tissues is high from infancy

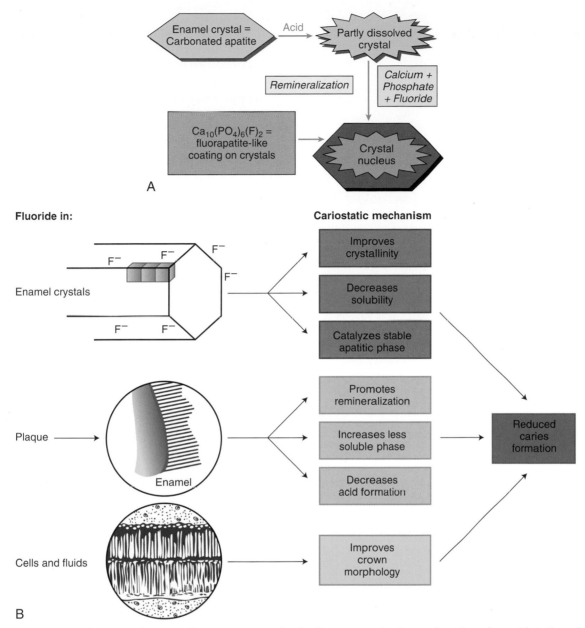

FIGURE 9-5 A, Demineralization and remineralization processes that lead to remineralized crystals with surfaces rich in fluoride and low in solubility. **B,** The mechanisms of cariostatic action of fluoride and their interrelationship. (**A,** Modified from Featherstone JDB: Prevention and reversal of dental caries: role of low level fluoride. *Community Dent Oral Epidemiol* 1999;27(1):31-40. **B,** Adapted from Nikiforuk G: Mechanism of cariostatic action of fluorides. In: Nikiforuk G, editor: *Understanding dental caries prevention: II,* Basel, Switzerland, 1985, S. Karger.)

until age 16, when mineralization of unerupted permanent teeth occurs. Compared with healthy enamel, demineralized enamel retains more fluoride.

Fluoride stimulates osteoblast proliferation and increases new mineral deposition in cancellous bone, improves bone integrity, and decreases bone resorption and bone solubility. Concurrent adequate intake of calcium, vitamin D, and fluoride is essential.

Requirements

Because of its toxicity, adequate intake of fluoride has been established at 3 mg/day for all women and 4 mg/day for men (Table 9-7). Average intake in the United States is 0.9 mg/day in areas with nonfluoridated water and 1.7 mg/day in areas with fluoridation. The tolerable upper intake level for healthy individuals age 9 years and older is 10 mg/day.

Absorption and Excretion

Most fluoride is absorbed in the stomach, with small amounts also absorbed in the intestine. The rate and degree of absorption depend on the solubility of the fluoride and amount ingested at a particular time. Absorption of fluoride from sodium fluoride in water is estimated to be 80% to 90%. Incorporation of fluoride into bones and enamel is proportional to total intake and need. Children retain a larger percentage of fluoride in developing bones and teeth,

Table 9-7	Institute of Medicine recommendations for fluoride		
	AI* (mg/day)		
Life Stage Group	Male	Female	UL†
Birth–6 months	0.01	0.01	0.7
7-12 months	0.5	0.5	0.9
1-3 years	0.7	0.7	1.3
4-8 years	1	1	2.2
9-13 years	2	2	10
14-18 years	3	3	10
>18 years	4	3	10
Pregnancy and Lactation			
≤50 years	—	3	10

Data from Institute of Medicine (IOM), Food and Nutrition Board: *Dietary reference intakes for calcium, phosphorus, magnesium, vitamin D, and fluoride*, Washington, DC, 1997, National Academy Press.

*AI (adequate intake)—the observed estimate of nutrient intake that reduces the incidence of dental caries maximally in a group of healthy people. For healthy infants fed human milk, AI is the mean intake. The AI is used if insufficient scientific evidence is available to derive an estimated average requirement. The AI is believed to cover their needs, but lack of data or uncertainty in the data prevents being able to specify with confidence the percentage of individuals covered by this intake.

†UL (tolerable upper intake level)—the highest level of daily nutrient intake that is likely to pose no risk of adverse health effects to almost all individuals in the general population. As intake increases above the UL, the risk of adverse effects increases. Unless specified otherwise, the UL represents total nutrient intake from food, water, and supplements.

whereas adults retain less in calcified structures. Protein-bound fluoride in foods is not as well absorbed.

Approximately 60% to 70% of fluoride intake is excreted by the kidneys; approximately 5% is excreted in the feces. Aluminum (aluminum-containing antacids) and soy (soy-based foods) bind with fluoride and increase fluoride excretion in the feces. Calcium and fluoride supplements given at the same time inhibit absorption of both.

Sources

Water

The Centers for Disease Control and Prevention recognizes water fluoridation as one of the most important public health measures.[13] Fluoride is available through community water supplies, food, beverages, dentifrices, and other dental products. Fluoridation of community water contributes to fluoride intake and is a practical, cost-effective means of achieving significant decreases in the prevalence of dental caries. Approximately 80% of fluoride consumed is provided from tap and bottled water and water-based beverages, especially teas. To ensure everyone receives adequate amounts of fluoride, the U.S. Department of Health and Human Services Agency and the U.S. Environmental Protection Agency suggest drinking water contain approximately 0.7 parts per million (ppm) of fluoride (equivalent to 1 mg/L).[14] In warmer climates where water consumption is higher, the optimal level of fluoride may need to be lower. Scientists do not all agree on the maximum acceptable fluoride level. Several

government agencies have suggested/recommended no more than 2 ppm. Additional studies are currently being conducted to determine appropriate guidelines.[15,16] Home water purification and filtration systems can reduce the fluoride content of tap water.

Approximately 74% of the U.S. population has access to optimally fluoridated drinking water; the goal, as stated by *Healthy People 2020*, targets 79.6% of the population. The *Healthy People 2010* objective of 75% was met by only 27 states.[17] Water fluoridation is particularly beneficial for children and adults in economically-depressed communities who have less access to oral healthcare and alternative fluoride resources. Children who do not regularly receive dental care or have no dental insurance are at high risk for dental caries.

Many households and businesses are using bottled water for various reasons, including taste preference and convenience. Bottled water may be chosen as a healthy alternative to soft drinks and alcoholic beverages. For water bottled in the United States, the U.S. Food and Drug Administration requires fluoride be listed on the label only if the manufacturer adds fluoride during processing. Fluoride amounts in bottled water may or may not be denoted on the label. Bottled water containing 0.6 to 1.0 mg/L fluoride may state on the packaging, "Drinking fluoridated water may reduce the risk of tooth decay."

In some areas of the United States, the water supply naturally contains much higher levels of fluoride than the recommended amounts. The U.S. Environmental Protection Agency allows a maximum level of 4 mg/L.[15] This level could possibly cause adverse health effects.

Food

Food is not a major source of fluoride for adults. All foods contain some fluoride, but the amounts provided in vegetables, meats, cereals, and fruits are insignificant (0.2 to 1.5 ppm of fluoride) (Table 9-8). Seafood may contain 5 to 15 ppm of fluoride. Brewed tea provides approximately 1 to 6 ppm of fluoride per cup, depending on the amount of tea, brewing time, and amount of fluoride in the water, but herbal tea has negligible fluoride levels. The process of mechanically deboning poultry results in poultry containing a high concentration of fluoride. Carbonated beverages can be a significant source of fluoride if the water used in the bottling process is fluoridated.

Because of varied levels of fluoride in the water supply, the amount of fluoride in infant formulas was reduced in 1979. Components in soy bind fluoride; soy-based formulas usually contain some fluoride.

Topical

Topical applications of fluoride include gels, foams, varnishes, dentifrices, prophylactic paste (polishing paste), and mouth rinses. These high-concentration fluoride sources prevent demineralization when oral pH decreases. When used in combination with other fluoride sources, a decline in prevalence or severity of dental caries occurs.

Table 9-8	Fluoride content of selected foods
Food	Fluoride (µg/100 g)
Black tea, brewed	373
Instant tea	335
Green tea, decaffeinated, brewed	272
Raisins	234
Crab, canned	210
Shrimp, canned	201
Carbonated water, fruit-flavored	105
Coffee, brewed	91
Oatmeal, cooked	72
Carrots, canned	47
Potatoes, baked	45
Cheese, American processed	35
Tomato sauce	35
Rice, white, long grain	33
Cottage cheese	32
Yogurt, plain	12

Data from U.S. Department of Agriculture, Agricultural Research Service. 2005. *USDA national nutrient database for standard reference, release 26.* Nutrient Data Laboratory Home Page. Accessed August 20, 2013: http://www.ars.usda/gov/ba/bhnrc/ndl

Hyper States and Hypo States

Fluorosis and Bone Health

Mottling of tooth enamel results from overexposure (approximately three to four times the amount necessary to prevent caries) during tooth formation. Ameloblasts are extremely sensitive to excessive fluoride ingestion. Dental fluorosis (hypomineralization of enamel) is directly related to fluoride exposure during tooth development and cannot occur after tooth development is complete. Fluorosed enamel contains a total protein content similar to normal enamel, but it contains a relatively high proportion of immature matrix proteins. Mild to moderate enamel fluorosis on early forming enamel surfaces was strongly associated with use of infant formula before 1979. Frequent brushing with fluoridated toothpaste was encouraged, and fluoride supplements were used.

Dental fluorosis varies from very mild cases characterized by whitish opaque flecks, to white or brown staining, to severe dental fluorosis with secondary, extrinsic, brownish discoloration and varying degrees of enamel pitting (Fig. 9-6). When drinking water contains 2 ppm or more of fluoride, teeth appear extremely white; brown stains appear when the fluoride level is greater than 4 ppm. Mild to moderate fluorosis is primarily cosmetic, but teeth are caries-resistant; severe dental fluorosis can result in increased caries rate.

Excessive fluoride intake for adults can result in adverse effects on skeletal tissue and kidney function. These changes may gradually increase in severity, eventually resulting in a general increase in bone fractures and calcification of ligaments in the neck and vertebral column.

Dental Caries.   A lack of fluoride may result in increased dental caries. The protective effect against caries is greatest during tooth formation. The American Dental Association

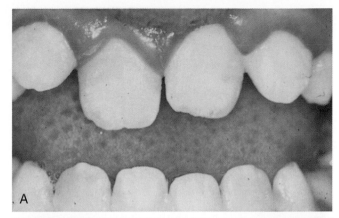

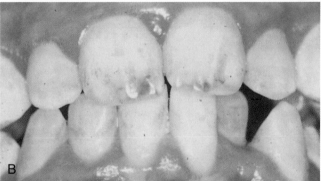

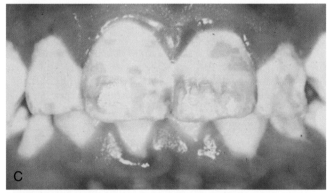

FIGURE 9-6 A, Mild fluorosis—white opaque areas in the enamel over less than 50% of the tooth. **B,** Moderate fluorosis—all enamel surfaces of the teeth are affected; brown stain frequently present. **C,** Severe fluorosis—hypoplasia affecting the general shape of the tooth; widespread brown stains, corroded-like appearance of teeth. (Courtesy of Alton McWhorter, DDS, MS, Associate Professor, Department of Pediatric Dentistry, The Texas A&M University System, Baylor College of Dentistry, Dallas, TX.)

and the American Academy of Pediatrics recommend exposure of the teeth to fluoride until calcification of all teeth is completed (about age 16 years). Dosages for fluoride supplements for children are presented in Table 14-2. Various conditions warrant topical fluoride treatment in adults, such as hypersensitivity, exposed root surfaces, white spot lesions, xerostomia, use of smokeless tobacco, and radiation therapy.

Continued use of fluoridated water by adults is beneficial in maintaining the integrity of teeth. Posteruption, systemic fluoride is present in saliva and plaque, creating an environment that inhibits demineralization and enhances remineralization of tooth surfaces.

Safety

The addition of fluoride in the U.S. water supply continues to be opposed by a small but vocal and aggressive minority of people. Antifluoridation groups have attempted to link water fluoridation to cancer, AIDS, Alzheimer disease, mental illness, CHD, and Down syndrome, but scientific evidence to support these allegations has not been provided. Regardless, a handful of communities in the U.S. have banned the addition of fluoride to their water.

Fluoridation is one of the most thoroughly researched health issues in recent history. No negative trends have been identified that could be attributed to the introduction or duration of fluoride in drinking water. In contrast, almost all professional health organizations have concluded that results of numerous long-term community trials of adding fluoride to public water supplies at optimal levels verify the effectiveness, safety, and cost-benefit of this public health measure in reducing the prevalence of dental caries. Water fluoridation is the most cost-effective method of preventing dental caries, providing the greatest benefit to individuals who can least afford preventive and restorative dentistry.

Dental Hygiene Considerations

- Educate patients about the purpose and value of fluoridation to oral and bone health.
- Contact the state or local health department to determine the fluoride content of the water system in the area. Encourage patients to send samples of well water or home water treatment systems to their state health department to determine fluoride content.
- 3M™ ESPE™ FluoriCheck Water Analysis System can also be used to determine the fluoride content of drinking water.
- Request the content of fluoride in bottled water from the manufacturer.
- Long-term use of infant formulas, particularly powdered formulas reconstituted with fluoridated water, can be a factor for mild fluorosis.
- Carefully estimate the total amount of fluoride the patient consumes daily in foods and water. Because fluoride is available from multiple sources, the possibility of toxic levels should be considered when recommending fluoride supplements or providing treatment, especially for children. Consider the number of carbonated beverages consumed and consumption of all beverages using fluoridated water. The fluoride content is not listed on the label, making it difficult to approximate the amount of fluoride being consumed.
- Educate patients about the caries process. Encourage patients to practice optimal oral hygiene. Plaque biofilm is the primary factor in caries formation. Appropriate oral hygiene when using topical fluorides at home also increases their effectiveness.

- Recommend fluoride supplements only when the fluoride level of the home water supply is known to be deficient.
- Fluoride supplements can be in liquid or tablet form. Tablet forms that dissolve slowly in the mouth also provide a topical effect.[18]
- An adequate fluoride intake is beneficial during development of skeletal tissue and teeth. Encourage fluoride-fortified foods, water, or supplements for breastfed infants, and fluoridated water for children and adolescents, if applicable.
- Growth of cariogenic bacteria is reduced by the presence of fluoride. Suggest use of dentifrices or mouthwashes with fluoride for oral self-care for individuals older than 3 years.
- Caution parents of children younger than 6 years of age to (a) use only small (pea size) amounts of fluoridated dentifrices, (b) minimize swallowing toothpaste, (c) avoid the use of fluoride mouth rinse, (d) keep fluoride products out of the reach of children, and (e) use a nonfluoridated toothpaste for children age 2 years and younger. Fluoride levels in children's toothpastes often equal the levels in adult fluoridated toothpastes.
- If fluoride and calcium supplements are given concurrently, absorption of both is decreased.
- For individuals living in an area where the fluoride content of water is naturally 2 to 4 ppm, recommend drinking bottled water without fluoride, or using commercially available filters to reduce the fluoride to safer levels.
- There is no risk of fluorosis after enamel has developed.
- Dental professionals need to be alert and active in their communities and prepared to present factual information to governing bodies.

Nutritional Directions

- A 2.2-mg amount of sodium fluoride contains 1 mg of fluoride ion.
- To provide maximum benefits, systemic fluoride is important before tooth eruption, when development of unerupted permanent teeth is occurring.
- Fluoride supplementation is recommended for patients 6 months to 16 years old with less than 0.6 ppm fluoride in their water source (home, child care settings, school, or bottled) if there is no other significant source of fluoride.
- Fluoride supplements are not recommended during pregnancy.
- If a child receives suboptimal levels of fluoride, an increase in dental caries may occur. Exposure to multiple sources of fluoride increases the risk of excess fluoride causing fluorosis.
- Fluoride supplements are inappropriate for individuals living in areas where the fluoride content of drinking water is optimal, unless the bottled or treated water does not contain fluoride.

- Topical availability of fluoride at low concentrations on a daily basis after tooth eruption is important to deter development of dental caries.
- If caries susceptibility is high, professionally applied and self-applied home fluoride therapies may be an integral component of dental hygiene care.
- When bottled water is being used, obtain the fluoride content from the distributor or the label.
- Studies have found no association between fluoride supplementation and cancer in humans.
- Aluminum antacids decrease fluoride absorption.
- High levels of calcium can interfere with the absorption of fluoride.

HEALTH APPLICATION **9**   **Osteoporosis**

Osteoporosis is a common and costly disease, increasing in prevalence in men and women. This condition is partly genetically determined. Ten million Americans are affected by osteoporosis, and another 34 million have low bone mass (osteopenia). Approximately 80% of individuals with osteoporosis are women (one in two women older than age 50 years); however, osteoporosis will also affect one in four men older than age 50 years. This condition could incur a financial burden of approximately $25.3 billion in medical costs by 2025.[1] Fractures resulting from osteoporosis are a significant source of bone pain, disability, and disfigurement.

Osteoporosis is more likely to develop in individuals with at least some of the risk factors listed in Box 9-3. The incidence of osteoporosis is greatest in white, Asian, Hispanic, and African American women, especially those who are small and thin. A woman's risk of osteoporosis starts around menopause (age 50 years or older). Women can lose 20% of their bone mass within 5 to 7 years after menopause. Bone loss in men increases after age 65 years. Men who fall and break a hip are twice as likely to die within a year after the incident.[1] For individuals at risk for osteoporosis, an objective of treatment is to slow or stop disease progression before irreversible structural changes have occurred. The National Osteoporosis Foundation recommends steps for preventing osteoporosis: [20]

1. Get the daily recommended amounts of calcium and vitamin D. Dietary modifications for patients at risk of developing osteoporosis should include at least two portions of dairy products daily (to provide 75% of RDAs). For patients who have inadequate intake of milk or milk products (including patients who are lactose intolerant), inclusion of calcium and vitamin D supplements may be indicated.[19]
2. Engage in regular weight-bearing and muscle-strengthening exercise.
3. Avoid tobacco use and excessive alcohol.
4. Talk to a healthcare provider about bone health and supplement use.
5. Take steps to prevent falling, such as regular vision and hearing exams, investigate neurological problems, and improve safety concerns at home.
6. Have a bone mineral density (BMD) test and take medication when appropriate. Specialized tests to assess BMD should be conducted on women older than 65 years, men older than 70 years, those older than 50 years with risk

factors for osteoporosis, and, all individuals who have broken a bone after age 50 years.[19]

The oral cavity (teeth, maxilla, and mandible) can be affected by osteoporosis. When identifying periodontal issues, such as tooth mobility or loss, resorption of alveolar bone, temporomandibular disorders, and clinical attachment loss, a relationship to osteoporosis should be considered.[19]

To date, osteoporosis cannot be cured, but medications can help prevent or deter bone loss. Medications used to slow bone loss include estrogen hormone, bisphosphonates (alendronate, alendronate plus D, ibandronate, risedronate, risedronate with 500 mg of calcium carbonate and zoledronic acid), calcitonin, estrogen agonists/selective estrogen receptor modulators, and PTH. A significant dental consideration for the use of bisphosphonates, particularly following intravenous bisphosphonate treatment for patients with cancer, is the risk for the development of osteonecrosis of the jaw.[21] Commonly used medications for other conditions have a documented effect on bone mineralization. Thiazide diuretics, principally used for blood pressure control, positively affect bone mineralization. Glucocorticoids, used to reduce inflammation, adversely affect bone mineralization. Antiandrogenic drugs for prostate cancer may lead to bone loss.

An adequate calcium intake is important at all stages of life, with a daily intake of a minimum of 1000 mg for all healthy adults and 1200 mg for women older than 51 years. Adequate exposure to sunlight and vitamin D intake are also important. The action of these two nutrients is complementary; calcium supports bone formation and repair, and vitamin D helps with calcium absorption. Other nutritional considerations include B vitamins and vitamin K, which may reduce fracture risk by improving BMD. Several studies have reported a positive association between the use of phytochemicals (plant chemicals) and preventing bone loss. Diets high in fruits, vegetables, and whole grains contribute nutrients that may reduce calcium excretion. However, high fiber intake (including oxalates and phytates) should be paired with increased calcium intake. High levels of phosphorus, sodium, or caffeine intake may increase calcium loss in urine. **Phytochemicals**, natural components of foods, found in soy products and flaxseed, stimulate estrogen secretion, which may boost BMD.[22] A healthcare provider or RDN can tailor the osteoporosis regimen to meet the patient's needs.

BOX 9-3   **Risk Factors for Osteoporosis**

Certain people are more likely to develop osteoporosis than others. Factors that increase the likelihood of developing osteoporosis and broken bones are called "risk factors." These risk factors include:

- Being female
- Older age
- Family history of osteoporosis or broken bones
- Being small and thin
- Certain races/ethnicities such as white, Asian, or Hispanic/Latino, although African Americans are also at risk
- History of broken bones
- Low sex hormones
  - Low estrogen levels in women, including menopause

  - Missing periods (amenorrhea)
  - Low levels of testosterone and estrogen in men
- Diet
  - Low calcium intake
  - Low vitamin D intake
  - Excessive intake of protein, sodium, and caffeine
- Inactive lifestyle
- Smoking
- Alcohol abuse
- Certain medications such as steroid medications, some anticonvulsants, and others
- Certain diseases and conditions such as anorexia nervosa, bulimia, rheumatoid arthritis, gastrointestinal diseases, and others

Data from National Osteoporosis Foundation. Prevention and healthy living. Accessed August 20, 2013: http://www.nof.org/learn/prevention

Case Application for the Dental Hygienist

During Annie's routine dental examination, her mother asked the dental hygienist whether she should start Annie (age 5 years) on a fluoride supplement. Annie's examination revealed a caries-free mouth. She had been brushing her teeth twice a day.

Nutritional Assessment
- Food consumption pattern
- Frequency of carbohydrate intake
- Fluoride content of water consumed; average amount of water/water-based beverages consumed
- Type and amount of toothpaste used

Nutritional Diagnosis
Health-seeking behaviors related to inadequate knowledge about fluoride supplementation.

Nutritional Goals
The patient will practice good oral self-care and receive adequate fluoride to prevent dental caries.

Nutritional Implementation
Intervention: Explain the benefits of fluoride.

Rationale: Fluoride is advantageous to dental health because of its systemic effect before tooth eruption and its topical effects after tooth eruption. The caries-preventive properties of systemic and topical fluoride are additive.

Intervention: Discuss the toxic effects of fluoride.

Rationale: Dental fluorosis is directly related to the level of fluoride exposure during tooth development. It can also have adverse effects on bone structure.

Intervention: Assess current fluoride consumption from (a) food, (b) water supply, (c) carbonated beverages, and (d) fluoridated dentifrices and mouth rinses.

Rationale: (a) All foods contain some fluoride, but the amounts provided in vegetables, meats, cereals, and fruits are insignificant unless large amounts of seafood, tea, or deboned poultry are consumed; (b) water is usually the main source of fluoride, but some municipal water supplies and bottled waters may contain negligible amounts of fluoride; and (c) fluoride is added to 90% of all dentifrices in the United States. Because younger children swallow most of the toothpaste used, they should be provided with a dentifrice without fluoride.

Intervention: Show Annie and her mother how much toothpaste to use, and discuss the importance of not swallowing it.

Rationale: Because fluoride in toothpaste can be readily absorbed, toothpaste should not be swallowed to prevent the harmful effects of systemically available fluoride.

Intervention: Encourage the patient and her mother to consume a well-balanced diet with limited amounts of fermentable carbohydrates at snack time.

Rationale: Not only is fluoride important, but also other nutrients are essential for dental health. Snacks, especially carbohydrate-containing foods, increase risk for dental caries.

Intervention: Suggest fluoride supplements only if fluoride intake seems to be low.

Rationale: In many cases, total fluoride exposure seems to be higher than necessary to prevent tooth decay. No more than the amount of fluoride necessary to provide the desired effect should be used.

Intervention: Recommend parental supervision and assistance for Annie's tooth brushing and flossing.

Rationale: Monitoring the child's brushing technique and assisting with flossing will ensure that effective biofilm removal occurs once a day.

Evaluation
If the patient and her mother can demonstrate the toothbrushing procedure, the patient says she will brush her teeth after every meal and will try to eat the foods her mother provides, and dental caries continues to be minimal, dental hygiene care was effective.

STUDENT READINESS

1. A patient claims that she dislikes milk. How would you advise her to obtain the calcium she needs?
2. What are the main physiological roles of calcium, phosphorus, magnesium, and fluoride?
3. How do minerals differ from vitamins?
4. How would you respond to a remark that milk is only for babies?
5. Discuss three dietary factors that affect calcium absorption.
6. Determine the level of fluoride in your community's drinking water.
7. If an adult patient (weight about 75 kg) is drinking only bottled water that does not contain fluoride, and the patient dislikes fish and tea, how much topical fluoride would be necessary to furnish the recommendation for fluoride?
8. List five types of over-the-counter calcium supplements available. Evaluate these items for primary sources of calcium and elemental calcium per unit consumed. Find how many tablets or units would have to be consumed daily to receive 1000 mg of elemental calcium.
9. Discuss how to deal with a patient who is opposed to community water fluoridation.
10. Why would you advise a patient to obtain his or her mineral requirement from food sources rather than mineral supplements (unless ordered by the healthcare provider)?

CASE STUDY

Mrs. J. M., a 69-year-old woman, fell and fractured her hip 6 months ago. She admits she is taking calcium supplements occasionally, when she can afford them. She does not like milk and has been unable to walk much since her fall.

1. What additional questions would you ask to clarify the situation?
2. What nutritional advice could you give her about her osteoporosis?
3. What is her RDA for calcium?
4. What foods could you suggest she consume to increase her calcium intake?
5. When should she take her calcium supplement to maximize its absorption?
6. What oral changes might you expect to find in your assessment?
7. What effect would increased vitamin D intake have on her condition?

References

1. National Osteoporosis Foundation: *Bone health basics: get the facts*. Available at http://www.nof.org/node/40. Accessed August 20, 2013.
2. U.S. Department of Agriculture, Agricultural Research Service: *What we eat in America, NHANES 2009-2010*. Available at http://www.ars.usda.gov/ba/bhnrc/fsrg. Accessed August 20, 2013.
3. Centers for Disease Control and Prevention, National Center for Health Statistics: *National Health and Nutrition Examination Survey Data*, Hyattsville, MD, 2007–2008, U.S. Department of Health and Human Services. Available at http://www.cdc.gov/nchs/nhanes/nhanes2007-2008/nhanes07-08.htm. Accessed August 20, 2013.
4. Bailey RL, Dodd KW, Goldman JA, et al: Estimation of total usual calcium and vitamin D intakes in the United States. *J Nutr* 140(4):817–822, 2010.
5. U.S. Preventive Services Task Force: *U.S. Preventive Services Task Force issues final recommendation on vitamin D and calcium supplements to prevent fractures*. Available at http://www.uspreventiveservicestaskforce.org. Accessed August 20, 2013.
6. Xiao Q, Murphy RA, Houston DK, et al: Dietary and supplemental calcium intake and cardiovascular disease mortality. *JAMA Intern Med* 173(8):639–646, 2013.
7. Reid IR: Cardiovascular effects of calcium supplements. *Nutrients* 5:2522–2529, 2013.
8. Committee to Review Dietary Reference Intakes for Vitamin D and Calcium, Food and Nutrition Board, Institute of Medicine: *Dietary reference intakes for calcium and vitamin D*, Washington, DC, 2010, National Academy Press.
9. Adegboye ARA, Christensen LB, Holm-Pedersen P, et al: Intake of dairy products in relation to periodontitis in older Danish adults. *Nutrients* 4(9):1219–1229, 2012.
10. Brzozowska MM, Sainsbury A, Eisman JA, et al: Bariatric surgery, bone loss, obesity and possible mechanisms. *Obes Rev* 14(1):52–67, 2013.
11. Takeda E, Yamamoto H, Yamanaka-Okumura H, et al: Dietary phosphorus in bone health and quality of life. *Nutr Rev* 70(6): 311–321, 2012.
12. Larsson SC, Orsini N, Wolk A: Dietary magnesium intake and risk of stroke: a meta-analysis of prospective studies. *Am J Clin Nutr* 95(2):362–366, 2012.
13. Centers for Disease Control and Prevention. Division of Oral Health: *2010 water fluoridation statistics*. Available at http://www.cdc.gov/fluoridation/statistics/2010stats.htm. Accessed August 20, 2013.
14. U.S. Department of Health and Human Services Agency, U.S. Environmental Protection Agency: *HHS and EPA announce new scientific assessments and actions on fluoride*. 2011. Available at http://www.hhs.gov/news/press/2011pres/01/20110107a.html. Accessed August 20, 2013.
15. Environmental Protection Agency: *Fluoride risk assessment and relative source contribution*. 2011. Available at http://water.epa.gov/action/advisories/drinking/fluoride_index.cfm. Accessed August 20, 2013.
16. National Research Council, Committee on Fluoride in Drinking Water: *Fluoride in drinking water: a scientific review of EPA's standards*, Washington, DC, 2006, National Academies Press.
17. Healthy People 2020: *Oral Health 2020 Topics and Objectives*. Available at http://www.healthypeople.gov/2020/topicsobjectives2020/objectiveslist.aspx?topicId=32. Accessed January 3, 2013.
18. Palmer CA, Gilbert JA, Academy of Nutrition and Dietetics: Position of the Academy of Nutrition and Dietetics: The impact of fluoride on health. *J Acad Nutr Diet* 112(9):1443–1453, 2012.
19. Prentice RL, Pettinger MB, Jackson RD, et al: Health risks and benefits from calcium and vitamin D supplementation: Women's Health Initiative clinical trial and cohort study. *Osteoporos Int* 24(2):567–580, 2013.
20. National Osteoporosis Foundation: *Clinician's guide to prevention and treatment of osteoporosis*, Washington, DC, 2010, National Osteoporosis Foundation.
21. Stewart S, Hanning R: Building osteoporosis prevention into dental practice. *J Can Dent Assoc* 78:c29, 2012.
22. Shen CL, von Bergen V, Chyu MC, et al: Fruits and dietary phytochemicals in bone protection. *Nutr Res* 32:897–910, 2012.

ⓔ EVOLVE RESOURCES

Please visit http://evolve.elsevier.com/Stegeman/nutritional for additional practice and study support tools.

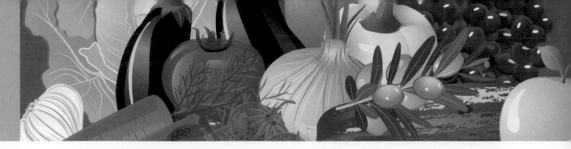

Chapter 10

Nutrients Present in Calcified Structures

Student Learning Outcomes

Upon completion of this chapter, the student will be able to achieve the following student learning outcomes:

- Describe the physiological roles of specific minerals and how these apply to oral health, along with sources of copper, selenium, chromium, and manganese.
- List ultratrace elements present in the body.

- Identify reasons why large amounts of one mineral may cause nutritional deficiencies of another.
- Apply dental hygiene considerations for trace elements present in calcified structures.
- Discuss nutritional directions for patients regarding the role of trace elements present in calcified structures.

Key Terms

Enteral feedings
Kayser-Fleischer ring
Keshan disease
Manganese madness

Neurotransmitters
Osteodystrophy
Stannous
Total parenteral nutrition (TPN)

 Test Your NQ

1. **T/F** The IOM has established tolerable upper intake levels (ULs) for copper, manganese, chromium, and molybdenum.
2. **T/F** Lead in dental enamel can be used to determine environmental exposure to lead.
3. **T/F** Copper is important in the formation of collagen.
4. **T/F** Aluminum toxicity causes Alzheimer disease.
5. **T/F** Selenium functions as an antioxidant.
6. **T/F** Refined foods are good sources of trace minerals.
7. **T/F** Aluminum is cariogenic.
8. **T/F** The function of many trace elements present in enamel and dentin is unknown.
9. **T/F** Sugar is a good source of chromium.
10. **T/F** Selenium supplements are a good way to increase longevity.

Table 10-1	Trace element concentrations in human enamel and dentin

	Enamel* (ppm)	Dentin* (ppm)
Aluminum	1.5-700	10-100
Boron	0.5-39	1-10
Cadmium	0.3-10	
Chromium	<0.1-100	1-100
Copper	0.1-130	0.2-100
Iron	0.8-200	90-1000
Lead	1.3-100	10-100
Lithium	0.23-3.40	
Manganese	0.8-20	0.6-1000
Molybdenum	0.7-39	1-10
Nickel	10-100	10-100
Selenium	0.1-10	10-100
Strontium	26-1000	90-1000
Sulfur	130-530	
Tin	0.03-0.9	
Vanadium	0.01-0.03	1-10
Zinc	60-1800	

Adapted from Gron P: Inorganic chemical and structural aspects of oral mineralized tissues. In Shaw JH, editors: Philadelphia, 1978, Saunders, pp 484-507.
*μg/g dry weight.

Table 10-2	Institute of Medicine recommendations for copper

	EAR (μg/day)*		RDA (μg/day)†		AI‡ (μg/day)
Life Stage	Male	Female	Male	Female	
Birth– 6 months	—	—	—	—	200
7-12 months	—	—	—	—	220
1-3 years	260	260	340	340	
4-8 years	340	340	440	440	
9-13 years	540	540	700	700	
14-50 years	685	685	890	890	
>50 years	700	700	900	900	
Pregnancy					
14-18 years		785		1000	
19-50 years		800		1000	
Lactation					
14-18 years		985		1300	
19-50 years		1000		1300	

Data from Institute of Medicine (IOM), Food and Nutrition Board: *Dietary reference intakes for vitamin A, vitamin K, arsenic, boron, chromium, copper, iodine, iron, manganese, molybdenum, nickel, silicon, vanadium, and zinc,* Washington, DC, 2001, National Academy Press.
*EAR (estimated average requirement)—the intake that meets the estimated nutrient needs of half of the individuals in a group, men and women combined.
†RDA (recommended dietary allowance)—the intake that meets the nutrient needs of almost all (97% to 98%) individuals in a group.
‡AI (adequate intake)—the observed average or experimentally set intake by a defined population or subgroup that seems to sustain a defined nutritional status, such as growth rate, normal circulating nutrient values, or other functional indicators of health. An AI is used if insufficient scientific evidence is available to derive an EAR. For healthy human milk–fed infants, the AI is the mean intake. *The AI is not equivalent to an RDA.*

Very small amounts of several minerals are essential for optimal growth and development. Many of these ultratrace elements (Table 10-1) are found in enamel and dentin. The role of minerals may not be obvious as you clinically assess patients; nevertheless, patients with inadequate amounts may exhibit deficiency symptoms.

Tolerable upper intake levels (ULs) have not been established for several of these nutrients because of the lack of data. The requirement for these nutrients should be obtained from food sources because even small amounts may be toxic. Available evidence suggests ultratrace minerals—especially arsenic, boron, nickel, and silicon—may be physiologically essential. Because no human deficiencies have been determined, their importance in humans can only be inferred from results of animal studies. Human requirements have not been quantified. If they are required, the amounts needed are easily met by naturally-occurring sources in food, water, and air. Other elements present in calcified structures, such as cadmium, lead, and tin, have no known function and may be contaminants.

COPPER

Physiological Roles

Copper is the third largest trace element found in the human body, following iron and zinc. Copper is essential for formation of red blood cells and connective tissue. Its function as a catalyst is important in the formation of collagen from a precollagenous stage. Copper is a component of many enzymes that function in oxidative reactions, and copper-containing enzymes encourage production of **neurotransmitters** (including norepinephrine and dopamine), which transmit messages through the central nervous system. Two other roles are nutrient metabolism and immune function.

Copper is readily incorporated into tooth enamel. X-ray fluorescence imaging of teeth shows an increased concentration of copper in carious portions of the tooth. Epidemiological data suggest that copper deficiency may induce caries, but in bacteriological studies, copper has proven to be cariostatic by reducing the acidogenicity of plaque.

Requirements

The IOM established the recommended dietary allowance (RDA) for copper as 900 μg/day for adults. The UL has been set at 10 g/day for adults (Table 10-2).

Absorption and Excretion

Approximately one third of dietary copper is absorbed, with absorption occurring in the stomach and duodenum. Absorption is enhanced by a low pH and is diminished by large amounts of calcium and zinc. Copper is stored mostly in the liver and muscle, and it is excreted through bile in feces.

Sources

Copper is widely distributed in foods. The richest sources include shellfish, oysters, crabs, liver, nuts, sesame and sunflower seeds, soy products, legumes, and cocoa.

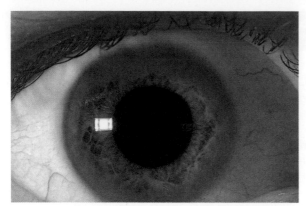

FIGURE 10-1 Cornea in Wilson disease. Copper deposits in the corneal periphery produce the characteristic Kayser-Fleischer ring. This is a complete or incomplete brown-to-green ring near the cornea, best seen in early stages of the disease. (Courtesy of Professor Dame S. Sherlock and J.A. Summerfield. In McLaren DS: *A colour atlas and text of diet-related disorders*, ed 2, London, 1992, Mosby-Year Book.)

Hyper States and Hypo States

Copper toxicity is seldom encountered. Copper taken orally is an emetic; 10 mg of oral copper can produce nausea. Serum copper levels are elevated in patients with rheumatoid arthritis, myocardial infarction, conditions requiring administration of estrogen, and pregnancy.

Wilson disease represents a special metabolic disorder in which large amounts of copper accumulate in the liver, kidney, brain, and cornea. The body cannot release copper from the liver at a normal rate due to a genetic abnormality. Copper concentrates in the cornea, causing a characteristic brown or green ring called the Kayser-Fleischer ring (Fig. 10-1).

Most copper deficiencies have been detected under unusual conditions, such as with zinc supplementation, malnutrition, malabsorption disorders, or in patients receiving total parenteral nutrition (TPN) (delivery of all nutritional needs intravenously). Copper deprivation results in profound effects on the bones, brain, arteries, and other connective tissues; decreased hair and skin pigmentation; and hematological abnormalities, such as a low white blood cell count. Seemingly, all these effects are ultimately caused by an inadequate supply of copper, which is required for enzyme synthesis and activity.

Copper deficiency causes a variety of lesions within connective tissues and bone, resulting in failure to grow (in children), spontaneous fractures, osteoporosis, arthritis, arterial disease, and ultimately marked bone deformities. These lesions have been attributed to abnormal formation of cross-linkages in collagen and elastin. Changes closely resemble those seen in vitamin C deficiency.

Dental Considerations

- Anemia that cannot be corrected with iron supplements may be caused by copper deficiency.
- High doses of zinc supplements decrease copper absorption, possibly leading to anemia-related fatigue.

Table 10-3	Institute of Medicine recommendations for selenium		
Life Stage	EAR (µg/day)*	RDA (µg/day)†	AI (µg/day)‡
0-6 months			15
7-12 months			20
1-3 years	17	20	
4-8 years	23	30	
9-13 years	35	40	
>13 years	45	55	
Pregnancy			
≤18-50 years	49	60	
Lactation			
≤18-50 years	59	70	

Data from Institute of Medicine (IOM), Food and Nutrition Board: *Dietary reference intakes for vitamin C, vitamin E, selenium, and carotenoids*, Washington, DC, 2000, National Academy Press.
*EAR (estimated average requirement)—the intake that meets the estimated nutrient needs of half of the individuals in a group, men and women combined.
†RDA (recommended dietary allowance)—the intake that meets the nutrient needs of almost all (97% to 98%) individuals in a group.
‡AI (adequate intake)—the observed average or experimentally set intake by a defined population or subgroup that seems to sustain a defined nutritional status, such as growth rate, normal circulating nutrient values, or other functional indicators of health. An AI is used if insufficient scientific evidence is available to derive an EAR. For healthy human milk–fed infants, the AI is the mean intake. *The AI is not equivalent to an RDA.*

Nutritional Directions

- High-fiber intake increases the dietary requirement for copper.
- Large amounts of vitamin C supplements decrease serum bioavailability of copper.
- Excess molybdenum produces a copper deficiency.

SELENIUM

Physiological Roles

Selenium functions mainly as a cofactor for an antioxidant enzyme that protects membrane lipids, proteins, and nucleic acids from oxidative damage. It also contributes to the maintenance of normal immune function. Selenium works hand in hand with vitamin E; a deficiency of either nutrient increases the requirement for the other. Although selenium has been suspected as a carcinogen, it may actually be an anticarcinogen.

Selenium is present in tooth enamel and dentin. It is probably incorporated into the enamel during amelogenesis. Large amounts during tooth formation may be detrimental to the mineralization process.

Requirements

The RDA establishes the adult requirement at 55 µg. The UL is 400 µg per day for adults (Table 10-3). Typical intake in the United States is 60 to 220 µg daily.

Sources

Animal products, especially seafood, kidney, liver, and other meats, are rich in selenium. Selenium intake correlates closely with caloric and protein consumption. Selenium in dairy products and eggs is more readily absorbed than selenium from other foods. Whole-grain products, nuts, and mushrooms are also good sources.

Hyper States and Hypo States

Toxicity and deficiency symptoms have occurred in animals from irregular distribution of selenium in soil, but these are rarely seen in humans. Routine ingestion of 2 to 3 mg of selenium can cause toxic symptoms, including nausea and vomiting, weakness, dermatitis, hair loss, white blotchy nails, and garlic-smelling breath. Cirrhosis of the liver also may develop. A moderate intake of selenium has been linked to reduced risks of prostate, lung, and colon cancers and heart disease because of its role as an antioxidant.

Animal studies indicate that excessive selenium may promote dental caries when given before eruption, whereas moderately high levels seem to have some cariostatic effects. Increased dental caries rates have been observed in areas where food and water contain higher levels of selenium. Whether this increase in caries is caused by a topical effect on plaque biofilm or by an effect on the structural composition of teeth is unknown.

In parts of China, an endemic cardiomyopathy called Keshan disease is associated with severe selenium deficiency. Oral selenium prophylaxis is extremely effective in reducing Keshan disease, but not in eradicating it.

Dental Considerations

- Decreased selenium levels may cause heart damage, resulting in a heart attack.
- Selenium is essential for health, but it can also be toxic.

Nutritional Directions

- Because of increased risk of toxicity, selenium supplements should not be taken by patients with cancer, CHD, arthritis, and HIV, unless recommended by a healthcare provider.
- Gastrointestinal disorders, such as Crohn disease, can impair selenium absorption.

CHROMIUM

Physiological Roles

Chromium is an odorless and tasteless metallic element. Chromium is involved in carbohydrate and lipid metabolism, especially in the use of glucose. Chromium potentiates the action of insulin, possibly by assisting cells in glucose uptake and energy release. Supplementation may improve systemic insulin sensitivity, but a cause-and-effect relationship has not

been established; consequently, more extensive research is needed.

Requirements

The adequate intake (AI) of a healthy adult has been estimated as 20 to 35 µg per day. No UL has been set (Table 10-4). The IOM reports the average chromium content in well-balanced diets as 13.4 µg/1000 kcal. Chromium is poorly absorbed; whether intestinal absorption compensates for increased demand is unclear. Chromium status decreases with age, suggesting that older adults may have an increased risk of deficiency.

Sources

Chromium is found in meats, whole-grain cereals, wheat germ, nuts, mushrooms, green beans, broccoli, brewer's yeast, beer, wine, and tap water. The refining process depletes chromium from grains and cereal. The Safe Drinking Water Act requires the U.S. Environmental Protection Agency (EPA) to review and update the national primary drinking water standards. The current EPA standard for chromium in public water systems is not to exceed 100 parts per billion (ppb).[1]

Chromium supplements are available as picolinate, nicotinate, or chloride (the form provided in most multivitamin-mineral supplements). The use of chromium supplements for individuals with diabetes is controversial.

Table 10-4	Institute of Medicine recommendations for chromium	
	AI* (µg/day)	
Life Stage Group	Male	Female
Birth-6 months	0.2	0.2
7-12 months	2.2	2.2
1-3 years	11	11
4-8 years	15	15
9-13 years	25	21
14-18 years	35	24
19-50 years	35	25
>50 years	30	20
Pregnancy		
14-18 years		29
19-50 years		30
Lactation		
14-18 years		44
19-50 years		45

Data from Institute of Medicine (IOM), Food and Nutrition Board: *Dietary Reference intakes for vitamin A, vitamin K, arsenic, boron, chromium, copper, iodine, iron, manganese, molybdenum, nickel, silicon, vanadium, and zinc,* Washington, DC, 2001, National Academy Press.
*AI (adequate intake)—the observed average or experimentally determined intake by a defined population or subgroup that seems to sustain a defined nutritional status, such as growth rate, normal circulating nutrient values, or other functional indicators of health. An AI is used if insufficient scientific evidence is available to derive an estimated average requirement. For healthy human milk–fed infants, the AI is the mean intake. *The AI is not equivalent to an RDA.*

Hyper States and Hypo States

Chromium deficiencies result in decreased insulin sensitivity, impaired glucose intolerance, neuropathy, and elevated plasma free fatty acid concentration. Patients on TPN are at risk of a chromium deficiency. Chromium toxicity has been caused by use of chromium supplements and by industrial exposure, resulting in liver damage and lung cancer.

Dental Considerations

- Assess patients employed in industrial settings or artists using supplies with high chromium content for chromium toxicity.
- Serum chromium levels decline with age.
- More research is needed regarding use of chromium supplements to enhance glycemic control in diabetes and to treat or prevent other health problems.
- Chromium supplements may cause serious renal impairment when taken in excess. This over-the-counter supplement is marketed for weight loss and in treating type 2 diabetes mellitus.

Nutritional Direction

- Do not take chromium supplements unless instructed by a healthcare provider. Currently, the evidence is unclear as to whether any type of supplemental chromium can help with fat loss or enhance lean body mass.

MANGANESE

Physiological Roles

Manganese is essential in several enzyme systems and is important for optimal bone matrix development; prevention of osteoporosis; insulin production; and amino acid, cholesterol, and carbohydrate metabolism. It is absorbed in the small intestine, transported to the liver, and excreted in bile.

Requirements

As shown in Table 10-5, an adequate intake is 1.8 to 2.3 mg per day for adults. The absorption of iron and manganese is inversely proportional, so a large amount of one reduces absorption of the other. The UL has been established as 11 mg per day for adults. Median intake in the United States is 2.1 to 2.3 mg per day for men and 1.6 to 1.8 mg per day for women.

Sources

Foods high in manganese include whole-grain cereals, legumes, nuts, tea, leafy vegetables, and infant formula. The bioavailability of manganese from meats, milk, and eggs makes these important sources despite their smaller quantities.

Hyper States and Hypo States

Manganese dust can be an environmental hazard. Manganese miners and welders have developed a syndrome similar to Parkinson disease called "manganese madness". Manganese miners are exposed to large amounts of manganese fumes, but other groups are at risk for manganese poisoning as well, including workers in factories manufacturing dry alkaline batteries and workers in facilities making manganese alloys. Symptoms of toxic exposure include ataxia, headache, fatigue, anxiety, hallucinations, psychosis and a syndrome similar to Parkinson disease (marked by memory loss, tremors, and rigid body posture).

Elevated concentrations of manganese in salivary plaque and enamel are associated with increased caries. Studies have not clarified whether this association is due to incorporation of manganese in enamel or due to its effects on oral bacteria.

Manganese deficiencies have never been reported in individuals consuming a normal diet. Signs of deficiency include abnormal formation of bone and cartilage, growth retardation, congenital malformations, hypercholesterolemia, impaired glucose tolerance, and poor reproductive performance.

Table 10-5	Institute of Medicine recommendations for manganese	
	AI* (mg/day)	
Life Stage Group	**Male**	**Female**
Birth-6 months	0.003	0.003
7-12 months	0.6	0.6
1-3 years	1.2	1.2
4-8 years	1.5	1.5
9-13 years	1.9	1.6
14-18 years	2.2	1.6
>18 years	2.3	1.8
Pregnancy		
14-50 years		2
Lactation		
14-50 years		2.6

Data from Institute of Medicine (IOM), Food and Nutrition Board: *Dietary reference intakes for vitamin A, vitamin K, arsenic, boron, chromium, copper, iodine, iron, manganese, molybdenum, nickel, silicon, vanadium, and zinc,* Washington, DC, 2001, National Academy Press.

*AI (adequate intake)—the observed average or experimentally determined intake by a defined population or subgroup that seems to sustain a defined nutritional status, such as growth rate, normal circulating nutrient values, or other functional indicators of health. The AI is used if insufficient scientific evidence is available to derive an estimated average requirement. For healthy infants receiving human milk, AI is the mean intake. *The AI is not equivalent to an RDA.*

Dental Considerations

- Inhaling manganese dust can be toxic. Patients whose occupations expose them to increased inhalation of manganese (i.e., factory workers, welders, or manganese miners) may exhibit psychotic symptoms or Parkinson-like symptoms.

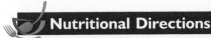

Nutritional Directions

- Phytate and fiber in bran, tannins in tea, and oxalic acid in spinach inhibit absorption of manganese.
- Consistent low iron intake results in more manganese absorption.
- Excess manganese can produce iron-deficiency anemia.[2]
- Manganese should not be confused with magnesium.

MOLYBDENUM

Physiological Roles

Molybdenum functions as an enzyme cofactor. Molybdenum, a trace element present in teeth, may inhibit caries formation. Studies with humans and animals have been inconsistent, however, and molybdenum is not clinically recommended for prevention of dental caries. No mechanism has been proposed for how molybdenum could inhibit caries formation, but rodent studies suggest that molybdenum affects crown morphology.

Requirements

The RDA for molybdenum is 45 µg per day for adults. The UL is set at 2000 µg per day for adults (Table 10-6).

Table 10-6	Institute of Medicine recommendations for molybdenum				
	EAR (µg/day)*		RDA (µg/day)†		AI (µg/day)‡
Life Stage	Male	Female	Male	Female	
Birth–6 months	—	—	—	—	2
7-12 months	—	—	—	—	3
1-3 years	13	13	17	17	
4-8 years	17	17	22	22	
9-13 years	26	26	34	34	
14-18 years	33	33	43	43	
>18 years	34	34	45	45	
Pregnancy					
14-50 years		40		50	
Lactation					
14-18 years		35		50	
19-50 years		36		50	

Data from Institute of Medicine (IOM), Food and Nutrition Board: *Dietary reference intakes for vitamin A, vitamin K, arsenic, boron, chromium, copper, iodine, iron, manganese, molybdenum, nickel, silicon, vanadium, and zinc,* Washington, DC, 2001, National Academy Press.
*EAR (estimated average requirement)—the intake that meets the estimated nutrient needs of half of the individuals in a group.
†RDA (recommended dietary allowance)—the intake that meets the nutrient needs of almost all (97% to 98%) individuals in a group.
‡AI (adequate intake)—the observed average or experimentally set intake by a defined population or subgroup that seems to sustain a defined nutritional status, such as growth rate, normal circulating nutrient values, or other functional indicators of health. An AI is used if insufficient scientific evidence is available to derive an EAR. For healthy human milk–fed infants, the AI is the mean intake. *The AI is not equivalent to an RDA.*

Sources

Legumes, whole-grain cereals, milk, liver, nuts, and many vegetables are good sources.

Hyper States and Hypo States

Except for deficiency reported during administration of TPN, molybdenum deficiency has not been documented in the United States.

Dental Considerations

- Consumption of large quantities of molybdenum may result in copper deficiency, making the patient prone to anemia and risk of gout.[2]

Nutritional Directions

- Milk and whole grains are good sources of molybdenum.

ULTRATRACE ELEMENTS

Many ultratrace elements have been studied for their potential influence on dental caries. Results of research investigations are complicated by many factors. Nevertheless, some studies suggest relationships between some ultratrace elements and the development of caries in humans or animals. Further research is warranted to determine the mechanism of their effects.

More attention has been given to ultratrace elements as contaminants in the environment and foods. Some are considered to have no harmful effects and are used therapeutically, such as aluminum in antacids.

Boron

Boron may have an effect on metabolism of calcium, phosphorus, magnesium, or vitamin D, and may be needed to maintain membrane structure. Inadequate amounts of vitamin D increase the boron requirement. Boron, along with fluoride, is necessary for development and maintenance of strong, healthy bones. Dietary intake may also have an association with inflammation.[3] Boron is principally present in foods of plant origin, especially fruits, vegetables, nuts, legumes, and wine.

Boron deficiency affects mineral metabolism. Patients with disturbed mineral metabolic disorders of unknown etiology, such as osteoporosis, may be deficient in boron.

Nickel

The physiological role of nickel is still unclear. It may be involved in the metabolism of vitamin B₁₂ and folic acid. Nickel deficiency results in suboptimal growth in animals. Inadequate nickel alters trace-element composition of bone and impairs iron use. Good sources of nickel include dried beans and peas, grains, nuts, and chocolate.

Silicon

Silicon contributes to the structure and resilience of collagen, elastin, and polysaccharides. Silicon is present in tooth enamel in larger amounts than most other trace elements, but its function, if any, is unknown. Deficiencies in animal studies result in depressed collagen in bone and long bone abnormalities, resulting in malformed joints and defective bone growth. Whole grains and root vegetables are good food sources.

Tin

Tin has no known function in development or maintenance of bone, but it may affect bone metabolism because tin accumulates in bone. The absorption of tin can alter use of calcium and zinc, affecting bone growth and maintenance. Animal studies show that a high dietary level of tin results in decreased collagen synthesis and decreased compressive strength of bones. Although results of studies are inconsistent, several investigators believe that stannous (chemical term for tin) fluoride exhibits more cariostatic activity than other fluoride compounds by reducing plaque biofilm and gingivitis.

Most Americans consume only minimal amounts of tin daily because most foods contain trace amounts of tin. Foods packed in tin cans that are totally coated with lacquer contain very little tin, but acidic foods, such as pineapple and orange juice and tomato sauce, packed in cans that are not coated with lacquer contain significant amounts of tin. Other sources of tin include stannous chloride, approved for use as a food additive, and stannous fluoride, the active ingredient in some self-applied dentifrices and mouth rinses.

Aluminum

Aluminum probably is not an essential nutrient; its presence in the body seems to be harmful. Under normal conditions, very little aluminum is absorbed; the kidneys excrete about the same amount as is absorbed.

Aluminum accumulates in bone and has been observed to cause osteodystrophy (defective bone formation) in patients who have received aluminum from routes other than through the gastrointestinal tract. Water used in intravenous solutions and dialysis fluid is sometimes contaminated with aluminum. The kidneys are frequently unable to remove the daily load of aluminum present in these fluids, causing undesirable effects. Aluminum content of these fluids has been reduced, but may still be high because of naturally-occurring aluminum in the water used to make the solutions. Aluminum accumulation can occur through oral ingestion of aluminum hydroxide antacids and from the diet.

Aluminum is also present in all dental tissues. Dental caries may be reduced because aluminum enhances the uptake and retention of fluoride and enhances the cariostatic activity of fluoride. Solubility of enamel is decreased, and plaque biofilm formation and acidogenicity are inhibited by aluminum.

Lead

Much information is available about the harmful effects of lead in the body, but little is known about its beneficial role or its essentiality. As a result of implementation of aggressive public health measures, blood lead levels have decreased markedly since the late 1970s.

Lead is more readily absorbed from the gastrointestinal tract during infancy and early childhood than in adulthood, meaning children are more susceptible to lead exposure. Lead is ingested from toddlers' normal hand-to-mouth activities; in older children, playing with dirt or lead-contaminated objects may result in lead ingestion. Milk intake results in reduced lead absorption. Nutritional status can influence susceptibility to lead toxicity. Lead is also a contaminant in water, most commonly resulting from corroding lead pipes. Therefore, it cannot be directly detected. The EPA requires water systems to control the level of lead to less than 15 ppb.[4]

Inorganic lead can have detrimental effects on children. Even low levels of lead exposure may impair intellectual performance. With elevated serum lead levels, general cognitive, verbal, and perceptual abilities are increasingly affected by slower learning aptitudes, which appear to be irreversible. Lead toxicity is most pronounced in children and fetuses because it can damage the central nervous system and kidneys. Lead also decreases normal production of red blood cells.

A large proportion of absorbed lead is incorporated into the skeleton and teeth. Lead deposited in the enamel matrix has been associated with pitting hypoplasia. The amount of lead in shed deciduous teeth can be used as an index of lead exposure. The effects of lead stored in the bones and teeth are unknown. Elevated levels of lead in the blood may be associated with periodontitis.

Lithium

Lithium is another ultratrace element found in calcified structures. As lithium accumulates in animal bones, calcium content decreases. When this substitution is made in apatite of bone and teeth, the structure and solubility properties are changed. A decreased calcium-to-phosphorus ratio of apatite caused by lithium substitution is accompanied by an increase in acid solubility.

Vanadium

Studies on the essentiality of vanadium have been inconsistent in their findings. Most research has not found that vanadium deficiency consistently impairs any biological function in animals. Vanadium is readily incorporated into areas of rapid mineralization of bones and tooth dentin, but its role in bones and teeth is unknown.

The cariostatic effect of vanadium has been studied. Although an inverse correlation between vanadium content in drinking water and caries incidence was observed in one study, animal experiments are inconclusive in their results. It has been hypothesized that vanadium may exchange for phosphorus in the apatite tooth substance. Shellfish, mushrooms, and parsley contain small amounts of vanadium.

Mercury

Mercury is not a nutrient, but this toxic substance is often found in the food and water supply either naturally in the environment or emitted by industrial pollution. Even a trace amount of mercury can cause neurological and developmental problems in infants and young children. It is also harmful to the kidney and cardiovascular system. The U.S. Food and Drug Administration (FDA) monitors the presence of contaminants in food and water, issuing warnings as needed. In 2001, the FDA advised women of childbearing age, pregnant

and nursing women, and young children to avoid shark, swordfish, mackerel, and tilefish because of the high levels of methyl mercury in them. In 2004, the FDA and EPA issued a warning to potentially vulnerable consumers (i.e., young children and pregnant and nursing women) to limit their intake of albacore tuna to less than 6 oz per week because of its mercury content. The EPA set 2 ppb as the maximum contaminant level for mercury in water.[5]

Nutritional Directions

- A diet low in boron increases calcium excretion, so patients with osteoporosis should be encouraged to consume recommended amounts of fresh fruits and vegetables.
- Acidic foods and foods with high nitrate content, such as tomatoes, can accumulate very high levels of tin if left in unlaquered, opened cans in the refrigerator for more than 3 days. Once opened, these foods should be stored in glass or plastic containers.
- Consumption of a variety of foods and fluids helps people obtain trace minerals and avoid excessive amounts.
- Unrefined foods generally provide more trace minerals than highly refined foods.
- Supplements of these trace elements are not encouraged.
- Some bone meal and oyster shell used for calcium supplementation may contain dangerous amounts of lead.
- Lead does not accumulate in fish, but does in some shellfish (e.g., mussels).[4]
- Those who obtain water from a well, can contact the local health department or water system for information on contaminants, or they may have the water tested for contaminants.[5]

Dental Considerations

- Boron deficiency signs may be related to abnormalities in vitamin D, calcium, phosphorus, or magnesium levels.
- Aluminum is a cariostatic agent, especially in combination with fluoride.
- Seafood is a good source of important nutrients, including omega-3 fats. The AHA recommends at least two servings of fish each week. Encourage fish and shellfish with lower mercury levels, such as salmon, clams, sardines, crabs, tilapia, scallops, catfish, perch, whitefish, canned tuna, cod, and mahi-mahi. (Large, older fish higher on the food chain, such as shark and swordfish, king mackerel, or tilefish, are the leading sources of mercury in the diet.)

HEALTH APPLICATION 10 Alzheimer Disease

Identified more than 100 years ago, Alzheimer disease is the most common type of dementia in individuals, comprising 60% to 80% of dementia cases. An estimated 5.4 million Americans have Alzheimer disease; 5.2 million of those individuals are older than 65 years. About half of those with Alzheimer disease may be undiagnosed. Alzheimer disease is the seventh leading cause of death. Direct and indirect healthcare costs together exceed $200 billion. The incidence increases with age: 13% of individuals older than 65 years and 45% of individuals older than 85 years have Alzheimer disease.[6] It is a slowly progressive disease, characterized by deterioration of judgment, orientation, memory, personality, and intellectual capability, typically with a period of 8 to 10 years between onset and death. Individuals progress through the disease at varying rates.

Known risk factors for developing Alzheimer disease include age, family history of Alzheimer disease, head trauma, and genetic disposition. Currently, there is no treatment available to delay or stop the progressive deterioration of brain cells in Alzheimer disease. Research suggests the health of the brain is a key to preventing Alzheimer disease. The Alzheimer's Association has compiled a list of 10 ways to "Maintain Your Brain" (Box 10-1).

Although much has been learned about the disease, a specific cause has not been determined. Different types of nerve

cells in the brain degenerate and die. Similarities observed between aluminum toxicity and Alzheimer disease led to the hypothesis that dietary or environmental aluminum might be involved. As a result, the public was inaccurately advised that aluminum cookware could be toxic. Chelation therapy was advocated to remove aluminum from the body as an unorthodox treatment for Alzheimer disease. However, brain lesions and neurotransmitter changes seen in aluminum toxicity and Alzheimer disease are different. In contrast to the subtle cognitive changes associated with Alzheimer disease, aluminum toxicity manifests with motor dysfunction.

A key element of disease management is early diagnosis to initiate therapy. Some causes of dementia can be treated, and some of the symptoms can possibly be reversed. A series of evaluations are used to make a clinical diagnosis of Alzheimer disease, including medical and behavioral assessments. Often, reports from family members and friends provide valuable information regarding mental status of the individual. The Alzheimer's Association has developed "warning signs" for detection of Alzheimer disease (Box 10-2).

The FDA has approved five medications to improve cognitive symptoms of Alzheimer disease. Behavioral and psychiatric symptoms, such as physical or verbal outbursts, restlessness, hallucinations, and delusions, are treated either with medications prescribed to control symptoms or with nondrug

Continued

HEALTH APPLICATION 10   Alzheimer Disease—cont'd

treatments. Vitamin E supplementation is sometimes pre-scribed by the healthcare provider because it is an antioxidant and may protect nerve cells. Although vitamin E may slightly delay the loss of ability to perform daily activities, it should only be used under the supervision of a healthcare provider.

Many herbal remedies, vitamins, and other nutrition sup-plements are promoted as memory enhancers or treatments. Studies involving these alternative therapies have not substan-tiated these claims. Currently, promoters of ginkgo biloba (a plant extract), huperzine A (a moss extract), coenzyme Q10 (an antioxidant naturally occurring in the body), coral calcium, omega-3 fatty acids, tramiprosate (an amino acid), and phos-phatidylserine (a phospholipid) claim these products can cure or prevent Alzheimer disease.[7] Further scientific studies are required not only to determine the effectiveness of alternative nutritional therapies, but also to observe their interaction with other drugs and nutrients.

Alzheimer disease has significant effects on nutrition and hydration status. Initially, individuals with Alzheimer disease may have problems with food purchasing and meal prepara-tion. Appetite and food intake fluctuate with mood swings and increasing confusion. Forgetting when they last ate, they may skip some meals, eat twice, or forget about food cooking on the stove. Changes in food preferences may be tied to a decline in olfactory function. Sweet and salty foods are preferred.

During the middle phase of the illness, individuals with Alzheimer disease often become agitated and may pace all night, increasing caloric expenditure. Weight loss is common. Energy requirements may increase by 1600 kcal per day, and frequent snacking is necessary to maintain body weight. Because of abnormal sleep patterns, caffeine may need to be discontinued to avoid further stimulation of the central nervous system,

Appetite is usually good, but caloric intake may be inade-quate to maintain body weight unless snacks or liquid nutri-tional supplements or both are provided. Food hoarding (to accumulate or stash food) or failure to chew food sufficiently increases the risk of choking. Ability to use utensils deterio-rates. Finger foods may be more appropriate to allow continu-ation of self-feeding. Foods should be cut up and offered in bite-size pieces. Serving foods one at a time helps decrease confusion. A larger meal at midday, when cognitive abilities are at their peak, is recommended.

During the final stage, which is characterized by severe intellectual impairment, food may not be recognized and may be refused. The individual also may forget how to swallow. Enteral feedings (the provision of nutrients through a tube placed in the nose, stomach, or small intestine) are usually indicated to maintain nutritional status as a result of impaired cognition.

BOX 10-1   Maintain Your Brain

- Stay physically active. Physical exercise is essential for main-taining good blood flow to the brain as well as to encour-age new brain cells. It also can significantly reduce the risk of heart disease, stroke and diabetes, thereby protecting against those risk factors for Alzheimer disease.
- Adopt a brain-healthy diet. Research suggests that high cho-lesterol may contribute to stroke and brain cell damage. A low fat, low cholesterol diet is advisable. There is growing evidence that antioxidants may help protect brain cells.
- Remain socially active. Social activity not only makes physical and mental activity more enjoyable, it can reduce stress levels, which helps maintain healthy connections among brain cells.
- Stay mentally active. Mentally stimulating activities strengthen brain cells and the connections between them, and may even create new nerve cells.

Data from Alzheimer's Association: *Brain health*. Accessed August 19, 2013. Available at: www.alz.org/we_can_help_brain_health_maintain_your_brain.asp

BOX 10-2   Warning Signs of Alzheimer Disease

- Memory loss that disrupts daily life
- Challenges in planning or solving problems
- Difficulty performing familiar tasks
- Confusion with time or place
- Trouble understanding visual images and spatial relationships
- New problems with words in speaking or writing
- Misplacing things or losing the ability to retrace steps
- Decreased or poor judgment
- Withdrawal from work or social activities
- Changes in mood or personality

Data from Alzheimer's Association: *Symptoms of Alzheimer's*. Accessed August 19, 2013. Available at: http://www.alz.org/alzheimers_disease_symptoms_of_alzheimers.asp

Case Application for the Dental Hygienist

A young female executive confides in you that she always feels tired and sometimes finds it difficult to get through the day. When you bring up the subject of nutrition, she tells you that she read a book about the importance of minerals and began taking supplements approximately one year ago. These self-prescribed supplements include selenium and zinc. She also takes a vitamin C supplement daily. She is concerned about a lack of energy, which she relates to her poor eating habits. Meals are frequently missed or eaten at her desk.

Nutritional Assessment
- Willingness to learn
- Knowledge level regarding food consumption guidelines, such as the *MyPlate* and the *Dietary Guidelines*
- Desire for improving nutritional and general health
- Cultural or religious influences
- Knowledge of the physiological roles of vitamins and minerals
- Recognition of the interactive effects of vitamins and minerals, especially when taken in excess of RDAs

Nutritional Diagnosis
Health-seeking behaviors related to inadequate knowledge of optimal nutrition, healthy eating habits, and the deleterious effects associated with consumption of excess vitamins and minerals.

Nutritional Goals
The patient will use the *Dietary Guidelines* and *MyPlate* to improve her eating pattern and dietary intake of nutrient-dense foods. The patient will recognize the health risks associated with improper supplementation and will decrease reliance on nutritional supplements.

Nutritional Implementation
Intervention: Review the *Dietary Guidelines* and discuss how these guidelines support healthy eating habits and disease prevention.
Rationale: Healthy dietary practices can improve energy reserves and overall nutritional status.
Intervention: Encourage consumption of a variety of foods from each of the five main food groups.
Rationale: A nutritious diet is composed of a variety of foods that together supply all the essential nutrients needed for good health.

Intervention: Review serving sizes and emphasize more servings of nutrient-dense foods. Encourage a meal timetable that is planned according to her daily schedule.
Rationale: Eating an inadequate number of kilocalories from foods that are limited in nutrients can contribute to fatigue and poor nutrition. Scheduled mealtimes throughout the day help to supply an adequate number of kilocalories when appropriate serving sizes of nutritious food are selected.
Intervention: Describe the body's metabolic need for vitamins and minerals. Inform the patient that a well-balanced diet can supply all the nutrients needed without supplementation.
Rationale: Vitamins and minerals are required for normal metabolic and physiological functions. When supplements are taken in excess of the RDAs, some nutrients can be harmful.
Intervention: Describe how zinc supplements interact with copper absorption and relate to fatigue. Inform the patient that large amounts of vitamin C in excess of the RDAs may decrease the availability of copper in the blood. List the toxic effects of selenium.
Rationale: Because most minerals are supplied by a varied diet, supplementation can result in toxic levels and harmful nutrient interactions.
Intervention: Advise the patient to see her healthcare provider if fatigue persists or worsens.
Rationale: Poor dietary intake may act as a contributing factor to fatigue when the actual cause may be related to a systemic disease or condition.

Evaluation
The patient will improve dietary habits by planning meals and snacks each day. Meal planning will accommodate the patient's work schedule. The patient will use *MyPlate* and the *Dietary Guidelines* to improve the nutritional quality and quantity of her diet. The patient can state the symptoms associated with large quantities of zinc, selenium, and vitamin C, and will stop taking supplements. Persistent or worsening symptoms of fatigue will prompt the patient to seek the advice of a healthcare provider.

STUDENT READINESS

1. List all nutrient interactions indicated in this chapter that decrease the absorption or alter the metabolism of another nutrient. Why would a dental hygienist advise a patient to obtain mineral requirements from food sources rather than mineral supplements (unless ordered by a healthcare provider)?
2. Which trace minerals incorporated into enamel are beneficial? Which weaken the tooth, or make it more susceptible to tooth decay?
3. Which element is involved in insulin metabolism?
4. If a patient is concerned about obtaining adequate amounts of trace elements, what are some suggestions that a dental hygienist can make?
5. Name some minerals that may be useful as well as toxic to patients.

References

1. U.S. Environmental Protection Agency: Basic information about chromium in drinking water. Available at www.epa.gov/drink/contaminants/basicinformation/chromium.cfm. Accessed August 19, 2013.
2. Keenan KP, Wallig MA, Haschek WM: Nature via nurture: effect of diet on health, obesity, and safety assessment. *Toxicol Pathol* 41(2):190–209, 2013.
3. Hunt CD: Dietary boron: progress in establishing essential roles in human physiology. *J Trace Elem Med Biol* 26:157–160, 2012.
4. U.S. Environmental Protection Agency: Factsheet on lead in drinking water. Available at http://water.epa.gov/lawsregs/rulesregs/sdwa/lcr/fs_consumer.cfm. Accessed August 19, 2013.
5. U.S. Environmental Protection Agency: Basic information about mercury (inorganic) in drinking water. Available at http://water.epa.gov/drink/contaminants/basicinformation/mercury.cfm. Accessed August 19, 2013.

6. Alzheimer's Association: 2012 Alzheimer's disease facts and figures. *Alzheimers Dement* 8(2):131–168, 2012.

7. Alzheimer's Association: Alternative treatments. Available at http://www.alz.org/professionals_and_researchers_alternative_ treatments_.asp. Accessed August 19, 2013.

ⓔ EVOLVE RESOURCES

Please visit http://evolve.elsevier.com/Stegeman/nutritional for additional practice and study support tools.

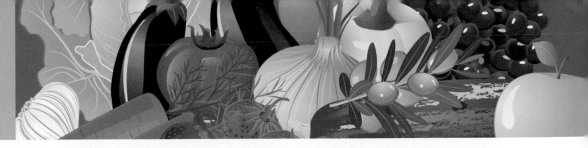

Chapter 11

Vitamins Required for Oral Soft Tissues and Salivary Glands

Student Learning Outcomes

Upon completion of this chapter, the student will be able to achieve the following student learning outcomes:

- Educate the patient on oral soft tissue changes that occur in a B-complex deficiency.
- Differentiate between scientifically-based evidence versus food fads concerning vitamins.
- Explain to a patient who is a vegan why vitamin B_{12} is important and identify appropriate sources.
- Compare and contrast the functions and sources of vitamins and minerals important for healthy oral soft tissues, as well as deficiencies, toxicities, and associated symptoms.

- Identify dental considerations for vitamins closely involved in maintaining healthy oral soft tissues.
- Discuss nutritional directions for vitamins closely involved in maintaining healthy oral soft tissues.
- Describe the association between beriberi and alcoholism.

Key Terms

Achlorhydria
Alternative medicine
Antigenic
Ariboflavinosis
Ataxia
Avidin
Beriberi
Bradycardia
Candida
Cheilosis
Cholinergic
Circumvallate lingual papillae
Complementary medicine
Epithelialization
Filiform papillae
Foliate papillae
Fungating
Fungiform papillae
Glossitis
Glossopyrosis
Herbs
Homeopathy
Hypotonic

Intrinsic factor
Keratinized epithelium
Megaloblastic anemia
Myelin
Naturopathy
Neoplasia
Neural tube defects
Nystagmus
Parasympathetic autonomic nerves
Pellagra
Periodontal disease
Pernicious anemia
Pyogenic
R-binder
Sensory neuropathy
Signs
Spices
Squamous metaplasia
Stomatitis
Sympathetic autonomic nerves
Symptoms
Tachycardia
Thiaminase

PHYSIOLOGY OF SOFT TISSUES

The oral cavity can reflect systemic disease before other **signs** (noticeable to the clinician) and **symptoms** (perceived by the patient) become evident; the condition in the oral cavity may also cause systemic problems by affecting the patient's nutrient intake. The oral cavity is the site of a wide variety of systemic disease manifestations for several reasons: (a) it has a rapid cellular turnover rate, (b) it is under constant assault by microorganisms, and (c) it is a trauma-intense environment.

The systemic circulation provides nutrients and removes metabolic waste products from underlying structures and the salivary glands via the blood supply. Figure 11-1 shows healthy gingiva; changes in color, size, shape, texture, and functional integrity of the oral tissues often reflect systemic nutritional disorders. Signs and symptoms in soft oral tissues can be caused by deficiencies of many of the B-complex vitamins, vitamins C and E, iron, and protein (Box 11-1). Nutritional deficiencies result in similar oral signs and symptoms, such as pain, erythema, atrophy of tissues, and infection. **Pyogenic** (producing pus) and **fungating** (skin lesions with ulcerations, necrosis, and foul smell) microorganisms cause local infections in cracked epithelial surfaces.

Approximately 90% of saliva is produced and secreted by three paired sets of major salivary glands: the parotid, submandibular, and sublingual glands (Fig. 11-2). Additionally, the lips and inner lining of the cheeks are equipped with hundreds of minor salivary glands.

Saliva keeps surfaces of the oral cavity healthy and lubricated and is necessary to maintain functional integrity of taste buds. Solid substances first must be dissolved in saliva to be tasted. Healthy adults produce approximately 1 to 1.5 L/day of saliva. **Sympathetic autonomic nerves** stimulate the body in times of stress and crisis; sympathetic impulses influence salivary composition. **Parasympathetic autonomic nerves** balance or slow down impulses from sympathetic nerves; parasympathetic stimulation increases the amount of saliva secreted.

Compared with plasma, saliva is hypotonic, with its main constituent being water. **Hypotonic** solutions have a lower solute concentration than plasma. Saliva contains more than 20 proteins and glycoproteins, and many electrolytes, including sodium, potassium, calcium, chloride,

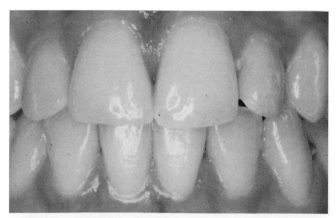

FIGURE 11-1 Normal gingiva. (Courtesy of Barbara D. Altshuler, BSDH, MS, Clinical Assistant Professor, Caruth School of Dental Hygiene, The Texas A&M University System, Baylor College of Dentistry, Dallas, TX.)

BOX 11-1	Vitamins and Minerals Required for Healthy Oral Soft Tissues

Water-Soluble Vitamins
B Vitamins
  Thiamin
  Riboflavin
  Niacin
  Vitamin B$_6$
  Folate
  Vitamin B$_{12}$
  Pantothenic acid
  Biotin
Vitamin C

Fat-Soluble Vitamins
Vitamin A
Vitamin E

Minerals
Iron
Zinc
Iodine

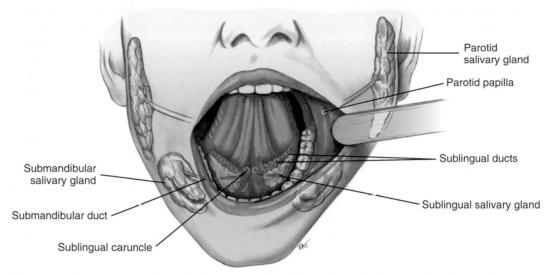

FIGURE 11-2 The major salivary glands and associated structures. (From Fehrenbach MJ, Herring SW: *Illustrated anatomy of the head and neck*, ed 4, Philadelphia, 2012, Elsevier Saunders.)

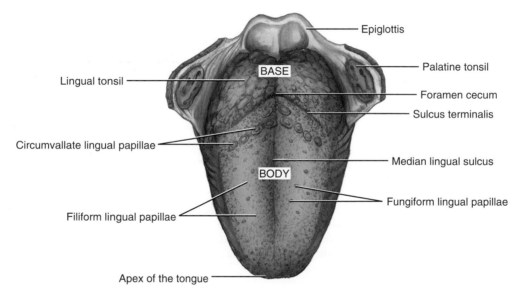

FIGURE 11-3 Papillae on the tongue with its landmarks noted. (From Fehrenbach MJ, Herring SW: *Illustrated anatomy of the head and neck*, ed 4, Philadelphia, 2012, Elsevier Saunders.)

bicarbonate, inorganic phosphate, magnesium, sulfate, iodide, and fluoride. Saliva functions as a buffer to maintain the oral pH. Buffering substances increase their acid or alkali content to change the pH of the solution. The pH of unstimulated saliva is approximately 6.1, but this can rise to 7.8 at high flow rates. Antimicrobial properties of saliva provide protection and remove toxins, such as tobacco smoke.

The oral cavity is lined with nonkeratinized mucosa except for the hard palate, dorsum of the tongue, and gingiva surrounding the teeth, which are covered with a **keratinized epithelium** (a protein, main component of epidermis and horny tissues). The oral cavity may contain **antigenic** (capable of inducing an immune response with specific

antibodies) substances; the oral mucosa separates a potentially adverse environment from underlying connective tissue.

Mucosal cells have a very rapid turnover rate, resulting in complete turnover in 3 to 5 days. Rapid generation of new cells in the oral epithelia provides replacement tissue for trauma resulting from friction of the teeth and mastication. Additionally, hundreds of cells in the filiform papillae and fungiform papillae are in constant transition, from their anabolism until their catabolism (Fig. 11-3). **Filiform papillae** are smooth, threadlike structures on the dorsum surface of the tongue, whereas **fungiform papillae** are red, mushroom-shaped structures scattered throughout the filiform papillae.

Taste buds are located on the foliate papillae (vertical grooves located on the lateral borders of the tongue), circumvallate lingual papillae (large, mushroom-shaped distinct structures forming a V) on the dorsal surface, and the fungiform papillae of the tongue. A loss of fungiform and foliate papillae leads to loss of taste buds and changes in taste acuity.

Many filiform papillae cover the anterior two-thirds of the tongue. If the filiform papillae become denuded or atrophied, the tongue appears red and pebbled, giving it a strawberry-like appearance. Fungiform papillae are bright red because of a rich vascular supply. Keratinized cells normally cover the fungiform papillae on the tongue surface. Chronic severe nutrient deficiencies result in loss of fungiform papillae and a smooth red tongue.

Dental Considerations

- Because of rapid turnover rate of oral tissues, the first signs of nutritional deficiency are frequently evident in the oral cavity. The glossal epithelium is usually the first to be affected, followed by areas around the lips. Assess patients for oral signs of nutritional deficiencies.
- The tongue may become edematous as a result of disease or nutritional deficiency.
- Angular cheilitis or **cheilosis** (cracks around the corners of the mouth) and **glossitis** (inflammation of the tongue) are commonly associated with deficiencies of several B-complex vitamins.
- Saliva aids in the ability to speak properly, and taste and swallow foods.
- The composition of saliva affects taste and can be a determining factor in food choices.
- Xerostomia may result in increased incidence of caries, **stomatitis** (inflammation of oral mucosa), gingival inflammation, and greater susceptibility to oral infections (see Chapter 19).
- Saliva may be used to diagnose some local and systemic diseases and heavy-metal toxicity, such as mercury toxicity.
- Salivary secretion is controlled primarily by **cholinergic** (nerves stimulated by acetylcholine) parasympathetic (autonomic) nerves; patients taking anticholinergic medications (which usually contain atropine) exhibit decreased salivary flow. These medications may be prescribed for **bradycardia** (low heart rate), diarrhea, peptic ulcers, and occasionally asthma.

Nutritional Directions

- Saliva helps maintain integrity of the teeth, tongue, and mucous membranes of the oral and oropharyngeal areas.
- Nutritional abnormalities affect oral soft tissues in a variety of ways (e.g., angular cheilitis and glossitis).

THIAMIN (VITAMIN B₁)

Physiological Roles

Thiamin functions as a coenzyme in metabolism of energy nutrients via the TCA cycle (or Krebs or citric acid cycle) to produce energy. This role makes it crucial for normal functioning of the brain, nerves, muscles, and heart. However, the main effects of thiamin deficiency are disturbances of carbohydrate metabolism, which is impossible without thiamin. Thiamin is a component necessary for the synthesis of niacin, and it also helps regulate appetite. It is a constituent of enzymes that degrade sucrose to organic acids that can ultimately dissolve tooth enamel.

Requirements

Thiamin is involved in using carbohydrates as kilocalories; the requirement is based on total caloric need. The recommended dietary allowance (RDA) for men (≥14 years old) is 1.2 mg/day and for women (≥19 years old) is 1.1 mg/day (Table 11-1). Participation in rigorous physical activity uses more energy, so more thiamin is required. Also, requirements are increased by pregnancy and lactation, hemodialysis or peritoneal dialysis, fever, hyperthyroidism, cardiac conditions, alcoholism, and the use of loop diuretics. No known adverse effects are evident from excessive thiamin intake, including supplements. Although a tolerable upper intake level (UL) is not established for thiamin, care should be taken when consumption routinely exceeds the RDA.

Sources

Thiamin is widely distributed in foods, and intake of a variety of foods, including enriched grains or whole grains, can

Table 11-1	Institute of Medicine recommendations for thiamin				
	EAR (mg/day)*		RDA (mg/day)†		
Life Stage	Male	Female	Male	Female	AI (mg/day)‡
0-6 months					0.2
7-12 months					0.3
1-3 years	0.4	0.4	0.5	0.5	
4-8 years	0.5	0.5	0.6	0.6	
9-13 years	0.7	0.7	0.9	0.9	
14-18 years	1	1	1.2	1	
≥19 years	1	0.9	1.2	1.1	
Pregnancy					
14-50 years		1.2		1.4	
Lactation					
14-50 years		1.2		1.4	

Data from Institute of Medicine (IOM), Food and Nutrition Board: *Dietary reference intakes for thiamin, riboflavin, niacin, vitamin B₆, folate, vitamin B₁₂, pantothenic acid, biotin, and choline*, Washington, DC, 1998, National Academy Press.

*EAR (estimated average requirement)—the intake that meets the estimated nutrient needs of half of the individuals in a group.

†RDA (recommended dietary allowance)—the intake that meets the nutrient needs of almost all (97% to 98%) individuals in a group.

‡AI (adequate intake)—the observed average or experimentally set intake by a defined population or subgroup that seems to sustain a defined nutritional status, such as growth rate, normal circulating nutrient values, or other functional indicators of health. An AI is used if insufficient scientific evidence is available to derive an EAR. For healthy human milk–fed infants, the AI is the mean intake. *The AI is not equivalent to a RDA.*

Table 11-2	Thiamin content of selected foods	
Food	**Portion**	**Thiamin (mg)**
Total, whole grain	1 cup	2.0
Wheaties	1 cup	1.0
Trail mix, tropical	1 cup	0.63
Lean pork chop, broiled	3 oz	0.44
Green peas, cooked	1 cup	0.41
Bagel, wheat	3½-4 inches	0.40
White rice, enriched, cooked	1 cup	0.26
Bread, white, enriched	1 slice	0.15
Bread, whole-wheat	1 slice	0.13
Sweet potato, baked	1 cup	0.12
Peanuts, dry roasted	1 oz	0.12

Data from U.S. Department of Agriculture, Agricultural Research Service. *USDA national nutrient database for standard reference, release 26, 2013.* Nutrient Data Laboratory Home Page. Accessed August 30, 2013. Available at: http://www.ars.usda.gov/nutrientdata

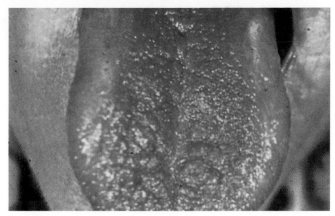

FIGURE 11-4 Glossitis associated with thiamin deficiency. (From American Dental Association Council on Dental Therapeutics: *Oral manifestations of metabolic and deficiency changes*, Chicago.)

ensure adequate amounts (Table 11-2). Approximately 40% of thiamin intake is provided by enriched breads, cereals, and pasta. (Because of enrichment, enriched breads may contain almost twice as much thiamin as whole grains). In the meat group, pork is an exceptionally good source. Other good sources include nuts and legumes. Following the guidelines for *MyPlate* and eating a variety of foods ensures adequate intake.

Hypo States

Thiamin is required for metabolism of carbohydrates, proteins, and fats; insufficient intake adversely affects most organ systems. Primary dietary deficiency usually occurs in developing countries where polished rice is the staple diet. In developed countries, thiamin deficiency is secondary to alcoholism, ingestion of raw fish containing microbial thiaminase (an enzyme that inactivates thiamin), chronic febrile states, and total parenteral nutrition (TPN). Cooking deactivates thiaminase.

Thiamin is called the "morale vitamin" because short-term deficiency causes patients to become depressed, irritable, anorexic, fatigued, and unable to concentrate. The brain and central nervous system, almost entirely dependent on glucose for energy, are seriously impaired when thiamin is unavailable.

Severe thiamin deficiency results in beriberi, which causes extensive damage to the nervous and cardiovascular systems. Beriberi means "I cannot"; patients with this severe thiamin deficiency cannot move easily. The classic chronic form of beriberi manifests with impairment of sensory and motor function without involvement of the central nervous system. Other symptoms include muscular wasting (dry beriberi), edema (wet beriberi), deep muscle pain in the calves, peripheral paralysis, tachycardia (rapid heartbeat), and an enlarged heart.

Whether or not a thiamin deficiency is evident in oral tissues is controversial. Some clinicians have associated a flabby, red, and edematous tongue with thiamin deficiency

(Fig. 11-4). The fungiform papillae become enlarged and hyperemic (engorged with blood).

Wernicke-Korsakoff syndrome is another thiamin deficiency disease, typically associated with alcoholism, which is characterized by mental confusion, nystagmus (involuntary rapid movement of the eyeball), and ataxia (a gait disorder characterized by uncoordinated muscle movements). These symptoms occur most frequently in malnourished alcoholics. Alcohol intake increases thiamin requirement, yet total nutrient intake is usually poor in alcoholics. Early diagnosis is essential to initiate thiamin therapy early in the course of the disease to prevent permanent damage and death.

Dental Considerations

- A careful medical, social, and dietary history, including a clinical assessment of the oral cavity, alcohol consumption, and activity level, help identify early stages of thiamin deficiency.
- Risk of alcohol abuse or dependence is based on how much and how often an individual drinks. Moderation is considered 4 to 14 drinks per week for men and 3 to 11 drinks per week for women; five or more drinks per occasion is considered excessive for any adult.
- Vitamin deficiencies seldom occur in isolation. If a deficiency is suspected, symptoms of other vitamin B deficiencies also may be present.
- Because thiamin is essential for carbohydrate metabolism, a thiamin deficiency is closely linked to aberrations of brain function. For patients who are confused or have altered thought processes, assess nutrient intake.
- Carbohydrate loading or a very-high-carbohydrate diet and high physical activity slightly increase the thiamin requirement. (Generally, increased food intake results in increased thiamin consumption.)
- Thiamin deficiency has been reported in patients after gastrectomy and bariatric surgery (gastric bypass) related to decreased absorption.
- Although immediate clinical response to thiamin therapy is often dramatic, ultimate recovery may be incomplete, and relapses may occur, especially if precipitating factors persist.
- Massive amounts (1000 times greater than the RDA) of thiamin suppress the respiratory system and cause death.

Table 11-3	Institute of Medicine recommendations for riboflavin				
	EAR (mg/day)*		RDA (mg/day)†		
Life Stage	Male	Female	Male	Female	AI (mg/day)‡
0-6 months					0.3
7-12 months					0.4
1-3 years	0.4	0.4	0.5	0.5	
4-8 years	0.5	0.5	0.6	0.6	
9-13 years	0.8	0.8	0.9	0.9	
14-18 years	1.1	0.9	1.3	1	
≥19 years	1.1	0.9	1.3	1.1	
Pregnancy					
14-50 years		1.2		1.4	
Lactation					
14-50 years		1.3		1.6	

Data from Institute of Medicine (IOM), Food and Nutrition Board: *Dietary reference intakes for thiamin, riboflavin, niacin, vitamin B₆, folate, vitamin B₁₂, pantothenic acid, biotin, and choline,* Washington, DC, 1998, National Academy Press.

*EAR (estimated average requirement)—the intake that meets the estimated nutrient needs of half of the individuals in a group.

†RDA (recommended dietary allowance)—the intake that meets the nutrient needs of almost all (97% to 98%) individuals in a group.

‡AI (adequate intake)—the observed average or experimentally set intake by a defined population or subgroup that seems to sustain a defined nutritional status, such as growth rate, normal circulating nutrient values, or other functional indicators of health. An AI is used if insufficient scientific evidence is available to derive an EAR. For healthy human milk–fed infants, the AI is the mean intake. *The AI is not equivalent to a RDA.*

Nutritional Directions

- Raw fish contains an active enzyme, thiaminase, which destroys thiamin.
- Baking soda added to cooking water to enhance the color of vegetables destroys thiamin.
- Overcooking and high temperatures destroy thiamin.
- Antacids reduce use of thiamin.
- Some diuretics can increase thiamin excretion.
- The RDA is higher than the average need for an individual. If the amount consumed is slightly under the listed RDA, most individuals will still be healthy. However, the lower the requirement of a vitamin or mineral, the greater the risk of a deficiency.

RIBOFLAVIN (VITAMIN B₂)

Physiological Roles

Riboflavin functions as a coenzyme in metabolism of carbohydrate, protein, and fat to release cellular energy. Closely related to the metabolism of protein, all conditions requiring increases in protein (e.g., growth spurts or burns) lead to additional riboflavin requirements. Riboflavin is also essential for healthy eyes and skin, and maintenance of mucous membranes. Along with thiamin, riboflavin is necessary for synthesis of niacin.

Requirements

As shown in Table 11-3, the Institute of Medicine (IOM) recommends an intake of 1.3 mg/day for men (14 years old and older) and 1.1 mg/day for women (19 years old and older). This level is influenced by individual energy

Table 11-4	Riboflavin content of selected foods	
Food	Portion	Riboflavin (mg)
Beef liver, braised	3 oz	3.08
Total, whole grain	1 cup	2.28
Wheaties	1 cup	1.12
Cheese, American	1 oz	0.67
Custard, egg	1 cup	0.67
Yogurt, low-fat, plain	8 oz	0.49
Milk, skim	1 cup	0.45
Cottage cheese, low-fat	1 cup	0.45
Spinach, cooked	1 cup	0.43
Pork loin, lean only, baked	3 oz	0.28
Egg, hard boiled	1	0.26
Cornbread	1 slice	0.19
Chicken breast, meat only, roasted	1	0.16
Cheese, cheddar	1 oz	0.11

Data from U.S. Department of Agriculture, Agricultural Research Service. *USDA national nutrient database for standard reference, release 26, 2013.* Nutrient Data Laboratory Home Page. Accessed August 30, 2013: http://www.ars.usda.gov/nutrientdata

requirements. Additionally, when nitrogen balance is positive, more riboflavin is retained. No UL has been established.

Sources

Although milk and milk products are excellent sources of riboflavin, approximately 30% of the dietary intake is furnished by foods in the grain group (Table 11-4). Meat, poultry, and fish also provide about one-fourth of the dietary requirement.

Hypo States

The body carefully guards its limited riboflavin stores. Even in severe deficiency, one-third of the normal amount is present in the liver, kidney, and heart. Primary riboflavin deficiency is uncommon, but is encountered in patients with multiple nutrient deficiencies as a result of poor nutrient absorption or use. Because riboflavin is essential in vitamin B₆ and niacin functions, riboflavin deficiency leads to symptoms related to secondary deficiency of these nutrients.

Symptoms associated with riboflavin deficiency, or **ariboflavinosis**, include angular cheilitis (Fig. 11-5), glossitis (Fig. 11-6), dermatitis, and anemia. With consistently inadequate intake, these symptoms may be observed within 8 weeks. Along with angular cheilosis, the lips may become extremely

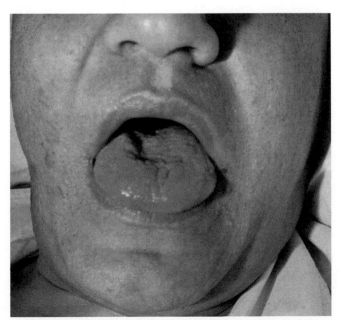

FIGURE 11-5 Angular cheilitis. (From Ibsen OAC, Phelan JA: *Oral pathology for the dental hygienist*, ed 6, St Louis, 2014, Elsevier Saunders.)

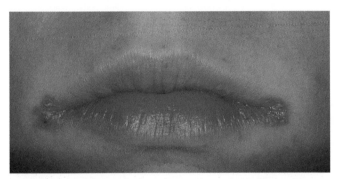

FIGURE 11-6 Glossitis associated with severe riboflavin deficiency. (From McLaren DS: *A colour atlas and text of diet-related disorders*, ed 2, London, 1992, Mosby-Year Book.)

red and smooth. Fungiform papillae become swollen and slightly flattened and mushroom-shaped during early stages of riboflavin deficiency; the tongue has a pebbly or granular appearance. Severe chronic deficiencies lead to progressive papillary atrophy and patchy, irregular denudation of the tongue. The tongue may become purplish red or magenta in color because of vascular proliferation and decreased circulation. In more advanced cases, the entire tongue may become atrophic and smooth (Fig. 11-6). These symptoms, especially glossitis and dermatitis, may be secondary to vitamin B₆ deficiency.

Dental Considerations

- Hyperthyroidism, fevers, the added stress of injuries or surgery, excessive alcohol consumption, and malabsorption syndromes increase riboflavin requirements. Assess patients with these conditions for signs of deficiency: cheilitis, papillary atrophy, glossitis, and dermatitis.
- Congenital facial abnormalities may occur if the mother is deficient in riboflavin at the time of conception.
- Bilateral cheilosis may not be due to riboflavin deficiency; consider improperly constructed dentures, fungal (candidiasis) or yeast infection, and aging that may contribute to cheilosis.
- Phenothiazines and antibiotics increase excretion of riboflavin, so monitor for a deficiency in patients on long-term therapy.

Nutritional Directions

- Enriched products provide more riboflavin than their whole-grain counterparts.
- Lighted display cases have the potential to cause decomposition of riboflavin when milk is marketed in translucent plastic containers.
- A mixed diet that contains a pint of low-fat milk and 4 to 6 oz of meat daily ensures adequate riboflavin intake.
- Vegans and those who consume minimal or no dairy products are at risk of developing riboflavin deficiency.
- Riboflavin is not known to be toxic, but there is no benefit from high doses.

NIACIN (VITAMIN B₃)

Physiological Roles

The term *niacin* is loosely used to refer to two compounds, nicotinic acid and nicotinamide. Both compounds are used by the body. Niacin is crucial as a coenzyme in energy (adenosine triphosphate) production. It functions with riboflavin in glucose production and metabolism and is involved in lipid and protein metabolism. Niacin also functions in enzymes involved in microbial degradation of sucrose to produce organic acids.

Requirements

The body obtains niacin not only directly from food, but also indirectly from conversion of an amino acid, tryptophan,

Table 11-5	Institute of Medicine recommendations for niacin					
	EAR (mg/day)*†		**RDA (mg/day)‡**			
Life Stage	Male	Female	Male	Female	AI (mg/day)§‖	UL (mg/day)
0-6 months					2	ND¶
7-12 months					4	ND¶
1-3 years	5	5	6	6		10
4-8 years	6	6	8	8		15
9-13 years	9	9	12	12		20
14-18 years	12	11	16	14		30
≥19 years	12	11	16	14		35
Pregnancy						
14-18 years		14		18		30
≥19 years		14		18		35
Lactation						
14-18 years		13		17		30
≥19 years		13		17		35

Data from Institute of Medicine (IOM), Food and Nutrition Board: *Dietary reference intakes for thiamin, riboflavin, niacin, vitamin B₆, folate, vitamin B₁₂, pantothenic acid, biotin, and choline*, Washington, DC, 1998, National Academy Press.

*EAR (estimated average requirement)—the intake that meets the estimated nutrient needs of half of the individuals in a group.
†Niacin equivalents.
‡RDA (recommended dietary allowance)—the intake that meets the nutrient needs of almost all (97% to 98%) individuals in a group.
§AI (adequate intake)—the observed average or experimentally set intake by a defined population or subgroup that seems to sustain a defined nutritional status, such as growth rate, normal circulating nutrient values, or other functional indicators of health. An AI is used if insufficient scientific evidence is available to derive an EAR. For healthy human milk–fed infants, the AI is the mean intake. *The AI is not equivalent to a RDA.*
‖Preformed niacin.
¶ND—not determinable because of lack of data of adverse effects in this age group and concern with regard to lack of ability to handle excess amounts. Source of intake should be from food and formula to prevent high levels of intake.

and from synthesis by intestinal microorganisms. RDAs are given in terms of niacin equivalents, which include dietary sources of niacin plus its precursor, tryptophan. Approximately 1 mg of niacin may be formed from 60 mg of dietary tryptophan. Niacin requirements are related to caloric intake. The RDA niacin equivalents for adults are 14 to 16 mg daily (Table 11-5). The UL for adults is 35 mg daily. There is no known adverse effect related to naturally-occurring niacin in foods.

Sources

Niacin is widely distributed in plant and animal foods. Good sources include meats, cereals, legumes, seeds, and nuts (Table 11-6). Approximately 65% of the niacin in the U.S. diet is obtained from meat and milk. Tryptophan is found mainly in milk, eggs, and meats. The RDA for niacin equivalents is easily met by consuming foods high in niacin and foods containing tryptophan.

Hyper States and Hypo States

Supplemental doses of nicotinic acid (3 to 6 g/day) are effective in reducing low-density lipoprotein (LDL) cholesterol and triglycerides, while increasing high-density lipoprotein (HDL) cholesterol. (Nicotinamide does not function in this role.) Despite positive changes in serum lipid levels, a large study funded by National Institutes of Health using a combination of niacin supplements and statin did not reduce risk

Table 11-6	Niacin content of selected foods	
Food	**Portion**	**Niacin (mg)**
Beef liver, braised	3 oz	15.77
Wheaties	1 cup	13.32
Chicken breast, skinless, cooked	3 oz	12.84
Salmon, cooked	3 oz	8.24
Halibut, broiled	3 oz	6.72
Tuna, white, canned in water	3 oz	4.93
Turkey, whole, cooked	3 oz	4.80
Peanuts, dry roasted	1 oz	3.83
Potato, white, baked	1 med	2.64
Mushrooms, raw	1 cup	2.53
Rice, enriched white, cooked	1 cup	2.33
Milk, skim	1 cup	0.23

Data from U.S. Department of Agriculture, Agricultural Research Service. *USDA national nutrient database for standard reference, release 26, 2013.* Nutrient Data Laboratory Home Page. Accessed August 30, 2013: http://www.ars.usda.gov/nutrientdata

of CHD (heart attacks and strokes), causing the study to be terminated early.[1,2]

The use of 50 mg of niacin taken daily can function as a vasodilator, producing flushing of the skin, itching, tachycardia, nausea and vomiting, and severe liver damage. Extended-release niacin is associated with few gastrointestinal symptoms without increasing liver damage. Because the body is able to store some niacin, larger doses associated with supplements may lead to serious problems, including abnormal liver function and gout.

Niacin deficiency is usually associated with a maize (corn) diet because corn products contain all the essential amino acids except tryptophan. This diet increases the body's requirements for tryptophan and niacin. A deficiency is also seen in alcoholics but is unlikely in individuals who consume adequate protein. Niacin deficiency results in degeneration of the skin, gastrointestinal tract, and nervous system, a condition known as **pellagra**. Symptoms of pellagra have been referred to as "the 4 Ds"—dermatitis, diarrhea, depression or dementia, and death. The term *pellagra* is derived from the Latin word for animal hide; the skin may become rough and resemble goose flesh. The most striking and characteristic sign of pellagra is a reddish skin rash, especially on the face, hands, or feet, which is always bilaterally symmetrical (i.e., appears on both sides of the body at the same time) (Fig. 11-7*A*). It flares up when skin is exposed to strong sunlight. Neurological symptoms include depression, apathy, headache, fatigue, and loss of memory. If untreated, it may lead to death.

Deficiency also affects mucous membranes: (a) painful stomatitis causes diminished food intake, and (b) lesions in the gastrointestinal tract result in diarrhea and less vitamin absorption. Pellagrous glossitis begins with swelling of the papillae at the tip and lateral borders of the tongue. The tongue becomes painful, scarlet, and edematous (Fig. 11-7*B*). Atrophic changes involve loss of filiform and fungiform papillae, and the tongue becomes smooth and shiny. The mucosa is also reddened. Fissures occur in the epithelium and along the sides of the tongue; these become infected rapidly. The gingiva may become inflamed, resembling ulcerative gingivitis. Corners of the lips are initially pale; fanlike fissuring occurs that radiates into the perioral epithelium and may leave permanent scars.

Dental Considerations

- Assess patients, especially alcoholics and immigrants from areas with a heavy dependence on corn or maize, for oral signs of niacin deficiency. Symptoms to watch for include complaints of a nonspecific burning sensation throughout the oral cavity; a smooth, shiny, bright red tongue swollen at the tip and lateral margins; stomatitis; and red and inflamed marginal and attached gingiva.
- Prolonged treatment with isoniazid for tuberculosis may lead to niacin deficiency. Niacin supplements may be prescribed by the healthcare provider to prevent deficiency.

Nutritional Directions

- Patients should understand a frequent side effect of a therapeutic dose of nicotinic acid is flushing. This should be discussed with the healthcare provider.
- Nicotinic acid, nicotinamide, and niacinamide are correct terms for niacin and should not be confused with nicotine.

PANTOTHENIC ACID (VITAMIN B₅)

Physiological Roles

Pantothenic acid is similar to other B vitamins in its metabolic roles. Pantothenic acid plays a key role in carbohydrate, fat, and protein metabolism. Additionally, it is important in synthesis and degradation of triglycerides, phospholipids, and sterols, and in formation of certain hormones and nerve-regulating substances.

Requirements

The estimated average requirement (EAR), RDA, or UL has not been determined for pantothenic acid for any age group. The adequate intake (AI) for adults is 5 mg/day (Table 11-7).

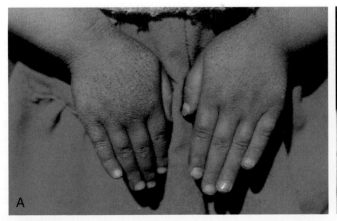

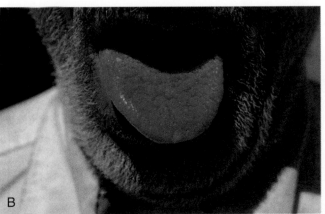

FIGURE 11-7 A, Symmetrical chapping of dorsum of hands. This is a common site for the skin changes of pellagra to occur. A careful history and full examination permit the diagnosis to be made. **B,** Scarlet tongue. The tongue in pellagra is frequently scarlet in appearance and extremely painful. However, this may occur in many nonnutritional conditions, and other signs, especially those in the skin, have to be present to make the clinical diagnosis. Fissuring of the tongue alone is not significant. (From McLaren DS: *A colour atlas and text of diet-related disorders,* ed 2, London, 1992, Mosby-Year Book.)

Table 11-7	Institute of Medicine recommendations for pantothenic acid
Life Stage	AI (mg/day)*
0-6 months	1.7
7-12 months	1.8
1-3 years	2
4-8 years	3
9-13 years	4
14-18 years	5
19->70 years	5
Pregnancy	
14-50 years	6
Lactation	
14-50 years	7

Data from Institute of Medicine (IOM), Food and Nutrition Board: *Dietary reference intakes for thiamin, riboflavin, niacin, vitamin B6, folate, vitamin B12, pantothenic acid, biotin, and choline,* Washington, DC, 1998, National Academy Press.

*AI (adequate intake)—the observed average or experimentally set intake by a defined population or subgroup that seems to sustain a defined nutritional status, such as growth rate, normal circulating nutrient values, or other functional indicators of health. An AI is used if insufficient scientific evidence is unavailable to derive an estimated average requirement. For healthy human milk–fed infants, the AI is the mean intake. *The AI is not equivalent to an RDA.*

Table 11-8	Pantothenic acid content of selected foods	
Food	Portion	Pantothenic Acid (mg)
Total, whole grain	1 cup	12.5
Beef liver, cooked	3 oz	5.6
Sunflower seeds	¼ cup	2.5
Egg, hard boiled	1	1.9
Trail mix, tropical	1 cup	1.7
Trout, cooked	3 oz	1.7
Corn, canned	1 cup	1.4
Pork loin chop, broiled	3 oz	1.4
Salmon, cooked	3 oz	1.3
Mushrooms, raw	1 cup	1.1
Chicken, skinless, cooked	3 oz	1.1
Yogurt, low-fat, plain	8 oz	1.0
Rice, enriched, cooked	1 cup	0.5
Lean beef, cooked	3 oz	0.4
Peanuts, dry roasted	1 oz	0.4

Data from U.S. Department of Agriculture, Agricultural Research Service. *USDA national nutrient database for standard reference, release 26, 2013.* Pantothenic acid (mg) content of selected foods per common measure. Accessed August 30, 2013: http://www.ars.usda.gov/nutrientdata

Sources

Pantothenic acid is synthesized by most microorganisms and plants. It is particularly abundant in animal foods and whole-grain cereals (Table 11-8). Bacteria in the digestive tract also produce pantothenic acid. The estimated average daily intake of pantothenic acid in the United States is 5 to 10 mg.

Hypo States

Naturally-occurring dietary deficiency of pantothenic acid is very rare. A deficiency results in dysfunctional lipid synthesis and energy production. Symptoms include burning sensations in the feet, depression, fatigue, insomnia, and weakness.

Dental Considerations

- Pantothenic acid deficiency rarely occurs alone, but may occur along with other B-vitamin deficiencies.
- Pantothenic acid may help in wound healing, so encourage patients undergoing oral or periodontal surgery to eat a well-balanced diet.

Nutritional Directions

- Distribution of pantothenic acid is widespread.
- Diets including whole-grain unprocessed foods contain more pantothenic acid.

VITAMIN B6 (PYRIDOXINE)

Vitamin B6 is the term commonly used for a group of three compounds: pyridoxine, pyridoxal, and pyridoxamine. All three forms can be used by the body in their role as coenzymes.

Physiological Roles

Several essential roles for vitamin B6 have been identified. In addition to (a) its role as a coenzyme in protein metabolism, vitamin B6 plays a part in (b) conversion of tryptophan to niacin, (c) hemoglobin synthesis, (d) synthesis of unsaturated fatty acids from essential fatty acids, (e) energy production from glycogen, (f) production of antibodies and immune cells, and (g) proper functioning of the nervous system including synthesis of neurotransmitters.

Requirements

The current RDA for vitamin B6 ranges from 1.1 to 1.7 mg daily for adults (Table 11-9). The requirement for vitamin B6 increases with protein intake because of its major role in amino acid metabolism. Limited amounts of vitamin B6 are produced by microorganisms in the digestive tract. The UL has been determined to be 100 mg/day for adults. Four groups in the U.S. population are frequently deficient in vitamin B6: women of childbearing age, especially current and former users of oral contraceptives; male smokers; non-Hispanic African American men; and individuals older than age 65 years.

Table 11-9	Institute of Medicine recommendations for pyridoxine/vitamin B_6					
	EAR (mg/day)*		RDA (mg/day)†			
Life Stage	Male	Female	Male	Female	AI (mg/day)‡	UL (mg/day)§‖
0-6 months					0.1	ND¶
7-12 months					0.3	ND¶
1-3 years	0.4	0.4	0.5	0.5		30
4-8 years	0.5	0.5	0.6	0.6		40
9-13 years	0.8	0.8	1	1		60
14-18 years	1.1	1	1.3	1.2		80
19-50 years	1.1	0.9	1.3	1.1		100
≥51 years	1.4	1.3	1.7	1.5		100
Pregnancy						
14-18 years		1.6		1.9		80
≥19 years		1.6		1.9		100
Lactation						
14-18 years		1.7		2		80
≥19 years		1.7		2		100

Data from Institute of Medicine (IOM), Food and Nutrition Board: *Dietary reference intakes for thiamin, riboflavin, niacin, vitamin B_6, folate, vitamin B_{12}, pantothenic acid, biotin, and choline,* Washington, DC, 1998, National Academy Press.

*EAR (estimated average requirement)—the intake that meets the estimated nutrient needs of half of the individuals in a group.

†RDA (recommended dietary allowance)—the intake that meets the nutrient needs of almost all (97% to 98%) individuals in a group.

‡AI (adequate intake)—the observed average or experimentally set intake by a defined population or subgroup that seems to sustain a defined nutritional status, such as growth rate, normal circulating nutrient values, or other functional indicators of health. An AI is used if insufficient scientific evidence is available to derive an EAR. For healthy human milk–fed infants, the AI is the mean intake. *The AI is not equivalent to a RDA.*

§UL (tolerable upper intake level)—the highest level of daily nutrient intake that is likely to pose no risk of adverse health effects to almost all individuals in the general population. As intake increases above the UL, the risk of adverse effects increases. Unless specified otherwise, the UL represents total nutrient intake from food, water, and supplements.

‖Vitamin B_6 as pyridoxine.

¶ND—not determinable because of lack of data of adverse effects in this age group and concern with regard to lack of ability to handle excess amounts. Source of intake should be from food and formula to prevent high levels of intake.

Sources

Meat, poultry, and fish are good sources of vitamin B_6. Other good sources include some fruits, nuts, fortified cereals, whole-grain products, and vegetables (Table 11-10). Vitamin B_6 from animal sources has greater bioavailability than that provided by plants. Pyridoxine in some plants (potatoes, spinach, beans and other legumes) is frequently bound to proteins, resulting in low bioavailability. Canning, roasting, boiling, or stewing meat and various food-processing techniques can reduce pyridoxine content of food as the vitamin is leached into the water.

Absorption and Excretion

Absorption of vitamin B_6 differs from other B-complex vitamins. All three forms of the vitamin are converted to an absorbable form by an intestinal enzyme. Body stores are small, and repletion is gradual.

Hyper States and Hypo States

Numerous studies suggest possible benefits of supplemental amounts of vitamin B_6 in CHD, sickness during pregnancy, premenstrual syndrome, carpal tunnel syndrome, and neuropathies. Because of inconsistent findings, supplemental amounts beyond the UL are not currently recommended. Acute pyridoxine toxicity is uncommon; however, routine supplementation with megadoses has documented

Table 11-10	Pyridoxine (vitamin B_6) content of selected foods	
Food	Portion	Pyridoxine (mg)
Total, whole grain	1 cup	2.67
Beef liver, braised	3 oz	0.92
Turkey, cooked	3 oz	0.64
Halibut, broiled	3 oz	0.63
Spinach, cooked	1 cup	0.44
Banana	1 med	0.43
Chicken, meat only, roasted	3 oz	0.42
Pinto beans, cooked	1 cup	0.39
Potato, white, baked	1 med	0.37
Baked beans	1 cup	0.33
Sunflower seeds	¼ cup	0.26
Tuna, white, canned in water	3 oz	0.18
Tomato, raw	1 med	0.10
Peanuts, dry roasted	1 oz	0.07

Data from U.S. Department of Agriculture, Agricultural Research Service. *USDA national nutrient database for standard reference, release 26, 2013.* Nutrient Data Laboratory Home Page. Accessed August 30, 2013: http://www.ars.usda.gov/nutrientdata

side effects, including ataxia and severe sensory neuropathy (impairment of the ability to feel) and, in some instances, bone pain, and muscle weakness. In most cases, complete recovery occurs with discontinuation of megadose supplementation.

Deficiency rarely occurs alone; vitamin B₆ deficiency is most commonly observed along with deficiency of several other B vitamins. Individuals with poor-quality diets in addition to overall low nutrient intake (e.g., alcoholics and elderly individuals) may experience a deficiency. Clinical signs include central nervous system abnormalities or convulsions, dermatitis with cheilosis and glossitis, impaired immune responses, and anemia. Pyridoxine deficiency–induced glossitis is denoted by pain, edema, and papillary changes. Initially, the tongue has a scalded sensation, followed by reddening and hypertrophy of filiform papillae at the tip, margins, and dorsum (Fig. 11-8).

Stores of vitamin B₆ in a mother's body are critical to the well-being of her newborn infant. Oral contraceptive agents (OCAs) taken before conception may reduce maternal vitamin B₆ levels during pregnancy and in breast milk. An increase in dietary intake of vitamin B₆ may be recommended for women taking OCAs, especially if a pregnancy is planned in the near future.

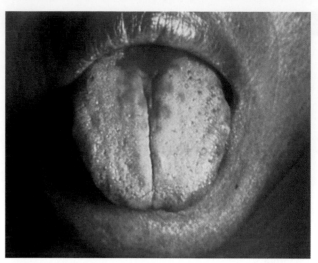

FIGURE 11-8 Fungiform papillary hypertrophy. The condition can be seen and felt as a tongue blade is drawn lightly over the anterior two-thirds of the tongue. The tongue may have a berrylike appearance. (Courtesy of Dr. H.H. Sandstead. From McLaren DS: *A colour atlas and text of diet-related disorders*, ed 2, London, 1992, Mosby-Year Book.)

Dental Considerations

- Patients may present with pain of the tongue, which precedes redness and swelling of the tip of the tongue. Eventually, atrophy of papillae results in a smooth, purplish tongue. Angular cheilitis, oral ulcers, and stomatitis also may be noted.
- Lower serum levels of vitamin B₆ are seen in women who are menstruating and those taking or have taken OCAs.
- Encourage foods high in vitamin B₆, and monitor for deficiency signs and symptoms, especially in women of child-bearing age, alcoholics, and elderly individuals.
- In animal studies, the presence of pyridoxine alters oral flora and reduces incidence of dental caries.
- Use of drugs affecting vitamin B₆ metabolism warrants supplementation to avoid secondary vitamin B₆ deficiency. These drugs include isoniazid and cycloserine (for tuberculosis), penicillamine (for Wilson disease, lead poisoning, kidney stones, and arthritis), theophylline (for asthma), and OCAs.
- Excessive pyridoxine can reduce clinical benefits of levodopa therapy in patients with Parkinson disease or other neurological problems. Encourage these patients to limit intake of foods fortified with vitamin B₆ and to avoid vitamin B₆ supplements. If desired effects of the drug are not seen, or if over-the-counter supplements are being taken, refer the patient to the healthcare provider.

Nutritional Directions

- Vitamin B₆ supplements should not be taken unless ordered by a healthcare provider.
- If supplements are needed, signs and symptoms improve within 1 week.
- Adequate daily intake of pyridoxine is important.
- Vitamin B₆ is removed during grain processing and not replaced during enrichment; whole-grain breads and cereals are better choices.

FOLATE/FOLIC ACID

The generic term folate encompasses several compounds that have nutritional properties similar to those of folic acid. Several different metabolically active forms have been identified. The terms *folate, folic acid,* and *folacin* are used interchangeably. Folate is the natural form found in foods, whereas folic acid is a synthetic form used in vitamin supplements and food fortification. The body converts folic acid to folate.

Physiological Roles

Folate functions as a coenzyme for approximately 20 enzymes. As such, it has an important role in synthesis of RNA and DNA. It functions in conjunction with vitamins B₁₂ and C in maintaining normal levels of mature red blood cells (RBCs). Folate has an important role in proper formation of the neural tube during the first month of fetal development.

Requirements

As shown in Table 11-11, the RDA is 400 µg for adults. Folate can be expressed as dietary folate equivalents, which are equivalent to 1 µg of folate. Requirements for folate are increased during periods of growth and development, such as adolescence, pregnancy, and lactation, because of its role in DNA formulation. The IOM established a UL for the synthetic forms of folic acid available in dietary supplements and fortified foods, but the UL does not pertain to folate from food because a high intake from food sources has not been reported to cause adverse effects.

Table 11-11	Institute of Medicine recommendations for folate*					
	EAR (μg/day)†		RDA (μg/day)‡			
Life Stage	Male	Female	Male	Female	AI (μg/day)§	UL (μg/day)‖¶
0-6 months					65	ND**
7-12 months					80	ND**
1-3 years	120	120	150	150		300
4-8 years	160	160	200	200		400
9-13 years	250	250	300	300		600
14-18 years	330	330	400	400		800
≥19 years	320	320	400	400		1000
Pregnancy						
14-18 years		520		600		800
≥19 years		520		600		1000
Lactation						
14-18 years		450		500		800
≥19 years		450		500		1000

Data from Institute of Medicine (IOM), Food and Nutrition Board: *Dietary reference intakes for thiamin, riboflavin, niacin, vitamin B₆, folate, vitamin B₁₂, pantothenic acid, biotin, and choline*, Washington, DC, 1998, National Academy Press.

*Dietary folate equivalents.

†EAR (estimated average requirement)—the intake that meets the estimated nutrient needs of half of the individuals in a group.

‡RDA (recommended dietary allowance)—the intake that meets the nutrient needs of almost all (97% to 98%) individuals in a group.

§AI (adequate intake)—the observed average or experimentally set intake by a defined population or subgroup that seems to sustain a defined nutritional status, such as growth rate, normal circulating nutrient values, or other functional indicators of health. An AI is used if insufficient scientific evidence is available to derive an EAR. For healthy human milk–fed infants, the AI is the mean intake. *The AI is not equivalent to a RDA.*

‖UL (tolerable upper intake level)—the highest level of daily nutrient intake that is likely to pose no risk of adverse health effects to almost all individuals in the general population. As intake increases above the UL, the risk of adverse effects increases. Unless specified otherwise, the UL represents total nutrient intake from food, water, and supplements.

¶Folate from fortified foods or supplements.

**ND—not determinable because of lack of data of adverse effects in this age group and concern with regard to lack of ability to handle excess amounts. Source of intake should be from food and formula to prevent high levels of intake.

Sources

Rich sources of folate include liver, green leafy vegetables, fortified cereals and grain products, legumes, and some fruits (grapefruit and oranges) (Table 11-12).

In 1996 the U.S. Food and Drug Administration (FDA) mandated the addition of specific amounts of folic acid to all enriched cereals and grain products. Since then, folate intake and serum folate levels have been monitored because of potential risks of some individuals consuming excessive amounts. The prevalence of low RBC folate among U.S. women of childbearing age declined from 37.6% in 1988-1994 to 4.5% in 2005-2006.[3]

Absorption and Excretion

Dietary folate must undergo changes to be absorbed. The intestinal enzyme that accomplishes this requires a slightly acidic pH and is activated by the presence of zinc. Folic acid from supplements and fortified foods is actually absorbed almost twice as well as that from naturally occurring folate in foods. Individuals needing larger amounts, especially menstruating women who may become pregnant, may need a supplement in addition to fortified folate-rich foods.

Table 11-12	Folate content of selected foods	
Food	Portion	Folate (DFE) (μg)
Total, whole grain	1 cup	901
Pinto beans, cooked	1 cup	294
Asparagus, cooked	1 cup	268
Spinach, cooked	1 cup	263
Navy beans	1 cup	255
Liver, beef, braised	1 slice	228
Noodles, enriched, cooked	1 cup	221
Turnip greens, cooked	1 cup	170
Broccoli, cooked	1 cup	168
Romaine lettuce	1 cup	64
Bread, white, enriched	1 slice	48
Orange juice	1 cup	47
Peanuts, dry roasted	1 oz	41
Orange	1 med	39
Tomato	1 med	18
Bread, whole-wheat	1 slice	13
Brown rice	1 cup	8

Data from U.S. Department of Agriculture, Agricultural Research Service. *USDA national nutrient database for standard reference, release 26, 2013.* Nutrient Data Laboratory Home Page. Accessed August 30, 2013: http://www.ars.usda.gov/nutrientdata
DFE, Dietary folate equivalent.

Hyper States and Hypo States

A high folic acid intake may be harmful for some people. Prolonged intake of excessive folic acid can cause kidney damage and mask symptoms of vitamin B_{12} deficiency, resulting in neurological and cognitive symptoms. Although an increased risk of cognitive decline has been reported in elderly individuals taking folic acid supplements, a systematic meta-analysis study found only a causal relationship between high folic acid intake and risk of developing dementia.[4]

Abundant intake of folate-rich foods may protect against some common cancers, particularly colorectal cancer. A meta-analysis of scientific studies found no significant effect of folic acid supplementation on incidence of cancer of the large intestine, prostate, lung, breast, or any other specific site.[5] Possibly, folic acid should be considered a "pharmaceutical" form of the vitamin; it may affect tumorigenesis (tumor formation) in a distinctively different way than the natural form of the vitamin. This complex relationship has impeded efforts to increase folic acid fortification.[6] The UL of 1000 μg/day for adults is applicable to supplements and fortified foods, not to naturally-occurring folate in food.

Folate deficiency, the most common vitamin deficiency among the B-complex vitamins, usually occurs with other nutrient deficiencies. Folate inadequacy may occur secondary to excessive alcohol consumption, malabsorptive disorders, pregnancy and lactation, kidney disease, inadequate dietary intake, or taking medications that interfere with folate absorption or metabolism (Box 11-2). Folate deficiency can produce soreness and shallow ulcerations on the tongue and oral mucosa, as well as swelling of the tongue.

Deficiency symptoms first appear in rapidly dividing cells, such as in the gastrointestinal tract, RBCs, and white blood cells. RBCs do not develop normally; they become pale and extremely large (megaloblastic), but cannot transport oxygen to cells, a condition known as megaloblastic anemia.

Folic acid deficiency during pregnancy is associated with an increased risk of spina bifida and other neural tube defects (birth defects of the skull, brain, and spinal cord), cleft palate and lip, low birth weight, and premature birth. Before fortification, approximately 4130 babies had neural tube defects each year in the United States, and nearly 1200 died. After folic acid fortification, the yearly number of pregnancies affected by neural tube defects dropped to approximately 3000, and the related deaths declined to 840.[7]

Glossitis is usually present in individuals with folic acid deficiency. The tongue becomes fiery red and papillae are absent (Fig. 11-9). Folic acid deficiency impairs immune responses and resistance of the oral mucosa to penetration by pathogenic organisms such as *Candida*.

Dental Considerations

- Evaluate oral status for folate deficiency. Observe for swelling and pallor or reddening of the tip of the tongue (depending on the degree of anemia) with atrophy of filiform papillae, reddening of the fungiform papillae at the tip and lateral border, and formation of small ulcers. Posterior progression eventually leads to complete atrophy of the filiform papillae and formation of bright red spots (fungiform papillae). Angular cheilitis (see Fig. 11-5) and painful ulcerations of the buccal mucosa and palatal and gingival epithelia may also occur.
- Factors increasing metabolic rate, such as infection and hyperthyroidism, or cellular turnover rate, such as a malignancy, increase folate requirement. Assess folate intake by questioning about dietary intake.
- Folic acid supplementation may improve resistance to periodontal inflammation in patients deficient in folate.
- A low serum folate level is associated with **periodontal disease** (infections and lesions affecting tissues that form the attachment apparatus of the teeth) in older adults and may warrant encouraging the patient to increase intake of folate-rich foods.[8]
- Folate is one of the most common nutrient deficiencies after bariatric surgery.[9] Encourage patients who have had this procedure to adhere to strict eating behavior guidelines and supplement prescriptions.
- Folate absorption is lower when folate is given to individuals taking anticonvulsants and OCAs.
- High doses of folic acid may interfere with the chemotherapy drug methotrexate and other drugs like it. A patient with cancer or who is undergoing chemotherapy should avoid folic acid supplements and large amounts of food enriched with folic acid. Refer this patient to a RDN.
- Increased gingival inflammation has been associated with OCAs; encourage women taking OCAs to increase their consumption of folate-rich foods.
- Phenytoin (Dilantin) is associated with gingival overgrowth (see Fig. 17-11). Certain studies have shown folate supplementation reduces severity and incidence of this overgrowth. However, patients taking anticonvulsants should be closely monitored if folate supplements are prescribed because high intakes can decrease effectiveness of the medication.

BOX 11-2	Drugs That May Negatively Affect Folate Status*

Anticonvulsants
Oral contraceptives
Analgesics
Metformin (antihyperglycemic)
Sulfasalazine (antiinflammatory, antiarthritic)
H_2-receptor blockers (decreased gastric acid secretion)
Antacids
Triamterene (diuretic)
Methotrexate (antiarthritic, antineoplastic)
Alcohol

*Nutritional status may be negatively affected because of interference with folate absorption or metabolism or both.

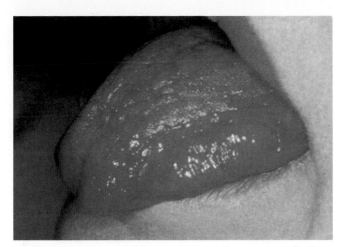

FIGURE 11-9 Folic acid deficiency. Fiery red tongue completely devoid of papillae. (Courtesy of Dr. W.R. Tyldesley. From McLaren DS: *A colour atlas and text of diet-related disorders*, ed 2, London, 1992, Mosby-Year Book.)

Nutritional Directions

- Folate may be called folic acid or folacin.
- Prolonged cooking destroys folate.
- The American Heart Association does not recommend folic acid supplements to reduce the risk of heart disease and stroke, but supports a healthy, balanced diet rich in high folate-containing foods.[10]
- Folate is easily destroyed by food processing; raw vegetables provide more folate than cooked ones.
- Adequate folic acid is important in the periconceptual period (400 μg/day before conception and 600 μg/day for pregnant women) because the critical time for neural tube formation is the first month of pregnancy.
- Orange juice is a good source of folate because vitamin C protects it from deterioration. Choosing fortified cereals and crackers also enhances folate intake.

VITAMIN B₁₂ (COBALAMIN)

Vitamin B_{12}, or cobalamin, represents a complex group of compounds that contain cobalt. (The only known physiological function of cobalt is as an integral component of vitamin B_{12}.) It is the only vitamin that contains a mineral.

Physiological Roles

Vitamin B_{12} functions as a coenzyme in conjunction with folate metabolism in DNA synthesis. It also functions in metabolism of certain amino acids, fatty acids, carbohydrates, and folate. Vitamin B_{12} is essential in formation and regeneration of RBCs, myelin synthesis, and cognitive function. Myelin is the lipid substance that insulates nerve fibers and affects transmission of nerve impulses. It is essential for a normal functioning nervous system.

Requirements

The RDA for adults is 2.4 μg daily (Table 11-13). A high vitamin B_{12} intake results in accumulation in the liver with

Table 11-13	Institute of Medicine recommendations for vitamin B₁₂				
	EAR (μg/day)*		**RDA (μg/day)†**		
Life Stage	**Male**	**Female**	**Male**	**Female**	**AI (μg/day)‡**
0-6 months					0.4
7-12 months					0.5
1-3 years	0.7	0.7	0.9	0.9	
4-8 years	1	1	1.8	2.4	
9-13 years	1.5	1.5	1.8	1.8	
≥70 years	2	2	2.4	2.4	
Pregnancy					
14-50 years		2.2		2.6	
Lactation					
14-50 years		2.4		2.8	

Data from Institute of Medicine (IOM), Food and Nutrition Board: *Dietary reference intakes for thiamin, riboflavin, niacin, vitamin B₆, folate, vitamin B₁₂, pantothenic acid, biotin, and choline*, Washington, DC, 1998, National Academy Press.
*EAR (estimated average requirement)—the intake that meets the estimated nutrient needs of half of the individuals in a group.
†RDA (recommended dietary allowance)—the intake that meets the nutrient needs of almost all (97% to 98%) individuals in a group.
‡AI (adequate intake)—the observed average or experimentally set intake by a defined population or subgroup that seems to sustain a defined nutritional status, such as growth rate, normal circulating nutrient values, or other functional indicators of health. An AI is used if insufficient scientific evidence is available to derive an EAR. For healthy human milk–fed infants, the AI is the mean intake. *The AI is not equivalent to a RDA.*

increasing age, but this may be desirable because serum vitamin B_{12} levels decline in elderly individuals because of lower absorption rates. No UL has been established, but caution of excessive intake is warranted.

Sources

Microorganisms (bacteria, fungi, and algae) can synthesize vitamin B_{12}. Vitamin B_{12} is not found in plants unless they are fortified or contaminated by microorganisms (legumes and root vegetables). More than 80% of dietary vitamin B_{12} is provided by meat and animal products (Table 11-14). Gastrointestinal flora produce small amounts of absorbable vitamin B_{12}.

Absorption and Excretion

Vitamin B_{12} from food is released from its protein bond by hydrochloric acid and enzymes in the stomach and intestine. Free vitamin B_{12} combines with salivary **R-binder** (protein produced by the salivary glands) in the stomach. In the small intestine, trypsin (pancreatic enzyme) removes the R-binder, and vitamin B_{12} combines with **intrinsic factor**, a glycoprotein secreted by the parietal cells in the stomach. Absorption of vitamin B_{12} occurs at specific receptor sites in the ileum and is possible only if it is bound to intrinsic factor. The vitamin is recycled from bile and other intestinal secretions. Excessive amounts are bound to a protein and stored for 3 to 4 years in the liver, or they are excreted.

Table 11-14	Vitamin B$_{12}$ content of selected foods	
Food	**Portion**	**Vitamin B$_{12}$ (μg)**
Beef liver, braised	3 oz	70.6
Oysters, cooked	3 oz	24.5
Total, whole grain	1 cup	8.0
Salmon, cooked	3 oz	4.8
Beef, ground (80/20), broiled	3 oz	2.3
Yogurt, low-fat, plain	8 oz	1.5
Shrimp	3 oz	1.4
Skim milk	1 cup	1.0
Lean pork chop, broiled	3 oz	0.6
Egg, hard boiled	1	0.6
Chicken breast, roasted	1	0.3

Data from U.S. Department of Agriculture, Agricultural Research Service. *USDA national nutrient database for standard reference, release 26, 2013.* Nutrient Data Laboratory Home Page. Accessed August 30, 2013: http://www.ars.usda.gov/nutrientdata

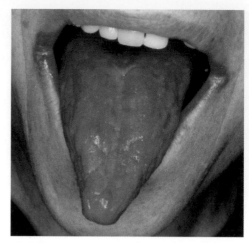

FIGURE 11-10 Pernicious anemia. (From Ibsen OAC, Phelan JA: *Oral pathology for the dental hygienist,* ed 6, St Louis, 2014, Elsevier Saunders.)

Hyper States and Hypo States

No benefits are seen from large quantities of vitamin B$_{12}$, but no harmful effects have been observed either. Approximately 1 in every 31 (3.2%) adults older than 51 years of age has a low vitamin B$_{12}$ serum level.[11] Excessive intake of folic acid from supplements delays the diagnosis of, or exacerbates the effects of, vitamin B$_{12}$ deficiency, causing anemia and cognitive impairment. Injections of vitamin B$_{12}$ are popular treatments for fatigue and weakness; oral administration of vitamin B$_{12}$ is as effective as intramuscular administration in correcting the deficiency, regardless of etiology.[12] Vitamin B$_{12}$ deficiency is rarely caused by insufficient dietary sources, unless strict vegan diets are followed. Lack of intrinsic factor, R-binder, or an enzyme needed for absorption of vitamin B$_{12}$, is the primary cause of deficiency. Pernicious anemia, which is characterized by abnormally large RBCs, glossitis, gastrointestinal disturbances, weakness, and neurologic manifestations, occurs frequently in elderly patients relative to achlorhydria (decreased hydrochloric acid production in the stomach) and decreased synthesis of intrinsic factor by the parietal cells. Rapid neuropsychiatric decline occurs with severe vitamin B$_{12}$ deficiency.[13]

Cobalamin malabsorption is caused by inability to release vitamin B$_{12}$ from food so it cannot be taken up by intrinsic factor for absorption. Patients develop a lemon-yellow tint of the skin and eyes as a result of concurrent anemia and jaundice from inability to produce RBCs; a smooth, beefy red tongue; and neurologic disorders. Deficiency symptoms develop very slowly.

Initial oral symptoms of vitamin B$_{12}$ deficiency include glossopyrosis (unexplained pain of the tongue), followed by swelling and pallor with eventual disappearance of the filiform and fungiform papillae. The tongue may be completely smooth, shiny, and deeply reddened with a loss or distortion of taste (Fig. 11-10). Bright red, diffuse, excruciatingly painful lesions may occur in the buccal and pharyngeal mucosa and undersurface of the tongue. An oral examination may reveal stomatitis or a pale or yellowish mucosa, xerostomia, cheilosis, hemorrhagic gingiva, and bone loss.

Neurological symptoms, such as numbness or tingling, occur as a consequence of demyelination of the nerves. Deficiency symptoms are rapidly corrected with vitamin B$_{12}$ supplements or intramuscular injections. The crystalline form of vitamin B$_{12}$ found in supplements does not require gastric acid or enzymes for initial digestion, and large oral doses (containing more than 200 times the RDA) can reverse biochemical signs of vitamin B$_{12}$ deficiency in older adults.

Children with vitamin B$_{12}$ deficiency (e.g., vegans) may have stunted growth. Other symptoms include anorexia (loss of appetite), altered taste sensation, abdominal pain, and general weakness. A vitamin B$_{12}$ deficiency is also associated with poor cognitive performance.[14,15]

Dental Considerations

- Assess for oral signs of deficiency; signs and symptoms of vitamin B$_{12}$ deficiency are similar to those of folic acid deficiency except that burning tongue pain precedes physical signs of vitamin B$_{12}$ deficiency.
- Without R-binder, absorption of vitamin B$_{12}$ is drastically reduced. Patients with xerostomia may have poor absorption of vitamin B$_{12}$.
- Patients older than age 50 years are encouraged to choose fortified sources of vitamin B$_{12}$ to meet their needs because the synthetic form is better absorbed than naturally-occurring vitamin B$_{12}$ in foods.
- Concomitant ingestion of megadoses of ascorbic acid via foods or supplements can destroy substantial amounts of vitamin B$_{12}$ and produce vitamin B$_{12}$ deficiency. If the patient is prone to or has vitamin B$_{12}$ deficiency and takes large amounts of vitamin C supplements, advise the patient to decrease vitamin C intake gradually to approximately the RDA level.
- Patients who have had permanent gastric surgery or ileal damage require other forms of vitamin B$_{12}$ for life. Vitamin B$_{12}$ injections and nasal gel do not require intrinsic factor.

Dental Considerations—cont'd

- Because of profound changes in digestive physiology after gastric bypass surgery, vitamin B$_{12}$ is one of the nutrients of concern.
- Vitamin B$_{12}$ deficiency is associated with metformin (an antihyperglycemic medication) therapy in patients with diabetes. A supplement containing the amount recommended by the IOM (2.4 μg) does not alleviate a biochemical deficiency.[16] Patients with diabetes taking metformin may need a supplement. Routine levels of vitamin B$_{12}$ should be assessed by the healthcare professional to determine the individual's need.
- Some antiulcer medications decrease the production of acid by the parietal cells, inhibiting vitamin B$_{12}$ absorption. Histamine receptor antagonists (H$_2$ blockers) (ranitidine [Zantac EFFERdose], famotidine [Pepcid], and cimetidine [Tagamet]) do not affect vitamin B$_{12}$ status, but prolonged use of proton-pump inhibitors (esomeprazole [Nexium], lansoprazole [Prevacid], omeprazole [Prilosec OTC], pantoprazole [Protonix], and rabeprazole [AcipHex]) by older adults negatively affects vitamin B$_{12}$ status. Oral supplementation with recommended amounts of vitamin B$_{12}$ does not prevent this decline. Encourage patients taking these medications to consult their healthcare provider if vitamin B$_{12}$ is not being addressed.

Nutritional Directions

- Because vitamin B$_{12}$ is found only in animal products, vegans (strict vegetarians) require vitamin B$_{12}$–fortified foods or a daily supplement.
- Vitamin B$_{12}$ shots are not a panacea for "tired blood."

BIOTIN (VITAMIN B$_7$)

Physiological Roles

Biotin functions as a coenzyme in metabolism of carbohydrates, proteins, and fats. It has an important biochemical role in every living cell in maintaining metabolic homeostasis. Biotin also plays an important role in regulating gene transcription, and metabolically functions closely with folic acid, pantothenic acid, and vitamin B$_{12}$.

Requirements

Because of insufficient data, only an adequate intake for biotin has been established for all age groups (Table 11-15). Intakes of 10 to 200 μg/day are considered safe and adequate. No UL has been established for biotin.

Sources

Although biotin is widely distributed in foods, its availability is low compared with that of other water-soluble vitamins. Rich sources of biotin include egg yolk, liver, and cereals. Microflora in the gastrointestinal tract probably provides part of the body's needs. Biotin is included in many dietary supplements, infant formulas, and baby foods. Food composition tables usually do not report biotin content of food.

Table 11-15	Institute of Medicine recommendations for biotin
Life Stage	**AI (μg/day)***
0-6 months	5
7-12 months	6
1-3 years	8
4-8 years	12
9-13 years	20
14-18 years	25
>18 years	30
Pregnancy	
14-50 years	30
Lactation	
14-50 years	35

Data from Institute of Medicine (IOM), Food and Nutrition Board: *Dietary reference intakes for thiamin, riboflavin, niacin, vitamin B$_6$, folate, vitamin B$_{12}$, pantothenic acid, biotin, and choline*, Washington, DC, 1998, National Academy Press.
*AI (adequate intake)—the observed average or experimentally set intake by a defined population or subgroup that seems to sustain a defined nutritional status, such as growth rate, normal circulating nutrient values, or other functional indicators of health. An AI is used if insufficient scientific evidence is unavailable to derive an estimated average requirement. For healthy human milk–fed infants, the AI is the mean intake. *The AI is not equivalent to a RDA.*

Hypo States

Biotin deficiency can be produced by the ingestion of avidin, the protein found in raw egg whites. Avidin is denatured by heat; cooked egg white does not present a problem. Twelve to 24 raw egg whites per day can produce anorexia, nausea, vomiting, glossitis, pallor, depression, and dry scaly dermatitis.

Oral signs of biotin deficiency are pallor of the tongue and patchy atrophy of the lingual papillae. Although the pattern resembles geographic tongue, it is confined to the lateral margins or is generalized to the entire dorsum.

Dental Considerations

- Assess patients for signs of deficiency: glossitis, lingual and pallor of the mucosal tissue, and papillary atrophy.
- Antibiotics reduce the production of biotin by intestinal bacteria.

Nutritional Directions

- Drinking or eating large amounts of raw egg whites over a long period may lead to biotin deficiency.
- Eggs should be cooked to decrease avidin's binding capacity and to minimize the danger of *Salmonella* poisoning.
- A balanced diet that includes a variety of foods contains adequate amounts of biotin.

OTHER VITAMINS

As you have already learned, most nutrients perform more than one physiological function. Although one nutrient may appear to be more important in calcified structures and of lesser importance in oral soft tissues, its roles actually are equally important. The following nutrients have been discussed in previous chapters, but they have important functions in soft oral tissues that the dental hygienist should not overlook.

Vitamin C

Vitamin C is involved in improving the host defense mechanism by ensuring optimal activity of white blood cells. It has an important role in protecting soft oral tissues from infections caused by bacterial toxins and antigens and protecting tooth enamel from plaque microorganisms.

The role of vitamin C in collagen formation is well known. Vitamin C deficiency causes weakened collagen, leading to gingivitis and poor wound healing (see Fig. 8-10).

Vitamin A

Vitamin A, necessary for maintaining the integrity of epithelial tissues, is a significant factor in the development and

maintenance of salivary glands. Large amounts of vitamin A have an antikeratinizing effect on epithelial cells. Vitamin A increases synthesis of cellular proteins that stimulate growth and influence metabolism.

Vitamin A deficiency produces squamous metaplasia (change in cell structure in the oral cavity) with keratin production in the duct cells of salivary glands. This results in decreased salivary secretion and xerostomia. Oral and oropharyngeal cancers have been associated with vitamin A deficiency in humans.

Vitamin E

As discussed in Chapter 8, cell membranes contain polyunsaturated fatty acids that are susceptible to peroxidation. Vitamin E plays a major role as an antioxidant to neutralize free radicals, especially in membranes that contain a large proportion of unsaturated fatty acids. It not only prevents inflammation of the periodontium, but also promotes integrity of cell membranes of the mucosa.

 Dental Considerations

- One of the first signs of vitamin C deficiency is increased susceptibility to infections. During later stages, the gingiva becomes reddened and swollen, and bleeds easily with an increased risk of candidiasis and petechiae; also, the collagenous structure is weakened, and wound healing is slow.
- When a deficiency exists, vitamin C supplementation decreases permeability of the sulcular epithelium and increases collagen synthesis.
- Parotid gland enlargement is associated with deficiencies of vitamins A and C and protein malnutrition.
- Vitamin A deficiency may result in retarded **epithelialization** (natural healing), impaired wound healing and tissue regeneration, and increased risk of candidiasis.

 Nutritional Directions

- Foods rich in antioxidants (vitamins E and carotene) may suppress chemically-induced **neoplasia** (abnormal growth of tissue) in the mouth, esophagus, and stomach. However, a meta-analysis indicated an increased risk of mortality related to supplementation of these nutrients. Encourage individuals with these neoplasias to choose nutrient-dense foods that are rich in vitamin E and beta-carotenes.
- Vitamin C functions in maintaining periodontal health. A varied and adequate diet including at least one vitamin C–rich food (Table 8-10) daily provides adequate amounts.

HEALTH APPLICATION 11   Vitamin, Mineral, and Herbal Supplements

Approximately one-half of the U.S. population consumes vitamins, minerals, herbal ingredients, amino acids, and other naturally-occurring products in the form of dietary supplements. One-third use a multivitamin-multimineral (MVM) supplement on a daily basis. Approximately 70% of adults 71 years of age or older used dietary supplements in 2003-2006.[17] An estimated $22.1 billion was spent on dietary supplements in 2006, running up a collective tab of over $28 billion in 2010.[18] Less than 25% of supplements were recommended by a healthcare provider. These supplements are subject to misrepresentation and misuse because they are misunderstood by most consumers.

The five most popular products are fish oil, multivitamins, vitamin D, calcium, and CoQ10. Most adults are taking dietary supplements to optimize their health and well-being and

prevent chronic diseases, cancer in particular, and as nutritional "insurance" to cover lifestyle choices.[19] Interesting is the fact that people who take dietary supplements generally are consuming more nutrient-dense foods, resulting in higher nutrient intakes than those who do not take a supplement.[20]

Rates of vitamin-mineral deficiencies involve less than 10% of the general population. The nutrients and their rates of deficiency are vitamin B_6 (10%); iron (9.5%); vitamin D (8.1%); vitamin C (6%); vitamin B_{12} (2%); and vitamins A and E, and folate (<1%).[21] MVM supplements usually contain 100% of the recommended intake for 10 vitamins and 10 minerals except for calcium (100% reference daily intake for calcium makes the pill too large). There is no standard or regulation governing which vitamins and minerals or how much are included in a MVM supplement.

Vitamins and supplements are drugs, but they are not subject to the same regulations as real drugs. The *Dietary Supplement Health and Education Act* (DSHEA) of 1994 defines dietary supplements (or dietary ingredient) as vitamins, minerals, amino acids, sports nutrition and weight loss supplements, homeopathic medicines, herbs and botanicals, and other products such as enzymes, organ tissues, and metabolites to supplement dietary intake. In other words, a dietary supplement is any product not meant for use as a conventional food or as a sole item of a meal or diet. DSHEA restricted FDA's ability to regulate products marketed as "dietary supplements." This act allows supplement manufacturers to market products without proving purity, strength, or effectiveness of supplements to the FDA. Manufacturers are responsible for ensuring that products are safe before they put them on the market. Once a product is marketed, the FDA is responsible for showing that a dietary supplement is "unsafe" before taking action to restrict the product's use or removal from the marketplace. Manufacturers of dietary supplements must record, investigate, then forward to FDA any reports they are aware of; however, a great majority of the estimated 50,000 adverse events that occur annually remain unreported, a situation referred to as "American Roulette."[22]

In 2007, the FDA implemented good manufacturing practices to ensure supplements are produced in a quality manner, do not contain contaminants or impurities, and are labeled accurately. The new mandate was intended to ensure that products are free of contamination and impurities. The law requires manufacturers to file a safety notification with the FDA before marketing dietary ingredients that were not on the market in 1994. But the FDA has received only about 700 notifications of new dietary ingredients. The FDA believes more than 55,000 dietary ingredients are currently marketed.[22]

The FDA has determined that many dietary supplements contain undeclared active pharmaceutical ingredients. Of particular concern are supplements contaminated with prescription medications, controlled substances, experimental compounds, or drugs rejected by the FDA because of safety concerns. Some products on the market contain ingredients used for patients with diabetes, high cholesterol, dementia, or insomnia; most of the products containing potentially hazardous ingredients are those promising sexual enhancement, optimal athletic performance, and weight loss.

Because there are no uniform manufacturing rules for these products, a MVM supplement may not contain what the bottle claims, could be contaminated with something from the manufacturing plant, or may have tainted ingredients. ConsumerLab.com, often called the "watchdog" of the supplement industry, is a private organization that provides independent evaluations of dietary products. In a recent evaluation, more than 30% of multivitamins tested contained significantly more or less of an ingredient than claimed, were contaminated with lead, or did not dissolve fast enough for maximum absorption.[23] The U.S. Government Accountability Office investigated retail outlets marketing herbal dietary supplements by hiring an accredited laboratory to examine 40 single-ingredient supplements for contaminants. None of the supplements were deemed as having toxic levels, but trace amounts of at least one contaminant were found in 37 of 40 products.[24]

Manufacturers can legally make three types of claims for a dietary supplement: health claims, structure/function claims, and nutrient content claims. Claims can describe the link between a food substance and disease or a health-related condition; intended benefits of using the product; or the amount of a nutrient or dietary substance present. The label on a product sold as a dietary supplement and promoted as a treatment, prevention, or cure for a specific disease or condition would not be allowed. Manufacturers must notify the FDA if they want to make a claim on the product and must include evidence of the product's effectiveness and safety.

If the FDA finds that supplements do not contain ingredients claimed, the agency can consider the products adulterated or misbranded. In minor cases, the FDA may ask the manufacturer to remove an ingredient or revise its label. In more serious cases, it could seize the product, file a lawsuit, or seek criminal charges.

The United States Pharmacopeia (USP), the National Sanitation Foundation International (NSF), and ConsumerLab.com (CL) are nonprofit groups that verify whether companies offer contamination-free products and use good manufacturing practices. The presence of a USP, NSF, or CL symbol on the label helps to ensure quality of a product because the symbols mean that the product has been tested to disintegrate and dissolve in the gastrointestinal tract, contains uniform quality (potency and purity), and contains ingredients as listed on the packaging. These organizations require an expiration date on the packaging. The symbols do not indicate that the supplement is safe for everyone or has any benefits. Not every brand has the seals; some manufacturers may not submit their products for testing.

In most instances, evidence does not indicate a need for most MVM supplements, but use of supplementation is endorsed when there is a demonstrated vitamin or mineral deficiency based on laboratory tests. Some nutrients are more likely to be inadequate during particular phases of life, as follows:

- Iron and folic acid—for adolescent girls and women during childbearing years, especially during pregnancy (see Chapter 13)
- Vitamin B_{12}—for people who are older than age 50 years (see Chapter 15)
- Vitamin D—for older adults, people with heavily pigmented skin, and people exposed to inadequate ultraviolet-B radiation (see Chapter 9)

Additionally during specific circumstances, typical nutritional needs or eating patterns change, so healthcare professionals should assess and determine whether a nutrient supplement is appropriate. Food intake patterns less than 1600 kcal daily are typically inadequate in vitamins and minerals. Supplements may be used to prevent, treat, or manage disease or other conditions. This would include supplementation with calcium and vitamin D for osteoporosis, and electrolyte replacement to treat acute diarrhea. Individuals who limit the variety of foods in their diet may need a MVM supplement, especially if whole food groups are omitted. Examples include vegans (inadequate amounts of calcium, iron, zinc, and vitamins D and B_{12}); people who eliminate all dairy foods (lack of calcium and vitamin D); and patients who severely restrict food choices because of allergies and food intolerances, such as celiac disease (malabsorption and

Continued

HEALTH APPLICATION 11   Vitamin, Mineral, and Herbal Supplements—cont'd

elimination of grain-based foods). In general, unless a health-care provider specifically indicates a need for more than 100% of the RDA of a particular nutrient, supplementation is probably not wise.

Patients may be taking amino acid and folic acid supplements, unconventional items, or herbal products described as "natural." These supplements may be deemed safe and desirable, but may adversely affect an existing medical condition or interact with other supplements or prescribed medications. Heroin, cocaine, and tobacco also can be considered "natural" plant-based substances, but lead to obvious health issues and are unsafe.

Megadoses of vitamins with intakes of 20 to 600 times the RDAs are sometimes advocated. Vitamin megadosage is defined as a dosage that is more than 10 times the RDA. A megadose of a vitamin is actually a misnomer because at these levels, the vitamin is functioning as a drug rather than a nutrient. This practice is dangerous and should be supervised by a healthcare provider to ensure toxicities do not occur. A well-established principle of pharmacological therapy is that all substances are potentially toxic at large enough doses. Taking more than the IOM's UL means risks likely outweigh benefits.

Complementary and alternative medicine (CAM) is using diverse medical and healthcare systems and products that are not generally considered part of conventional medicine. Complementary medicine utilizes CAM medicine together with conventional medicine, such as using acupuncture to alleviate pain. Alternative medicine pertains to use of CAM in place of conventional medicine. CAM practices often utilize herbal medicines and other "natural products." Many are available over-the-counter as dietary supplements. Interest in and use of CAM products have grown considerably in the past few decades.

Medical systems that have evolved from different cultures apart from conventional or Western medicine include homeopathy (treatment of diseases with minute doses of drugs that cause symptoms of a disease in healthy people to cure similar symptoms in sick people) and naturopathy (support of the body's inherent ability to maintain and restore health, using noninvasive treatments with minimal use of surgery and drugs). Theoretically, if a certain substance causes a symptom in a healthy person, a very small amount of the same substance may cure the symptoms. However, the website of the National Center for Complementary and Alternative Medicine (NCCAM) of the National Institutes of Health notes that most rigorous clinical trials and systematic analyses of research on homeopathy have concluded that "there is little evidence to support homeopathy as an effective treatment for any specific condition."[25] Some studies suggest the results are similar to a placebo effect, whereas others have found positive effects not readily explained in scientific terms. In general, homeopathics are benign because they are so dilute, they are unlikely they cause harm if used properly.

As with any medical treatment, risks are associated with CAM therapies. Several general precautions to help minimize risks are: (a) "natural" does not always mean "safe"; (b) herbal supplements may contain dozens of compounds and some active ingredients may not be known; (c) ingredients indicated on the label and actual ingredients in the product may be different; (d) some active ingredients may be lower or higher than indicated on the label; (e) the product may be contaminated with other herbs, pesticides, or metals; (f) some dietary supplements may interact with medications or nutrients, and may have their own side effects; and (g) inform all healthcare providers about use of any complementary and alternative practices. Research-based information about specific CAM treatments is available on the NCCAM website: http://nccam.nih.gov/health/atoz.htm.

Herbal medicines were used in initial attempts to improve health. Emerging evidence indicates commonly used botanicals (herbs and spices) may help protect against certain chronic conditions, such as cancer, diabetes, and heart disease. (Herbs are considered leafy green parts of a plant, whereas spices are from another part of the plant—seeds, berries, bark, or roots). Many botanicals contain high levels of antioxidants. In the amounts currently used, no negative side effects are expected. Because herbs and spices are not actual nutrients, when used for health benefits, they are considered CAMs. NCCAM's Herbs at a Glance (http://nccam.nih.gov/health/herbsataglance .htm?nav=gsa) has reliable information about botanicals—research, potential side effects and cautions, and resources for more information. By seasoning foods with herbs and spices, less salt, sugar, and fat may be necessary for taste appeal and may help with weight control and other conditions.

The body processes essential nutrients from food differently than pill form, probably because substances in foods interact with each other in a way that may affect nutrient absorption and utilization. High-dose dietary supplements may not only fail to prevent chronic disease but may actually do harm. For example, kidney stones may occur with high doses (500 mg/day) of vitamin C.

Patients become their own diagnosticians by self-prescribing MVM or herbal supplements without consulting their healthcare provider. The potencies of these self-prescribed supplements vary widely, containing from insignificant amounts to more than 5000% of the Dietary Reference Intake. Consumers use dietary supplements to achieve their self-care goals. Dietary supplements are, in their opinion, an easy means to ensure good health; treat and prevent serious illnesses, colds, and flu; increase mental acuity; and alleviate depression. These individuals may delay seeking medical attention for various health problems. Dietary supplements are not intended to treat disease. Many patients consider vitamins safe to take in any amount, but each year thousands of supplement toxicities occur, especially in children.

Public health nutrition would be served best by insisting on a scientifically sound basis for dietary supplementation. Despite consensus of public opinion, healthy patients do not need dietary supplements if they eat a well-balanced diet 80-90% of the time using a variety of foods. Vitamin and mineral supplements are not recommended as a preventive measure in a well-nourished population. Foods are the best source of nutrients. Only a few supplements are likely to help, some may do more harm than good, and many are expensive disappointments. Many research and observational studies have shown little or no evidence of protection regarding associations of MVM use for CHD (myocardial infarction or stroke), or cancers, or mortality from these.[26,27]

The long-term impact of supplementation is unknown. Supplements do not replace or improve the benefits of eating fruits and vegetables, and they may cause unwanted health consequences. In most situations, money is better spent on fresh fruits and vegetables. Obtaining nutrients from dietary sources rather than supplements reduces risk for nutrient deficiencies, excesses, and potential interactions with other drugs or medical conditions. A vast body of observational and epidemiological studies has associated an increased dietary intake of antioxidants from fruits and vegetables with reduced risks of a range of diseases, including cancer. Despite this, when such antioxidants have been extracted and put into supplements, numerous randomized clinical trials have shown they do not produce the same benefits and may cause harm. Health benefits associated with eating broccoli require consumption of the whole vegetable. Without specific enzymes found in whole foods, phytonutrients are poorly absorbed and are of far less value if taken as a supplement.[28]

Conservative, evidence-based information is often hard to balance against dramatic claims for health in a pill. Whereas the scientific community has reached a consensus about the overall lack of scientific evidence for healthy Americans needing a supplement, several cautions, shown in Box 11-3, are offered for decision making.

One of the biggest dangers is the effect supplements may have on people's attitudes: "I'm taking vitamins; I don't have to exercise, I can continue to smoke, and I can eat however I like." For patients who choose to self-prescribe supplements, low levels of nutrients that do not exceed the RDA are recommended. Amounts greater than 100% of the RDA should be limited to treatment of specific circumstances under medical supervision.

Store brands of vitamins are often identical to name brands; expensive supplements are no better than less costly supplements. Except for vitamin E, "natural" vitamins are no more beneficial than synthetic vitamins. (An all-natural vitamin E should contain only d-α-tocopherol.) Also, food folate is not as well absorbed as synthetic folic acid, and some individuals have difficulty absorbing naturally-occurring vitamin B_{12}. Other components in foods, however, may help with the absorption and use of some nutrients.

Daily MVM supplements are most effective when taken with a meal. It takes longer for a full stomach to empty, allowing more time for the supplement to dissolve and be absorbed.

Some nutrients may compete or block the action or absorption of another nutrient; taking single supplements at different meals may be necessary to avoid potential interactions. Chelated supplements are marketed to have superior absorption ability, but they are broken down by gastric acids and absorbed similar to other supplements. Most supplements marked "time release" also have no value. The body does not need to maintain a constant level of vitamins as it does for some medications, such as antibiotics.

In addition, herbs or supplements can be found in many oral health products (Box 11-4) that may cause adverse reactions when taken with over-the-counter or prescription medications. The dental professional should be cognizant of products containing herbs or supplements when recommending them to patients. Look for the American Dental Association Seal of Acceptance on the product.

A medical history should include specific queries about dietary and herbal supplements because many patients typically do not inform healthcare professionals of their usage. Document the type of supplement, amount, potential interactions, and dental implications (Box 11-5). By asking additional questions to determine why the patient is taking the supplement, the dental hygienist can discuss the benefits of a balanced diet, fluids, exercise, and smoking cessation (see Chapter 19, *Health Application 19*). More importantly, a careful investigation of peer-reviewed literature and use of scientifically based, current, quality research with valid clinical trials would provide dental hygienists with accurate information to help assess a patient's intake and provide advice.

All health professionals are responsible for reporting any damaging effects or illness resulting from nutritional supplements to the FDA (http://www.fda.gov/medwatch), and submitting complaints to the Federal Trade Commission regarding misleading advertising (http://www.ftc.gov/ftc/complaint.htm). Dental hygienists must consider whether or not their academic training and scope of practice qualifies them to provide advice regarding dietary supplement usage. Promoting healthy eating patterns and lifestyles according to national guidelines is appropriate advice to provide patients. A complete nutritional assessment of the patient needs to be conducted to validate the use of a supplement.

BOX II-3   Buyer Beware!!

- Beware of extravagant claims; if it sounds too good to be true, it is usually not true.
- Beware of testimonials and endorsements, especially from celebrities. Even the most sincere, all-meaning success stories offered by friends and relatives without financial incentives can't establish a product's safety or efficacy.
- Beware of the idea that if a little is good, more is better. Although vitamin A is essential for health, for example, doses that exceed the UL (3000 IU a day) increase risk of fractures. And a high intake of folic acid may increase risk for certain tumors.
- Beware of meaningless terms such as all-natural, antioxidant-rich, clinically proven, antiaging, and other vague but seductive claims that a product will promote heart health, prostate health, sexual prowess, energy, weight loss, fat loss, muscle power, and the like.
- Beware of interactions between supplements and medication. Always inform all healthcare providers, including pharmacists, about supplements taken, and ask specifically about potential interactions with prescription and over-the-counter medications.

- Beware of adulterated products. Do not assume all supplements are safe. More than 140 products laced with undisclosed pharmaceutical ingredients have been recalled because of FDA intervention. Products touted for sexual performance, weight loss, and athletic performance are most likely to be contaminated with medications.
- Beware of products that do not contain the amounts indicated on the label (more than or less than). In general, products that have been approved by the USP or NSF are safest.
- Beware of overconsumption of nutrients. In spite of all the publicity regarding the need for calcium to prevent osteoporosis, several recent studies have linked high dose calcium supplements with cardiovascular health. Estimate how much calcium and vitamin D is provided from usual food intake, then determine if supplementation is needed. Calcium from food is the ideal way of obtaining calcium.
- Beware of products marketed via the Internet. Whereas the FDA oversight seen by many as overly obtrusive, other countries have no regulations for manufacturing dietary supplements. Most of the recalled supplements are produced in other countries.

Adapted from Harvard Men's Health Watch: *Supplements: a scorecard*. Harvard Health Publications Harvard Medical School 2012 Apr. Accessed August 27, 2013: http://www.health.harvard.edu/newsletters/Harvard_Mens_Health_Watch/2012/April/supplements-a-scorecard

---

BOX II-4   "ABCD" Approach to Asking Patients about Use of Dietary Supplements

Ask
- What do you take: what form, what brand, what dose, and what else?
- How long have you been taking it, how much do you take, and how often?
- Why do you take it, why was it recommended, and by whom?
- Does it do what you thought it would?

Be
- Wary of any single nutrient used (e.g., vitamin C, E, or B_{12}) not recommended by a healthcare provider or RDN, and of doses exceeding the National Academy of Sciences, Institute of Medicine, Food and Nutrition Board dietary reference intakes.
- Sure to look up supplements used in a reliable resource.

Communicate
- Any concerns or risks about safety, drug–nutrient interactions, toxicity to the patient.

Document
- Supplements used, risks of concern, communication with patient, interaction.

Do
- Not get into the supplement business; when in doubt or wanting to refer a patient, contact the credentialed nutrition professional, a RDN.

From Touger-Decker R: Vitamin and mineral supplements: what is the dentist to do? *J Am Dent Assoc* 2007;138(9):1222-1226.

BOX II-5   Selected Ingredients Used in Oral Healthcare Products

- Bloodroot
- Calendula
- Cayenne
- Chamomile
- Clove oil
- Coenzyme Q10
- Echinacea
- Eucalyptus
- Fennel
- Garlic
- Ginger
- Goldenseal
- Grape seed extract
- *Lactobacillus acidophilus*
- Lemon balm
- Licorice root
- Lycopene
- Lysine
- Myrrh
- Nettle leaves
- Prickly ash
- Rhatany
- Sage
- Soy
- Tea
- Tea tree oil (*Melaleuca alternifolia*)
- Vitamin C
- Watercress
- Witch hazel
- Zinc

From Goldie MP: Dietary supplements and herbs: implications for client care. *Access* 2002;16:28-35.

Case Application for the Dental Hygienist

A young mother of a 3-year-old says she has heard that she should be taking folate supplements because she is considering discontinuing her birth control pills. She is concerned about the effects of the birth control pills on her nutritional status and their effect on a fetus should she become pregnant.

Nutritional Assessment
- Types of foods consumed
- Knowledge base of foods rich in folate
- Current use of any dietary supplements
- Motivation to change eating habits
- Knowledge of physiological values and absorption of folate

Nutritional Diagnosis
Health-seeking behavior related to nutritional status and effects on fetus.

Nutritional Goals
The patient will consume foods rich in folate and ask her healthcare provider about the need to take a multivitamin supplement or a folate supplement.

Nutritional Implementation
Intervention: Evaluate the oral area for symptoms of folate or other nutrient deficiencies.

Rationale: This will help determine whether or not she is currently deficient and help determine whether or not she should consult her healthcare provider immediately.

Intervention: Teach the following about folate: (a) different names used, (b) functions, (c) requirements, and (d) sources.

Rationale: This provides the patient with a sound base of knowledge about folic acid.

Intervention: Discuss symptoms of folate deficiency and harmful effects of too much folic acid.

Rationale: Although it is important that the patient obtain adequate amounts of folic acid to prevent neural tube defects, too much can also be harmful.

Intervention: Discuss the stability of folate during cooking and processing.

Rationale: Knowing folate can easily be destroyed during food preparation allows the patient to make decisions based on her eating habits and to determine whether or not her diet provides adequate amounts of folate.

Intervention: Explain her requirement for folic acid is increased because of the birth control pills, and because of the needs of the fetus and other physiological changes occurring early during pregnancy.

Rationale: This knowledge will help her realize the importance of changing dietary patterns consistently.

Evaluation
The patient should increase her intake of folate-rich foods (cereal products that are fortified with folate; oranges; liver; raw, green, leafy vegetables). Additionally, she should consult her healthcare provider before she discontinues the OCA and begins taking a multivitamin. She can state why she has an increased requirement for folic acid and why it is important not to take excessive amounts.

STUDENT READINESS

1. Name the two water-soluble vitamins most involved in the metabolism of fats, proteins, and carbohydrates to form energy (adenosine triphosphate) through the TCA cycle.
2. Match the conditions associated with the appropriate vitamin deficiency:

Thiamin	Cheilosis
Riboflavin	Scurvy
Iodine	Pellagra
Niacin	Megaloblastic anemia
Vitamin B_{12}	Beriberi
Ascorbic acid	Graves disease

3. Why is it important that water-soluble vitamins be consumed daily?
4. Define "vitamin megadose." What are the disadvantages of taking vitamin megadoses?
5. Name three foods that are good sources of each of the following nutrients: thiamin, riboflavin, vitamin B_{12}, and folate.
6. What would you teach a vegan about vitamin B_{12}?
7. Discuss why signs and symptoms of deficiencies of water-soluble vitamins appear periorally. List signs and symptoms of deficiencies you should be alert for, and list vitamins that might be implicated.
8. What recommendations could you offer to a patient to ensure the availability of folate? Why is folate so important before and during pregnancy?
9. Evaluate five of the stress or megavitamin supplement preparations in a drugstore or health food store. List the amounts of vitamin C, niacin, and vitamin B_6 (pyridoxine) in them, and compare those amounts with the RDAs for children younger than 10 years old, men 19 to 24 years old, and women 25 to 50 years old.

CASE STUDY

A 32-year-old man presents with the following symptoms: swollen tongue with reddening at the tip, small oral ulcerations, and gingival hyperplasia. The patient is being treated with long-term anticonvulsant medication.

1. Is a dietary assessment indicated? Explain your answer.
2. What are possible effects of the patient's medication on his nutritional and oral status?
3. If a deficiency exists, which vitamins/minerals are most likely lacking? Why?
4. Which types of foods and food preparation methods should be suggested? Why?
5. What advice should you give regarding oral care?

References

1. National Institutes of Health: *NIH stops clinical trial on combination cholesterol treatment.* NIH News, May 26, 2011. Accessed August 30, 2013: http://www.nih.gov/news/health/may2011/nhlbi-26.htm.

2. AIM-HIGH Investigators, Boden WE, Probstfield JL, Anderson T, et al: Niacin in patients with low HDL cholesterol levels receiving intensive statin therapy. *N Engl J Med* 365(24):2255–2267, 2011.

3. McDowell MA, Lacher DA, Pfeiffer CM, et al: Blood folate levels: the latest NHANES results. *NCHS Data Brief* (6):1–8, 2008. Hyattsville, MD: National Center for Health Statistics, May 2008. Last updated January 19, 2010. Accessed August 30, 2013: http://www.cdc.gov/nchs/data/databriefs/db06.htm.

4. Ho RC, Cheung MW, Fu E, et al: Is high homocysteine level a risk factor for cognitive decline in elderly? A systematic review, meta-analysis and meta-regression. *Am J Geriatr Psychiatry* 19(7):607–617, 2011.

5. Vollset SE, Clarke R, Lewington S, et al: Effects of folic acid supplementation on overall and site-specific cancer incidence during the randomised trials: meta-analyses of data on 50,000 individuals. *Lancet* 381(9871):1029–1036, 2013.

6. Mason JB: Folate, cancer risk, and the Greek god, Proteus: a tale of two chameleons. *Nutr Rev* 67(4):206–212, 2009.

7. Centers for Disease Control and Prevention (CDC): *Global initiative to eliminate folic acid-preventable neural tube defects.* Division of Birth Defects, National Center on Birth Defects and Developmental Disabilities, Centers for Disease Control and Prevention, Atlanta GA. Last updated November 14, 2011. Accessed August 30, 2013: http://www.cdc.gov/ncbddd/folicacid/global.html.

8. Yu YH, Kuo HK, Lai YL: The association between serum folate levels and periodontal disease in older adults: data from the National Health and Nutrition Examination survey 2001-02. *J Am Geriatr Soc* 55(1):108–113, 2007.

9. Saltzman E, Karl JP: Nutrient deficiencies after gastric bypass surgery. *Ann Rev Nutr* 33:183–203, 2013.

10. American Heart Association: *Homocysteine, folic acid and cardiovascular disease.* Updated January 20, 2012. Accessed August 30, 2013: http://www.heart.org/HEARTORG/GettingHealthy/NutritionCenter/Homocysteine-Folic-Acid-and-Cardiovascular-Disease_UCM_305997_Article.jsp.

11. Centers for Disease Control and Prevention (CDC): *Natural history and prevalence of vitamin B$_{12}$ deficiency.* Atlanta, GA. Last updated June 29, 2009. Accessed August 30, 2013: http://www.cdc.gov/ncbddd/b12/history.html.

12. Langan RC, Zawistoski KJ: Update on vitamin B$_{12}$ deficiency. *Am Fam Physician* 83(12):1425–1430, 2011.

13. Morris MS, Selhub J, Jacques PF: Vitamin B$_{12}$ and folate status in relation to decline in scores on the mini-mental state examination in the Framingham heart study. *J Am Geriatr Soc* 60(8):1457–1464, 2012.

14. Moore E, Mander A, Ames D, et al: Cognitive impairment and vitamin B$_{12}$: a review. *Int Psychogeriatr* 24(4):541–556, 2012.

15. Tangney CC, Aggarwal NT, Li H, et al: Vitamin B$_{12}$, cognition and brain MRI measures: a cross-sectional examination. *Neurology* 77(13):1276–1282, 2011.

16. Reinstatler L, Qi YP, Williamson RS, et al: Association of biochemical B$_{12}$ deficiency with metformin therapy and vitamin B$_{12}$ supplements: the National Health and Nutrition Examination Survey, 1999-2006. *Diabetes Care* 35(2):327–333, 2012.

17. Gahche J, Bailey R, Burt V, et al: Dietary supplement use among U.S. adults has increased since NHANES III (1988-1994). *NCHS Data Brief* (61):1–8, 2011.

18. Cohen PA: Assessing supplement safety—the FDA's controversial proposal. *N Engl J Med* 366(5):389–391, 2012.

19. Bailey RL, Gahche JJ, Miller PE, et al: Why US adults use dietary supplements. *JAMA Intern Med* 173(5):355–361 2013.

20. Moshfegh AJ: Monitoring the U.S. population's diet: the third step—the national "What We Eat in America" survey. *Agric Res* March 60(3):16–21, 2012. Accessed August 30, 2013: http://www.ars.usda.gov/is/AR/archive/mar12/diet0312.htm.

21. Centers for Disease Control and Prevention (CDC): *CDC's second nutrition report: a comprehensive biochemical assessment of the nutrition status of the U.S. population.* March 2012. Accessed August 30, 2013: http://www.cdc.gov/nutritionreport/.

22. Cohen PA: American roulette—contaminated dietary supplements. *N Engl J Med* 361:1523–1525, 2009.

23. ConsumerLab: *Multivitamin and multimineral supplements review.* Updated May 31, 2013. Accessed August 30, 2013: https://www.consumerlab.com/reviews/review_multivitamin_compare/multivitamins/.

24. U.S. Government Accountability Office: *Herbal dietary supplements—examples of deceptive or questionable marketing practices and potentially dangerous advice.* GAO-10-662T, May 26, 2010. Accessed August 30, 2013: http://www.gao.gov/new.items/d10662t.pdf.

25. National Center for Complementary and Alternative Medicine (NCCAM): *Homeopathy: an introduction.* Last updated May 2013. Accessed August 30, 2013: http://nccam.nih.gov/health/homeopathy.

26. Sesso HD, Christen WG, Bubes V, et al: Multivitamins in the prevention of cardiovascular disease in men: the physicians' health study II randomized controlled trial. *JAMA* 308(17):1751–1760, 2012.

27. Neuhouser ML, Wassertheil-Smoller S, Thomson C, et al: Multivitamin use and risk of cancer and cardiovascular disease in the Women's Health Initiative cohorts. *Arch Intern Med* 169(3):294–304, 2009.

28. Clarke JD, Riedl K, Bella D, et al: Comparison of isothiocyanate metabolite levels and histone deacetylase activity in human subjects consuming broccoli sprouts or broccoli supplement. *J Agric Food Chem* 59(20):10955–10963, 2011.

ⓔ EVOLVE RESOURCES

Please visit http://evolve.elsevier.com/Stegeman/nutritional for additional practice and study support tools.

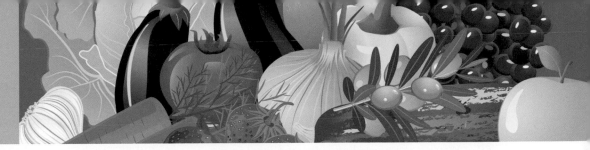

Chapter 12

Fluids and Minerals Required for Oral Soft Tissues and Salivary Glands

Student Learning Outcomes

Upon completion of this chapter, the student will be able to achieve the following student learning outcomes:

- Describe the process of osmosis.
- Explain how electrolytes affect hydration status.
- List normal fluid requirements and identify factors that may affect these requirements.
- Discuss the roles, imbalances, and sources of water, sodium, potassium, iron, zinc, and iodine.
- Discuss with patients how to decrease dietary sources of sodium and increase potassium intake and state why these are important.

- Identify oral signs and symptoms of fluid and electrolyte imbalances.
- Discuss areas of nutritional concern with patients who have fluid and electrolyte imbalances.
- Determine which diseases and medications may require patients to restrict sodium intake.
- Identify the most prominent oral symptoms or signs of iron, zinc, and iodine deficiency.

Key Terms

Aldosterone
Anions
Antidiuretic hormone (ADH)
Cations
Coliforms
Cretinism
Diaphoresis
Essential hypertension
Extracellular fluid (ECF)
Fluid volume deficit (FVD)
Fluid volume excess (FVE)
Ginseng
Goiter
Goitrogens
Guarana
Heme iron
Hemochromatosis
Hyperkalemia

Hypernatremia
Hypodipsia
Hypokalemia
Hyponatremia
Intracellular fluid (ICF)
Longitudinal fissures
Myxedema
Nonheme iron
Osmoreceptors
Osmosis
Peripheral edema
Quercetin
Renin
Solutes
Solvent
Taurine
Theanine
Transferrin

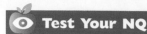

Water and several mineral elements are essential for maintenance of healthy oral tissues, including tooth enamel. Visual signs of these nutrient deficiencies in the gingiva, mucous membranes, and salivary glands are less obvious than signs observed with the B-vitamin complex and vitamin C deficiencies discussed in Chapters 9 and 11. Nevertheless, water and several minerals have a significant effect on integrity of the oral cavity and, ultimately, nutritional status. Oral problems associated with hyper states or hypo states of the minerals discussed in this chapter are slow to develop and may not be critical immediately. Chronically decreased salivary flow attributable to inadequate body fluids may lead to rampant tooth decay and eventually loss of teeth.

FLUIDS

Water is the most abundant component in the body. At birth, water constitutes approximately 75% to 80% of body weight. Because such a large percentage of the infant's body weight consists of water, fluid loss is more significant in infants than in adults. Total body water decreases with age, representing 50% to 60% of the total body weight of an adult. Adipose tissue contains less water than muscle; a person with a large amount of fat has a lower percentage of total body water. Women's bodies, with inherently larger fat stores, contain less water than do men's bodies, which have a higher percentage of lean muscle tissue.

Body fluids are distributed intracellularly and extracellularly. **Intracellular fluid (ICF)**, which constitutes 60% of the body's fluid weight, includes all the fluid within cells (chiefly in muscle tissue). **Extracellular fluid (ECF)** consists of fluid outside the cells. Fluid compartments are separated from one another by semipermeable membranes. These membranes serve as barriers by preventing movement of certain substances from one compartment to another; however, they do not completely isolate the compartments. Water is essentially unrestricted in its movement from compartment to compartment. Certain dissolved substances, or **solutes**, such as glucose, amino acids, and oxygen, also cross membranes freely. The cellular membranes allow maintenance of solute concentration by their selectivity.

When two compartments are separated by semipermeable membranes, and the movement of some solutes is restricted, osmosis occurs. **Osmosis** is the movement of water from an area of lower solute concentration to one of a higher solute concentration. Osmotic pressure within the body equalizes the solute concentration of ICFs and ECFs by shifting small amounts of water in the direction of higher concentration of solute, as shown in Chapter 3, Figure 3-6.

Physiological Roles

Water has several important physiological roles: (a) it acts as a **solvent** (fluid in which substances are dissolved), enabling chemical reactions to occur by entering into some reactions, such as hydrolysis; (b) it maintains stability of all body fluids, as principal component and medium for fluids (blood and lymph), secretions (saliva and gastrointestinal fluids), and excretions (urine and perspiration); (c) it enables transport of nutrients to cells and provides a medium for excretion of waste products; (d) it acts as a lubricant between cells to permit movement without friction; and (e) it regulates body temperature by evaporating as perspiration from skin and vapor from the mouth and nose. Negative fluid balance has serious detrimental effects on many physiological functions. A few days without water can be fatal.

Requirements and Regulation

Water requirements are based on experimentally-derived intake levels that are expected to meet nutritional needs of a healthy population. To maintain normal hydration, the Institute of Medicine (IOM) established an adequate intake (AI) for total fluid (beverages, water, and food). As shown in Table 12-1, men require 3.7 L/day (15 to 16 cups), and women require 2.7 L/day (11 to 12 cups). No tolerable upper intake level (UL) is established for water.

Overconsumption and underconsumption of fluids can occur over short periods. However, if adequate amounts of fluids are available, consumption matches physiological needs over an extended period. Loss of 1% of body water is usually compensated within 24 hours.[1] Individuals who consume a high-protein or high-fiber diet, have diarrhea or vomiting, or are physically active or exposed to warm or hot weather, require more fluids.

Water is lost by a variety of routes: (a) urination, (b) perspiration, (c) expiration, and (d) defecation. Urine production depends on the amount of fluid intake and type of diet

Table 12-1	Institute of Medicine recommendations for water	
	AI[a]	
Life Stage	Male (L/d)[b]	Female (L/d)[b]
0-6 months	0.7[c]	0.7[c]
7-12 months	0.8[d]	0.8[d]
1-3 years	1.3[e]	1.3[e]
4-8 years	1.7[f]	1.7[f]
9-13 years	2.4[g]	2.1[h]
14-18 years	3.3[i]	2.3[g]
>18 years	3.7[j]	2.7[k]
Pregnancy		
14-50 years		3[l]
Lactation		
14-50 years		3.8[m]

Data from Institute of Medicine (IOM), Food and Nutrition Board: *Dietary reference intakes for water, potassium, sodium, chloride, chloride, and sulfate,* Washington, DC, 2005, National Academies Press.

[a]AI (adequate intake)—the observed average or experimentally set intake by a defined population or subgroup that seems to sustain a defined nutritional status, such as growth rate, normal circulating nutrient values, or other functional indicators of health. An AI is used if insufficient scientific evidence is available to derive an estimated average requirement. For healthy human milk–fed infants, the AI is the mean intake. *The AI is not equivalent to a recommended dietary allowance.*

[b]L = liter; 1 L = 4.2 cups.

[c]Assumed to be from human milk.

[d]Assumed to be from human milk, complementary foods, and beverages. This includes ~0.6 L (~3 cups) as total fluid, including formula or human milk, juices, and drinking water.

[e]Total water. This includes ~0.9 L (~4 cups) as total beverages, including drinking water.

[f]Total water. This includes ~1.7 L (~5 cups) as total beverages, including drinking water.

[g]Total water. This includes ~1.8 L (~8 cups) as total beverages, including drinking water.

[h]Total water. This includes ~1.6 L (~7 cups) as total beverages, including drinking water.

[i]Total water. This includes ~2.6 L (~11 cups) as total beverages, including drinking water.

[j]Total water. This includes ~3 L (~13 cups) as total beverages, including drinking water.

[k]Total water. This includes ~2.7 L (~9 cups) as total beverages, including drinking water.

[l]Total water. This includes ~3 L (~10 cups) as total beverages, including drinking water.

[m]Total water. This includes ~3.1 L (~13 cups) as total beverages, including drinking water.

eaten. However, waste products must be kept in solution; minimum urine output to eliminate waste products is 400 to 600 mL/day.

Water losses in the form of sweat can vary greatly. An increase in body temperature (fever) is accompanied by increased sweating and respiration. Strenuous exercise can greatly affect the amount of water lost through the skin. Vapor in expired air varies with the rate of respiration. The presence of respiratory inflammation also elevates respiration rate. Approximately 100 to 200 mL of water is lost each day in feces; this is dramatically increased in individuals with diarrhea.

Water losses result in stimulation of water (thirst) and decreased kidney output to maintain fluid balance. Saliva also may help maintain water balance because saliva flow is reduced in dehydration, leading to drying of the mucosa and sensation of thirst.

Normal fluid requirements (Fig. 12-1) can be drastically changed in different climatic environments, with various exercise levels, diet, and social activities, and with illnesses resulting in (or are accompanied by) diarrhea or vomiting. The body cannot store water, so the amount lost must be replaced.

In healthy adults, thirst is an early sign of the body's need for fluids, but is often mistaken for hunger. The ability to regulate water balance is not as precise in infants and older adults. Older patients often have a reduced sensation of thirst. When 2% of body water is lost, osmoreceptors are stimulated, creating a physiological desire to ingest liquids. **Osmoreceptors** are neurons in the hypothalamus that are sensitive to changes in serum osmolality levels. Stimulation of osmoreceptors not only causes thirst, but also increases release of **antidiuretic hormone (ADH)** from the pituitary gland (Fig. 12-2). ADH causes the body to retain fluid by decreasing urinary output. Conversely, if there is too much water in the body, ADH secretion is inhibited, and excess water is eliminated.

Decreased blood pressure also stimulates release of the enzyme **renin**, which ultimately leads to increased release of the hormone **aldosterone** by the adrenal cortex. This release of aldosterone results in retention of sodium and water by the kidneys, and excretion of potassium and hydrogen ions, causing blood pressure to increase.

Absorption

No digestion is necessary for water absorption; it is transported easily in both directions across the intestinal mucosa by osmosis. Within an hour, 1 L can be absorbed from the small intestine. Normally, almost all fluid is absorbed with a small amount excreted in feces.

Sources

Water

Water is the only liquid nutrient that is essential for body hydration. During the process of metabolism, liquids and solid foods provide water. Some fruits and vegetables have a higher percentage of water than does milk, and meats are more than half water (Table 12-2). Regardless of its source, fluids act the same physiologically. Water liberated in the process of metabolism is also available. Metabolism of fat produces approximately twice as much water as the metabolism of protein or carbohydrate; metabolism of these macronutrients supplies about 300 to 350 mL daily.

Plain tap water is the most natural source of fluids, best for quenching thirst, most economical, and healthiest. However, many Americans have become disenchanted with tap water. Although not perfect, the United States has one of the safest public water supplies in the world. During the past century, many improvements in Americans' health can be

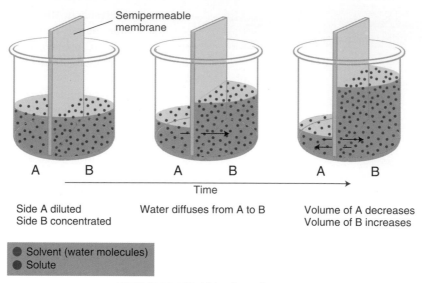

Side A diluted   Water diffuses from A to B   Volume of A decreases
Side B concentrated   Volume of B increases

● Solvent (water molecules)
● Solute

FIGURE 12-1 Fluid intake and output.

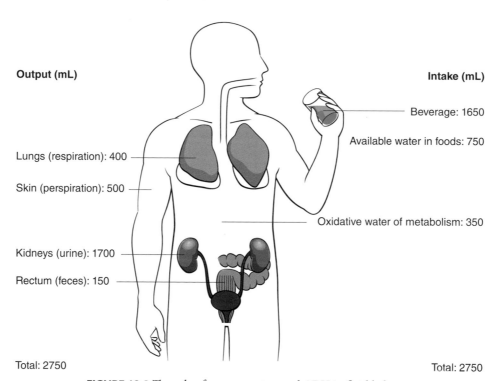

Output (mL)   Intake (mL)

Beverage: 1650

Available water in foods: 750

Lungs (respiration): 400

Skin (perspiration): 500

Oxidative water of metabolism: 350

Kidneys (urine): 1700

Rectum (feces): 150

Total: 2750   Total: 2750

FIGURE 12-2 The role of osmoreceptors and ADH in fluid balance.

attributed to improvements in drinking water, such as community fluoridation and controlling infectious diseases. When ground water becomes polluted, it is no longer safe to drink. Naturally occurring arsenic and radon in the environment can contaminate water. Some of the ways water can become contaminated is from use of fertilizers and pesticides, microbial contamination, and manufacturing processes. Drugs have been detected in drinking water of several major metropolitan areas. This contamination could be from medications not absorbed by individuals and eliminated through physiological discharges or numerous other reasons. Many pharmaceuticals pass through sewage and drinking

water treatment plants. Some gastrointestinal illnesses occur from small or individual water systems.

The U.S. Environmental Protection Agency regulates levels of contaminants allowed in drinking water in public water systems. Water utility companies are required to provide Consumer Confidence Reports to their customers annually. Private well owners are responsible for ensuring their water is safe from contaminants of high concern. Wastewater is treated, but most treatments do not remove all drug residues and other contaminants. In some cases, contaminants are not monitored. Although present in very low amounts, the effect of these drugs and contaminants on

Table 12-2 Percentage of water in foods	
Food Item	**% Water**
Beer and wine	90-95
Milk, fruit juice, fruit drinks	85-90
Cooked cereals	85-90
Fruits (strawberries, melons, grapefruit, peaches, pears, oranges, apples, grapes, cucumbers, tomatoes)	80-85
Vegetables (lettuce, celery, cabbage, broccoli, onions, carrots)	80-85
Cottage cheese and yogurt	75-80
Liquid drinks for weight loss, muscle gain, meal replacement	70-85
Fish and seafood	70-80
Vegetables (potatoes, corn)	70-75
Rice and pasta	65-80
Eggs	65-80
Stew, pasta and meat dishes, casseroles (with meat and meatless), meatloaf, tacos, enchiladas, macaroni and cheese	60-80
Sauces and gravies	50-85
Ice cream	50-60
Beef, chicken, lamb, pork, turkey, veal	45-65
Cheese	40-50
Breads, bagels, biscuits	30-45
Ready to-eat breakfast cereals	2-5
Chips, pretzels, candies, crackers, dried fruit, popcorn	1-5

Adapted from Grandjean A, Campbell S: *Hydration: fluids for life*, Washington, DC, 2004, ILSI North America.

health is unknown. The U.S. Environmental Protection Agency is continually looking at methods to detect and quantify pharmaceuticals and other contaminants in wastewater.

Because of mistrust of the water supply, and a desire for a safer and more convenient form of fluid intake, consumers frequently choose bottled water. The bottled water market has been increasing, with an annual per capita consumption of 11 gallons in 2011.[2] However, as a result of environmental concerns (energy required to produce plastic nonbiodegradable plastic bottles, bisphenol A [BPA] content of bottles, cost of marketing and shipping bottles containing water), and the revelation that approximately 75% of reputable bottlers utilize groundwater (same source as the public water supply) or tap water, the rate of increase has declined.[3]

Bottled water is regulated by the U.S. Food and Drug Administration (FDA). Bottled waters come with many labels: drinking water, sparkling water, mineral water, Artesian water, and purified water (distilled, demineralized, deionized, and reverse osmosis). Bottled water also includes flavored waters and nutrient-added water beverages. In 2009, the FDA mandated that all manufacturers of bottled water test their water source for the presence of coliforms (a bacterial indicator of sanitation, universally present in the feces of animals) on a weekly basis. If further tests prove positive for *Escherichia coli*, companies must take measures to eliminate the bacteria and retest samples before use. The FDA also established the U.S. Environmental Protection Agency's maximum levels for contaminants (except for a lower maximum amount of lead) and disinfection by-products (e.g., bromate, chlorite, etc.), and disinfectants (e.g., chlorine) in bottled water.[4]

This trend has resulted in increased water intake, but numerous problems are associated with this practice. Many consumers think bottled water is healthier, but most bottled waters do not contain fluoride. Fluoride does not have to be listed on the label unless it is added.

In addition to plain bottled water, manufacturers are adding other ingredients; many of these are nutrients. Supermarket shelves are filled with ready-to-serve coffees and teas, carbonated beverages, sports and energy drinks; vitamin water; and drinks containing amino acids, B vitamins, caffeine, green tea, vitamin C, ginger, cranberry extracts, or ginkgo (*Ginkgo biloba*). These drinks are often expensive.

Many of these flavored beverages contain additional kilocalories, which are consumed in excessive amounts by most Americans. Kilocalories in drinks are not hidden, and the body does not treat them differently from energy provided in foods. But kilocalories in beverages go down so smoothly, significant amounts can be consumed without realizing how much is being consumed. Studies have produced conflicting results as to whether or not people compensate for kilocaloric intake from sugar-sweetened beverages. Sugar-containing beverages are at least questionable for individuals needing to control their energy intake and weight.[5,6]

Water has been recommended for weight loss, despite the fact that fluids satisfy thirst and not hunger. Water consumed with a meal does not affect caloric consumption at mealtime, but water incorporated into food (as in soup) increases satiety, ultimately leading to less caloric intake. Basically, foods that incorporate water tend to appear larger; more volume provides greater oral stimulation; and water bound to food slows absorption and increases satiety.[7]

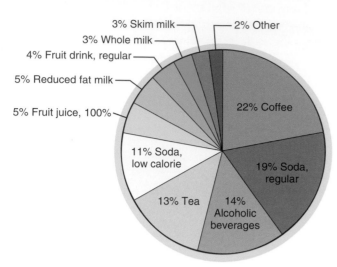

FIGURE 12-3 Distribution of intake (grams) across beverage types, U.S. adults (age 19+ years). Other beverages include fruit drink (low calorie), milk substitute/evaporated milk, and vegetable juice, each contributing less than 2%. Percentages do not add to 100% as a result of rounding. Data source: NHANES 2005-2006. Available at: http://riskfactor.cancer.gov/diet/foodsources/beverages/figure4.html

Although water is the only fluid truly needed by the body, many other liquids are acceptable, and some, such as low-fat milk, contribute significant amounts of important nutrients. Figure 12-3 depicts the beverage intake pattern of adults in the United States; beverages in these amounts and proportions represent almost 400 kcal daily. A recommended healthier intake would include at least 100 fl oz total intake with approximately 50% from water, approximately 16 oz of unsweetened tea or coffee, at least 8 oz low fat milk, approximately 24 oz of beverages with some kilocalories and nutrients (fruit juice), and approximately 12 oz of calorically sweetened and diet beverages.

Coffees and Teas

For many Americans, coffee tastes good and helps "jump start" the morning. Coffee, without added sugars or creamers, contains negligible kilocalories. In addition to contributing to fluid intake, coffee has some health benefits. Coffee contains literally a thousand different substances, including healthful antioxidants. It is not a significant source of vitamins and minerals, but it does contain small amounts of magnesium, chromium, and potassium, nutrients many Americans are lacking.

Although research has not yet produced definite answers, a growing body of research suggests that moderate coffee drinkers, compared to nondrinkers, are less likely to have type 2 diabetes;[8] Parkinson and Alzheimer disease;[9,10] dementia;[11] certain cancers (liver and prostate);[12] heart failure;[13] arrhythmia problems;[14] and strokes.[15] However, coffee has not been shown to prevent these conditions. A large prospective study found an inverse relationship between coffee consumption and total and cause-specific mortality, but this study was unable to determine whether this was a causal or associative finding.[16] Both regular and decaffeinated coffee

contain acids that may aggravate heartburn. Because of the addition of caffeine to many new products, the U.S. FDA is investigating the safety of caffeine.

Polyphenols in tea appear to possess health benefits, specifically antioxidant and anti-inflammatory actions as key mechanisms in preventing certain types of cancer, CHD, and diabetes.[17-19] Teas also contain multiple flavonoids and have virtually no kilocalories unless sugar or milk are added. It is fairly well established that flavonoids in tea have health benefits, and tea may be a better alternative beverage to coffee, partly because of its lower caffeine content (Box 12-1). Highly processed tea leaves provide less polyphenols or flavonoids: oolong and black teas are oxidized or fermented, resulting in lower concentrations of polyphenols than green tea. Green tea has been more widely studied than other teas.

All green, black, and white teas contain caffeine and **theanine** (an amino acid used to treat anxiety and high blood pressure and other things). These chemicals affect the brain and appear to heighten mental alertness.[20,21] Limited studies support the theories that compounds in tea may help encourage weight loss,[22] lower cholesterol, and improve resistance to infections.[23] One drawback to tea consumption is its tannin content, which inhibits iron absorption, particularly when tea and iron are consumed at the same time.

Herbal teas are made from herbs, fruits, seeds, or roots steeped in hot water. Although their chemical composition varies widely depending on the plant used, they have lower concentrations of antioxidants than green, white, black, and oolong teas. Research on health benefits (weight loss and resistance to infections) of herbal teas has been limited.

Most teas are benign, but the FDA has issued warnings regarding those that contain senna, aloe, buckthorn, and other plant-derived laxatives. The FDA has granted permission for unauthorized health claims for some teas and requested some manufacturers remove health claims on their labels.

Energy Drinks

Energy drinks were introduced in the United States in 1997. Sales of energy drinks and shots have more than doubled in the past 5 years; they are especially appealing to teenagers and young adults, especially young men. Sales in the United States increased to almost $9 billion in 2011.[24] Energy drinks are marketed to provide a higher energy level, make a person feel more awake, and boost attention span.

Energy drinks contain ingredients that act as stimulants, such as caffeine, **guarana** (a seed containing four times as much caffeine as coffee beans), and **taurine** (an amino acid with antioxidant properties). Coffee-energy drinks blend coffee extract with milk, taurine, and **ginseng** (allegedly improves concentration and thinking, physical stamina, athletic endurance; causes abdominal pain and headaches). Energy shots (approximately 2 oz) contain the same stimulants as energy drinks but are more concentrated. Decaffeinated energy drinks have eliminated caffeine but are packed with B vitamins and **quercetin** (bioflavonoid reported to energize muscles). Whereas quercetin improved performance of mice on a treadmill, human studies failed to improve athletic performance.[25] One popular liquid shot contains 8333% of the RDA for vitamin B_{12} and 2000% for vitamin B_6, 150% for niacin, and 100% for folic acid.

Contrary to what commercial advertisements claim, B vitamins are not little packets of energy. Vitamins help the body use energy from foods, but extra B vitamins do not provide additional energy bursts. Almost all Americans get adequate amounts of B vitamins in their diets, yet marketers would lead people to believe that a megadose of B vitamins energizes. Energy drinks usually contain 140 kcal/8 oz from carbohydrates. These beverages may include some nutrients, but lack principal nutrients deficient in Americans' diets.

Several of these energy drinks have been linked to unexpected deaths in apparently healthy adults and children, possibly leading to closer scrutiny and regulation by FDA. Energy drinks have contributed to increases in emergency department visits resulting from excessive caffeine intake especially when these drinks are combined with alcohol.[26,27] Many in the medical community are concerned about potential negative problems associated with stimulants in beverages and lack of disclosure about the amount. Use of energy drinks may increase risk for caffeine overdose in caffeine abstainers, as well as habitual consumers of caffeinated coffee, soft drinks, and tea.

The amount of caffeine in a product is not required on labels because it is not a nutrient. If energy drinks contain "natural" ingredients, such as ginkgo or guarana, the FDA considers them a dietary supplement rather than a food or medication. One major corporation has recently decided to

---

BOX 12-1   Caffeine Myths and Facts*

Caffeine occurs naturally in many plants including coffee beans, tea leaves, kola nuts (used to flavor carbonated beverages), and cacao pods (used for chocolate products). Caffeine is sometimes added to medications and foods but is most frequently found in beverages. Most Americans consume about 300 mg/day. Caffeine is a central nervous system stimulant, affecting the brain, spinal cord, and other nerves. The FDA considers caffeine both a drug and a food additive. Caffeine reaches a peak level in the blood within 1 hour after consumption and remains at these levels for 4 to 6 hours.

Although caffeine is beneficial for physical and mental performance in some cases, very little research has been conducted to validate the benefits of very high caffeine intake. Caffeine increases a person's metabolic rate and may be associated with increased wakefulness. Very high caffeine intake (>500 mg/day) is associated with nervousness, restlessness, anxiety, insomnia, arrhythmia, gastrointestinal upset, tremors, and psychomotor agitation. Moderate amounts of caffeine (about 300 mg/day) do not cause these effects in most individuals.

1. Caffeine is not addictive. As a central nervous system stimulant, it can cause mild physical dependence, but it does not threaten physical, social, or economic health as addictive drugs do. Abruptly stopping caffeine may cause withdrawal symptoms such as headache, fatigue, anxiety, and depressed mood and concentration for a day or two.
2. Caffeine consumed within 6 hours of going to bed may cause insomnia. Caffeine is quickly absorbed but has a relatively short half-life. Drinking 1 or 2 cups of coffee in the morning will not interfere with nighttime sleep for most people.
3. Moderate amounts of caffeine do not increase risk for conditions such as osteoporosis, CHD, and cancer. High levels (more than 700 mg/day) do not increase risk for bone loss if adequate amounts of calcium are consumed. (The addition of 2 tbsp of milk to 1 cup of coffee can offset calcium loss). However, older adults may be more sensitive to the effects of caffeine on calcium metabolism and, to be cautious, postmenopausal women should limit caffeine intake to less than 300 mg/day. Several large studies do not link caffeine to high cholesterol, irregular heartbeat, or increased risk of CHD. People who have been diagnosed with hypertension should discuss caffeine intake with their doctor. Studies involving 20,000 people revealed no relationship between cancer and caffeine and suggested caffeine may even have a protective effect.
4. Low amounts of caffeine (less than 200 mg caffeine/day) have not been found to interfere with the ability to get pregnant, or cause miscarriages, birth defects, premature birth, or low birth rate. One cup of coffee (containing approximately 200 mg caffeine) is considered safe during pregnancy.
5. Caffeine is not dehydrating. Caffeine acts as a mild diuretic, but fluid in caffeinated beverages offsets the effect of fluid loss, and does not cause dehydration.
6. Caffeine has been linked to a number of harmful health effects in children, including effects on the developing neurologic and cardiovascular systems. The American Academy of Pediatrics recommends children avoid caffeine-containing beverages, including carbonated beverages, and adolescents limit caffeine to less than 100 mg caffeine daily.† Health Canada has issued the following maximum levels of intake: 4-6 year olds–45 mg/day; 7-9 year olds—62.5 mg/day; 10-12 year olds—85 mg; adolescents 13 and older—no more than 2.5 mg/kg; healthy adults—400 mg; pregnant or breastfeeding women—300 mg.‡ Popular drinks (carbonated beverages, energy drinks, and sweetened teas) put children at higher risk for obesity due to the empty calories and dental caries because of their low pH.
7. Caffeine has no effect in helping people under the influence of alcohol to sober up. Reaction time and judgment are still impaired.
8. Caffeine has some health benefits: improved alertness, concentration, and energy, slower decline in cognitive ability, possible improvement in immune function, and relief from allergic reactions. Limited evidence suggests caffeine may reduce the risk of Parkinson and liver diseases, colorectal cancer, type 2 diabetes, and dementia.

However, high levels of caffeine have adverse effects. More studies are needed to confirm the benefits and potential risks from caffeine. Energy drinks and sodas may contain sugar and/or caffeine. In general, sodas contain less caffeine than energy drinks per ounce. Caffeine content of many beverages, candies, over-the-counter medications, and energy drinks are listed on next page.

Continued

BOX 12-1	Caffeine Myths and Facts—cont'd		

CAFFEINE CONTENT OF BEVERAGES AND OTHER PRODUCTS§

ENERGY DRINKS	CAFFEINE CONTENT (mg)	ENERGY DRINKS	CAFFEINE CONTENT (mg)
5-Hour Energy, 2 oz	207	Tea, green, (brewed), 8 oz	24-40
Amp, 8 oz	74	Coffee (brewed), 8 oz	95-200
Cran-Energy, 8 oz	58	Coffee, espresso, restaurant-style, 1 oz	40-75
Full Throttle, 8 oz	79		
Monster, 8 oz	86	Coffee, McDonalds, brewed, 16 oz	100
Red Bull, 8.4 oz	76-80		
Rockstar, 8 oz	79-80	Coffee, McDonalds, Mocha Frappe, 16 oz	125
Vault, regular or sugar-free, 8 oz	47		
Sodas		Coffee, Starbucks Latte, 16 oz	150
Coca-Cola, Classic or Zero, 12 oz	30-35	Coffee, Starbucks Pike Place Brewed, 16 oz	330
Dr Pepper, 12 oz	36	Milk, chocolate (whole, or reduced/low fat)	2
Mountain Dew, 12 oz	46-55		
Pepsi, 12 oz	32-39	Excedrin Extra Strength, 2 pills	130
A&W Root Beer, 7Up, or Sprite, 12 oz	0	NoDoz Maximum Strength, 1 pill	200
Other		StayAlert Gum, 1 piece	100
Tea, Arizona iced, green, 8 oz	11	Vivarin, 1 pill	200
Tea, black (brewed), 8 oz	14-61		

*Adapted from Kiefer D: Caffeine myths and facts. WebMD February 27, 2011. Accessed August 31, 2013. Available at: http://www.webmd.com/balance/caffeine-myths-and-facts

†American Academy of Pediatrics: Kids should not consume energy drinks, and rarely need sports drinks, says AAP. May 30, 2011. Accessed August 31, 2013: http://www.aap.org/en-us/about-the-aap/aap-press-room/pages/Kids-Should-Not-Consume-Energy-Drinks,-and-Rarely-Need-Sports-Drinks,-Says-AAP.aspx?nfstatus=401&nftoken=00000000-0000-0000-0000-000000000000&nfstatusdescription=ERROR%3a+No+local+token

‡Health Canada reminds Canadians to manage their caffeine consumption, June 11, 2013. Accessed August 31, 2013: http://www.ers.usda.gov/data-products/chart-gallery/detail.aspx?chartId=36247&ref=collection#.UVC5s1fB98E

§Data from Mayo Clinic staff: Caffeine content for coffee, tea, soda and more. Accessed August 31, 2013. Available at: http://www.mayoclinic.com/health/caffeine/AN01211; U.S. Department of Agriculture, Agricultural Research Service. 2013. USDA national nutrient database for standard reference, release 26. Nutrient Data Laboratory. Accessed August 31, 2013. Available at: http://www.ars.usda.gov/ba/bhnrc/ndl

reclassify their energy-boosting products as a conventional food rather than a dietary substance because of what they call erroneous and misguided criticism. They have indicated they will include caffeine content on labels.

Sports Drinks

Recent emphasis on Americans increasing their physical activity appears to have sparked an interest in supplemental products by sports enthusiasts and people who are attempting to maintain their health. Sports nutrition products are now available in super markets and convenience stores in addition to their previous availability in gyms and health food stores.

Sports drinks and energy drinks are significantly different products, but the terms are confusing and used interchangeably by many consumers. Sports drinks (e.g., Gatorade and Powerade), popular among children and sports enthusiasts, are designed to restore fluid balance, to replace fluid and electrolytes lost in sweat during physical activity, and ultimately, to optimize athletic performance. Sports drinks often contain carbohydrates (a source of kilocalories), minerals (e.g., calcium and magnesium), electrolytes (e.g., sodium and potassium), and sometimes vitamins or other nutrients, such as protein and/or amino acids. Flavorings are added to

enhance the taste. Protein in energy drinks has not been found to improve athletic performance, but protein enhances muscle recovery when ingested promptly after exercise. Specific amino acids added to sports drinks are reported to enhance immune function and enhance lipolysis; this claim has not been supported by clinical trials. There is no advantage to consuming vitamins and/or the minerals calcium and magnesium in sports drinks; these are readily available in a well-balanced diet.

Most research on sports products has been conducted using highly trained endurance athletes who exercise at high intensity for long periods. Sports nutrition recommendations are sometimes extrapolated to recreational athletes who have very different reasons for exercising, and therefore different nutritional needs. Most endurance athletes can benefit from a sports beverage that contains carbohydrates and electrolytes, and sometimes protein, but for most people engaged in routine physical activity, sports drinks offer little to no advantage over plain water. Sports drinks can be helpful for young athletes engaged in prolonged, vigorous physical activities; they are probably unnecessary during school physical education or in the school lunchroom. Sports drinks containing 6% to 8% carbohydrate are recommended when exercise is longer than 1 hour. These drinks can easily meet carbohydrate and fluid needs as well as sodium and potassium lost in sweat.[28]

Scientific studies do not support claims about improved performance and recovery for many sports drinks and protein shakes. Rather, researchers feel that it is virtually impossible for the public to make informed choices about the benefits and harms of advertised sports products.[29]

Sodas

Beverages provide approximately 15% to 21% of Americans' total daily kilocalories. Approximately 46% of 35- to 54-year olds say they drink at least one glass of soda daily as compared to 56% of 18- to 34-year olds reporting equivalent amounts.[30] Approximately 20% of the U.S. population consumed diet sodas during 2009-2010.[31] Soda consumption decreased among adolescents and young adults, whereas sports and energy drink consumption tripled among adolescents.[32,33] Approximately half of the increase in energy intake occurring over the past 20 years is contributed to sweetened beverages. Most people are unaware of how many kilocalories are in the beverages they drink, but these kilocalories may be a major contributor to the alarming increase in obesity.

Dental Erosion

Most sports and energy drinks have a pH in the acidic range (pH 3 to 4) which is associated with enamel demineralization. The increase in use of sports and energy drinks by children and adolescents causes irreversible damage to teeth because high acidity levels (citric acid) in drinks erode tooth enamel. Damage to tooth enamel is evident after just 5 days of exposure to sports or energy drinks. Energy drinks cause twice as much damage to teeth as sports drinks.[34] Calcium added to sports drinks lessens the erosive potential to teeth. Research suggests enamel erosion with various beverages occurs in the following order (from greatest to least): energy drinks, sports drinks, regular soda, and diet soda.[35]

Hyper States and Hypo States

Regulation of fluid intake and excretion by the kidneys usually maintain fluid balance in the body despite a wide range of intake. Imbalances may occur, however. **Fluid volume excess (FVE)** is the relatively equal gain of water and sodium in relation to their losses; **fluid volume deficit (FVD)** results from relatively equal losses of sodium and water.

Fluid Volume Excess

FVE mainly occurs in ECF compartments secondary to an increase in total body sodium content (Fig. 12-4, *C*). Because water follows sodium, an excess of sodium leads to an increase in total body water. Excess fluid moves into interstitial compartments, located between cells and in body cavities such as joints, pleura, and gastrointestinal tract, causing edema.

Congestive heart failure, chronic renal failure, chronic liver disease, and high levels of steroids may predispose an individual to FVE because of sodium retention. Diseases causing a loss of protein and reduced serum albumin levels (e.g., malnutrition and renal diseases) may contribute to FVE because osmotic forces ordinarily exhibited by proteins and albumin are lacking. Common manifestations of FVE include rapid weight gain, puffy eyelids, distended neck veins, and elevated blood pressure. **Peripheral edema** is commonly observed in the legs and feet. Treatment involves correction of underlying problems, or therapy for the specific disease; fluid or sodium may be restricted (or both), or diuretics prescribed.

Fluid Volume Deficit

In FVD (Fig. 12-4, *A*), the sodium-to-water ratio remains relatively equal; ADH and aldosterone secretions are not activated. Prolonged inadequate fluid intake can result in FVD. However, FVD is usually associated with excessive loss of fluids from the gastrointestinal tract (vomiting, or diarrhea, drainage tubes), urinary tract (diuretics, polyuria, or excessive urination), or skin (sweating). Fever increases the need for electrolytes, increases fluid losses in dehumidified air (e.g., in an airplane), and causes **diaphoresis** (excessive sweating).

Dehydration temporarily leads to weight loss, but more importantly, adversely influences cognitive function and motor control.[36] Decreased food and fluid intake can result from dementia, anorexia, nausea, or fatigue. Other, less obvious reasons are an inability to (a) obtain water, such as with impaired movement; (b) activate the thirst mechanism, as in **hypodipsia** (diminished thirst); or (c) swallow, as in neuromuscular problems or unconsciousness. Excessive fluid losses occasionally occur with prolonged exercise.

Common characteristics of FVD include weight loss, confusion and fatigue, sunken eyes, hypotension, and orthostatic hypotension. Classic signs are dry tongue with **longitudinal fissures** (slits or wrinkles that extend lengthwise on the tongue) (Fig. 12-5), xerostomia, shrinkage of oral mucous membranes, decreased skin turgor, dry skin, and decreased urinary output. A diminished salivary flow is associated with inadequate fluid intake. Pale yellow or almost colorless urine indicates adequate hydration. Dark yellow urine with a strong odor, advancing to painful urination, and (eventually) cessation of urine formation are progressive signs of inadequate water intake and dehydration. Treatment involves replacing lost fluid. If FVD is mild, oral fluids are likely to be sufficient. Intravenous solutions are needed with significant FVD.

Dental Considerations

- Small to moderate amounts of caffeine are not a concern for most individuals, but excessive consumption can cause insomnia, headaches, irritability, and nervousness.
- Direct measurement of the total amount of body water is impossible. Evaluation of physical signs of fluid deficit or excess is vital to diagnosis and treatment.

Continued

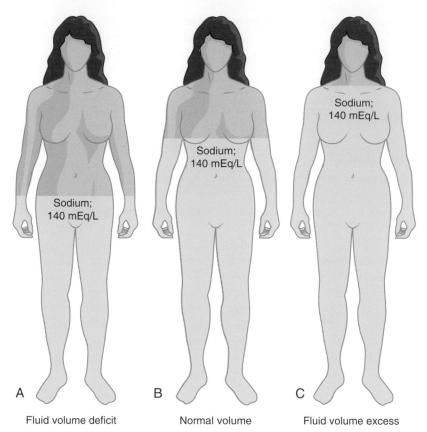

A   Fluid volume deficit

B   Normal volume

C   Fluid volume excess

FIGURE 12-4 A to **C,** Fluid-volume disturbances. Compared with normal body fluids (**B**), in FVD (**A**), equal percentages of water and sodium losses occur, producing an isotonic depletion. In FVE (**C**), water and sodium are retained, producing an isotonic expansion. (Adapted from Davis JR, Sherer K: *Applied nutrition and diet therapy for nurses*, ed 2, Philadelphia, 1994, Saunders Elsevier.)

Dental Considerations—cont'd

- Assess patients for puffy eyelids or distended neck veins; inquire about recent unintentional weight changes, check blood pressure, and refer to a healthcare provider if necessary. A rapid weight loss or gain of 3% or greater of total body weight is significant.
- Observe for dry tongue with longitudinal fissures, xerostomia, or shrinkage of oral mucous membranes; adequacy of salivary flow; decreased skin turgor; and dry skin. Inquire about frequency and amount of urine output and fluid intake.
- Salivary flow measurements may be indicated for patients who present with FVD.
- Reduced total body water, decreased renal function, renin activity, and aldosterone secretion in geriatric patients place them at risk for dehydration. In addition, this population may drink less fluid because of dementia, immobility, or fear of incontinence.
- The greater surface area-to-body mass ratio in infants places this group at risk for FVD.
- Rapid weight changes generally indicate loss or gain of water rather than fatty tissue; a loss or gain of 480 mL (2 cups) of fluid is equivalent to a loss or gain of 1 lb.
- Because of the sensitivity of oral mucosa to the body's fluid volume, increases and decreases in body fluid affect the fit of a denture. FVD generates a loose-fitting prosthesis, whereas FVE may create a tight-fitting prosthesis. Patients may present with ulcerations in each situation and find the prosthesis uncomfortable to wear.
- Remain alert for new caffeine guidelines recommended by Health Canada and the FDA.

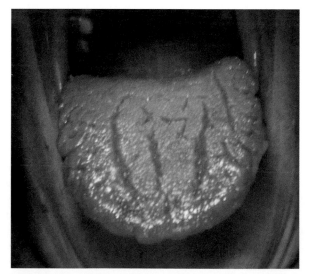

FIGURE 12-5 Fissured tongue. (From Ibsen OAC, Phelan JA: *Oral pathology for the dental hygienist*, ed 6, St Louis, 2014, Saunders Elsevier.)

- Do not encourage patients with iron-deficiency anemia to consume tea, particularly with meals or an iron supplement.
- Question patients regarding use of herbal supplements. Ma-huang (ephedra) and products containing this herb can cause xerostomia.

Nutritional Directions

- To help with conversion of total water intake: 1 L = 33.8 fluid oz and 1 cup = 8 fluid oz.
- Encourage patients experiencing a "dry mouth" to increase fluid intake and salivary production by chewing sugarless gum, preferably gum containing xylitol.
- Habitual intake of caffeinated beverages (coffee, tea, soft drinks, and other caffeinated beverages) contributes to the daily total water intake similar to that contributed by noncaffeinated beverages.
- Encourage beverages to satisfy nutritional and hydration needs and fluid preferences.
- Energy drinks are inappropriate for children and athletic activities, especially if they contain caffeine.
- FDA has suggested that up to 400 mg/day of caffeine (4 to 5 cups of coffee) is a safe amount for adults, except for pregnant women who should limit caffeine intake to 200-300 mg, but they are conducting a review of its safety because of its addition to so many new products.
- Based on limited data, moderate amounts of alcohol ingestion increase fluid excretion and do not result in appreciable fluid losses.
- High-protein diets, such as diets in which fruit and vegetable intake is minimal, require larger amounts of water to eliminate higher levels of urinary waste products.
- Because of fluid loss through perspiration, patients need to drink fluid during exercise. (Loss of 1 lb of body weight during exercise means that at least 2 cups of water have been lost.) In most cases, water is the most appropriate choice.
- To make wise beverage choices, read labels on bottled waters to see what ingredients they contain.
- Most tap water is safe and economical.
- Water is the preferred beverage to fulfill daily fluid needs and should be served with most meals. Beverages with no or few kilocalories should take precedence over consumption of beverages with more kilocalories.
- Make water more exciting by adding slices of lemon, lime, cucumber, or watermelon, or add a splash of 100% juice to plain sparkling water.
- When selecting a sugar-sweetened beverage, choose a small size. Some companies now market 8-oz containers of soda.

ELECTROLYTES

Electrolytes are compounds or ions that dissociate in solution; they are also known as **cations** if they have a positive charge, and **anions** if they have a negative charge. Cations in the body include sodium, potassium, calcium, and magnesium; anions include chloride, bicarbonate, and phosphate. The body's hydration status depends on an electrolyte balance of equal concentrations of cations to anions. Because the electrolyte concentration in plasma is so low, it is expressed as milliequivalents per liter (mEq/L). Electrolytes are important in water balance and acid–base (pH) balance.

Electrolyte distribution is different in ICF and ECF compartments. The principal cation in plasma and interstitial fluid is sodium; the principal anion is chloride. The principal cation in ICF is potassium; the principal anion is phosphate. The major difference between intravascular fluid and interstitial fluid is the large amount of protein in the former.

Because sodium and potassium are the major cations, these are discussed in more detail.

SODIUM
Physiological Roles

The important physiological roles of sodium include (a) maintaining normal ECF concentration by affecting the concentration, excretion, and absorption of potassium and chloride, and water distribution; (b) regulating acid–base balance; and (c) facilitating impulse transmission in nerve and muscle fibers. Sodium is present in calcified structures in the body; its function in bones and teeth is unclear. It is also present in saliva. Sodium concentration in saliva determines one's recognition of salt in food.

Requirements and Regulation

Because sodium is so readily available in foods, no RDA has been established. The IOM estimates a safe minimum intake might be 500 mg/day. This amount is increased in the face of abnormal losses. Sodium regulation involves several mechanisms. To keep the ECF concentration normal, the sodium-potassium pump is constantly moving sodium from the cell to ECF. Aldosterone released by the adrenal cortex results in sodium reabsorption or excretion by the kidneys depending on the body's need (Fig. 12-6). The kidneys can adjust sodium excretion to match sodium intake despite large variations in intake. If serum sodium is high, aldosterone is inhibited, and sodium is excreted; the opposite is true for depressed serum sodium levels.

For most adults, the AI for sodium is 1500 mg/day with the UL being 2300 mg/day (Table 12-3). This AI does not apply to highly active individuals, such as endurance athletes, who lose large amounts of sodium through sweat.

Average consumption of salt is approximately 3400 mg/day. The *Dietary Guidelines* and *MyPlate* encourage most Americans to decrease salt intake to 2300 mg daily; adults older than age 50 years, all African Americans, and individuals with high blood pressure, diabetes, or chronic kidney disease should further reduce sodium intake to 1500 mg a day. More than 90% of adults exceed the recommendation of consuming more than 2300 mg of sodium (more than the UL). Although the IOM recommends a daily sodium intake of 1500 mg/day for many Americans, more than 98% of adults routinely consume greater amounts.[37] In comparison with sodium intakes in 1988-1994, average intake in 2003-2008 has not changed significantly. The World Health Organization recommends a maximum intake of 2000 mg a day for adults.[38]

Scientific studies irrefutably agree that reducing salt intake reduces blood pressure. However, numerous well-designed studies and even systematic review of studies indicate conflicting outcomes as to whether or not lower sodium intake will prevent blood pressure-related cardiovascular events.[39,40] Nevertheless, the current public health recommendation in many countries is to reduce salt intake by about half.

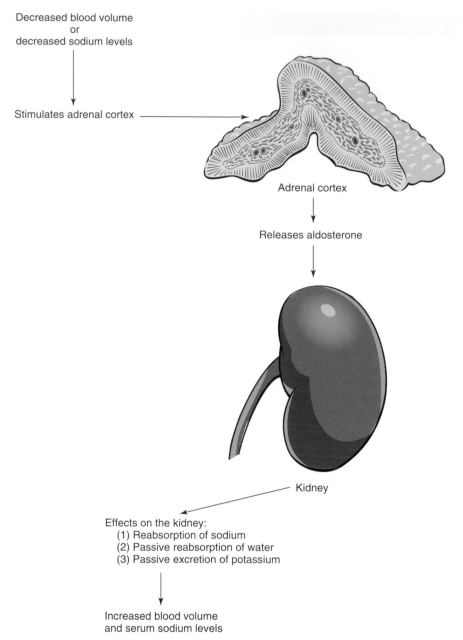

Decreased blood volume
or
decreased sodium levels

Stimulates adrenal cortex

Adrenal cortex

Releases aldosterone

Kidney

Effects on the kidney:
(1) Reabsorption of sodium
(2) Passive reabsorption of water
(3) Passive excretion of potassium

Increased blood volume
and serum sodium levels

FIGURE 12-6 Effects of aldosterone on sodium levels. (Adapted from Davis JR, Sherer K: *Applied nutrition and diet therapy for nurses*, ed 2, Philadelphia, 1994, Saunders Elsevier.)

Sources

Approximately 10% of the sodium consumed comes from the natural content of foods and fluids regularly ingested. Sodium is a natural constituent of most foods (Table 12-4); animal foods such as meat, saltwater fish, eggs, dairy products, and some vegetables (beets, carrots, celery, spinach, and other dark green leafy vegetables) contain measurable amounts of sodium. Bread and rolls are the number one source of salt in the American diet. The large quantity of bread products consumed accousnt for more than twice as much sodium as snack foods like potato chips and pretzels.[41]

Most consumers believe that sea salt is lower in sodium than regular salt.[42] Sea salt has been marketed as containing "natural" nutrients and more minerals than table salt. Trace elements in sea salt are minuscule and meaningless with no known health benefits. Far more relevant is the fact that unlike table salt, sea salt is not fortified with iodine, which is important for thyroid health, especially during pregnancy. Taste intensity of sea salt is generally the same as regular salts and does not appear to be a viable sodium reduction strategy.[43]

Approximately 75% to 80% of the sodium consumed is added to processed foods (Box 12-2) and foods prepared in restaurants and fast food establishments. Foods purchased at restaurants with wait staff have the highest sodium density (2151 mg sodium/1000 kcal) followed by fast food establishments (1864 mg/1000 kcal),[44] as shown in Figure 12-7. Processed, cured, canned, pickled, convenience, and fast

Table 12-3	**Institute of Medicine recommendations for sodium and chloride**							
	AI* for Sodium		UL† for Sodium		AI for Chloride		UL for Chloride	
Life Stage	Male (g/day)	Female (g/day)	Male (g/day)	Female (g/day)	Male (g/day)	Female (g/day)	Male (g/day)	Female (g/day)
0-6 months	0.12	0.12	ND‡	ND‡	0.18	0.18	ND‡	ND‡
7-12 months	0.37	0.37	ND‡	ND‡	0.57	0.57	ND‡	ND‡
1-3 years	1	1	1.5	1.5	1.5	1.5	2.3	2.3
4-8 years	1.2	1.2	1.9	1.9	1.9	1.9	2.9	2.9
9-14 years	1.5	1.5	2.2	2.2	2.3	2.3	3.4	3.4
14-50 years	1.5	1.5	2.3	2.3	2.3	2.3	3.6	3.6
51-70 years	1.3	1.3	2.3	2.3	2	2	2.3	2.3
>70 years	1.2	1.2	2.3	2.3	1.8	1.8	2.3	2.3
Pregnancy								
14-50 years		1.5		2.3		2.3		3.6
Lactation								
14-50 years		1.5		2.3		2.3		3.6

Data from Institute of Medicine (IOM), Food and Nutrition Board: *Dietary reference intakes for water, potassium, sodium, chloride, chloride, and sulfate,* Washington, DC, 2005, National Academies Press.

*AI (adequate intake)—the observed average or experimentally set intake by a defined population or subgroup that seems to sustain a defined nutritional status, such as growth rate, normal circulating nutrient values, or other functional indicators of health. An AI is used if insufficient scientific evidence is available to derive an estimated average requirement. For healthy human milk–fed infants, the AI is the mean intake. *The AI is not equivalent to a RDA.*

†UL (tolerable upper intake level)—the highest level of daily nutrient intake that is likely to pose no risk of adverse health effects to almost all individuals in the general population. As intake increases above the UL, the risk of adverse effects increases. Unless specified otherwise, the UL represents total nutrient intake from food, water, and supplements.

‡ND—not determinable because of lack of data of adverse effects in this age group and concern with regard to lack of ability to handle excess amounts. Source of intake should be from food and formula to prevent high levels of intake.

Table 12-4	**Where's the sodium?**		
Food Groups	**Sodium (mg)**	**Food Groups**	**Sodium (mg)**
Whole and Other Grains and Grain Products*		Natural cheeses, 1½ oz	110-450
Cooked cereal, rice, pasta, unsalted, ½ cup	0-5	Process cheeses, 2 oz	600
Ready-to-eat cereal, 1 cup	0-360	**Nuts, Seeds, and Legumes**	
Bread, 1 slice	110-175	Peanuts, salted, ⅓ cup	120
Vegetables		Peanuts, unsalted, ⅓ cup	0-5
Fresh or frozen, cooked without salt, ½ cup	1-70	Beans, cooked from dried or frozen, without salt, ½ cup	0-5
Canned or frozen with sauce, ½ cup	140-460		
Tomato juice, canned, ½ cup	330	Beans, canned, ½ cup	400
Fruit		**Lean Meats, Fish, and Poultry**	
Fresh, frozen, canned, ½ cup	0-5	Fresh meat, fish, poultry, 3 oz	30-90
Low-Fat or Fat-Free Milk or Milk Products		Tuna canned, water pack, no salt added, 3 oz	35-45
Milk, 1 cup	107	Tuna canned, water pack, 3 oz	230-350
Yogurt, 1 cup	175	Ham, lean, roasted, 3 oz	1,020

From U.S. Department of Health and Human Services, National Institutes of Health: *Your guide to lowering your blood pressure with Dash.* NIH Publication No 06-4082. Revised April 2006. Accessed August 31, 2013: http://www.nhlbi.nih.gov/health/public/heart/hbp/dash/new_dash.pdf
*Whole grains are recommended for most grain servings.

foods, and condiments are significant sources of sodium. "Hidden" sources include softened and bottled water, baking powder, baking soda, dentifrices (including toothpastes containing baking soda or sodium fluoride), antibiotics, chewing tobacco, and over-the-counter medications (e.g., antacids, cough medicines, and laxatives).

Representatives from the food industry complain that lower sodium products are less palatable and are not competitive with higher-sodium products on the market, so a reduction of sodium in their products is not economically viable. The flavor of a food is the major determinant of food choices, overriding other factors, such as healthy choices. The U.S. government and Health Canada are working with food manufacturers to lower sodium content of products. The goal is to slowly, and without loss of consumers' acceptance, achieve safer levels of sodium that are consistent with

> **BOX 12-2   Guidelines for Implementing the Dietary Guidelines for Americans for Sodium Intake (2400 mg)**
>
> - Avoid foods with concentrated sources of sodium, and do not add salt to foods.
> - Avoid adding salt to food at the table or in recipes. Flavor foods with herbs, spices, wine, lemon, lime, or vinegar (see Table 12-5 for additional ideas).
> - Salt substitutes can contain sodium, potassium, and other minerals. Salt substitutes should not be used unless approved by a healthcare provider or RDN.
> - Sodium is found naturally in most foods. Animal products such as meat, fish, poultry, milk, and eggs are naturally higher in sodium than fruits and vegetables.
> - Restaurant meals should be selected carefully because of their high sodium content.
> - Limit the following high-sodium processed foods:
>   *Meats:* Smoked, cured, salted, or canned meats, fish, or poultry, including bacon, cold cuts, ham, frankfurters, and sausages; sardines, anchovies, and marinated herring; pickled meats or pickled eggs
>   *Dairy products:* Processed cheese, blue cheese, buttermilk
>   *Vegetables:* Sauerkraut, pickled vegetables prepared in brine, commercially frozen vegetable mixes with sauces
>
>   *Breads and cereals:* Breads, rolls, and crackers with salted tops
>   *Soups:* Canned soups, dried soup mixes, broth, bouillon (except salt-free)
>   *Fats:* Salad dressings containing bacon bits, salt pork, dips made with instant soup mixes or processed cheese
>   *Beverages:* Commercially softened water, cocoa mixes, club soda, sports drinks, tomato or vegetable juice
>   *Miscellaneous:* Casserole and pasta mixes; salted chips, popcorn, and nuts; olives; commercial stuffing; gravy mixes; seasoning salts (garlic, celery, onion), light salt, monosodium glutamate (MSG); meat tenderizer; catsup, prepared mustard, prepared horseradish, soy sauce
> - Read food labels. Compare the sodium content of products.
> - Use reduced sodium or no-salt-added products. Read the ingredient list on food labels to identify and avoid sources of sodium additives such as salt, sodium chloride (NaCl), sodium caseinate, MSG, trisodium phosphate, sodium ascorbate, and sodium bicarbonate.
> - Foods making nutrient claims must meet certain labeling guides (see Chapter 1, Box 1-3).

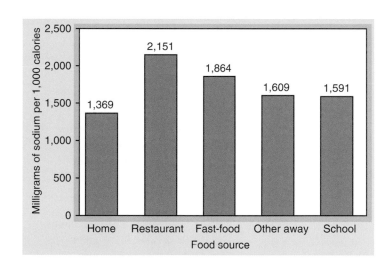

Note: All food sources are statistically different from each other at the 1% probability level, except for school foods and other away foods.

FIGURE 12-7 Restaurants offered the most sodium-dense foods in 2005-2008. (From Guthrie J, Bing-Hwan L, Okrent A, Volpe R: Americans' food choices at home and away: how do they compare with recommendations? *Amber Waves* February 21, 2013. Accessed August 31, 2013: http://www.ers.usda.gov/data-products/chart-gallery/detail.aspx?chartId=36247&ref=collection#.UVC5s1fB98E)

public health recommendations. Reformulation by the food industry, rather than individual dietary advice, is the most cost-effective strategy for salt reduction.

Hyper States and Hypo States

Serum sodium concentration is an index of water deficit or excess, not an index of total sodium levels in the body. Sodium levels in the blood are significantly higher than potassium levels because sodium is the major cation in intravascular fluid. **Hypernatremia** (elevated serum sodium level) and **hyponatremia** (low serum sodium level) are usually a result of hormonal imbalances or increased fluid loss or retention. "True" hypernatremia or hyponatremia, or imbalances caused by too much or too little sodium intake,

Table 12-5	Herbs and spices to complement foods
Food	**Herbs/Spices**
Beef	Onion, bay, chives, cloves, cumin, garlic, pepper, marjoram, rosemary, thyme, ginger
Bread	Caraway, marjoram, oregano, poppy seed, rosemary, thyme
Carrots	Cinnamon, cloves, nutmeg, marjoram, sage
Cheese	Basil, chives, curry, dill, fennel, garlic, marjoram, oregano, parsley, sage, thyme
Fish	Dill, curry powder, paprika, fennel, tarragon, garlic, parsley, thyme
Fruit	Cinnamon, coriander, cloves, ginger, mint
Green beans	Dill, oregano, tarragon, thyme
Lamb	Garlic, marjoram, oregano, rosemary, thyme
Other vegetables	Basil, chives, dill, tarragon, marjoram, mint, parsley, pepper, thyme
Pork	Onion, coriander, cumin, garlic, ginger, hot pepper, pepper, sage, thyme, ginger
Potatoes, rutabaga	Dill, garlic, paprika, parsley, sage
Poultry	Garlic, ginger, oregano, rosemary, sage, tarragon
Salads	Basil, chives, French tarragon, garlic, parsley, arugula, sorrel (best if fresh or added to salad dressing, or use herbs and vinegars for extra flavor)
Soups	Bay, tarragon, marjoram, parsley, rosemary
Winter squash/sweet potatoes	Cloves, nutmeg, cinnamon, ginger

rarely occur in adults. If renal and hormonal mechanisms for sodium retention and excretion function efficiently, and water intake is adequate, the amount of dietary sodium causes little change in total body sodium; sodium fluctuations do affect plasma volume.

Because water and sodium are closely related, a change in one causes a change in the other. Hypernatremia can be associated with FVD or FVE. A very high sodium intake can be toxic, especially if intake is insufficient.

Water deprivation (as occurs in unconscious, debilitated individuals or infants), insensible water loss (as a result of exposure to dry heat, sweating, or hyperventilation), and watery diarrhea lead to a loss of water in excess of sodium. Infants are more prone to watery diarrhea, whereas older patients are susceptible to water deprivation. If polyuria is not balanced with increased water intake, hypernatremia may occur.

Symptoms of hypernatremia are a result of fluid moving from the ICF to the ECF in an attempt to equalize sodium and water balance. This movement of fluid causes atrophy of tissue cells. Cells in the central nervous system shrink, producing hallucinations, disorientation, lethargy, and possibly coma. Other signs are extreme thirst; dry, "sticky" tongue and oral mucous membranes; fever; and convulsions. A sticky tongue can be identified by slowly rolling a tongue depressor over the lateral side of the tongue; tacky filiform papillae stick to the tongue depressor and rise up.

Hyponatremia may develop when sodium losses exceed water losses, or when fluids are retained, leading to a greater concentration of water than sodium. Because of the decrease in ECF concentration, sodium moves from the ECF to the ICF, and water enters the ICF, causing cellular edema. This can cause problems, especially in the cranium where there is no room for expansion. Sodium deficiency may lead to a decrease in salivary flow or a decrease in sodium concentration of saliva.

Water intoxication or hyponatremia can occur when individuals drink too much water (many liters a day). The blood sodium level decreases to a dangerously low level, causing headaches, blurred vision, cramps, swelling of the brain, coma, and possibly death.

Heat exhaustion in unacclimated individuals may result in a sodium deficit. Hyponatremia also may occur in individuals who drink excessive quantities of water as part of a psychiatric disorder, or when excessive amounts of diuretics are given. Hyperglycemia may precipitate hyponatremia because an elevated blood glucose draws water into the vascular space (edema), causing a dilutional effect. Excessive vomiting and diarrhea, especially in infants, can also lead to a sodium deficit.

Early symptoms of hyponatremia are nausea and abdominal cramps. Other symptoms—headache, confusion, lethargy, and coma—are the result of cellular edema. Even though there is cellular edema, peripheral edema is not present. This is because water is primarily retained within cells rather than in the interstitial compartment. Chronic hyponatremia is usually well tolerated. It may or may not be treated, depending on the precipitating cause and severity.

Dental Considerations

- Assess patients for signs and symptoms of hypernatremia (thirst; dry, sticky tongue; xerostomia) and hyponatremia.
- The salt recognition threshold is determined by sodium concentration of saliva (i.e., the lower the level of sodium in saliva, the easier it is to detect a small amount of salt in food).
- Patients with hypertension who are salt sensitive need to consume 1500 mg or less of sodium daily. Encourage these patients to use herbs and spices to flavor food instead of high-sodium seasonings (see Table 12-5).
- A low salt recognition threshold is desirable for patients who need to curtail salt intake for health reasons, but in a hyponatremic patient, diminished salt consumption could contribute further to sodium depletion.
- Sodium deficiency may lead to a decreased salivary flow rate.
- High levels of sodium (greater than 2 g/day) cause calcium loss in the urine.

Continued

Dental Considerations—cont'd

- Identify "hidden" sources of sodium in a patient's diet. Educate the patient regarding sodium intake reduction.
- Refer patients who would benefit by reducing sodium intake to 1500 mg/day to a RDN.

Nutritional Directions

- Stress the importance of appropriate sodium intake, as recommended by the healthcare provider.
- Dietary sodium restriction is rarely the cause of hyponatremia. Sodium depletion may occur in combination with excessive losses as a result of vomiting, diarrhea, surgery, or profuse perspiration from exercise or fever.
- To convert milligrams of sodium to milliequivalents, divide the number by 23 (the atomic weight of sodium). For example, 1000 mg of sodium ÷ 23 = 43 mEq of sodium.
- Table salt contains sodium and chloride (40% sodium and 60% chloride); 1 tsp of salt is equivalent to 2000 mg of sodium.
- Many low-sodium or reduced-sodium foods are available as alternatives to foods processed with salt and other sodium-containing ingredients. Compare labels for the sodium content of these foods to find the lowest value.
- The water supply and use of water softeners are "hidden" sources of sodium.
- Read the Nutrition Facts label to compare sodium content of prepared foods such as soups, broths, breads, and frozen dinners, and choose the healthiest option.
- Fresh fruits and vegetables, fresh meats, poultry, and fish, home-prepared beans and peas, unsalted nuts, eggs, and low-fat or fat-free milk and dairy products are wiser choices providing only naturally-occurring sodium.

CHLORIDE

Physiological Roles

Chlorine is the primary anion connected with sodium in ECF to help maintain ECF balance, osmotic equilibrium, and electrolyte balance. Large concentrations of chloride are present in gastric secretions, which are important for protein digestion and creating an acidic environment to inhibit bacterial growth and enhance iron, calcium, and vitamin B_{12} absorption.

Requirements and Regulation

The AI for chloride has been established by the IOM at 2300 mg/day (see Table 12-3). Chloride intake and losses parallel those of sodium.

Sources

Most chloride intake is from salt (sodium chloride). Sources of chloride are the same as those for sodium, including processed foods. Water is an additional source of chloride.

Hyper States and Hypo States

Toxicity from chloride can be caused by excessive intakes of salt (NaCl), dehydration, renal failure, diarrhea, and Cushing syndrome. Conditions associated with sodium

Table 12-6	Institute of Medicine recommendations for potassium	
	AI*	
Life Stage	Male (g/day)	Female (g/day)
0-6 months	0.4	0.4
7-12 months	0.7	0.7
1-3 years	3	3
4-8 years	3.8	3.8
9-13 years	4.5	4.5
≥14 years	4.7	4.7
Pregnancy		
≥18 years		4.7
Lactation		
≥18 years		5.1

Data from Institute of Medicine (IOM), Food and Nutrition Board: *Dietary reference intakes for water, potassium, sodium, chloride, chloride, and sulfate,* Washington, DC, 2005, National Academies Press.
*AI (adequate intake)—the observed average or experimentally set intake by a defined population or subgroup that seems to sustain a defined nutritional status, such as growth rate, normal circulating nutrient values, or other functional indicators of health. An AI is used if insufficient scientific evidence is unavailable to derive an estimated average requirement. For healthy human milk–fed infants, the AI is the mean intake. *The AI is not equivalent to a RDA.*

depletion, such as persistent heavy sweating, chronic diarrhea, vomiting, or chronic renal failure, may precipitate hypochloremia and an acid-base imbalance.

POTASSIUM

Physiological Roles

Potassium has the following important physiological roles: (a) maintains cellular (ICF) concentration, (b) directly affects muscle contraction (especially cardiac) and electrical conductivity of the heart, (c) facilitates transmission of nerve impulses, and (d) regulates acid–base balance. Potassium is important to maintain good muscle function for physically active individuals.

Requirements and Regulation

Similar to sodium, there is no RDA for potassium. As shown in Table 12-6, the AI for potassium has been established by the IOM at 4700 mg/day for all adults. This is equivalent to approximately 10 servings of fruits and vegetables. No UL has been set for healthy adults.

Poor food choices result in diets deficient in potassium. Additionally, high intake of meats and other animal proteins cause further depletion of this mineral. Average potassium intake of the U.S. population has declined; the average dietary potassium intake is 2640 mg/day.[45] Intake of potassium is low because insufficient amounts of fruits and vegetables are chosen. Low potassium consumption can cause sensitivity to salt, further increasing risk of hypertension.

The sodium-potassium pump regulates potassium levels. Depending on cellular needs, potassium is constantly moving either into or out of cells. Aldosterone indirectly affects serum potassium levels. If aldosterone is released,

Table 12-7	Potassium content of selected foods	
Food	Portion	Potassium (mg)
Beet greens, cooked	1 cup	1309
Lima beans, cooked	1 cup	969
Potato, baked with skin	1 med	952
Pinto beans	1 cup	746
Spinach, cooked from frozen	1 cup	664
Yogurt, low fat, plain	8 oz	573
Beets, cooked	1 cup	518
Cantaloupe	1 cup	473
Banana	1 med	422
Milk, 1%	1 cup	366
Sirloin steak, broiled	3 oz	323
Raisins	¼ cup	302
Tomato, fresh	1 med	292
Salmon, canned	3 oz	255
Carrots, baby, raw	10	240
Orange	1 med	237
Gatorade sports beverage	8 oz	31

U.S. Department of Agriculture, Agricultural Research Service: *USDA national nutrient database for standard reference, release 26, 2013.* Accessed August 31, 2013: http://www.ars.usda.gov/nutrientdata

sodium is reabsorbed, but potassium is excreted. Subsequently, if aldosterone is inhibited, potassium is retained in the body (see Fig. 12-6). Approximately 92% of ingested potassium is excreted in urine. Some is lost through feces or sweat.

Sources

Potassium is naturally available from foods and fluids regularly consumed (Table 12-7). Dairy, meat, and grains contribute 31%, and fruits and vegetables contribute 20% of total dietary potassium. Milk is the number one single food source of potassium for all age groups in the United States.[46] Processed foods usually contain less potassium than fresh products. Potassium supplements and salt substitutes are another source; salt substitutes (potassium chloride [KCl]) often replace sodium with potassium.

Hyper States and Hypo States

Minor deviations in serum potassium levels can be life-threatening. Abnormal levels are referred to as either **hyperkalemia** (elevated serum potassium level) or **hypokalemia** (low serum potassium level).

Hyperkalemia has three causes: (a) impaired renal excretion, (b) increased shift of potassium out of cells, and (c) increased potassium intake. Acute or chronic renal failure impairs potassium excretion, resulting in potassium being retained in the body. This is logical because a large percentage is excreted through the kidneys. Increased serum potassium levels can result from an increased dietary intake, excessive administration of potassium supplements orally or intravenously, or excessive use of potassium-containing salt

substitutes. Burns, trauma, crushing injuries, myocardial infarction, Addison disease, insulin deficiency, hypoaldosteronism, increased catabolism, and acidosis can allow secretion of potassium by the distal nephron.

Hyperkalemia is life-threatening because cardiac arrest may occur. Elevated potassium levels are irritating to the body; symptoms include muscle weakness (the first sign), tingling and numbness in the extremities, diarrhea, bradycardia, abdominal cramps, confusion, and electrocardiographic changes. Treatment for hyperkalemia involves potassium restriction or using medications to remove potassium.

Potential consequences of chronic potassium deficiency are often unrecognized. Problems include hypertension, heart attacks, strokes, kidney stones, and a loss of bone minerals that can lead to osteoporosis. Potassium deficiency can cause individuals to feel tired, weak, and irritable, while unable to pinpoint a cause.

Excessive loss or inadequate intake of potassium can result in hypokalemia. Potassium loss occurs through the gastrointestinal and renal tracts and by excessive sweating. Because potassium is contained in gastric and intestinal secretions, vomiting and diarrhea may cause hypokalemia. Some potassium is lost through sweat; excessive perspiration can lead to hypokalemia. Drugs, such as diuretics (e.g., furosemide and hydrochlorothiazide) and antibiotics (e.g., carbenicillin and amphotericin B), are major offenders. Cushing syndrome, hyperaldosteronism, an excess of insulin, hypomagnesemia, alcoholism, and alkalosis also cause hypokalemia.

Potassium is the major ICF cation; deficits can affect every body system. Death from cardiac or respiratory arrest can occur. Clinical manifestations are anorexia, absence of bowel sounds, muscle weakness in the legs, leg cramps, and electrocardiographic changes.

Dental Considerations

- Be aware of factors that can cause potassium to increase or decrease. Refer the patient to the healthcare provider or RDN as needed.

Nutritional Directions

- Stress the importance of increasing potassium intake for healthy patients.
- Read labels; salt substitutes may be high in potassium. Consult a healthcare provider or RDN before using potassium-containing salt substitutes.
- Encourage patients taking potassium-wasting diuretics to consume high-potassium foods if they are not taking a potassium supplement.
- Medical conditions that can interfere with excretion of potassium include diabetes, renal failure, severe heart events, and adrenal insufficiency.
- Medications that can interfere with excretion of potassium are angiotensin-converting enzyme inhibitors, angiotensin receptor blockers, and potassium-sparing diuretics.

IRON

Physiological Roles

Every cell contains iron; approximately 4 g (less than 1 tsp) is present in the entire body. Iron is a major component of hemoglobin, which transports oxygen from the lungs to the tissues, including both oral soft and hard tissues. It also catalyzes many oxidative reactions within cells and participates in the final steps of energy metabolism. Other roles include (a) conversion of beta-carotene to vitamin A, (b) synthesis of collagen, (c) formation of purines as part of nucleic acid, (d) removal of lipids from the blood, (e) detoxification of drugs in the liver, and (f) production of antibodies. Lactoferrin, a salivary glycoprotein, is capable of binding iron. It has an antibacterial action by competing with iron-requiring organisms in the mouth for limited amounts of available iron.

Requirements

The IOM recommends 18 mg/day for women 19 to 50 years old, and 8 mg/day for women 51 years old and older and men 19 years old and older (Table 12-8). The RDA is higher for premenopausal women than for men or postmenopausal women because of blood loss during menstruation. During the reproductive phase of a woman's life, iron loss is at least twice that of a man or of a postmenopausal woman.

Although premenopausal women need more iron, they tend to consume less than men. Iron requirements also increase during times of impaired absorption (e.g., diarrhea), periods of rapid growth, and heavy physical activity because of the increased need for oxygen transport and energy production.

The RDA is based on the approximation that 10% of dietary iron is absorbed. The demand for iron replenishment is constant because cells are continually being replaced; the life of a red blood cell is 120 days. When a cell dies, iron is recycled, being released and transported to various storage sites to be used again. A UL for iron was established at 45 mg/day for adults.

Absorption and Excretion

Similar to calcium, iron is poorly absorbed. Most of the iron in food is in the oxidized form of ferric iron (Fe^{3+}). Gastric acid in the stomach helps promote iron absorption. By binding to the serum protein transferrin, iron is continuously transported through the body because transferrin functions to recycle iron.

Absorption of heme iron parallels the body's need; absorption of nonheme iron depends on intraluminal and meal composition and physiological need. Heme iron is provided by meat sources containing hemoglobin from red blood cells and myoglobin from muscle cells. The RDA is

Table 12-8	Institute of Medicine recommendations for iron						
	EAR (mg/day)*		RDA (mg/day)†		AI (mg/day)‡		
Life Stage	Male	Female	Male	Female	Male	Female	UL (mg/day)§
0-6 months					0.27	0.27	40
7-12 months	6.9	6.9	11	11			40
1-3 years	3	3	7	7			40
4-8 years	4.1	4.1	10	10			40
9-13 years	5.9	5.7	8	8			40
14-18 years	7.7	7.9	11	15			45
19-50 years	6	8.1	8	18			45
≥51 years	6	5	8	8			45
Pregnancy							
14-18 years		23		27			45
19-50 years		22		27			45
Lactation							
14-18 years		7		10			45
19-50 years		6.5		9			45

Data from Institute of Medicine (IOM), Food and Nutrition Board: *Dietary reference intakes for vitamin A, vitamin K, arsenic, boron, chromium, copper, iodine, iron, manganese, molybdenum, nickel, silicon, vanadium, and zinc,* Washington, DC, 2001, National Academy Press.

*EAR (estimated average requirement)—the intake that meets the estimated nutrient needs of half of the individuals in a group.

†RDA (recommended dietary allowance)—the intake that meets the nutrient needs of almost all (97% to 98%) individuals in a group.

‡AI (adequate intake)—the observed average or experimentally set intake by a defined population or subgroup that seems to sustain a defined nutritional status, such as growth rate, normal circulating nutrient values, or other functional indicators of health. An AI is used if insufficient scientific evidence is available to derive an EAR. For healthy human milk–fed infants, the AI is the mean intake. *The AI is not equivalent to a RDA.*

§UL (tolerable upper intake level)—the highest level of daily nutrient intake that is likely to pose no risk of adverse health effects to almost all individuals in the general population. As intake increases above the UL, the risk of adverse effects increases. Unless specified otherwise, the UL represents total nutrient intake from food, water, and supplements.

based on consumption of at least 75% of iron intake from heme sources. Nonheme iron is present in eggs, milk, and plants. Acidic conditions enhance iron absorption, but calcium and manganese interfere with its absorption. Figure 12-8 lists factors affecting iron absorption. Combinations of food can enhance iron absorption. A meal of roast beef (rich in iron) with potatoes (rich in vitamin C) increases iron absorption.

Sources

Iron is probably the most difficult mineral to obtain in adequate amounts in the American diet. Although liver is often considered the best source of iron, meats (especially beef), egg yolk, dark green vegetables, and enriched breads and cereals all contribute significant amounts (Table 12-9). Iron supplements come in two forms; the ferrous form is better

absorbed than the ferric form. Even though iron can be considered toxic because of the body's inability to excrete excess iron, supplementation is a safe and effective treatment for iron-deficiency anemia.

Hyper States and Hypo States

The body cannot easily eliminate excess iron; this may explain why iron absorption rates are poor. The body seldom overcomes its regulation of intestinal absorption. Iron overload may occur, however, if ingestion of iron is extremely elevated. **Hemochromatosis** is an uncommon disorder in which iron is absorbed at a high rate despite elevated iron stores in the liver. Accumulation of iron throughout the body may develop with excessive iron intake or multiple blood transfusions. Inexpensive red wines contain wide variations in iron content (10 to 350 mg/L) and have been associated

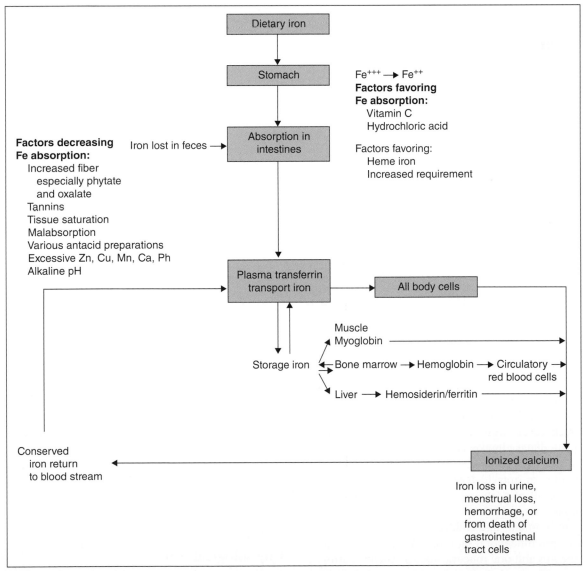

FIGURE 12-8 Iron absorption and use. (Adapted from Davis JR, Sherer K: *Applied nutrition and diet therapy for nurses,* ed 2, Philadelphia, 1994, Saunders Elsevier.)

Table 12-9 Iron content of selected foods		
Food	Portion	Iron (mg)
Total, whole grain	1 cup	24.0*
Multi Bran Chex	1 cup	21.6*
Chicken liver, pan-fried	3 oz	11.0†
Raisin Bran	1 cup	10.8*
Oatmeal, instant, fortified, prepared with water	1 packet	10.6*
Lentils, boiled	1 cup	6.6*
Beef liver, pan-fried	3 oz	5.9†
Kidney beans, mature, boiled	1 cup	5.2*
Oysters, canned	3 oz	4.6
Lima beans, mature, boiled	1 cup	4.5*
Spinach, frozen, boiled	1 cup	4.3*
Pinto beans, mature, boiled	1 cup	3.6*
Beef, chuck roast, lean only, cooked	3 oz	2.7†
Beef, ground, 85% lean, broiled	3 oz	2.2†
Turkey, dark meat, roasted	3 oz	1.3†
Molasses	1 tbsp	0.9*
Raisins, seedless	¼ cup	0.7*
Turkey, light meat, roasted	3 oz	0.6†

U.S. Department of Agriculture, Agricultural Research Service. *USDA national nutrient database for standard reference, release 26, 2013.* Accessed August 31, 2013: http://www.ars.usda.gov/nutrientdata
*Nonheme iron.
†Heme iron.

Dental Considerations

- Despite the prevalence of iron-deficiency anemia, supplements are not recommended without laboratory testing to indicate a deficiency.
- The most prominent sign of iron deficiency in the oral cavity is pallor and swelling of the tongue. The patient also may complain of soreness and a "burning" tongue. Atrophic changes progress from a patchy denudation of papillae to a smooth, reddened tongue.
- Hemochromatosis is common among chronic alcoholics, usually men, who may drink more than 1 L of inexpensive wine daily. Do not recommend iron-rich and iron-fortified foods to patients with this condition.
- Iron-containing supplements are the leading cause of poisoning deaths in children younger than 6 years old in the United States. Encourage storing iron supplements in a place inaccessible to children.
- Assess food intake of patients with renal failure, individuals experiencing periods of rapid growth (e.g., pregnant women, infants, toddlers, and teenage girls), and vegans for Al of iron-rich foods.
- Encourage good oral hygiene practices when iron supplements are taken to prevent extrinsic staining of teeth. The abrasive effect of baking soda can help reduce staining. Liquid forms of iron can be taken through a straw.
- Because older adults may have a reduced production of gastric acid, this can interfere with iron absorption, increasing the risk of an iron deficiency. A referral to the healthcare provider may be necessary.

Nutritional Directions

- A food rich in vitamin C with supplements or meals increases iron absorption, especially nonheme iron. Take iron with orange juice, tomato juice, or vitamin C–enriched juices such as apple juice.
- If nonheme-containing grains or vegetables are consumed with small amounts of heme iron, absorption of the nonheme iron doubles.
- Because iron provided in a vegan diet is the nonheme form, iron absorption is lower than for individuals consuming animal foods. Iron requirements may double for vegans.
- Chemicals (not caffeine) intrinsic to tea and coffee decrease iron absorption. No decrease in iron absorption occurs when tea or coffee is drunk 1 hour before or 2 hours after a meal.
- Vitamin A deficiency can cause iron deficiency because vitamin A helps to transport iron from the storage sites.
- Taking iron supplements with food and in divided doses reduces gastrointestinal symptoms associated with these supplements.
- A common treatment of hemochromatosis or iron overload is to donate blood regularly.
- For maximum absorption, avoid taking an iron supplement with a large calcium supplement (>800 mg).[47]

with hemochromatosis. Initially, it is difficult to diagnose because of its resemblance to other conditions in which fatigue and general weakness are symptoms. Elevated iron stores have been associated with increased risk of CHD and liver disease. Iron supplements should not be taken indiscriminately and without a comprehensive laboratory workup.

Inadequate dietary iron intake, chronic and acute inflammatory conditions, and obesity are individually associated with iron-deficiency anemia. As the leading nutrient deficiency in both developed and developing countries, iron-deficiency anemia continues to be a global health issue. Anemia has been linked to unfavorable outcomes of pregnancy and infants born to women experiencing anemia. A deficiency can lead to various symptoms, such as microcytic anemia, fatigue, faulty digestion, blue sclerae, pale conjunctivae, and tachycardia. Iron-deficiency anemia may be caused by inadequate dietary intake; accelerated demand or losses; and inadequate absorption secondary to diarrhea, decreased acid secretions, or antacid therapy. Iron deficiency is frequently the result of postnatal feeding practices and has a serious impact on growth and mental and psychomotor development in infants and children.

The most prominent oral signs of iron deficiency include pallor of the lips and oral mucosa, angular cheilitis, atrophy of filiform papillae, and glossitis (see Chapter 17, Figs. 17-1 and 17-2). Oral candidiasis and a reduced resistance to infection are frequently associated with iron deficiency.

ZINC

Physiological Roles

Zinc is a component in more than 200 enzymes that perform a variety of functions affecting cell growth and replication; sexual maturation, fertility, and reproduction; night vision;

immune defenses; and taste, smell, and appetite. Zinc is required for DNA, RNA, and protein synthesis. In this role, zinc is essential for bone growth and mineral metabolism. Zinc-containing enzymes are important in collagen synthesis and bone resorption and remodeling.

Requirements

The IOM recommends a daily intake of 11 mg for men and 8 mg for women (Table 12-10). Although some concerns have been expressed about marginal intakes, zinc deficiencies have not been reported in Americans consuming a variety of foods. Vegans absorb less zinc than individuals who consume animal products. The zinc requirement for vegans is definitely higher, and may be twice the RDA for individuals consuming meats. (The RDA is based on the traditional American diet in which most people consume meat.) The UL for zinc is 40 mg/day.

Absorption and Excretion

Bioavailability of zinc varies widely; approximately 25% to 40% of dietary zinc is absorbed. Absorption depends on several factors, including body size; total dietary zinc; and the presence of other potentially interfering substances, such as calcium, fiber, and phosphate salts. Higher quality protein improves zinc absorption. Many substances in plant products (e.g., fiber and phytate) interfere with zinc absorption. Zinc is lost in the feces; abnormal losses from diarrhea increase zinc requirements.

Sources

Protein-rich foods are good sources of zinc. Lamb, beef, crustaceans (especially oysters), eggs, and peanuts contain significant amounts of zinc (Table 12-11).

Hyper States and Hypo States

Consumption of high levels of zinc normally causes vomiting and diarrhea, epigastric pain, lethargy, and fatigue, and can result in renal damage, pancreatitis, and death. There is a connection with an excess of zinc and reduced copper status, altered iron function, decreased immune function, and decrease in high-density lipoproteins. Supplementation is recommended only under medical supervision.

In developing countries, severe zinc deprivation has been related to excessive consumption of inhibitors, which adversely affect zinc absorption, rather than inadequate zinc intake. In North America, overt zinc deficiency is uncommon. Individuals at particular risk of zinc deficiency include those whose zinc requirements are high (e.g., during periods of rapid growth and during pregnancy and lactation), alcoholics, total vegetarians whose diet consists primarily of cereal protein or is generally nutrient deficient, and individuals with severe malabsorption (ulcerative colitis, chronic diarrhea), sickle cell disease, or other chronic health problems.

Oral manifestations of zinc deficiency include changes in the epithelium of the tongue, such as thickening of

Table 12-10	**Institute of Medicine recommendations for zinc**						
	EAR (mg/day)*		RDA (mg/day)†		AI (mg/day)‡		UL (mg/day)§
Life Stage	Male	Female	Male	Female	Male	Female	
0-6 months					2	2	4
7-12 months	2.5	2.5	3	3			5
1-3 years	2.5	2.5	3	3			7
4-8 years	4	4	5	5			12
9-13 years	7	7	8	8			23
14-18 years	8.5	7.5	11	9			34
≥19 years	9.4	6.8	11	8			40
Pregnancy							
14-18 years	10		12				34
19-50 years	9.5		11				40
Lactation							
14-18 years	10.9		13				34
19-50 years	10.4		12				40

Data from Institute of Medicine (IOM), Food and Nutrition Board: *Dietary reference intakes for vitamin a, vitamin k, arsenic, boron, chromium, copper, iodine, iron, manganese, molybdenum, nickel, silicon, vanadium, and zinc*, Washington, DC, 2001, National Academy Press.
*EAR (estimated average requirement)—the intake that meets the estimated nutrient needs of half of the individuals in a group.
†RDA (recommended dietary allowance)—the intake that meets the nutrient needs of almost all (97% to 98%) individuals in a group.
‡AI (adequate intake)—the observed average or experimentally set intake by a defined population or subgroup that seems to sustain a defined nutritional status, such as growth rate, normal circulating nutrient values, or other functional indicators of health. An AI is used if insufficient scientific evidence is unavailable to derive an EAR. For healthy human milk–fed infants, the AI is the mean intake. *The AI is not equivalent to a RDA.*
§UL (tolerable upper intake level)—the highest level of daily nutrient intake that is likely to pose no risk of adverse health effects to almost all individuals in the general population. As intake increases above the UL, the risk of adverse effects increases. Unless specified otherwise, the UL represents total nutrient intake from food, water, and supplements.

Table 12-11	Zinc content of selected foods	
Food	**Portion**	**Zinc (mg)**
Oysters, canned	3 oz	77.3
Total, whole grain	1 cup	20.0
Baked beans, canned, plain or vegetarian	1 cup	5.8
Beef, chuck roast, braised	3 oz	5.4
Beef, hamburger, 85% lean, broiled	3 oz	5.4
Lobster, cooked	3 oz	3.4
Crab, canned	3 oz	3.2
Yogurt, plain, low fat	8 oz	2.2
Kidney beans, cooked, mature	1 cup	1.9
Cashews, dry roasted	1 oz	1.6
Cheese, Swiss	1 oz	1.2
Oatmeal, instant, plain prepared with water	1 packet	1.1
Peas, green, frozen, cooked	1 cup	1.1
Milk, low-fat or skim	1 cup	0.9
Almonds, dry roasted	1 oz	0.9
Chicken breast, roasted, skinless	3 oz	0.8
Flounder or sole, cooked	3 oz	0.3

U.S. Department of Agriculture, Agricultural Research Service. *USDA national nutrient database for standard reference, release 26, 2013.* Accessed August 31, 2013: http://www.ars.usda.gov/nutrientdata

epithelium; increased cell numbers; impaired keratinization of epithelial cells; increased susceptibility to periodontal disease; and flattened filiform papillae. Zinc deficiency in humans is associated with loss of taste and smell acuity, poor appetite, and impaired wound healing. Decreased linear growth and hypogonadism in adolescent boys are principal manifestations of zinc deficiency.

Zinc deficiency also results in congenital defects, such as skeletal abnormalities, especially cleft palate and lip. Collagen synthesis defects are seen in zinc-deficient animals. Even when adequate amounts of zinc are provided for an extended time, abnormalities in mineral metabolism are not completely reversed. When zinc deficiency is diagnosed, zinc supplementation is vital.

Dental Considerations

- Patients with abnormalities of taste because of zinc deficiency may respond to supplementation, but additional zinc is ineffective in reversing abnormal taste acuity associated with other conditions.
- Supplementation in zinc-depleted patients is beneficial for wound healing, but unnecessary for healthy individuals.
- Zinc supplementation interferes with use of iron and copper and adversely affects high-density lipoprotein levels. Do not advocate indiscriminate use of zinc.
- Zinc lozenges and zinc supplements are marketed to treat cold symptoms. If taken at onset of cold symptoms, zinc seems to reduce the duration of a cold. However, care should be taken when treating common cold symptoms with zinc. Notable side effects are bad taste and nausea. Currently zinc formulations are not standardized and the best dosage is unknown.[48]

Nutritional Directions

- Small amounts of animal protein can significantly improve bioavailability of zinc from a legume-based meal.
- Fruits and vegetables are low in zinc, whereas peanuts and peanut butter have higher amounts.
- Meat, fish, and poultry are the preferred sources of zinc because of its bioavailability from plant foods.
- If a well-balanced diet is consumed, zinc supplements are rarely needed, and may be harmful.
- Large amounts of iron can decrease zinc absorption from food. Iron supplements between meals allow greater zinc absorption from foods.

IODINE

Physiological Role

Iodine is required for production of thyroxine, a hormone secreted by the thyroid gland. Thyroxine regulates the basal metabolic rate; an altered metabolic rate affects other nutrient requirements. Thyroid hormones are essential for normal brain development.

Requirements

The adult RDA for iodine is 150 µg daily. Because iodine is related to the metabolic rate, needs are increased during periods of accelerated growth, especially during pregnancy and lactation. As shown in Table 12-12, the RDA for pregnant and lactating women is higher because of critical needs of the fetus and infant during this period. The UL for iodine is 1100 µg/day.

Currently, iodine nutrition of the average American adult is adequate. However, iodine levels for pregnant and breast-feeding women are less than desirable.[49]

Sources

A major source of iodine is seafood and plants grown near the ocean. Other natural sources include seaweed, dairy products, grain products, and eggs. Breast milk contains iodine and is added to infant formulas. The iodine content of common foods varies significantly, ranging from as little as 10 µg/kg to 1 mg/kg dry weight. The iodine content of meat and animal products depends on iodine content of foods consumed by animals; iodine content of fruits and vegetables is affected by the iodine content of soil and fertilizer and by irrigation practices. The iodine content of foods is not reflected on package labeling and is not available in the U.S. Department of Agriculture's Nutrient Database.

The best safeguard for acquiring an AI is the use of iodized salt. Until the 1920s, endemic iodine deficiency disorders were prevalent in the Great Lakes, Appalachian, and Northwestern regions of the United States. Iodized salt virtually eliminated endemic goiter and remains the mainstay of eradicating iodine deficiency in the United States and worldwide. Iodide in salt will remain stable for many months if kept dry, preferably in a cool place away from light.

Table 12-12   Institute of Medicine recommendations for iodine

Life Stage	EAR (µg/day)* Male	EAR (µg/day)* Female	RDA (µg/day)† Male	RDA (µg/day)† Female	AI (µg/day)‡ Male	AI (µg/day)‡ Female	UL (µg/day)§
0-6 months					110	110	ND¶
7-12 months					130	130	ND¶
1-3 years	65	65	90	90			200
4-8 years	65	65	90	90			300
9-13 years	73	73	120	120			600
14-18 years	95	95	150	150			900
≥19 years	95	95	150	150			1100
Pregnancy							
≥14 years	160		220				900
Lactation							
≥14 years	209		290				900

Data from Institute of Medicine (IOM), Food and Nutrition Board: *Dietary reference intakes for vitamin A, vitamin K, arsenic, boron, chromium, copper, iodine, iron, manganese, molybdenum, nickel, silicon, vanadium, and zinc*, Washington, DC, 2001, National Academy Press.

*EAR (estimated average requirement)—the intake that meets the estimated nutrient needs of half of the individuals in a group.

†RDA (recommended dietary allowance)—the intake that meets the nutrient needs of almost all (97% to 98%) individuals in a group.

‡AI (adequate intake)—the observed average or experimentally set intake by a defined population or subgroup that seems to sustain a defined nutritional status, such as growth rate, normal circulating nutrient values, or other functional indicators of health. An AI is used if insufficient scientific evidence is available to derive an EAR. For healthy human milk–fed infants, the AI is the mean intake. *The AI is not equivalent to a RDA.*

§UL (tolerable upper intake level)—the highest level of daily nutrient intake that is likely to pose no risk of adverse health effects to almost all individuals in the general population. As intake increases above the UL, the risk of adverse effects increases. Unless specified otherwise, the UL represents total nutrient intake from food, water, and supplements.

¶ND—not determinable because of lack of data of adverse effects in this age group and concern with regard to lack of ability to handle excess amounts. Source of intake should be from food and formula to prevent high levels of intake.

Hyper States and Hypo States

Very high levels of iodine may cause adverse effects in some individuals. Excessive amounts of iodine can result in enlargement of the thyroid gland similar to the condition produced by deficiency. Thyroiditis, hypothyroidism, hyperthyroidism, goiter (enlargement of the thyroid gland), and sensitivity reactions have occurred in relation to excessive iodine intake through foods, dietary supplements, topical medications, and iodinated contrast media.

With insufficient iodine intake, the thyroid cannot produce adequate amounts of thyroxine. The pituitary gland continues to secrete thyroid-stimulating hormone, resulting in further hypertrophy and engorgement of the thyroid gland. Goiter is usually associated with iodine deficiency, but may be caused by excessively high intake of goitrogens contained in cabbage, cauliflower, brussels sprouts, broccoli, kale, raw turnips, and rutabagas.

Goiter is the main disorder resulting from low iodine intake. Other iodine-deficiency disorders include stillbirths, spontaneous abortions (e.g., miscarriages), and congenital anomalies; endemic cretinism, usually characterized by impaired mental development and deaf mutism related to fetal iodine deficiency; and impaired mental function. Children born to mothers with severe iodine deficiency have delayed eruption of primary and secondary teeth and an enlarged tongue. Craniofacial growth and development are altered; malocclusion is common.

An iodine deficiency may cause profound metabolic and emotional influences ranging from a mild deceleration of catabolic functions, with sensitivity to cold, dry skin, and mildly elevated blood lipids, to mild depression of mental functions. Endemic goiter occurs where the soil or water is low in iodine content (Fig. 12-9).

A deficiency of iodine remains the most frequent cause worldwide, after starvation, of preventable mental retardation in children. Even a mild deficiency during pregnancy is related to mild and subclinical cognitive and psychomotor deficits in neonates, infants, and children.[50] Severe iodine deficiency usually leads to infertility and increased risks for miscarriage or congenital anomalies. Because of the prevalence of marginal iodine status of pregnant women in the United States, the American Thyroid Association, Neurobehavioral Teratology Society, and the American Medical Association recommend daily iodine supplementation containing 150 to 200 µg.[51] Currently, about half of prenatal vitamins do not contain iodine.[52] With public health efforts to limit salt intake, and increasing use of sea salt, further decreases in iodine nutriture may develop.

Iodine repletion in moderately iodine-deficient school-age children is beneficial by improving cognitive and motor function, increasing concentrations of growth factors, and improving somatic growth.

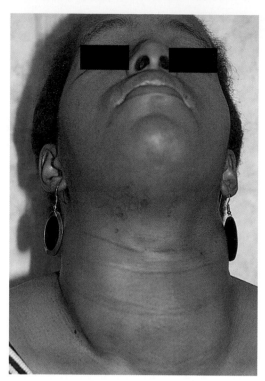

FIGURE 12-9 Goiter resulting from iodine deficiency. (From Swartz M: *Textbook of physical diagnosis: history and examination,* ed 6, St Louis, 2009, Saunders Elsevier.)

Dental Considerations

- Assess patients for possible thyroid problems.
- Enlargement of the thyroid gland can indicate hyperthyroidism or hypothyroidism. Refer these patients to a healthcare provider.
- The American Thyroid Association recommends a supplement of 150 µg of iodine/day during pregnancy and lactation. For women who are pregnant or breastfeeding, stress the importance of taking a prenatal multivitamin that contains at least 150 µg iodine.
- Severe hypothyroidism is termed **myxedema**; hyperthyroidism is also called Graves disease.

Nutritional Directions

- Sea salt has been advocated by health food promoters, but its iodine content is negligible. Purchase salt that is fortified with iodine, which is indicated on the label.
- Individuals consuming large amounts of seaweed, a rich source of iodine, may be at risk for iodine toxicity.

HEALTH APPLICATION 12   Hypertension

Of the more than 76 million Americans who have hypertension warranting some form of treatment, only 60% to 86% are aware of it, and 46% to 77% of hypertensive individuals receive treatment. Hypertension has been called mankind's most common disease. Approximately 1 in 3 adult Americans has hypertension.[53] Hypertension is common in individuals who are of African American descent, are 60 years old and older, have a family history of hypertension, have sedentary lifestyles, consume a large amount of alcohol, have dyslipidemia and/or diabetes, and are obese. Individuals who are normotensive at age 55 years have a 90% lifetime risk of developing hypertension.

Hypertension is defined as a persistent elevation of systolic blood pressure greater than 140 mm Hg and diastolic pressure greater than 90 mm Hg (Table 12-13). For patients with diabetes and chronic kidney disease, the goal is 130/80 mm Hg or less. For every increment of blood pressure above normal levels, there is a commensurate increase in risk of cardiovascular complications, stroke, peripheral vascular disease, and renal insufficiency. Hypertension may result in myocardial infarction, cerebrovascular accident, or heart failure. Uncontrolled hypertension can affect blood vessels in the eyes, kidneys, and nervous system. Hypertension cannot be cured, but it can be controlled. One of the goals of *Healthy People*

2020 is to reduce the proportion of adults with hypertension from 29.9% to 26.9%.[54]

Causes
Several important causal factors for hypertension have been identified, including excess body weight, excess sodium intake, minimal physical activity, inadequate intake of fruits and vegetables and potassium, and excess alcohol intake. Body fat deposited in the trunk increases risk of developing essential hypertension independent of the overall level of obesity, whereas peripherally deposited fat does not. Essential hypertension is elevated blood pressure of unknown cause.

A weight loss of 10% is as effective at reducing blood pressure as pharmacological treatment. Despite the fact that sodium restriction alone does not always result in lower blood pressure for all patients with hypertension, sodium reduction is effective in lowering mean blood pressure in salt-sensitive adults. There is no precise method of identifying salt sensitivity. Sodium restriction enhances effectiveness of diuretics and other pharmacological treatments. The American Heart Association recommendations are consistent with the *Dietary Guidelines* in reducing sodium (see Box 12-2). Generally, when sodium must be restricted, hidden sources of sodium should be considered: (a) sodium bicarbonate and other sodium products used as leavening agents; (b) sodium benzoate, used as a preservative in margarine and relishes; (c) sodium citrate and monosodium glutamate, used to enhance flavors in gelatin desserts, beverages, and meats; (d) sodium bicarbonate or sodium fluoride added to dentifrices or used in place of commercial dentifrices and mouth rinses; (e) some medications, particularly when taken regularly and frequently, such as antacids, laxatives, and cough medicines; and (f) chewing tobacco.

High potassium intake has a protective effect against hypertension, has no adverse effect on blood lipids, and is associated with a lower risk of stroke.[55] Potassium increases urinary sodium excretion. A customary high sodium-to-low potassium ratio consumed when most foods are highly processed may be detrimental to normal blood pressure regulation. Increasing dietary potassium intake from natural foods is a factor in reducing blood pressure and development of CHD. Compared with carbohydrate, dietary protein intake is associated with a significantly lower blood pressure, regardless of the source of protein (vegetable or animal).[56] Overall, a diet rich in protein, potassium, magnesium, and calcium; whole grains; fruits and vegetables; and low-fat and nonfat foods, and low in sodium can lead to a 15% decrease in CHD and 27% fewer strokes.

Drug therapy is effective, but for prehypertensive and treated hypertensive individuals, lifestyle changes are also important. Dietary modifications reduce blood pressure for many individuals with mild to moderate hypertension. Health-promoting lifestyle modifications are recommended to prevent the progressive increase in blood pressure and CHD. Looking at the overall dietary pattern instead of one single nutrient is the key for assessing risk. The dental hygienist can continue to monitor blood pressure, and educate and support the patient's efforts toward reducing blood pressure values. The DASH (Dietary Approaches to Stop Hypertension) approach to prevention and treatment of hypertension combines all the dietary and lifestyle factors related to hypertension.

Dietary Approaches to Stop Hypertension

By combining an eating plan with lifestyle modifications designed to prevent and treat hypertension, the DASH approach has been proven to be effective in reducing high blood pressure and other chronic health conditions. DASH focuses on a dietary pattern instead of decreasing kilocalories or restricting specific nutrients. It emphasizes fruits, vegetables, low-fat or nonfat dairy products, whole grains, nuts, fish,

and poultry, and it reduces and limits saturated fat, total fat, cholesterol, red meats, and sweets. The dietary pattern is rich in nutrients commonly lacking in American diets—fiber, potassium, magnesium, and calcium (Box 12-3 and Table 12-14). Participants with hypertension in the DASH study had greater decreases in blood pressure than nonhypertensive participants. Blood pressure improvement occurred within 2 weeks after beginning the study. Adherence to the DASH diet is associated with reduced risks of strokes and other concerns linked to hypertension.

To reduce sodium intake, patients need to retrain their taste buds by gradually reducing salt intake. For example, patients should remove the salt shaker from the table and refrain from using the salt packet included with fast foods. Eventually, individuals will adjust to a 2300-mg sodium intake and find it acceptable.

The National High Blood Pressure Education Program recommends the DASH diet for preventing and managing hypertension. In addition, the DASH diet is a dietary pattern–based template for all healthy individuals to implement the *Dietary Guidelines* and meet their nutrient recommendations. Individuals following the DASH diet achieve at least two-thirds of the Dietary Reference Intake recommendations for most nutrients despite reduced energy intake. The pattern offers individualization and flexibility in food choices.

Nonpharmacological treatment of hypertension can work if supported by the healthcare provider, and the patient is strongly motivated. When applied together, salt restriction (less than 6 g/day), moderate alcohol intake (less than two servings per day for men and less than one serving per day for women), weight loss for individuals whose body mass index is greater than 25, regular exercise, and following a DASH diet (providing >3500 mg of potassium) can achieve decreases of approximately 10 to 15 mm Hg systolic blood pressure.

For the past 3 years, many health and wellness experts have named the DASH diet as the best for helping with weight loss and improvement of overall health; *U.S. News and World Report* rated the DASH diet as the best diet in their 2013 rankings.[57] In addition to promoting lower blood pressure and cholesterol, research studies confirm that the DASH diet is beneficial in lowering risk of stroke, heart failure, osteoporosis, several types of cancer, kidney stones, type 2 diabetes, and preventing and delaying disease progression for kidney disease. The DASH dietary pattern has also been shown to improve glucose control in individuals with type 2 diabetes.[58]

Table 12-13   Classification of blood pressure for adults

Category	Systolic Pressure (mm Hg)	Diastolic Pressure (mm Hg)
Normal	<120	and <80
Prehypertension	120-139	or 80-89
Stage 1 hypertension	140-159	or 90-99
Stage 2 hypertension	≥160	or ≥100

Data from U.S. Department of Health & Human Services, National Institutes of Health: The seventh report of the Joint National Committee on prevention, detection, evaluation and treatment of high blood pressure. NIH Publication No. 04-5230. Washington, DC, August 2004. Accessed August 31, 2013: http://www.nhlbi.nih.gov/guidelines/hypertension/jnc7full.pdf

BOX 12-3   Tips for Beginning Implementation of the DASH Eating Plan

Implement 1 or 2 of the following suggestions each week.
- Make gradual changes like adding a vegetable as a snack or choosing fruit as a dessert.
- Reduce total fat intake by using half the butter or margarine currently used. (Be sure it does not contain *trans* fats).
- Reduce sodium intake by not adding salt at the table (for other suggestions see Box 12-2).
- Maintain calcium intake using low fat or nonfat dairy products. For lactose intolerance, try lactase enzyme pills or drops or buy lactose-free milk or milk with lactase enzyme added.
- Increase potassium intake by choosing more fresh fruits and vegetables.
- Consume rich sources of magnesium by selecting one serving of nuts as a snack, or dried beans or peas at mealtime.
- Increase dietary fiber by eating edible skins on fruits and/or vegetables.
- Get recommended amounts of minerals and fiber by choosing at least 1 whole grain food (cereal or bread) daily.
- Treat meat as a part of the meal, instead of the focal point; try casseroles, pasta, and stir-fry dishes. Have at least one meatless meal a week; reduce the portion size of meat.
- Increase intake of omega-3 fatty acids by choosing at least one serving of fatty fish (e.g., mackerel, herring, salmon) weekly.
- Consume 3 smaller meals a day plus one or more snacks.

Table 12-14   The DASH eating plan*

Food Group	Daily Servings (Except as noted)	Serving Sizes
Grains and grain products	7-8	1 slice bread 1 cup ready-to-eat cereal† 1/2 cup cooked rice, pasta, or cereal
Vegetables	4-5	1 cup raw leafy vegetable 1/2 cup cooked vegetable 6 oz vegetable juice
Fruits	4-5	1 medium fruit 1/4 cup dried fruit 1/2 cup fresh, frozen, or canned fruit 6 oz fruit juice
Lowfat or fat free dairy foods	2-3	8 oz milk 1 cup yogurt 1 1/2 oz cheese
Lean meats, poultry, and fish	2 or fewer	3 oz cooked lean meat, skinless poultry, or fish
Nuts, seeds, and dry beans	4-5/week	1/3 cup or 1 1/2 oz nuts 1 tbsp or 1/2 oz seeds 1/2 cup cooked dry beans
Fats and oils‡	2-3	1 tsp soft margarine 1 tbsp lowfat mayonnaise 2 tbsp light salad dressing 1 tsp vegetable oil
Sweets	5/week	1 tbsp sugar 1 tbsp jelly or jam 1/2 oz jelly beans 8 oz lemonade

Nutrient Target Totals/2000-kcal Dietary Pattern***

3932 mg potassium
450 mg magnesium
1131 mg calcium
18% protein
55% carbohydrates
28 g dietary fiber
27% fat
6% saturated fat
150 mg cholesterol

*The DASH (Dietary Approaches to Stop Hypertension) Eating Plan is based on 2000 kcal/day. The number of daily servings per food group may vary depending on caloric needs. It closely follows the *Dietary Guidelines for Americans* and *MyPlate* with a few modifications.
†Serving sizes vary between 1/2 cup and 1 1/4 cups. Check the product's nutrition label.
‡Fat content changes serving counts for fats and oils: For example, 1 tablespoon of regular salad dressing equals 1 serving, 1 tablespoon of lowfat salad dressing equals 1/2 serving, and 1 tablespoon of fat free salad dressing equals 0 servings.
***Lin PH, Appel LJ, Funk K, et al: The PREMIER intervention helps participants follow the Dietary Approaches to Stop Hypertension dietary pattern and the current Dietary Reference Intakes recommendations. *J Am Diet Assoc* 2007; 107(9):1541-1551.U.S. Department of Health and Human Services, National Institutes of Health: Your Guide to Lowering Blood Pressure. NIH Publication No 03-5232, May 2003. Accessed August 31, 2013: http://www.nhlbi.nih.gov/health/public/heart/hbp/hbp_low/hbp_low.pdf

Case Application for the Dental Hygienist

Your patient, an older gentleman, complains of a dry mouth and sore tongue. He states that he has not been thirsty, and his intake of fluids has been poor for 4 days. His healthcare provider recently prescribed a diuretic for hypertension and told him to eliminate salt and add more fruits and vegetables to his diet. He complains that "nothing tastes good."

Nutritional Assessment
- Blood pressure value
- Oral mucous membranes, tongue characteristics
- Fluid likes and dislikes
- Mental changes

Nutritional Diagnosis
Fluid volume deficit related to diuretic and poor fluid or food intake.

Nutritional Goals
Patient will have good skin turgor, moist oral mucous membranes, and increase his intake of liquids and food.

Nutritional Implementation
Intervention: Explain the need for fluid intake.
Rationale: Knowledge and involvement in self-care increase compliance.
Intervention: Encourage the patient to drink his favorite fluids, preferably water, on a regular schedule.
Rationale: The patient is more apt to drink his favorite fluid, and, in doing so, he will replace fluids lost because of the diuretic.
Intervention: Identify methods to increase salivary flow and oral lubrication.
Rationale: The patient's degree of oral comfort will improve, and soft tissue will heal.
Intervention: Explain the importance of oral hygiene and how to perform oral self-care procedures.

Rationale: Less saliva allows more food debris to remain on teeth, which may increase caries risk. Because oral mucosa and gingival tissues are more susceptible to trauma, an extra-soft bristle brush may be appropriate for plaque removal, and the patient should be cautioned against aggressive oral hygiene. Other oral physiotherapy aids may be warranted for optimal plaque biofilm removal.
Intervention: Explore challenges the patient will encounter with foods low in salt and discuss ways to enhance flavors of food without using sodium (see Box 12-2 and Tables 12-4 and 5). Explain that as his salt intake decreases, salt in the saliva will also decrease so that after about 3 months of moderately low intake, his preferred salt level in foods will decrease, and his taste for food will gradually improve.
Rationale: Most Americans consume about four to seven times the recommended amount of sodium. Sodium concentration in saliva determines a patient's recognition of salt in food; higher levels of sodium in saliva means higher levels of sodium are needed for it to be detected.
Intervention: Discuss types of dentifrices consistent with the healthcare provider's order to eliminate salt.
Rationale: Sodium bicarbonate or sodium fluoride is added to some dentifrices and mouth rinses; these would increase his sodium intake, especially if oral hygiene is practiced several times a day, and the patient ingests the dentifrice or mouth rinse.
Intervention: Have the patient record his dietary intake for 1 to 3 days. Compare this record with the DASH diet.
Rationale: Suggestions can be tailored to the patient's needs. The patient can set a goal based on the information presented.

Evaluation
Desired outcomes include the patient's adequate consumption of preferred beverages each day, moist oral mucous membranes, and no dental caries.

STUDENT READINESS

1. Define ICF and ECF. What are the principal electrolytes found in each?
2. Record your daily fluid intake. How does this record compare with the required intake? What percentage is water?
3. Fluid is essential for survival. Discuss advantages and disadvantages of water intake versus other fluids, such as milk, carbonated beverages, tea, and coffee.
4. List five clinical observations indicating FVD. What type of medication is frequently prescribed that affects hydration status?
5. What can cause hypernatremia? Hyponatremia? Why is altering salt intake of patients with these conditions not usually the mode of treatment?
6. What can cause FVD or FVE?
7. What is the general effect of food processing on sodium and potassium content of foods?
8. Explain the physiological change that occurs when salt intake is decreased, and why adding large amounts of salt to foods is unwise. Would you consider salt addictive?
9. Discuss dental hygiene interventions for iron-deficiency anemia. Discuss factors affecting iron absorption.
10. A patient asks you why he has to take zinc when his iron stores are depressed. How would you respond?
11. Which two nutrients discussed in this chapter are important for collagen formation?
12. Name the electrolyte(s) or mineral(s) discussed in this chapter associated with the following symptoms:
    - Shrinkage of mucous membranes
    - Thirst
    - Oral pallor
    - Taste abnormalities
    - Lethargy
    - Enlargement of thyroid
    - Poor wound healing
    - Swollen tongue
    - Loss of appetite
13. The *Dietary Guidelines* and the American Heart Association recommend restricting red meat and eggs. Their recommendations also include increasing fiber intake from cereal and vegetable sources to help reduce blood lipid levels. Discuss how these two recommendations

affect the known deficiency of iron stores in the U.S. population in general. Would you anticipate that long periods of compliance with cholesterol-reducing protocols might necessitate use of iron supplements in affected individuals?

14. Identify guidelines in the DASH diet that would be beneficial to the older adult in the Case Application box in this chapter.

CASE STUDY

A 17-year-old boy complains of a dry mouth; difficulty in swallowing food; dry, sticky tongue; and dry skin. The patient reports he has just recovered from the flu with fever, diarrhea, and vomiting. He also informs you he is currently training for an athletic competition and exercises 3 to 4 hours a day. A 24-hour diet recall reveals the patient's fluid intake includes 48 to 72 oz of caffeinated soft drinks without any other beverages and a high protein intake.

1. What other information should you obtain about the patient's dietary intake?
2. Could the patient's oral symptoms be attributed to his current fluid intake?
3. Is salivary analysis indicated for this patient?
4. What suggestions could you make that would decrease his symptoms of xerostomia? Identify ideas to increase his fluid intake.
5. What oral self-care practices would you recommend to relieve his oral discomfort and facilitate swallowing?

CASE STUDY

A 15-year-old girl comes into the dental office reporting a history of iron-deficiency anemia. She has clinical symptoms typical of this anemia: glossitis; smooth, shiny, red tongue; and painful cracks at the corners of her mouth. Her healthcare provider has prescribed ferrous sulfate and zinc to correct this deficiency.

1. When evaluating dietary intake, what are some foods you would need to watch for to assess iron intake?
2. If the patient is having problems with the ferrous sulfate supplement (e.g., constipation or nausea), would it be advisable to resolve the anemia by just increasing dietary iron intake? Why or why not?
3. Why has the healthcare provider ordered zinc supplements?
4. What should you tell her about iron from plant or animal foods?
5. What can she do to help increase absorption of iron?

References

1. Jaquier E, Constant F: Water as an essential nutrient: the physiological basis of hydration. *Eur J Clin Nutr* 64(2):115–123, 2010.
2. International Bottled Water Association (IBWA): *Bottled water market.* Accessed August 31, 2013: http://www.bottledwater.org/economics/bottled-water-market.
3. Block B: *Bottled water demand may be declining.* Worldwatch Institute, Washington, DC. Updated February 19, 2013. Accessed August 31, 2013: http://www.worldwatch.org/node/5878.
4. U.S. Food and Drug Administration (FDA): *Regulation of bottled water.* July 8, 2009. Accessed August 31, 2013: http://www.fda.gov/NewsEvents/Testimony/ucm170932.htm.
5. Malik VS, Pan A, Willett WC, et al: Sugar-sweetened beverages and weight gain in children and adults: a systematic review and meta-analysis. *Am J Clin Nutr* 2013: (Epub ahead of print) PMID:23966427.
6. Chen L, Appel LJ, Loria C, et al: Reduction in consumption of sugar-sweetened beverages is associated with weight loss: the PREMIER trial. *Am J Clin Nutr* 89(5):1299–1306, 2009.
7. Rolls BJ: Plenary Lecture 1: dietary strategies for the prevention and treatment of obesity. *Proc Nutr Soc* 69(1):70–79, 2010.
8. Bhupathiraju SN, Pan A, Malik VS, et al: Caffeinated and caffeine-free beverages and risk of type 2 diabetes. *Am J Clin Nutr* 91:155–166, 2013.
9. Costa J, Lunet N, Santos C, et al: Caffeine exposure and the risk of Parkinson's disease: a systematic review and meta-analysis of observational studies. *J Alzheimers Dis* 20(Suppl 1):S221–S238, 2010.
10. Eskelinen HM, Kivipelto M: Caffeine as a protective factor in dementia and Alzheimer's disease. *J Alzheimers Dis* 20(Suppl 1):S167–S174, 2010.
11. Gelber RP, Petrovitch H, Masaki KH, et al: Coffee intake in midlife and risk of dementia and its neuropathologic correlates. *J Alzheimers Dis* 23(4):607–615, 2011.
12. Geybels MS, Neuhouser ML, Stanford JL: Associations of tea and coffee consumption with prostate cancer risk. *Cancer Causes Control* 24(5):941–948, 2013.
13. Mostofsky E, Rice MS, Levitan EB, et al: Habitual coffee consumption and risk of heart failure: a dose-response meta-analysis. *Circ Heart Fail* 5(4):401–405, 2012.
14. Glatter KA, Myers R, Chiamvimonvat N: Recommendations regarding dietary intake and caffeine and alcohol consumption in patients with cardiac arrhythmias: what do you tell your patients to do or not to do? *Curr Treat Options Cardiovasc Med* 14(5):529–535, 2012.
15. Kim B, Nam Y, Kim J, et al: Coffee consumption and stroke risk: a meta-analysis of epidemiologic studies. *Korean J Fam Med* 33(6):356–365, 2012.
16. Freedman ND, Park Y, Abnet CC, et al: Association of coffee drinking with total and cause-specific mortality. *N Engl J Med* 366(20):1891–1904, 2012.
17. Fritz H, Seely D, Kennedy DA, et al: Green tea and lung cancer: a systematic review. *Integr Cancer Ther* 12(1):7–24, 2013.
18. Serafini M, Del Rio D, N'Dri Yao D, et al: Health benefits of tea. In: Benzie IFF, Wachtel-Galor S, editors. *Herbal medicine: herbal medicine: biomolecular and clinical aspects*, ed 2, Boca Raton, FL, 2011, CRC Press. PMID: 22593935. Accessed August 31, 2013: http://www.ncbi.nlm.nih.gov/books/NBK92768/.
19. Steinmann J, Buer J, Pietschmann T, et al: Anti-infective properties of epigallocatechin-3-gallate (EGCG), a component of green tea. *Br J Pharmacol* 168(5):1059–1073, 2013.
20. Borgwardt S, Hammann F, Scheffler K, et al: Neural effects of green tea extract on dorsolateral prefrontal cortex. *Eur J Clin Nutr* 66(11):1187–1192, 2012.
21. Hügel HM, Jackson N: Redox chemistry of green tea polyphenols: therapeutic benefits in neurodegenerative diseases. *Mini Rev Med Chem* 12(5):380–387, 2012.
22. Vernarelli JA, Lambert JD: Tea consumption is inversely associated with weight status and other markers for metabolic syndrome in US adults. *Eur J Nutr* 52(3):1039–1048, 2013.
23. van Dam RM, Naidoo N, Landberg R: Dietary flavonoids and development of type 2 diabetes and cardiovascular diseases: review of recent findings. *Curr Opin Lipidol* 24(1):25–33, 2013.

24. Wolk BJ, Ganetsky M, Babu KM: Toxicity of energy drinks. *Curr Opin Pediatr* 24(2):243–251, 2012.

25. Bigelman KA, Chapman DP, Freese EC, et al: Effects of 6 weeks of quercetin supplementation on energy, fatigue, and sleep in ROTC cadets. *Mil Med* 176(5):565–572, 2011.

26. Howland J, Rohscnow D: Risks of energy drinks mixed with alcohol. *JAMA* 309(3):245–246, 2013.

27. Meier B: FDA posts injury data for 3 drinks. *New York Times* November 16, 2012. Accessed August 31 2013: http://topics .nytimes.com/top/reference/timestopics/organizations/f/food_ and_drug_administration/index.html?inline=nyt-org.

28. Rosenbloom C: Food and fluid guidelines before, during, and after exercise. *Nutr Today* 47(2):63–69, 2012.

29. Heneghan C, Howick J, O'Neill B, et al: The evidence underpinning sports performance products: a systematic assessment. *BMJ Open* 2(4):pii: e001702, 2012. Accessed August 31, 2013: http://bmjopen.bmj.com/content/2/4/e001702.full.

30. Saad L: *Nearly half of Americans drink soda daily*. July 23, 2012. Accessed August 31, 2013: http://www.gallup.com/poll/156116/ nearly-half-americans-drink-soda-daily.aspx.

31. Fakhouri THI, Kit BK, Ogden CL: *Consumption of diet drinks in the United States, 2009-2010*. NCHS Data Brief, No. 109, October 2012. Accessed August 31, 2013: http://www.cdc.gov/ nchs/data/databriefs/db109.pdf.

32. Han E, Powell LM: Consumption patterns of sugar-sweetened beverages in the United States. *J Acad Nutr Diet* 113(1):43–53, 2013.

33. Welsh JA, Sharma AJ, Grellinger L, et al: Consumption of added sugars is decreasing in the United States. *Am J Clin Nutr* 94(3):726–734, 2011.

34. Jain P, Hall-May E, Golabek K, et al: A comparison of sports and energy drinks–physiochemical properties and enamel dissolution. *Gen Dent* 60(3):190–197, 2012.

35. Oliver MM, Drause PR: Powering up with sports and energy drinks. *J Pediatr Health Care* 21(6):413–416, 2007.

36. Armstrong LE, Ganio MS, Casa DJ, et al: Mild dehydration affects mood in healthy young women. *J Nutr* 142(2):382–388, 2012.

37. Cogswell ME, Zhang Z, Carriquiry AL, et al: Sodium and potassium intakes among US adults: NHANES 2003-2008. *Am J Clin Nutr* 96(3):647–657, 2012.

38. World Health Organization: *WHO issues new guidance on dietary salt and potassium*. January 31, 2013. Accessed August 31, 2013: http://www.who.int/mediacentre/news/notes/2013/ salt_potassium_20130131/en/.

39. Dinicolantonio JJ, Pasquale PD, Taylor RS, et al: Low sodium versus normal sodium diets in systolic heart failure: systematic review and meta-analysis. *Heart* 2013 Mar 12. doi:10.1136/ heartjnl-2012-302337 [Epub ahead of print]

40. Taylor RS, Ashton KE, Moxham T, et al: Reduced dietary salt for the prevention of cardiovascular disease. *Cochrane Database Syst Rev* (7):CD009217, 2011.

41. Centers for Disease Control and Prevention (CDC): *Vital Signs: Where's the sodium?* February 2012. Accessed on August 31, 2013: http://www.cdc.gov/vitalsigns/Sodium/index.html.

42. American Heart Association: *A grain of salt*. Updated January 2, 2013. Accessed August 31, 2013: http://www.heart .org/HEARTORG/GettingHealthy/NutritionCenter/Healthy Cooking/A-Grain-of-Salt_UCM_430087_Article.jsp.

43. Vella D, Marcone M, Duizer LM: Physical and sensory properties of regional sea salts. *Food Res Int* 45(1):415–421, 2012.

44. Guthrie J, Biing-Hwan L, Okrent A, et al: *Americans' food choices at home and away: how do they compare with recommendations?* Amber Waves February 21, 2013. Accessed August 31, 2013: http://www.ers.usda.gov/amber-waves/2013 -february/americans-food-choices-at-home-and-away.aspx# .UfaFDUrD_kg.

45. Hoy MK, Goldman JD: *Potassium intake of the U.S. population: what we eat in America, NHANES 2009-2010*. Food Surveys Research Group Dietary Data Brief No. 10. September 2012. Accessed August 31, 2013: http://www.ars.usda.gov/ SP2UserFiles/Place/12355000/pdf/DBrief/10_potassium _intake_0910.pdf

46. Ibid.

47. Gaitán D, Flores S, Saavedra P, et al: Calcium does not inhibit the absorption of 5 milligrams of nonheme or heme iron at doses less than 800 milligrams in nonpregnant women. *J Nutr* 141(9):1651–1656, 2011.

48. Singh M, Das RR: Zinc for the common cold. *Cochrane Database Sys Rev* (2):CD001364, 2011. doi: 10.1002/14651858. CD001364.pub3.

49. Centers for Disease Control and Prevention (CDC): *Second National Report on Biochemical Indicators of Nutrition and Nutrition in the U.S. Population*. Atlanta, 2012, CDC. Accessed August 31, 2013: http://www.cdc.gov/nutritionreport/pdf/ Nutrition_Book_complete508_final.pdf#zoom=100.

50. Trumpff C, De Schepper J, Tafforeau J, et al: Mild iodine deficiency in pregnancy in Europe and its consequences for cognitive and psychomotor development of children: A review. *J Trace Elem Med Biol* 27(3):174–183, 2013.

51. Stagnaro-Green A, Sullivan S, Pearce EN: Iodine supplementation during pregnancy and lactation. *JAMA* 308(23):2463–2464, 2012.

52. Leung AM, Pearce EN, Braverman LE: Iodine content of prenatal multivitamins in the United States. *N Engl J Med* 360(9): 939–940, 2009.

53. American Heart Association: Executive Summary: Heart disease and stroke statistics—2013 update: a report from the American Heart Association. *Circulation* 127:143–152, 2013.

54. U.S. Department of Health and Human Services: *Progress toward Healthy People 2020 targets & objectives: heart disease and stroke*. Accessed August 31, 2013: http:// www.healthypeople.gov/2020/topicsobjectives2020/ objectiveslist.aspx?topicId=21.

55. Aburto NJ, Hanson S, Gutierrez H, et al: Effect of increased potassium intake on cardiovascular risk factors and disease: systematic review and meta-analyses. *BMJ* 346:f1378, 2013.

56. Rebholz CM, Friedman EE, Powers, LJ, et al: Dietary protein intake and blood pressure: a meta-analysis of randomized controlled trials. *Am J Epidemiol* 176(Suppl 7):S27–S43, 2012.

57. U.S. News Staff: *U.S. News best diets: how we rated 29 eating plans*. January 7, 2013. Accessed February 23, 2013: http:// health.usnews.com/health-news/articles/2013/01/07/us -news-best-diets-how-we-rated-29-eating-plans.

58. Shirani F, Salehi-Abargouei A, Azadbakht L: Effects of dietary approaches to stop hypertension (DASH) diet on some risk for developing type 2 diabetes: a systematic review and meta-analysis on controlled clinical trials. *Nutrition* 29(7-8):939–947, 2013.

ⓔ EVOLVE RESOURCES

Please visit http://evolve.elsevier.com/Stegeman/nutritional for additional practice and study support tools.

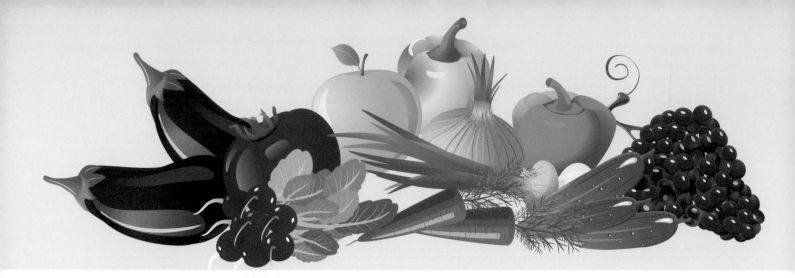

PART II
Application of Nutrition Principles

13 **Nutritional Requirements Affecting Oral Health in Women, 243**
14 **Nutritional Requirements During Growth and Development and Eating Habits Affecting Oral Health, 265**
15 **Nutritional Requirements for Older Adults and Eating Habits Affecting Oral Health, 292**
16 **Food Factors Affecting Health, 308**
17 **Effects of Systemic Disease on Nutritional Status and Oral Health, 339**

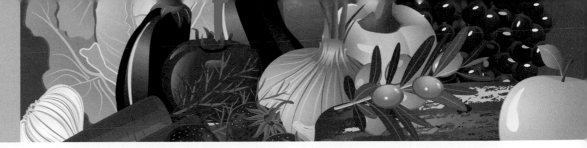

Chapter 13

Nutritional Requirements Affecting Oral Health in Women

Student Learning Outcomes

Upon completion of this chapter, the student will be able to achieve the following student learning outcomes:

- Assess nutrients commonly supplemented during pregnancy and lactation.
- Use recommended guidelines to assess food intake of pregnant and lactating women for adequate nutrients.

- Discuss each factor affecting fetal development.
- Implement nutrition and oral health considerations for patients who are pregnant or breastfeeding.
- Apply nutritional directions for patients who are pregnant or breastfeeding.

Key Terms

Anencephaly
Atrophic gingivitis
Dysesthesia
Erythropoiesis
Gravidas
Hormone replacement therapy (HRT)
Listeriosis
Low birth weight (LBW)

Menopausal gingivostomatitis
Menopause
Nutritional insult
Perimenopause
Pica
Preeclampsia
Premature
Toxoplasmosis

Test Your NQ

1. **T/F** All efforts should be made to satisfy a pregnant woman's food cravings because cravings reflect an innate need for certain nutrients.
2. **T/F** The fetus is nourished from the mother's nutrient stores.
3. **T/F** After pregnancy, most mothers have at least one carious lesion because calcium was pulled from teeth for use by the developing fetus.
4. **T/F** A woman should eat twice as much food when she is pregnant because she is eating for two.
5. **T/F** Most women should gain 25 to 35 lb during a pregnancy.

6. **T/F** Vitamin A is the only nutrient warranting global supplementation during pregnancy.
7. **T/F** Virtually all women can produce enough milk to support nutritional needs of the infant.
8. **T/F** Breast milk that is too thin must be nutritionally inadequate.
9. **T/F** If breast milk supply is inadequate, a feeding should be omitted to have more milk available later.
10. **T/F** WIC is a governmental program that provides supplemental foods for women, infants, and children.

HEALTHY PREGNANCY

Although there is no specific definition of a healthy pregnancy, the health of the mother and infant is important. In addition to continued preservation of the mother's physical health, her emotional and psychological well-being is important. Goals for the infant include being (a) full term (born between the 39th and 41st week of gestation) and (b) mature (weighing more than 6 lb). Infants with a **low birth weight (LBW)** (weighing less than 5½ lb) or who are **premature** (gestational age less than 37 weeks, especially those with a gestational age of less than 32 weeks) have more long-term health and developmental problems and increased mortality. Mortality rates are highest for infants born at 22 to 23 weeks of gestation (70%) and decline sharply to 8% with increasing gestational age more than 32 weeks.[1] The number of infants born prematurely has dropped from 12.8% in 2006 to 11.7% in 2011.[2] Primary factors for a successful pregnancy are nutritional status before conception, appropriate weight gain, and adequate intake of essential nutrients during pregnancy. If the mother's nutritional status is poor, the placenta apparently does not perform its function well.

A classic report published in 1970 by the National Academy of Sciences established a basis for increased nutritional requirements during pregnancy. The consensus of a more recent workshop acknowledged that the report was written when undernutrition and inadequate weight gain were principal concerns, whereas current primary concern has shifted to obesity and excess weight gain.[3]

Factors Affecting Fetal Development
Preconceptional Nutritional Status

"Getting healthy" before pregnancy is important. One of the most important times for prenatal care is before a pregnancy begins. Ideally, weight adjustments of overweight or underweight women should be achieved before conception. Because of the detrimental influence of maternal overweight and obesity on pregnancy outcomes, the Academy of Nutrition and Dietetics and the American Society for Nutrition recommend that all overweight and obese women of reproductive age should receive counseling prior to the pregnancy on the role of diet and physical activity to ameliorate adverse outcomes from an RDN.[4] Losing 15 to 20 lb before conception may be enough to avoid some weight-related pregnancy complications (e.g., preeclampsia, cesarean delivery, and large-for-gestational-age infants). **Preeclampsia** is a potentially serious complication of pregnancy involving high blood pressure that often leads to premature delivery. Preconceptual obesity or underweight not only hampers fertility, but also can set the stage for metabolic problems during pregnancy. Infant deaths are much more likely to occur when the mother is obese.[5]

Maternal health and fetal growth and development are affected by nutrient intake, not only during the pregnancy, but also before conception. By the time a woman has her first prenatal visit, fetal development has already progressed beyond a critical period during which a lack of folic acid or certain exposures may have already compromised the health and well-being of the mother and/or fetus. In addition to eating a well-balanced diet, prenatal vitamins are encouraged in anticipation of a pregnancy to ensure a good environment for the fetus from the beginning. Low levels of iron and folic acid before the pregnancy have been linked to premature births and stunted growth. Research suggests prenatal food choices may have enduring effects on the child's lifelong food preferences and negative metabolic outcomes.[7]

When a pregnancy occurs less than 1 year after a previous pregnancy, the woman may not have adequate maternal nutritional reserves; this may contribute to increased incidence of preterm births and fetal growth retardation, and risk of maternal mortality and morbidity. Because of the rapid development of body parts and organs during the first trimester, birth defects are likely to occur if usual dietary habits are poor, or if drugs are used during this critical period. Infant birth weights are affected more by nutrient intake during the second and third trimesters.

Although poor maternal nutrient intake can result in an infant with a LBW, it is commonly believed the fetus is protected at the mother's expense. With some nutrients, such as calcium and iron, higher requirements are met by more efficient maternal absorption to meet fetal needs, but for others, inadequate maternal intake may deplete the mother's stores (e.g., folic acid), and the infant's stores may be suboptimal at birth as well.

Unusual Dietary Patterns

Pica, or an abnormal consumption of specific food and nonfood substances, such as dirt, clay, baking soda, paint chips, stones, cloth, baby powder, starch (laundry and corn), large quantities of ice/frost, or other inedible items, affects 20% to 75% of American women. Women practicing pica behaviors are usually from lower socioeconomic groups or have less than a high school education; are in poor nutritional health; may be an adolescent having clinical problems, such as pregnancy-induced hypertension; or are affected by behavioral/environmental factors, such as alcohol or substance abuse. Pica is more frequently practiced by African American women living in rural areas with a childhood and family history of pica. Micronutrient deficiencies, especially iron and zinc, may result from these abnormal behaviors; however, scientific literature provides conflicting results between pica and iron and zinc status.[8] Pica may result in lead poisoning, and, depending on the nonfood item, the substance consumed can cause teeth to wear down quickly.

Beliefs about cravings and folklore that could influence dietary selections are cultural and regional. These beliefs may not be supported by scientific information and may be detrimental. Familiarity with local beliefs is needed to talk with **gravidas** (pregnant women) about beliefs that are potentially detrimental to good nutrition during pregnancy. Special dietary restrictions may be practiced based on food fads, or ethnic, cultural, or religious customs. In addition to assessing the effects of these on nutritional status, an awareness of these practices allows the dental hygienist to provide guidance about desirable food choices that are within these constraints.

Healthcare

Availability and use of healthcare services are related to problems in pregnancy. Inadequate prenatal care leads to problems for both mother and fetus. Prenatal care is important to protect the embryo from effects of chronic health problems later in life, such as diabetes and hypertension.

Age

Maternal age can be a factor in the increased number of LBW infants among gravidas younger than 18 years old. Most adolescent girls do not complete linear growth and achieve gynecological maturity until age 17. Nutritional requirements are quite high to meet the growth needs for both adolescent and fetus. Not only are many of these girls still growing and storing nutrients in their own bodies, but also most have an inadequate intake of numerous crucial nutrients. Approximately one of every three teenage mothers shows signs of significant bone loss after giving birth, but greater calcium and vitamin D consumption during pregnancy may protect against bone loss.

Intake of calorie-dense foods and erratic eating may preclude adequate intake of required nutrients. Socioeconomic disadvantages of these young mothers may affect their diet as a result of the amount of food available and their uninformed selections. Increased energy requirements are usually met without concentrated effort as a result of an increased appetite.

More women are choosing to become pregnant at an older age. Pregnancy after age 35 years is influenced by the woman's overall health. Maternal risks involve chronic conditions, such as diabetes, hypertension, and cardiovascular problems. These conditions are closely supervised to lessen their impact on the fetus. A woman needs to be particularly aware of maintaining her nutritional health if a pregnancy after age 35 years is anticipated.

Weight Gain

Successful pregnancies depend on ideal preconceptional weight plus appropriate weight gain during gestation. However, weight gain during pregnancy influences birth weight more than prepregnancy weight. Approximately 58% of women of reproductive age are overweight and almost 33% are obese.[9] The goal for women who are overweight before pregnancy is to avoid excessive weight gain, but to consume adequate kilocalories to allow optimal fetal growth.

Current recommendations take into consideration factors that affect pregnancy before conception and continue through the first year post-partum with regard to health of both infant and mother. These new guidelines are based on body mass index (BMI) categories and include a relatively narrow range of recommended gain for obese women (to determine BMI, see pg v). A range of weight gain is recommended to accommodate differences such as age, race/ethnicity, and other factors that affect pregnancy outcomes. The guidelines are intended to be used along with good clinical judgment and a discussion between the woman and her healthcare provider about diet and exercise. Women whose prepregnancy weight is within a normal BMI should have a total weight gain of 25 to 35 lb, or 0.8 to 1 lb/week during the second and third trimesters (Table 13-1). More research is needed to determine appropriate weight gain for adolescents. Women with a normal BMI who are pregnant with twins should gain between 37-54 lb; overweight women 31-50 lb; and obese women, 25-42 lb.[10] These new guidelines are not significantly different from the previous ones, but the committee believes that with full implementation, lower health risks can be expected for mothers and infants.

Some women are concerned about gaining too much weight during pregnancy, whereas others, recognizing the need to eat for two, consume excessive amounts of food. Too little or too much weight gain can harm the mother and fetus. Most women are physically inactive resulting in excess weight gain.

Excessive weight gain during pregnancy can increase risk of gestational diabetes, pregnancy-induced high blood

Table 13-1	Recommendation for total and rate of weight gain during pregnancy, by prepregnancy body mass index (BMI)		
Prepregnancy BMI	BMI* (kg/m^2) (WHO)	Total Weight Gain Range (lb)	Rates of Weight Gain† Second and Third Trimester (Mean Range in lb/wks)
Underweight	<18.5	28-40	1 (1-1.3)
Normal weight	18.5-24.9	25-35	1 (0.8-1)
Overweight	25.0-29.9	15-25	0.6 (0.5-0.7)
Obese (includes all classes)	≥30.0	11-20	0.5 (0.4-0.6)

From Institute of Medicine (IOM) and National Research Council (NRC): *Weight gain during pregnancy: reexamining the guidelines*, Washington, DC, 2009, National Academies Press.
*To determine BMI, go to www.nhlbisupport.com/bmi/ or use this formula: BMI = (weight in pounds/[height in inches × Height in inches]) × 703
†Calculations assume a 0.5-2 kg (1.1-4.4 lb) weight gain in the first trimester.

pressure, miscarriage or stillbirth, eclampsia, large-for-gestational-age infants, difficulties during delivery requiring cesarean delivery, and postpartum hemorrhage, and maternal morbidity.[11-13] Most women are physically inactive resulting in excess weight gain. Walking briskly for 30 minutes a day can help avoid putting on too many pounds.

More than 20% of U.S. women gain more than 40 lb during pregnancy.[14] Women who gain more than 22 lb during pregnancy are more likely to retain the weight and gain additional weight over time. Infants born to mothers who gain more than 50 lb during pregnancy are more than twice as likely to be heavier at birth, a predictor for a higher BMI later in life, excluding the effects of weight gain from genetic components.

On the other hand, underweight women are at increased risk for spontaneous preterm birth. LBW, which is associated with health problems for the infant, is more likely to occur with an inadequate amount of maternal weight gain.

Oral Health

Studies indicate that more than one-third of women do not receive dental care during their pregnancy. Even when an oral problem exists, most women do not see their dentist.[15] Hormonal changes occur during pregnancy that increase the risk of developing pregnancy gingivitis, which can affect health of the fetus. Women who do not receive routine dental care either before or during pregnancy are at markedly increased risk of receiving no information regarding the importance of oral healthcare during this period. Even though a gravida may not have overt dental problems, maintaining proper oral hygiene care is important. Attitudes and behaviors about dental care during pregnancy may be influenced by fear of harm to the woman or fetus. Routine dental care received during pregnancy is not associated with an increased risk of serious medical events, preterm deliveries, spontaneous abortions, or fetal deaths or anomalies.

Numerous factors contribute to increased incidence of oral changes observed in most pregnant women. Pregnancy gingivitis (Fig. 13-1A) usually becomes evident in the second month of pregnancy. Hormonal changes (estrogen and progesterone) associated with pregnancy contribute to an increased susceptibility to gingivitis and periodontitis. If plaque biofilm is allowed to accumulate and irritate the gingiva, gingivitis occurs and may result in large lumps called "pregnancy tumors" (Fig. 13-1B). Numerous studies indicate that periodontal disease during pregnancy is a significant risk factor for preeclampsia or delivering a premature or LBW infant, or both.[16]

Nausea is common during pregnancy; recurring vomiting increases oral exposure to gastric acid secretions, which may erode tooth enamel. In addition to nausea and vomiting, gastroesophageal reflux disease is common during pregnancy because of normal physiologic changes that affect the lower esophageal sphincter. Evidence shows a strong association between gastroesophageal reflux disease and dental erosion. Acidity from repeated regurgitation should be treated by rubbing a paste of baking soda and water on the

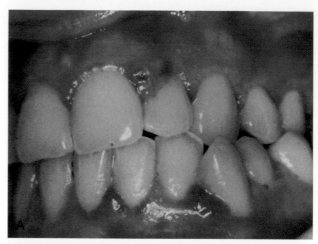
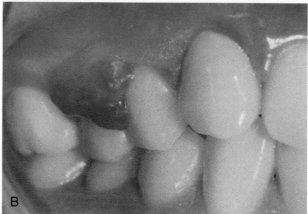

FIGURE 13-1 A, Pregnancy gingivitis. **B,** Pregnancy tumor. (From Perry DA, Beemsterboer PL: *Periodontology for the dental hygienist*, ed 4, St Louis, 2014, Saunders.)

teeth to neutralize oral pH, rinsing after 30 seconds, then brushing and flossing.

Drugs and Medications

Use of tobacco, alcohol, caffeine, some medications, megadoses of nutrients, and illegal drugs can harm the fetus. Results from many studies over the past three decades regarding effects of caffeine on pregnancy have produced conflicting results and caused much confusion. Caffeine is a stimulant and a diuretic, and it crosses the placenta. Recent studies found no association between maternal caffeine consumption during pregnancy and the risk of preterm birth. However, the current recommendation is to eliminate caffeine during pregnancy or limit it to less than 300 mg/day.[17] Brewed coffee, for example, can contain 150 to 500 mg caffeine per 16-oz cup. Considering the popularity of coffee, sodas, and energy drinks, minimizing caffeine intake may be challenging for some pregnant women.

Alcohol is a folic acid antagonist and can cross the placenta. For decades, doctors and researchers have known that heavy alcohol intake during pregnancy may cause birth defects, especially fetal alcohol syndrome (discussed in *Health Application 13*). The effects of a small amount of alcohol on the fetus are not well understood. Recent research has explored the effects of various amounts of alcohol consumption by pregnant women on their children at 5 years of age.[18-21] Overall, results indicate that low weekly drinking (1 to 4 drinks/week) or binge drinking in early pregnancy had no significant effect on birth weight or preterm birth,[22] or neurodevelopment (intelligence, executive functions, attention span),[23] or motor function[24] of children age 5 years. A single binge episode of alcohol during the first trimester results in low risk for adverse effects on the fetus if alcohol is discontinued for the duration of the pregnancy.[25] Nevertheless, researchers feel that conservatively, women should abstain from alcohol during pregnancy.[26-28]

Artificial Sweeteners

Nonnutritive sweeteners, while classified as generally safe, have received little attention regarding their safety during pregnancy. The FDA has approved aspartame, acesulfame-K, rebaudioside (Stevia), and sucralose for moderate consumption during pregnancy. Saccharin crosses the placenta so its use is questionable during pregnancy. Pregnant women with the genetic disorder phenylketonuria should not use aspartame throughout their life span.

Food Safety

During pregnancy, women are at high risk for foodborne illness because of physiological changes that may increase exposure of the mother and fetus to hazardous substances. Pregnant women should avoid unpasteurized juices; unpasteurized milk and dairy products; raw sprouts; and meat, poultry, eggs, fish, and shellfish that are raw or undercooked. Pregnant and breastfeeding women, in particular, should heed food-handling precautions discussed in Chapter 16, in addition to the other precautions discussed here.

Certain foodborne illnesses can be especially dangerous; for example, listeriosis can cause miscarriage, premature birth, stillbirth, or acute illness in newborns. **Listeriosis** is a serious infection usually caused by food contaminated with the bacterium *Listeria monocytogenes,* which principally affects infants and adults with weakened immune systems. Harmful bacteria grow slowly at refrigerated temperatures. Symptoms include gastrointestinal problems followed by fever and muscle aches. To reduce risk of listeriosis, pregnant women should heat leftovers and ready-to-eat foods (e.g., deli meats, hot dogs, and luncheon meats) until steaming hot (165° F); and avoid unpasteurized (raw) milk, soft cheeses (Brie, feta, blue, Camembert, and Mexican-style) and homemade cheese unless made with pasteurized milk; and smoked fish, pâtés, and meat spreads from a meat counter or refrigerated section of the store, and store-prepared salads such as ham, chicken, egg, tuna, and seafood salads.[29]

Toxoplasmosis is caused by a parasite and is a leading cause of death related to foodborne illness in the United States. This infection may be symptom-free because the immune system prevents the parasite from causing illness, but the infection is passed on to the fetus by the carrier gravida. In addition to observing safe food handling precautions listed in Box 16-3, gravidas should be especially mindful of cooking meat, poultry, and seafood to safe minimum internal temperatures, avoiding drinking untreated water, and washing hands with soap and water after touching soil, sand, cat litter, raw meat, or unwashed vegetables.[30]

Pregnant women are encouraged to consume at least 8 oz of cooked seafood weekly, especially salmon, herring, mussels, trout, sardines, and pollock, which are rich in omega-3 fatty acids, but limit total intake of acceptable fish, including shrimp and catfish, to 12 oz/week. Raw fish should be avoided. Mercury can affect the developing nervous system in a fetus or young baby. Therefore, the U.S. Food and Drug Administration (FDA) advises pregnant women to avoid consuming large fish, including shark, swordfish, king mackerel, and tilefish, because they may contain large amounts of methyl mercury. Albacore (white) tuna is higher in mercury than the "light" variety; white tuna should be limited to less than 6 oz/week. State and local health departments have information relevant to fish caught locally or sold in a particular location. If the information is unavailable, pregnant women should limit consumption of fish from local water to 6 oz/week.[31]

Lead, present in tap water leached from plumbing and in dust from deteriorating lead-based paint, can negatively affect socialization and behaviors. Absorbed lead accumulates and is stored in bones. Much later, it can be released from maternal bones into the bloodstream. Regardless of the source, lead is absorbed by fetal brain cells in place of calcium needed for thought processes. This results in lifelong developmental problems, such as reduced attention span, increased impulsive behavior, and lower intelligence.

Factors Affecting Oral Development

In general, potential arrangement of teeth, their eruption time, and pits and fissures on enamel are attributed to heredity. However, availability of nutrients in utero is closely associated with whether teeth achieve their optimum genetic potential.

Tooth development begins by the sixth week of gestation. Calcification of deciduous teeth begins about the fourth month; development of more than 60% of the 52 deciduous and permanent teeth is initiated during gestation (Table 13-2). By the fourth month of pregnancy, the mandible is calcified. All primary teeth and many permanent teeth are at various stages of development when the infant is born. Critical periods for various stages of tooth development occur at different times. Nutrients supplied by the mother must be available for development of pre-eruptive teeth and soft tissues in proper sequence.

Severe and irreversible damage results if **nutritional insult** (deficiency or excessive amounts of specific nutrients) or infection occurs during critical stages, especially in dentin or enamel formation (Table 13-3). After eruption, the tooth has no mechanism to repair itself. Severe nutrient deficiencies can result in malformations such as cleft palate, cleft lip, and shortened mandible. Less-severe nutrient deficiencies can reduce the size of the tooth, interfere with tooth formation, delay time of tooth eruption, and increase susceptibility

Table 13-2 — Chronology of development of the human dentition

Tooth	Hard Tissue Formation Begins	Amount of Enamel Formed at Birth	Enamel Completed	Eruption	Root Completed
Primary Dentition					
Maxillary					
Central incisor	4 months in utero	Five-sixths	1½ months	7½ months	1½ years
Lateral incisor	4½ months in utero	Two-thirds	2½ months	9 months	2 years
Canine	5 months in utero	One-third	9 months	18 months	3¼ years
First molar	5 months in utero	Cusps united	6 months	14 months	2½ years
Second molar	6 months in utero	Cusp tips still isolated	11 months	24 months	3 years
Mandibular					
Central incisor	4½ months in utero	Three-fifths	2½ months	6 months	1½ years
Lateral incisor	4½ months in utero	Three-fifths	3 months	7 months	1½ years
Canine	5 months in utero	One-third	9 months	16 months	3¼ years
First molar	5 months in utero	Cusps united	5½ months	12 months	2¼ years
Second molar	6 months in utero	Cusp tips still isolated	10 months	20 months	3 years
Permanent Dentition					
Maxillary					
Central incisor	3-4 months	—	4-5 years	7-8 years	10 years
Lateral incisor	10-12 months	—	4-5 years	8-9 years	11 years
Canine	4-5 months	—	6-7 years	11-12 years	13-15 years
First premolar	1½-1¾ years	—	5-6 years	10-11 years	12-13 years
Second premolar	2-2¼ years	—	6-7 years	10-12 years	12-14 years
First molar	At birth	Sometimes a trace	2½-3 years	6-7 years	9-10 years
Second molar	2½-3 years	—	7-8 years	12-13 years	14-16 years
Mandibular					
Central incisor	3-4 months	—	4-5 years	6-7 years	9 years
Lateral incisor	3-4 months	—	4-5 years	7-8 years	10 years
Canine	4-5 months	—	6-7 years	9-10 years	12-14 years
First premolar	1¾-2 years	—	5-6 years	10-12 years	12-13 years
Second premolar	2-2¼ years	—	6-7 years	11-12 years	13-14 years
First molar	At birth	Sometimes a trace	2½-3 years	6-7 years	9-10 years
Second molar	2½-3 years	—	7-8 years	11-13 years	14-15 years

Adapted and slightly modified by Massler and Shour from Logan WAG, Kronfeld R: *J Am Dent Assoc* 1933;20:420. From Touger-Decker R, Radler DR, Depaola DP: Nutrition and dental medicine. In: Ross AC, Caballero B, Cousins, RJ, et al, editors: *Modern nutrition in health and disease*, ed 11, Philadelphia, 2014, Wolters Kluwer/Lippincott Williams & Wilkins, pp 1016-1040.

Table 13-3 — Nutrient deficiencies and tooth development

Nutrient	Effect on Tissue
Protein	Delayed tooth eruption; increased caries susceptibility; dysfunctional salivary glands
Vitamin A	Disturbed keratin matrix of enamel; increased enamel hypoplasia; increased caries susceptibility; decreased epithelial tissue development; dysfunction of tooth morphogenesis
Vitamin D	Poor calcification; pitting
Calcium/phosphorus	Decreased calcium concentration; hypomineralization (hypoplastic defects)
Ascorbic acid	Disturbed collagen matrix of dentin; alterations of dental pulp
Fluoride/iron/zinc	Increased caries susceptibility
Iodine	Delayed tooth eruption
Magnesium	Hypoplasia of enamel

Compiled from information in Touger-Decker R, Radler DR, Depaola DP: Nutrition and dental medicine. In: Ross AC, Caballero B, Cousins RJ, et al, editors: *Modern nutrition in health and disease*, ed 11, Philadelphia, 2014, Wolters Kluwer/Lippincott Williams & Wilkins, pp 1016-1040; Nizel AE: Preventing dental caries: the nutritional factors. *Pediatr Clin North Am* 1977; 24:144-155; and Shaw JH, Sweeney EA: Oral health. In: Schneider HA, Anderson CD, Coursin DB, et al, editors: *Nutritional support of medical practice*, Philadelphia, 1983, Harper & Row.

of teeth to caries. Most nutrient deficiencies that occur in utero affecting developing teeth result in increased susceptibility to dental caries for the child.

When an infection in a gravida causes a fever, the resultant disruption of calcium and phosphorus balance affects developing fetal tooth structure. This disruption in tooth structure formation continues until the body regains calcium-phosphorus equilibrium.

Dentin and enamel depend on many nutrients: vitamin C for formation of collagen matrix, and calcium, magnesium, phosphorus, and vitamin D for mineralization. Infants whose mothers have low levels of vitamin D during pregnancy may be at increased risk for tooth enamel defects and early childhood tooth decay.[32] Keratin in enamel depends on vitamin A for its synthesis. An inadequate amount of any of these nutrients during tooth development results in an imperfect matrix, with subsequent imperfection of mineralization (see Table 13-2). Folate deficiency, known to cause neural tube defects, can result in incomplete formation of cranial bones.

Benefits of fluoride supplements during pregnancy in preventing dental caries in infants are uncertain. Fluoride passes through the placenta to the fetus and is incorporated into fetal bones and teeth. Whether the placenta can filter excess fluoride is unknown. Although fluoride supplements are considered safe for the mother and fetus, oral fluoride supplements during pregnancy seem to have minimal benefits on the developing fetus and are not indicated. Use of fluoridated products, such as toothpaste and mouth rinses, and fluoridated water are recommended.

Nutritional Requirements for Pregnancy

Dietary Reference Intakes for pregnancy indicate advisable nutrient intake for optimal health of the mother and fetus. Accelerated growth and metabolism increases most nutrient requirements to some extent. Each vitamin and mineral is not separately discussed in this chapter; Table 13-4 shows the increased amounts recommended for each of the nutrients. Based on several national studies, healthcare workers should be aware that adolescent females with childbearing potential may have inadequate intakes of nutrients, potentially affecting pregnancy outcomes.[33] The following mean nutrient intakes are commonly below the recommended dietary allowances (RDAs) for pregnant women: fiber, vitamin D, folate, iron, and polyunsaturated fatty acids.[34] In addition to low intake of these nutrients, gravidas on vegan diets frequently

Table 13-4	Vitamin and mineral recommended dietary allowances						
			Pregnant (19-30 Years Old)			Lactating (19-30 Years Old)	
Nutrient	Nonpregnant Women (19-30 Years Old)	Pregnant (14-18 Years Old)	Amount of Nutrient	Percent Increase†	Lactating (14-18 Years Old)	Amount of Nutrient	Percent Increase†
Vitamin A	700 µg	750 µg RE	770 µg RE	10	1200 µg RE	1300 µg RE	71
Vitamin D	15 µg	15 µg	15 µg	0	15 µg	15 µg	0
Vitamin E	15 α-TE	15 α-TE	15 α-TE	0	19 α-TE	19 α-TE	27
Vitamin K	90 µg*	75 µg*	90 µg*	0	75 µg*	90 µg*	0
Vitamin C	75 mg	85 mg	85 mg	13	115 mg	120 mg	60
Thiamin	1.1 mg	1.4 mg	1.4 mg	27	1.4 mg	1.4 mg	27
Riboflavin	1.1 mg	1.4 mg	1.4 mg	27	1.4 mg	1.6 mg	45
Niacin	14 mg NE	18 mg NE	18 mg NE	28	17 mg NE	17 mg NE	21
Vitamin B_6	1.3 mg	1.9 mg	1.9 mg	46	2.0 mg	2 mg	54
Folate	400 µg	600 µg	600 µg	50	500 µg	500 µg	25
Vitamin B_{12}	2.4 µg	2.6 µg	2.6 µg	8	2.8 µg	2.8 µg	17
Calcium	1000 mg	1300 mg	1000 mg	0	1300 mg	1000 mg	0
Phosphorus	700 mg	1350 mg	700 mg	0	1250 mg	700 mg	0
Magnesium	310 mg	400 mg	350 mg 360 mg¶	9	360 mg	310 mg	0
Fluoride	3 mg*	3 mg*	3 mg*	0	3 mg*	3 mg*	0
Iron	18 mg	27 mg	27 mg	50	10 mg	9 mg	[-50%]
Zinc	8 mg	12 mg	11 mg	38	13 mg	12 mg	50
Iodine	150 µg	220 µg	220 µg	47	290 µg	290 µg	93
Selenium	55 µg	60 µg	60 µg	9	70 µg	70 µg	27
Copper	900 µg	1000 µg	1000 µg	11	1300 µg	1300 µg	44

Data from National Research Council: *The guide to nutrient requirements*, Washington, DC, 2006, National Academies Press; and National Research Council: *Dietary reference intakes for calcium and vitamin D*, Washington, DC, 2011, National Academies Press. *Note:* This table presents recommended dietary allowances (RDAs) in **bold type** and adequate intakes (AIs) in regular type followed by an asterisk (*).
†Percent increase for pregnant women above nonpregnancy recommendation.
¶Ages 31-50 years old.

consume inadequate amounts of vitamin B_{12} and are at increased risk of inadequate intake of iron and vitamin D.

Energy and Kilocalories

During pregnancy, kilocalorie requirements increase slightly to ensure nutrient and energy needs. The estimated energy requirement does not increase during the first trimester of pregnancy, allows an additional 340 kcal/day during the second, and an additional 452 kcal during the third trimester. This additional energy is needed (a) to build new tissues, including added maternal tissues and growth of the fetus and placenta, (b) to support increased metabolic expenditure, and (c) to enable physical movement of additional weight. Appropriate weight gain reflects adequacy of energy intake and influences birth weight. When caloric intake is slightly inadequate, physiological adaptations spare energy for fetal growth. With adequate or generous kilocalories, energy balance is achieved in different ways depending on individual behavioral changes in food intake or energy expenditures and on adjustments in basal metabolism or fat stores.

Dieting for weight loss is not recommended during pregnancy even though studies indicate interventions can improve some outcomes for the mother and baby.[35] Dietary interventions are effective to control the amount of weight gain. Severe dietary restrictions are inappropriate when a woman is trying to conceive even though she is attempting to lose weight in anticipation of the pregnancy. Avoidance of carbohydrate-rich foods from enriched breads and cereals to reduce kilocalories, either preconceptionally or during pregnancy, negatively affects folic acid intake; this situation may be detrimental to the fetus. However, added sugars and excess saturated fat should be avoided in favor of nutrient-dense foods (Fig. 13-2).

Unless the gravida is significantly underweight before conception, additional kilocalories are not needed during the first trimester. Because requirements for many nutrients are increased, it is more important that foods be chosen wisely, using principally nutrient-dense foods. Studies indicate that poor food choices during pregnancy predispose the fetus to genetic changes that affect fat storage and increase risk of age-related diseases such as diabetes.[36]

Fat

The vitamin and mineral requirements during pregnancy increase proportionately higher than caloric needs; consequently, fats should be limited because of their minimal nutrient contribution. Hormonal changes result in significant elevations of serum cholesterol and triglycerides during the second trimester of pregnancy.

Polyunsaturated fatty acids reduce serum lipids, and omega-3 fatty acids may lessen some obstetrical complications.[37] Omega-3 fatty acids (docosahexaenoic acid) and omega-6 fatty acids (arachidonic acid) are important for central nervous system growth and visual development of infants. Docosahexaenoic acid accumulates rapidly in the fetal brain and retina during the latter part of gestation and early postnatal life, but evidence does not conclusively support that supplementation in pregnancy improves cognitive or visual development.[38] Requirements for omega-3 fatty acids have not been established, but they are thought to exceed that of a nonpregnant woman.

Protein

Protein is the basic nutrient for growth; an additional 21 g of protein, or a total of 67 g daily, is recommended. This can be accomplished with an additional 3 oz of meat or meat substitute (21 g protein), or by adding 2 oz of meat and 8 oz of milk (24 g protein) (see Fig. 13-2). Because Americans normally consume more than 65 g of protein daily, additional amounts are not required.

Calcium and Vitamin D

Calcium and vitamin D work together in the formation of skeletal tissue and teeth. During pregnancy, hormonal and physiological adjustments promote increased calcium absorption and retention. This extra calcium is thought to be stored in maternal bone for fetal availability in the third trimester when fetal bone growth is rapid. Because of enhanced calcium absorption and use, additional calcium supplementation is believed to be unnecessary. Pregnant women should consume the same amount of calcium as others in their age group.

The recommended 1000 mg/day of calcium for women older than 19 years of age can be met by three servings of milk or dairy products. Pregnant women younger than 19 years of age may need 4 cups of milk to provide the necessary 1300 mg/day. Dairy products may be incorporated into cooking or eaten in different forms, such as cheese, ice cream, or yogurt, for variety (see Table 9-2 and Box 9-2). A commonly reiterated erroneous myth is that a fetus removes calcium from the mother's teeth. If the gravida has sufficient calcium in her diet, problems do not develop. If the diet is deficient in calcium, the embryo's requirements are met first; some of the calcium may come from the mother's bones, not from her teeth.

Vitamin D intake during pregnancy is associated with infant growth, bone ossification, tooth enamel formation, and neonatal calcium homeostasis. Suboptimal vitamin D status has been documented in many urban populations, including those with adequate sunlight, which suggests maternal vitamin D insufficiency during pregnancy is more common than previously realized. Severe vitamin D deficiency during pregnancy has been associated with congenital rickets and fractures in the newborn.

In the past, doctors feared that too much vitamin D could cause birth defects; the current tolerable upper intake level (UL) established by the Institute of Medicine (IOM) is 4000 IU (100 µg). Recent clinical studies have established relationships between vitamin D levels and adverse pregnancy outcomes such as preeclampsia, gestational diabetes, low birthweight, preterm labor, cesarean delivery, and infectious diseases. Provision of vitamin D supplements improves serum vitamin D levels, but whether supplementation during pregnancy safely improves pregnancy and infant

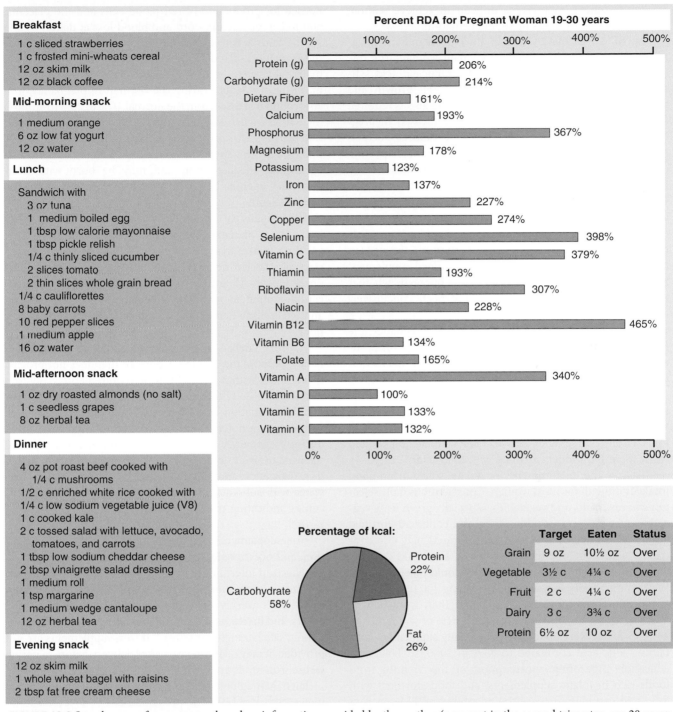

Breakfast

1 c sliced strawberries
1 c frosted mini-wheats cereal
12 oz skim milk
12 oz black coffee

Mid-morning snack

1 medium orange
6 oz low fat yogurt
12 oz water

Lunch

Sandwich with
  3 oz tuna
  1 medium boiled egg
  1 tbsp low calorie mayonnaise
  1 tbsp pickle relish
  1/4 c thinly sliced cucumber
  2 slices tomato
  2 thin slices whole grain bread
1/4 c cauliflorettes
8 baby carrots
10 red pepper slices
1 medium apple
16 oz water

Mid-afternoon snack

1 oz dry roasted almonds (no salt)
1 c seedless grapes
8 oz herbal tea

Dinner

4 oz pot roast beef cooked with
  1/4 c mushrooms
1/2 c enriched white rice cooked with
  1/4 c low sodium vegetable juice (V8)
1 c cooked kale
2 c tossed salad with lettuce, avocado,
  tomatoes, and carrots
1 tbsp low sodium cheddar cheese
2 tbsp vinaigrette salad dressing
1 medium roll
1 tsp margarine
1 medium wedge cantaloupe
12 oz herbal tea

Evening snack

12 oz skim milk
1 whole wheat bagel with raisins
2 tbsp fat free cream cheese

Percent RDA for Pregnant Woman 19-30 years

Nutrient	Percent
Protein (g)	206%
Carbohydrate (g)	214%
Dietary Fiber	161%
Calcium	193%
Phosphorus	367%
Magnesium	178%
Potassium	123%
Iron	137%
Zinc	227%
Copper	274%
Selenium	398%
Vitamin C	379%
Thiamin	193%
Riboflavin	307%
Niacin	228%
Vitamin B12	465%
Vitamin B6	134%
Folate	165%
Vitamin A	340%
Vitamin D	100%
Vitamin E	133%
Vitamin K	132%

Percentage of kcal:

Protein 22%
Carbohydrate 58%
Fat 26%

	Target	Eaten	Status
Grain	9 oz	10½ oz	Over
Vegetable	3½ c	4¼ c	Over
Fruit	2 c	4¼ c	Over
Dairy	3 c	3¾ c	Over
Protein	6½ oz	10 oz	Over

FIGURE 13-2 Sample menu for pregnancy based on information provided by the mother (pregnant in the second trimester; age 28 years; height 5 ft, 7 in; prepregnancy weight 140 lb; and moderately active [30 to 60 minutes of physical activity 5 days a week]).

outcomes has not been determined. At this time, there is insufficient evidence to recommend screening all pregnant women for vitamin D deficiency, but for those thought to be at increased risk of vitamin D deficiency, an assessment can be considered and interpreted in the context of the individual circumstance.[39] Further research is needed to determine whether higher levels of vitamin D prove beneficial. Most American and Canadian women consume less than the recommended amount. The American College of

Obstetrics and Gynecology and the IOM currently recommend 600 IU (15 μg) daily vitamin D supplementation during pregnancy to support maternal and fetal bone metabolism.[40-42]

B Vitamins

Several of the B-vitamin requirements are based on energy or caloric intake; usually, their intake increases automatically with intake of additional kilocalories. However, adequate intake of some B vitamins is difficult to achieve without careful selection of foods or supplementation.

The RDA for folate (600 μg) during pregnancy is significantly more than for the nonpregnant woman. The role of folate as a coenzyme is essential for nucleic acid synthesis. A folate deficiency that impairs cell growth and replication may cause fetal anomalies. Folate also is required for red blood cell formation, which is increased in pregnancy. Orofacial clefts and neural tube defects, such as spina bifida and anencephaly (absence of a major portion of the brain and skull), are attributed to inadequate folate intake before conception and during the first trimester. Ideally, attention should be focused on folate intake when a woman is considering a pregnancy because 50% to 70% of neural tube defects can be prevented if sufficient amounts of folic acid are consumed before conception and throughout the first trimester of the pregnancy. Continued supplementation throughout the pregnancy is encouraged; whether the effects' benefit outcomes have not been conclusively established.[43]

Because of the crucial effects affecting a pregnancy, the FDA requires supplementation of all enriched grain products with specific amounts of folic acid. Since implementation of folic acid fortification in the United States in 1996, neural tube defects have almost been cut in half.[45] To promote increased consumption of folic acid, the March of Dimes and the Grain Foods Foundation have created a new Folic Acid for a Healthy Pregnancy seal to help women quickly and easily identify products fortified with folic acid.

Meeting the requirement for folate solely from food intake is difficult for most women. Conscientious daily selections of raw fruits and vegetables, especially green leafy vegetables, can help ensure adequate intake. Folic acid–fortified grains and cereals and whole-grain products may also contribute significant amounts (see Tables 1-4 and 11-12). Every woman who might become pregnant should be encouraged to consume a daily supplement containing 400 μg folic acid; absorption from supplements is better than from natural folate in foods. In 2007, approximately 61% of women 18 to 24 years of age were not consuming a daily supplement containing folic acid compared to 45% in 2006.[44,45] Folic acid education promoting consumption of the vitamin from foods rich in folate, supplements, and foods fortified with folic acid can help increase the possibility of all women of childbearing age consuming adequate amounts and preventing neural tube defects.

Although folate intake is essential, some women take supplements providing eight times the RDA. High intakes may be transferred to the fetus. The downside of taking excessive amounts of folic acid is that other nutrients (especially vitamin B_{12}) may be adversely affected by excess supplementation (see Chapter 11).

Iron

A common problem among nonpregnant women is iron-deficiency anemia, so many women begin pregnancy with diminished iron stores. Increased iron during gestation is needed for production of red blood cells and the placenta, and to compensate for cord and blood loss at delivery.

The fetus acts as a parasite in that fetal erythropoiesis, the formation of red blood cells, occurs at the expense of maternal iron stores. Iron-deficiency anemia is seldom seen in full-term infants. During the last half of pregnancy, iron absorption increases from the normal 10% to 20% to approximately 25% when adequate iron is available. Fetal accumulation of iron occurs principally in the last trimester. Premature infants, having a shortened gestation, have insufficient time to acquire adequate iron and may be born with iron-deficiency anemia; however, premature infants absorb iron very efficiently.

When maternal iron-deficiency anemia is diagnosed on initiation of prenatal care, it is associated with low caloric and iron intake; inadequate gestational gain; and increased risks of preterm delivery, LBW, and impaired intellectual development. Maternal iron deficiency requires increased cardiac output to maintain adequate oxygen for maternal and fetal cells; if hemorrhage occurs at delivery, prognosis is poor.

Approximately 27 mg of iron is needed daily during pregnancy. Because the average American diet does not provide this amount within normal caloric requirements, daily iron supplements (30 mg elemental iron) are usually recommended. Initiation of supplements before gestational week 24 prevents iron deficiency. Low-dose iron supplementation during pregnancy, even if the gravida is not anemic, improves the woman's iron status and seems to protect the infant from iron-deficiency anemia. Evidence has linked infant iron status with subsequent cognitive and neurobehavioral outcomes, indicating the importance of optimal iron status at birth.[46]

Iron supplements frequently cause nausea and constipation, and occasionally high hemoglobin levels. Research on the effects of intermittent iron supplementation on maternal and infant status indicates that taking supplements one to three times weekly on nonconsecutive days reduces side effects, and increases acceptance and adherence, while maintaining safe hemoglobin levels.[47] If iron supplements are not provided, it may take two years after delivery before maternal serum iron levels are normal.

High hemoglobin levels have been associated with an increased risk of LBW and premature births, so levels should be routinely monitored.

Zinc

Zinc is crucial early in pregnancy during the formation of fetal organs, but requirements are highest in late pregnancy for fetal growth and development. The RDA for zinc is 12 mg during pregnancy. An increase in high-protein foods, especially meats, improves zinc intake.

Iodine

Dietary iodine requirements are higher during pregnancy as a result of increased maternal thyroid hormone production and fetal iodine requirements. In the United States, iodine nutritional status has declined among women of childbearing age over the last three decades. Adherence to the recommendations in *Dietary Guidelines* to decrease use of salt (usually iodized), and increased popularity of sea salt (contains no iodine), may be affecting iodine intake. Adverse effects of iodine deficiency in pregnancy include maternal and fetal goiter; cretinism; fetal brain development and intellectual impairments; neonatal hypothyroidism; and infant mortality, and it is a significant global public health problem.[48,49]

The IOM recommends a daily iodine intake of 220 µg during pregnancy. The American Thyroid Association has stressed that adequate maternal iodine is necessary to assure the health of the mother and the offspring; the addition of 150 µg of potassium iodide in prenatal vitamins does not pose a risk.[50] A study of nonprescription and prescription prenatal multivitamins currently on the market in the United States indicated a mean level of 119 µg iodine per daily dose, despite the amount indicated on the label.[51]

Although an infrequent occurrence, congenital hypothyroidism may also result from excess prenatal intake of iodine supplements.[52] IOM has not determined a safe upper limit for iodine in pregnancy and lactation.

Vitamin-Mineral Supplements

In the United States, vitamin and mineral supplementation is commonly recommended during pregnancy. Supplementation should be based on evidence of a benefit and lack of harmful effects. Food is considered to be the optimal vehicle for providing nutrients, but supplements may be warranted during this period. Supplement composition should be based on the nature of an identified nutritional need. Excessive amounts of many nutrients may have detrimental effects on the fetus (Table 13-5). Even if recommended by a healthcare provider, a supplement should not reduce the woman's motivation to maintain or improve the quality of her diet because, in most instances, nutrients in foods are better absorbed than those available in pills (except for folic acid).

The IOM subcommittee concluded that iron is the only known nutrient warranting global supplementation during pregnancy. A goal for *Healthy People 2020* is to reduce iron-deficiency anemia among pregnant females. Approximately 16% of pregnant females may be iron deficient.[53] Consequently, 30 mg of ferrous iron is recommended to provide adequate amounts of iron during the second and third trimesters of pregnancy.

Dietary folate intake does not usually meet the RDA, but since folate enrichment of cereal products began in 1998, maternal folate status has improved significantly. A supplement containing folate may be prudent if adequacy of intake is questionable. It should be initiated before conception because birth defects from inadequate folate intake may occur before the gravida realizes the pregnancy. Because of the number of unintentional pregnancies in women 15 to 24 years old, a multivitamin supplement containing folic acid is recommended for all young women.

As a result of several studies showing a relationship between high doses of vitamin A supplements and birth defects, the FDA issued recommendations for women of childbearing age. Ordinary multivitamins typically contain 5000 IU, but some brands can contain much more—sometimes 25,000 IU. Excess vitamin A (10,000 IU of vitamin A preformed from animal sources) during the first trimester can result in severe craniofacial and oral clefts and limb defects. Intake of preformed vitamin A should be limited to approximately 100% of the daily value (5000 IU). Liver and other animal products and fortified foods and vitamin supplements listing retinyl palmitate and retinyl acetate as ingredients contain preformed vitamin A. Beta-carotene, which the body converts to vitamin A, is much less

Table 13-5	**Nutrient supplementation associated with deleterious fetal outcomes**
Nutrient	**Effects on Fetus**
Vitamin A	Pharmacologic use of vitamin A analogues has resulted in major congenital defects (malformation of cranium, face, heart, thymus, and central nervous system) and spontaneous abortion, especially during first trimester
Vitamin D	Excessive intake of vitamin D can result in hyperabsorption of calcium, hypercalcemia, calcification of soft tissues, and mental retardation
Vitamin E	Associated with higher incidence of spontaneous abortions
Vitamin K	Menadione administered parenterally has been associated with hemolytic anemia, hyperbilirubinemia, and kernicterus in the newborn
Vitamin C	Megadoses of vitamin C have been reported to cause vitamin C dependency with symptoms of conditional scurvy observed postpartum
Iodine	Large amounts of iodides have resulted in infants with congenital goiter, hypothyroidism, and mental retardation
Zinc	Large amounts of zinc supplements during third trimester were implicated in premature delivery and stillbirth
Fluoride	Well water containing 12 to 18 parts/million (ppm) fluoride produced offspring with significant mottling of deciduous teeth

Data from Worthington-Roberts B: Nutrition deficiencies and excesses: impact on pregnancy, part 2. *J Perinatol* 1985;5(4):12. Reprinted by permission from Macmillan Publishers Ltd.

toxic. Fortified foods containing beta-carotene and fruits and vegetables that contain natural beta-carotene should be chosen whenever possible.

Nutritional supplementation may be warranted in high-risk pregnancies, including adolescent pregnancies; multiple gestations (carrying more than one fetus); and pregnancies in women who use cigarettes, alcohol, or other drugs. Women who are younger than 25 years of age or who do not routinely consume milk, dairy products, or foods fortified with calcium and vitamin D, should take a calcium supplement. Supplementation of vitamin D may be beneficial for some women living in northern latitudes with limited exposure to sunlight. Research suggests higher intakes of vitamin D may be required, but more study is needed to determine the most effective dosage. Iron supplements containing more than 30 mg of iron necessitate supplemental amounts of zinc and copper.[54]

If supplementation is warranted for a gravida of any age, the specific nutrient amounts for a daily multivitamin-mineral preparation are shown in Table 13-6. Compliance with taking the nutrition supplement is poor; only about half of the vitamins are taken. Many women do not take the supplement because of nausea and vomiting or previous adverse effects, whereas others indicate the size of the pill is a factor. Patients should be encouraged to take the prescribed supplement and informed of the importance and reasons why it is needed. Compliance with use of prenatal supplements is enhanced by convenient supply, affordability, and reinforcement by healthcare providers.

Dietary Intake and Education

Prenatal nutritional care improves outcome by saving lives, averting LBW, and decreasing costs of care that are consequences of LBW. Although adequate weight gain is the most reliable measurable tool for assessing adequacy of energy intake, food choices can provide adequate kilocalories, yet be deficient in vital nutrients. Nutrient intake warrants more attention than weight gain. For this reason, the IOM subcommittee recommends routine assessment of dietary practices for all gravidas in the United States to determine the need for improved diet or vitamin-mineral supplementation. Most women are highly motivated to make dietary changes during their pregnancy.

Because maternal nutrition has profound effects on infant health, the *MyPlate* website (http://www.choosemyplate.gov/pregnancy-breastfeeding) has links that provide a myriad of information for pregnant and breastfeeding mothers, including calculations for a healthy weight gain and other tips for making healthy food choices. Dental hygienists can use this tool to obtain nutrition guidance for their patients. *Super-Tracker* can be used to personalize a food plan based on age, height, prepregnancy weight, physical activity level, and due date (see Fig. 13-2). Through links on this website, other information available for the gravida includes issues such as dietary supplements, food safety, and special health needs.

Pregnant women may have little or no nutritional knowledge. Although knowledge is the key to wise food choices, nutrition counseling is often unavailable or ignored during pregnancy. The Academy of Nutrition and Dietetics recommends that women, especially overweight and obese women, receive information during pregnancy to avoid risk of adverse outcomes.[55] In many cases, low-income expectant mothers have more opportunities to receive nutritional information through established programs such as the Supplemental Nutrition Program for Women, Infants, and Children (WIC) than more affluent women receive through the private sector.

Identification of poor and desirable food habits and dietary patterns can serve as the foundation for appropriate nutrition education and intervention. Identified nutritional problems, such as pica or fad dieting, or risk factors, such as alcohol abuse, may require special attention. Most importantly, it must be determined whether the gravida understands what foods she should be eating. Breastfeeding should also be promoted during pregnancy.

Dental Considerations

Assessments

- *Physical:* level of education, income status, culture, religion, prenatal healthcare, medical history (including drugs taken), dental history, oral examination, feelings about weight gain.
- *Dietary:* health and nutritional knowledge and skills; adequacy of intake based on a well-balanced diet using a variety of foods, including enriched grain products; vegetarianism; food budget; food cravings and aversions; fad diets; beliefs about nutrition during pregnancy; pica, alcohol use, and caffeine intake.

Interventions

- Become familiar with local nutritional practices and beliefs about pregnancy; these beliefs are regional and may be affected by cultural beliefs.
- During routine dental recare for women of childbearing age, discuss the importance of maintaining oral health and dental appointments during pregnancy.
- Refer patients at risk of inadequate intakes of specific nutrients to an RDN or healthcare provider.
- Emphasize consumption of a well-balanced diet with three to six meals throughout the day to ensure optimal intake of nutrients.
- Patients who might become pregnant should have a high folate intake. If a woman of childbearing age is not taking a multivitamin

Table 13-6	Nutrient supplementation during pregnancy
Nutrient	**Amount of Supplement Recommended**
Vitamin C	50 mg
Vitamin B$_6$	2 mg
Folate	300 µg
Iron	30 mg
Zinc	15 mg
Copper	2 mg

Data from Institute of Medicine, Food and Nutrition Board: *Nutrition during pregnancy*, Washington, DC, 1990, National Academy Press.

Dental Considerations—cont'd

supplement and is following a carbohydrate-restricted diet, refer her to a healthcare provider or an RDN.

- Ask pregnant patients whether they are taking a prenatal supplement. If not, refer them to a healthcare provider.
- Seize pregnancy as the ideal opportunity to discuss good nutritional and oral hygiene habits needed during this period and for the newborn infant. Proper oral tissue development of the fetus depends on adequate maternal nutrition.
- Encourage foods high in calcium. Low calcium intake may impair bone mineral deposition, especially in women younger than 25 years of age. Consuming the recommended 1300 mg of calcium daily is particularly important for pregnant teens to meet calcium demands. The use of dietary calcium is preferred because these foods also provide other valuable nutrients—protein, riboflavin, and vitamin D and other components that enhance calcium absorption.
- Snacking is acceptable for pregnant women. Provide information on avoidance of acid attacks and resultant tooth decay by recommending appropriate oral hygiene techniques after snacking and encouraging foods such as nuts, raw vegetables, yogurt, and popcorn.
- If the mother has a strong preference for sweets, the infant's diet is also likely to be high in sugar. Review the gravida's diet for the form and frequency of sugar-containing foods, and suggest modifications or substitutions as indicated. This could create a healthier pattern for the patient and alleviate potential dental problems for the infant.
- Discuss the risk of early childhood caries with all pregnant women (see Chapter 14).
- Encourage pregnant patients to use iodized salt, and choose good dietary sources of iodine (e.g., milk and dairy products and fish). Avoid kelp supplements because of excessive levels of iodine.
- Because of increased risk of preterm or LBW infants associated with pregnancy gingivitis and other periodontal issues, encourage excellent oral hygiene habits throughout the day.
- Encourage pregnant women to enroll in educational breastfeeding classes that address benefits, techniques, common problems, myths, and skills training.

Nutritional Directions

- Pregnant women should consult their healthcare provider before taking any drug, including nonprescription drugs and herbal products.
- Preventive oral care, including limiting frequency of fermentable carbohydrate intake and adequate oral hygiene care, is important for the mother and fetus.
- Nutrient needs must be met by deliberate preplanning and informed food choices.
- Encourage sexually active women of childbearing age who drink alcohol to use reliable methods to prevent pregnancy, plan their pregnancies, and stop drinking before becoming pregnant.
- Low-fat or skim milk may be used to control weight, decrease saturated fat intake, and provide equivalent nutrients.
- Although the pregnant patient is "eating for two," her energy requirements are not double.
- Moderate increases in whole grains, milk, and legumes can provide additional protein and other important nutrients.

- Calcium, vitamin D, and vitamin B_{12} supplements are advisable for vegans, because they exclude all animal products. Pregnant vegans should be referred to an RDN.
- Vitamin D may be a special concern for women with minimal exposure to sunlight or routine use of sunscreens. Regular exposure to sunlight and foods fortified with vitamin D (e.g., milk and cheese) are recommended.
- Powdered milk (one-third cup) can be added to soups, cooked cereals, mashed potatoes, or casseroles if the gravida has an aversion to drinking milk.
- Adverse symptoms, such as nausea or constipation, frequently occur from iron supplementation. Rather than discontinuing the supplement, take it with meals, or consult the healthcare provider about possibly decreasing the dosage or taking it three to four times a week.
- Absorption of iron from supplements or foods is enhanced if taken between meals with vitamin C–rich foods, such as orange juice, while avoiding milk, tea, or coffee.
- Moderately intense exercise during pregnancy (such as 30-minute brisk walks) is beneficial if medical reasons do not prevent it. Exercise at this time enhances blood flow, which delivers nutrients to the fetus, improves mood and energy level, and increases cardiovascular fitness and endurance.

LACTATION

Exclusive breastfeeding for 4 to 6 months and continuing until 12 months is the ideal method of feeding infants. Complementary foods should begin at least by 6 months. U.S. health authorities began to promote breastfeeding about 25 years ago, a healthy practice that has been slowly gaining in popularity. In 2010, approximately 76% of mothers breastfed newborns, with 49% still breastfeeding 6 months later.[56] The target for breastfeeding established in *Healthy People 2020* is 81.9%.[57] Breastfeeding rates vary by race/ethnicity, participation in the WIC supplemental nutrition program, mother's age and education, and geography. Overall, 54% of African American mothers, 74% white mothers, and 80% of Hispanic mothers initiate breastfeeding.[58] This increase in breastfeeding rates shows outstanding gains, particularly for groups less likely to breastfeed—women who are African American, are younger than 20 years of age, have less than a high school education, are in their first pregnancy, and are employed. A new breastfeeding initiative, "It's Only Natural," launched in 2013 by the U.S. Department of Health & Human Services, is designed to provide materials uniquely designed for African American women to raise awareness of the importance and benefits of breastfeeding infants.

Despite extensive evidence for short-term and long-term health benefits for both mother and baby, and practical benefits, such as lower cost, many women choose to bottle feed. Personal and social biases (such as attitudes of family and close friends, and problems with breastfeeding in public and employment practices) are principal factors in this decision. A mother's decision to breastfeed can be positively influenced by health education and peer support; her success is greatly improved through active support from her family, friends, communities, clinicians, healthcare providers, employers, and policymakers. Peer counseling, lactation consultation, and formal breastfeeding education during pregnancy appear to increase both initiation and duration of breastfeeding.[59] The WIC supplemental program has attempted to increase the rate of participants breastfeeding by enhancing the food package for mothers who breastfeed and providing less formula for formula-fed infants.

Reports indicate that virtually all women are able to produce enough breast milk providing essential nutrients to support the growth and health of infants.[60] Breastfeeding has many advantages for the infant and mother (Box 13-1). Further discussion can also be found in Chapter 14.

Breast milk provides all the infant needs for about the first 6 months of life to support optimal growth and development, with rare exceptions. The principal reasons given by mothers for stopping breastfeeding is they perceive the infant is not satisfied by breast milk alone, pain associated with breastfeeding, and returning to work. Breastfeeding continues to provide important nutrition and protection from illness and infection beyond the first 6 months of life. There is no specific age when breastfeeding should be terminated, and mothers are encouraged to continue breastfeeding beyond the minimum of 6 months as long as they feel it is needed.

Nutritional Recommendations for Breastfeeding

For most nutrients, recommendations for lactating women are similar to the recommendations for pregnant women. Energy requirements are proportional to the quantity of milk produced. Approximately 85 kcal are needed for every 100 mL of milk produced, requiring approximately a 500-kcal daily increase. Although this increase may not be fully adequate to cover the needs for milk production, the 2 to 4 kg of fat accumulated during pregnancy is available to supply additional kilocalories. Return to prepregnancy weight is accelerated. The major determinant of milk production is the infant's demand for milk, not maternal energy intake. Weight loss during lactation has no apparent deleterious effects on milk production.

Carbohydrate intake from whole grains, dairy, fruits, and vegetables is important for maintaining lactose synthesis and milk volume. The amount of protein recommended is slightly higher than for pregnancy—an additional 25 g or a total of 70 g daily. Breastfeeding is positively related with mental development of the infant, but this may be influenced more by maternal education, social class, and intelligence of the parents than diet. Long-chain polyunsaturated fatty acids, especially docosahexaenoic acid, seem to play a beneficial role in children's mental development, but this area remains controversial in regards to the benefits of supplementation.[61] Other nutrients needed in larger quantities than during pregnancy include vitamins A, E, C, riboflavin, B_6, and B_{12}, and the minerals copper, zinc, iodine, and selenium. Maternal vitamin B_6 status affects amounts found in breast milk, and adequacy affects infant growth. A source of vitamin B_{12} intake, from either foods or supplements, is crucial for optimal infant nutriture. Neurological impairments have

---

BOX 13-1 | **Advantages of Breastfeeding**

For the Mother
- Maternal hormones produced as a result of lactation facilitate contractions of the uterus and control postpartum bleeding.
- Prepregnancy weight is achieved sooner because breast-feeding burns kilocalories.
- Breastfeeding is less expensive than formula feeding.
- Mother–infant bonding is enhanced with breastfeeding.
- Breastfeeding saves time because there are no bottles to clean, prepare, warm, or sterilize.
- Working mothers who breastfeed miss less work because of a sick infant.
- Prolactin, the hormone that helps the milk "come down," relaxes the mother.
- The mother is at reduced risk of premenopausal breast and ovarian cancer.

For the Infant
- Human milk is nutritionally balanced with maximum bioavailability for infants. It is easy for the infant to digest.
- Breast milk has immunological properties that help reduce infant morbidity (especially certain infectious gastrointestinal and respiratory diseases, and earaches) and mortality. Within 4 hours after exposure to germs, antibodies in the milk change to meet the needs of the infant.
- Breast milk constantly changes in composition to meet the changing needs of the infant, especially a premature infant.
- Human milk reduces the risk of food allergies and asthma (wheezing) and prevents or delays the occurrence of atopic dermatitis in early childhood.
- Breastfeeding promotes infant oral–motor and structural development; this can mean fewer dental bills or a decreased need for orthodontic work.
- Incidence of thumb sucking and tongue thrusting is lower in breastfed infants.
- Breastfed infants are exposed to a variety of tastes through the mother's milk.
- Breast milk reduces a child's risk for diabetes.
- Breast milk provides better brain development. Longer periods of exclusive breastfeeding during an infant's first year increase some measures of a child's cognitive development; this may lead to a smarter child and adult.
- Prolonged breastfeeding may reduce the risk of overweight in childhood. Breastfeeding has an indirect influence on body fat accumulation and selectively protects against extremes in body size and fat deposition.
- Breastfeeding longer than 6 months provides health benefits well beyond the breastfeeding period. A quantitative review of the evidence indicates that exclusively breastfed infants may have lower blood cholesterol concentrations in later life.
- Breastfeeding is associated with a reduction in risk for post-neonatal death.

---

occurred in children of breastfeeding vegan mothers who were eating no or very limited foods of animal origin, which is the source of vitamin B_{12}. A lactating woman also requires additional fluids to replace those secreted in the milk. An additional 1000 mL/day (4 cups) of fluids is needed.

Dietary Patterns for Lactating Women

The dietary pattern of a lactating woman is similar to that of a pregnant woman (Fig. 13-3). Consumption of 3 cups of milk or dairy products fortified with vitamin D daily provides approximately 1000 mg of calcium and 300 IU of vitamin D, which are adequate amounts for women older than 19 years. Much higher doses of vitamin D would be needed to achieve adequate concentrations in exclusively breastfed infants, so vitamin D supplementation in these infants is recommended.[62,63] Other high-calcium foods may also be used. High-protein foods may include 6 to 8 oz of meat daily, depending on the quantity of milk consumed. Adequate servings of fresh fruits, vegetables, and whole-grain products help provide the additional caloric requirement.

Repletion of iron stores is important, and a prenatal vitamin is encouraged for postpartum women to provide adequate iron and folate to replenish stores. Women who have mild iron deficiency are less sensitive to their infants' cues and have more difficulty bonding with their infants. Women who are anemic are more likely to experience postpartum depression.

Many substances consumed by the mother have been thought to affect breast milk. Certain foods, especially strongly flavored foods such as raw onion, garlic, curry, chili peppers, and chocolate, may cause gastrointestinal distress, rash, or irritability in the infant. These foods only need to be omitted if they affect the infant.

Many nonnutritive substances and drugs may be secreted in breast milk. Alcohol may impair milk flow and is transmitted in breast milk in approximately the same proportions as in the mother's blood. Intake should be limited to less than 0.5 g/kg daily. Large amounts of coffee and tea intake may adversely affect the iron content of human milk. Caffeine can be transferred to the infant in breast milk, so caffeine intake should be moderate (300 mg).

Because of the risk of medications being passed into breast milk, all drugs, including over-the-counter medications and herbal remedies, should be used cautiously and only if essential. Medications that are less likely to be secreted into the milk can be prescribed by the healthcare provider.

MyPlate (http://www.choosemyplate.gov) provides a plethora of health and nutrition information for breastfeeding women. Individualized nutrition guidance is available on the Internet consistent with the *Dietary Guidelines* to assist breastfeeding mothers (see Fig. 13-3). Nutrition information is provided for exclusively breastfeeding, or partially breastfeeding mothers. Tips are provided for eating a balanced diet, healthy weight maintenance or weight loss, physical activity, and use of dietary supplements.

Dietary assessment of routine food intake by an RDN is suggested, followed by nutrition counseling regarding foods rich in nutrients deficient in the diet. Continued use of the prenatal vitamin or a multivitamin supplement is recommended to ensure an adequate supply of folate if the woman may become pregnant again.

Dental Considerations

Assessments
- *Physical*: socioeconomic status, types of drugs, over-the-counter medications, supplements, and herbals used.
- *Dietary*: adequacy of kilocalories, nutrients, and fluid intake; alcohol and caffeine intake.

Interventions
- For a postpartum patient, encourage a gradual return to prepregnancy weight (maximum weight loss of 4 lb/month for lactating women) through a balanced diet and moderate exercise.
- Encourage lactating women to obtain their nutrients from a well-balanced diet.
- Stress the importance of nutrients from fruits and vegetables, enriched and whole-grain breads and cereals, calcium-rich dairy products, and protein-rich and carbohydrate-rich foods.
- Encourage intake of at least 10 to 12 cups of fluid each day.
- Encourage increased intake of nutrient-dense foods to achieve a caloric intake of at least 1800 kcal daily.
- Discourage the use of strict weight loss diets and appetite suppressants.
- Emphasize the importance of reduced-fat milk, cheese, or other calcium-rich dairy products.
- Encourage intake of vitamin D–fortified foods, such as fortified milk or cereal, for women with limited exposure to ultraviolet light.
- To support women during lactation, use the Internet to access *MyPlate* to provide nutrition education.
- For vegans who are breastfeeding, stress the importance of a balanced diet with appropriate supplements, especially vitamin B_{12}, in sufficient quantities. Offer a referral to an RDN.

Nutritional Directions

- Breastfeeding helps with weight loss.
- Intake of coffee (regular and decaffeinated), other caffeine-containing beverages, and medications should be limited. Encourage fluids such as juice, milk, and water.
- The *SuperTracker* can be an effective tool for improving dietary intake and promoting weight loss during lactation.[64]

ORAL CONTRACEPTIVE AGENTS

Many nutrients (especially folate, vitamin B_6, zinc, and magnesium) are affected by oral contraceptive agents (OCAs). Low-estrogen preparations currently on the market do not adversely affect the woman's vitamin levels as much as earlier preparations. Lower levels of water-soluble vitamins are a result of decreased intestinal absorption and increased metabolism. However, vitamin deficiencies have only been identified with marginal diets.

Low levels of vitamins B_6 and B_{12} have been noted in women using OCAs. Increased amounts of pyridoxine may be indicated because estrogen increases the production of tryptophan, which uses pyridoxine in its metabolism. Low levels of vitamin B_6 also are independently associated with the risk for chronic inflammation which may be associated with health problems including CHD, stroke, and type 2

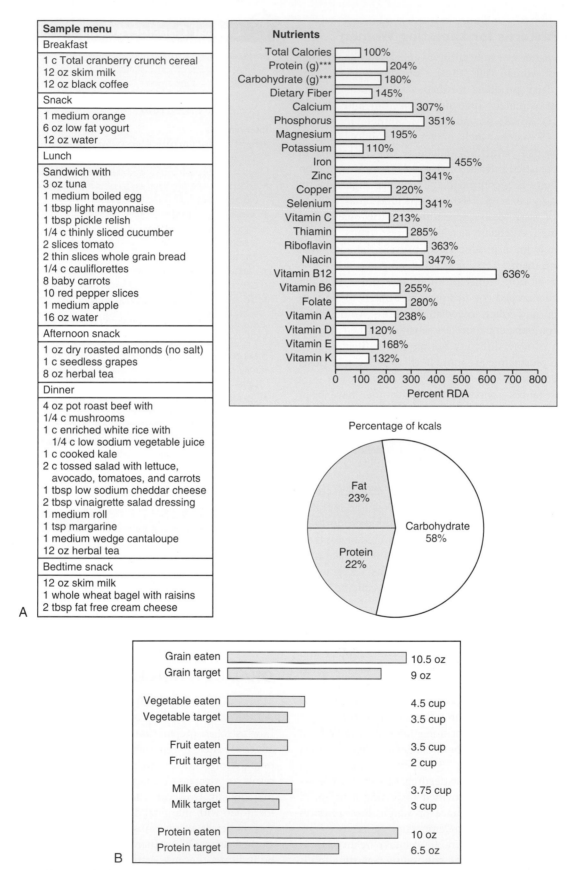

Sample menu
Breakfast
1 c Total cranberry crunch cereal
12 oz skim milk
12 oz black coffee
Snack
1 medium orange
6 oz low fat yogurt
12 oz water
Lunch
Sandwich with
3 oz tuna
1 medium boiled egg
1 tbsp light mayonnaise
1 tbsp pickle relish
1/4 c thinly sliced cucumber
2 slices tomato
2 thin slices whole grain bread
1/4 c cauliflorettes
8 baby carrots
10 red pepper slices
1 medium apple
16 oz water
Afternoon snack
1 oz dry roasted almonds (no salt)
1 c seedless grapes
8 oz herbal tea
Dinner
4 oz pot roast beef with
1/4 c mushrooms
1 c enriched white rice with
1/4 c low sodium vegetable juice
1 c cooked kale
2 c tossed salad with lettuce,
avocado, tomatoes, and carrots
1 tbsp low sodium cheddar cheese
2 tbsp vinaigrette salad dressing
1 medium roll
1 tsp margarine
1 medium wedge cantaloupe
12 oz herbal tea
Bedtime snack
12 oz skim milk
1 whole wheat bagel with raisins
2 tbsp fat free cream cheese

A

Nutrients

	Percent RDA
Total Calories	100%
Protein (g)***	204%
Carbohydrate (g)***	180%
Dietary Fiber	145%
Calcium	307%
Phosphorus	351%
Magnesium	195%
Potassium	110%
Iron	455%
Zinc	341%
Copper	220%
Selenium	341%
Vitamin C	213%
Thiamin	285%
Riboflavin	363%
Niacin	347%
Vitamin B12	636%
Vitamin B6	255%
Folate	280%
Vitamin A	238%
Vitamin D	120%
Vitamin E	168%
Vitamin K	132%

Percentage of kcals

Fat 23%
Protein 22%
Carbohydrate 58%

Grain eaten	10.5 oz
Grain target	9 oz
Vegetable eaten	4.5 cup
Vegetable target	3.5 cup
Fruit eaten	3.5 cup
Fruit target	2 cup
Milk eaten	3.75 cup
Milk target	3 cup
Protein eaten	10 oz
Protein target	6.5 oz

B

FIGURE 13-3 Sample menu for lactation based on information provided by the mother (100% breastfeeding 3-month-old infant; age 29 years; height 5′, 7″; weight 150 lb; and moderately active [30 to 60 minutes of physical activity 5 days a week]).

diabetes.[65] Supplements are appropriate if a deficiency is diagnosed by laboratory evaluation; increasing intake of vitamin B_6 foods is more appropriate to avoid side effects of excessive amounts. Depression and impaired glucose tolerance attributed to OCAs may be alleviated with pyridoxine supplementation. Megaloblastic anemia reported in women taking OCAs may be related to decreased folate absorption or to low levels of vitamin B_{12}.

Progestins can cause weight gain related to increased appetite and altered carbohydrate metabolism. Estrogens may lead to an increase in subcutaneous fat and fluid retention.

Use of OCAs is associated with increased risk of CHD related to changes in serum lipids. Progestin seems to cause an undesirable decrease in high-density lipoprotein cholesterol levels and elevation of low-density lipoprotein and total cholesterol levels (discussed in Chapter 6). The net effect on serum lipids depends on the amount and ratio of progestin and estrogens. OCAs containing progestin and estrogen have been shown to have little or no effect on high-density lipoprotein cholesterol levels, but may increase fasting triglyceride levels.

Various drugs and herbal medications can either increase or decrease the effect of OCAs. Grapefruit products (fruit and/or juice) increase the bioavailability of estradiol in OCAs, so total avoidance of grapefruit is recommended.

MENOPAUSE

During different stages of life, hormonal changes have many repercussions on general health. Female hormonal changes seem to be related to increased incidence of osteoporosis, which may be accompanied by some oral conditions, CHD, and certain cancers that occur later in life.

Perimenopause and menopause usually begin in the late 40s, but genetics, general health, and the age of menarche influence when it actually occurs in a particular woman. For several years before menopause, a range of symptoms may be experienced, including changes in menstruation, fatigue, night sweats, hot flashes, insomnia, loss of bone density, and mood swings; this cluster of symptoms is called **perimenopause**. **Menopause** (decreased production of estrogen and progesterone by the ovaries resulting in termination of menses) occurs between the ages of 35 and 58 years. Estrogen production decreases approximately 60%. Loss of the beneficial effects of estrogen causes health and nutrition issues.

Lower estrogen levels affect the natural process of bone turnover, resulting in a decrease of bone mass. Estrogen receptors on the bone-resorbing osteoclasts increase activity in response to the estrogen level, whereas estrogen receptors on the bone-forming osteoblasts decrease their activity. Bone resorption exceeds bone formation, with significant trabecular and cortical bone loss. Rate of bone loss is rapid in early menopause, then slows and gradually decreases for 8 to 10 years after menstruation ceases. This bone loss may result in osteopenia or osteoporosis (discussed in "*Health Application 9*" in Chapter 9). The alveolar bone provides a potential labile source of calcium; changes in the alveolar process may be used for early diagnosis of osteoporosis.[66] A referral to the healthcare provider should be offered.

Reduced salivary gland secretion is a possible cause for increased dental caries and may lead to increased prevalence of oral **dysesthesia** (impairment of the sense of touch) and taste alterations. Senile **atrophic gingivitis** (abnormally pale gingival tissues) may develop concurrently. **Menopausal gingivostomatitis** (dry and shiny gingivae and edematous mucosa) results in easily bleeding gingiva that may be abnormally pale to quite erythematous. Postmenopausal women with osteoporosis exhibit an exaggerated response to dental plaque biofilm, including increased bleeding on probing, loss of dentoalveolar bone height, and decreased bone mineral density of the alveolar crestal and subcrestal bone. Uncontrolled osteoporosis may lead to edentulism; markedly resorbed residual alveolar ridges may be unsuitable for conventional dentures.

Declines in estrogen and progesterone production are accompanied by unfavorable changes in body composition (increased abdominal fat and decreased lean tissue).[67] Weight gain is one of the major health concerns of women aged 55 to 65 years. Weight loss becomes more difficult because body metabolism is lower, and physical activity may be reduced. Also, blood lipid levels are negatively affected. Total and low-density lipoprotein cholesterol levels may increase with a concurrent decrease in high-density lipoprotein cholesterol levels.

Medically, symptoms of perimenopause and menopause may be treated with **hormone replacement therapy (HRT)**, which consists of low levels of estrogen and progesterone. This treatment is controversial, but when HRT treatment is initiated at the onset of menopause, increased osteoblastic activity reduces risk of osteoporosis and promotes oral health by inhibiting gingival inflammation, periodontitis, and the consequent loss of teeth. If symptoms significantly affect the quality of life, decisions regarding HRT should involve the woman's genetic and medical history. Because of increased risk of some chronic diseases attributed to HRT, low doses are recommended for the shortest time possible.[68]

Plant-based foods, such as legumes and soybeans, provide phytoestrogens and soluble fiber that may potentially reduce menopausal symptoms (i.e., hot flashes and night sweats), as well as regulate blood cholesterol levels. Foods containing phytoestrogens include soy products or isoflavone extracts. Herbal supplements also used to decrease menopausal symptoms include *Ginkgo biloba,* black cohosh, and flaxseed. Studies acknowledge that soy isoflavone supplements, derived by extraction or chemical synthesis, are effective in reducing the frequency and severity of hot flashes. Yet, further studies are needed to determine dose, isoflavone form, and treatment duration.[69]

Nutritional approaches to reduce menopausal symptoms continue to focus on quality of dietary choices and healthy weight maintenance. Adequate amounts of calcium, vitamins D and K, and magnesium are important for protecting bone health. Intake of adequate amounts of fruits, vegetables, and grains, following the *Dietary Guidelines,* are effective in possibly reducing risk of cancer and CHD. Although women need to reduce total energy consumption to prevent weight gain, adequate protein intake is important—at least three servings of iron-rich foods daily. Physical exercise, including aerobic activity and resistance and weight-bearing exercise, is beneficial for bone and cardiovascular health and weight control.

Dental Considerations

Assessments

- *Physical:* age, medical history (including drugs taken), dental history, oral examination, physical activity, oral radiographic findings.
- *Dietary:* health and nutritional knowledge and skills, adequacy of calcium and vitamin D intake from food and supplements, caffeine intake.

Interventions

- Maintain meticulous daily oral self-care to reduce the risk for periodontal disease resulting from an exaggerated response to plaque biofilm.
- For patients with xerostomia, provide information on preventive strategies, such as home and therapeutic fluoride applications; use of xylitol gum or mints; and minimizing choices of cariogenic snacks and beverages, to reduce caries risk (see Chapter 18).
- Patients not prescribed HRT or other medications to deter progressive bone loss may exhibit increased alveolar bone loss, and their periodontal condition should be carefully monitored at regular intervals with the use of oral radiographs.

Nutritional Directions

- Encourage a minimum of three servings of low-fat dairy products or foods fortified with calcium and vitamin D to maintain bone mass. Consumption of greater than 90 mg/day of isoflavones in soy products may be effective in increasing bone mass of menopausal women.
- Calcium and vitamin D supplementation beyond the UL should be discouraged unless taken under supervision of a healthcare provider.
- Encourage good sources of lean protein and regular exercise to maintain muscle mass.
- Choose whole grains, vegetables, fruit, low-fat dairy products, and lean meat or soy substitutes to minimize risk of CHD and to maximize bone health.
- If xerostomia is present, recommend avoidance of alcohol and alcohol-containing products to minimize burning and discomfort in the oral tissues.
- Provide nutritional advice about noncariogenic snack choices.

HEALTH APPLICATION 13　Fetal Alcohol Spectrum Disorder

The Centers for Disease Control and Prevention, American College of Obstetricians and Gynecologists, American Academy of Pediatrics, and March of Dimes all recommend no alcohol intake during pregnancy. Although some recent findings indicate moderate alcohol intake is not harmful to the fetus, this area needs further research to confirm findings. The effect of alcohol on a developing fetus may be determined by genetic variants of the mother.[70] No prenatal period has proven to be safe from the deleterious effects of alcohol.

Fetal alcohol syndrome (FAS) is a cluster of birth defects resulting from prenatal alcohol exposure. An infant with FAS is born exhibiting full effects of the alcohol (Box 13-2), characterized by a pattern of minor facial anomalies, prenatal and postnatal growth retardation, and functional or structural central nervous system abnormalities. Fetal alcohol spectrum disorder (FASD) is a combination of irreversible birth defects and behavioral challenges in infants and children whose mothers consumed alcohol during pregnancy. Based on more recent studies, prevalence of FAS in the general population of the United States is estimated to be 2 to 7/1000 births.[71]

The prevalence of FASD may be as high as 2% to 5% in the United States and some Western European countries, but may be higher in some Native American communities with high levels of alcohol use.[72] Small amounts of alcohol consumption may be associated with adverse effects such as spontaneous abortion, growth retardation, cleft palate, or some of the neurological and behavioral effects of FASD without the physical abnormalities. Prenatal alcohol exposure can cause damage to the brain resulting in significant problems with regulating behavior and optimal thinking and learning. This condition, called fetal alcohol effects, is difficult to diagnose.

FASD is totally preventable by abstaining from the use of alcohol. The first trimester, especially the first month, is the most vulnerable time for the fetus because the woman may not even be aware of the pregnancy. Four to five drinks a day, or at least 45 drinks per month, can produce the full FAS syndrome (see Box 13-2). The FAS child has specific physiological deformities (Fig. 13-4), but how alcohol affects the fetus is not fully understood. Accumulation of toxic levels of alcohol may interfere with cell formation. Several nutrients, especially folic acid, magnesium, and zinc, may be involved. The mental and physical abnormalities cannot be reversed.

Even with adequate nutrition, normal development of fetal organs is jeopardized. Other habits that usually accompany alcohol consumption (e.g., smoking, excessive amounts of coffee the "morning after," poor eating habits with little attention to needed nutrients, and perhaps use of tranquilizers) may also adversely affect the unborn child. Ethanol is a source of energy; chronic alcoholics may have a relatively low intake of protein, essential fats, vitamins, and minerals. Alcohol may impair placental transport of amino acids, calcium, and some vitamins.

Because the brain has a special affinity for alcohol, it is one of the first organs affected. Intellectual impairment is

HEALTH APPLICATION 13 Fetal Alcohol Spectrum Disorder—cont'd

frequently reported in children with FAS. Even at birth, the circumference of the head is small (microcephaly), indicating abnormal brain capacity (i.e., weight of 140 g in an infant with FAS compared with a normal brain weighing 400 g). Fewer brain cells exist, with damaged cells preventing normal functioning; fewer neurons result in disorganized thought. The thinking ability of the brain is permanently disturbed. The average IQ is 68; maladaptive behaviors are common. Additionally, as a result of fewer total body cells, abnormal weight gain affects normal cell development and growth.

Because of global adverse effects of alcohol intake, healthcare providers should advise pregnant women and women who might become pregnant to abstain from alcohol. Nutritional information and other efforts to improve food intake, such as referral to a social worker for food or monetary resources, are warranted. The IOM subcommittee recommended multivitamin-mineral supplements for heavy substance abusers who have difficulty changing their habits to improve nutrient intake.

BOX 13-2 Signs of Fetal Alcohol Syndrome

Fetal alcohol syndrome is a cluster or pattern of related problems, not just a single birth defect. The severity of symptoms varies, but the symptoms are irreversible. Facial features are more difficult to identify in preschool-age children. Signs of fetal alcohol syndrome may include the following:

- Small head circumference and brain size (microcephaly)
- Distinctive facial features: small eyelid openings; eyes close together; a sunken nasal bridge; a short, upturned, undefined nose; an exceptionally thin upper lip; and a smooth skin surface between the nose and upper lip
- Oral cavity: small teeth with faulty enamel, prominent ridges in palate, cleft lip or palate, and small jaws
- Ears poorly formed and incorrectly positioned
- Heart defects
- Deformities of joints, limbs, and fingers
- Weak skeletal muscles (hypotonia) and poor coordination
- Slow physical growth before and after birth
- Vision difficulties, including nearsightedness (myopia)
- Intellectual disabilities and delayed development
- Abnormal behavior such as poor judgment, distractibility and short attention span, hyperactivity, poor impulse control, extreme nervousness and anxiety, and social interaction problems

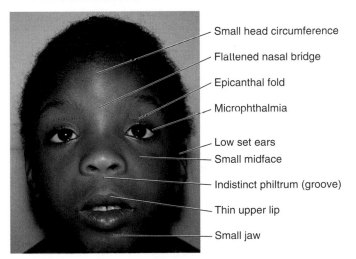

- Small head circumference
- Flattened nasal bridge
- Epicanthal fold
- Microphthalmia
- Low set ears
- Small midface
- Indistinct philtrum (groove)
- Thin upper lip
- Small jaw

FIGURE 13-4 Facial anomalies of a child with fetal alcohol syndrome. (From Zitelli BJ, Davis HW: *Atlas of pediatric physical diagnosis*, ed 6, St Louis, 2012, Mosby.)

Case Application for the Dental Hygienist

Your regular patient, Betty, a 16-year-old, confides to you on her 6-month recare appointment that she is 3 months pregnant. Even though she and her parents have decided to keep the infant, she has not seen a healthcare provider yet. Betty indicates that her mother lost a tooth with each child so she expects the same thing will happen to her.

Nutritional Assessment

- Knowledge about nutrition during pregnancy
- Special dietary restrictions; food fad practices; ethnic, cultural, or religious customs
- Adequacy of diet, especially kilocalories, protein, calcium, vitamin D, iron, and folate
- Medications (including vitamin supplements), drug, and tobacco use
- Support of parents, living arrangements, and social support
- Psychological status and feelings about the reality of becoming a mother at such a young age

Nutritional Diagnosis

Altered nutrition: less than body requirements related to lack of nutritional information and weight concerns.

Nutritional Goals

The patient will consume a well-balanced diet (based on *MyPlate* for pregnant and breastfeeding women) with additional kilocalories during the second and third trimesters, and verbalize ways to increase protein, iron, calcium, and folate intake.

Nutritional Implementation

Intervention: Encourage Betty to visit a healthcare provider as soon as possible.

Rationale: Fetal outcome is affected by nutrient intake during pregnancy; birth defects are likely to occur if dietary habits are poor, or if drug use occurs early in the pregnancy. Inadequate prenatal care leads to poor outcomes for the mother and fetus.

Continued

Case Application for the Dental Hygienist—cont'd

Intervention: Clarify nutritional misconceptions by providing written material and discussing the principal nutrients needing to be increased. Provide the name of an RDN with whom she can discuss these concerns.

Rationale: Nutritional requirements are quite high to meet the growth needs of the adolescent and the fetus because Betty is still growing and storing nutrients in her own body.

Intervention: Teach Betty about the importance of consuming enough calcium and vitamin D during the pregnancy.

Rationale: Calcium and vitamin D are important in formation of skeletal tissue and teeth.

Intervention: Discuss fermentable carbohydrates, and determine how frequently Betty consumes them.

Rationale: Fermentable carbohydrates, especially soft foods, stick to teeth, enhance plaque formation and increase severity of periodontal issues. Parental food selections reflect the foods a child is exposed to and accepts.

Intervention: Talk to Betty about gingivitis during pregnancy, why it occurs, and risks associated with it.

Rationale: Hormonal changes during pregnancy lead to an increased risk of oral problems affecting pregnancy outcome.

Intervention: Discuss nutrients needing to be increased during pregnancy. Provide snack ideas (cheese, nuts, yogurt, milkshakes, popcorn, raw vegetables, and fruits) that contain these nutrients.

Rationale: Most teenagers have an inadequate intake of calcium, iron, and vitamins A and D. Adequate intake of kilocalories, protein, calcium, iron, B vitamins, and zinc is essential for a healthy infant and to protect fetal stores.

Intervention: Explain the effects of her nutritional status on oral development of her infant.

Rationale: Nutrition can determine whether teeth achieve their optimum genetic potential.

Intervention: Explain why she should limit her intake of coffee, tea, and especially carbonated beverages containing caffeine. Explain why she should abstain from alcohol use.

Rationale: Large amounts of caffeine could be responsible for malformations and increased susceptibility to decay of the primary first molars. Alcohol consumption may cause FASD.

Evaluation

Betty should improve eating habits to consume at least the number of food groups recommended in *MyPlate* for pregnant and breastfeeding women. Other behaviors, such as decreasing sugar intake, consuming milk and dairy products (for calcium and vitamin D intake), and consuming raw fruits and green leafy vegetables (for folate intake), will increase intake of nutrients needed during pregnancy. Betty has been taking appropriate action toward oral hygiene self-care to prevent or minimize periodontal problems.

STUDENT READINESS

1. Plan food intake for 1 day with two snacks for a gravida who has four new carious lesions. What reasons would you give her for restricting sugar intake?
2. Explain what pica is, and the type of individuals who may be practicing this behavior.
3. Why is it undesirable to lose weight during pregnancy?
4. List five effects on oral development of the fetus when maternal nutrient intake is inadequate.
5. Why is oral healthcare especially important during pregnancy?
6. Which nutrients may be needed if dietary assessment indicates deficient intake that cannot be corrected by changing eating habits?
7. List advantages of breastfeeding, especially on oral–motor development.

CASE STUDY

A 32-year-old mother of two children (3 years old and 6 months old) who is breastfeeding complains of bleeding and sore gums and tongue. She has not visited her healthcare provider since the birth of her younger child because of lack of time. She has returned to her job as a clerk at a local department store. When questioned about her diet, she reports she drinks a cup of coffee on her way to work; she usually takes a peanut butter and jelly sandwich and soft drink for lunch; and during the evening, she grabs something fast and easy to eat such as hot dogs, canned soup, crackers, cookies, chips, or soft drinks. She complains she is tired and irritable and feels this is because of the stress imposed on her by the two children and her work.

1. List probable causes of the mother's symptoms.
2. Discuss the added stress of pregnancy and lactation on her nutritional needs.
3. Determine other foods that should be readily available for her to consume, such as cottage cheese, yogurt, nuts, fresh fruit, and raw vegetables.
4. Discuss possible nutrition-related causes of the "bleeding and sore gums and tongue."
5. As a dental hygienist, outline the steps to take to reach your recommendations.

References

1. MacDorman MF, Matthews TJ: *Behind international ranking of infant mortality: how the United States compares with Europe.* NCHS data brief, No 23. Hyattsville MD, 2009, National Center for Health Statistics.
2. Federal Interagency on Child and Family Statistics: *America's children: Key national indicators of well-being, 2013.* Accessed September 1, 2013: http://www.childstats.gov/americaschildren/health1.asp.
3. Board on Children, Youth and Families, Food and Nutrition Board: *Influence of pregnancy weight on maternal and child health: Workshop Report.* Washington, DC, 2007, National Academies Press.
4. American Dietetic Association: Position of the American Dietetic Association and American Society for Nutrition:

Obesity, reproduction, and pregnancy outcomes. *J Am Diet Assoc* 109(5):918–926, 2009.

5. Nohr EA, Villamor E, Vaeth M, et al: Mortality in infants of obese mothers: Is risk modified by mode of delivery? *Acta Obstet Gynecol Scand* 91(3):363–371, 2012.

6. Chen A, Feresu SA, Fernandez C, et al: Maternal obesity and the risk of infant death in the United States. *Epidemiology* 2009; 20(1):74–81.

7. Gugusheff JR, Ong ZA, Muhlhausler BS: A maternal "junk food" diet reduces sensitivity to the opioid antagonist naloxone in offspring postweaning. *FASEB* 27(3):1275–1284, 2013.

8. Young SL: Pica in pregnancy: new ideas about an old condition. *Annu Rev Nutr* 30:403-422, 2010.

9. Patterson T, Tita AT, Cliver SP, et al: Maternal body mass index: effect on pregnancy outcomes over a 10 year period. *Am J Obstet Gynecol* 204(Suppl 1):S80, 2011.

10. Institute of Medicine (IOM) and National Research Council (NRC): *Weight gain during pregnancy: reexamining the guidelines.* Washington DC, 2009, National Academy Press.

11. Yazdani S, Yosofniyapasha Y, Nasab BH, et al: Effect of maternal body mass index on pregnancy outcome and newborn weight. *BMC Res Notes* 5:34, 2012.

12. Sujatha VV, Sharma KVLN, Rajesh K: High body mass index in pregnancy, its effects on maternal and fetal outcome. *J Clin Gynecol Obstet* 1(1):15–18, 2012.

13. Patterson T, Tita AT, Cliver SP, et al: Maternal body mass index: effect on pregnancy outcomes over a 10 year period. *Am J Obstet Gynecol* 204(Suppl 1):S80, 2011.

14. Martin JA, Hamilton BE, Ventura SJ, et al: *Births: Final Data for 2010. National Vital Statistics Reports 2012 61 No 1.* Hyattsville MD, 2012, National Center for Health Statistics. Accessed August 27, 2013: http://www.cdc.gov/nchs/data/nvsr/nvsr61/nvsr61_01.pdf.

15. Committee on Health Care for Underserved Women: Committee Opinion No. 549: Oral health care during pregnancy and through the lifespan. *Obs Gynecol* 1122(2, part 1):417–422, 2013. Accessed September 1, 2013: http://www.acog.org/About_ACOG/News_Room/News_Releases/2013/Dental_X-Rays_Teeth_Cleanings_Safe_During_Pregnancy.

16. Babalola DA, Omole F: Periodontal disease and pregnancy outcomes. *J Pregnancy* 2010; Article ID 293439. Accessed August 27, 2013. Available at: http://www.hindawi.com/journals/jp/2010/293439/cta/.

17. Maslova E, Bhattacharya S, Lin SW, et al: Caffeine consumption during pregnancy and risk of preterm birth: a meta-analysis. *Am J Clin Nutr* 92(5):1120–1132, 2010.

18. Kesmodel US, Bertrand J, Støvring H, et al; Lifestyle During Pregnancy Study Group: The effect of different alcohol drinking patterns in early to mid-pregnancy on the child's intelligence, attention, and executive function. *BJOG* 119(10):1180–1190, 2012.

19. Falgreen Eriksen HL, Mortensen EL, Kilburn T, et al: The effects of low to moderate prenatal alcohol exposure in early pregnancy on IQ in 5-year-old children. *BJOG* 119(10):1191–1200, 2012.

20. Kesmodel US, Bertrand J, Støvring H, et al: The effect of alcohol binge drinking in early pregnancy on general intelligence in children. *BJOG* 119(10):1222–1231, 2012.

21. Underbjerg M, Kesmodel US, Landrø NI, et al: The effects of low to moderate alcohol consumption and binge drinking in early pregnancy on selective and sustained attention in 5-year-old children. *BJOG* 119(10):1211–1221, 2012.

22. Patra J, Bakker R, Irving H, et al: Dose–response relationship between alcohol consumption before and during pregnancy and the risks of low birthweight, preterm birth and small for gestational age (SGA)—a systematic review and meta-analyses. *BJOG* 118:1411–1421, 2011.

23. Skogerbø Å, Kesmodel US, Wimberley T, et al: The effects of low to moderate alcohol consumption and binge drinking in early pregnancy on executive function in 5-year-old children. *BJOG* 119(10):1201–1210, 2012.

24. Bay B, Kesmodel US: Prenatal alcohol exposure—a systematic review of the effects on child motor function. *Acta Obstet Gynecol Scand* 90(3):210–226, 2011.

25. Conover EA, Jones KL: Safety concerns regarding binge drinking in pregnancy: a review. *Birth Defects Res A Clin Mol Teratol* 94(8):570–575, 2012.

26. Kelly Y, Iacovou M, Quigley M, et al: Light drinking versus abstinence in pregnancy—behavioural and cognitive outcomes in 7-year-old children: a longitudinal cohort study. *BJOG* 2013; 2013 Apr 17. doi: 10.1111/1471-0528.12246. [Epub ahead of print]

27. Powell G: Danish studies suggesting low and moderate prenatal alcohol exposure has no adverse effects on children aged 5 years did not use appropriate or effective measures of executive functioning. *BJOG* 119(13):1669–1670, 2012.

28. Astley S, Grant T: Another perspective on 'the effect of different alcohol drinking patterns in early to mid pregnancy on the child's intelligence, attention, and executive function. *BJOG* 119(13):1672, 2012.

29. USDA: *Health and nutrition information for pregnant and breastfeeding women—Food Safety for Pregnant and breastfeeding women.* Accessed August 27, 2013. Available at: http://www.choosemyplate.gov/pregnancy-breastfeeding/food-safety.html.

30. Ibid.

31. U.S. Food and Drug Administration: *What you need to know about mercury in fish and shellfish,* updated 10/25/2011. Accessed August 27, 2013. Available at: http://www.fda.gov/Food/ResourcesForYou/Consumers/ucm110591.htm.

32. Schroth R: *Ever wonder why some kids never get cavities? The Dental Essentials for a cavity-free childhood.* Accessed September 1, 2013: http://www.thedentalessentials.com/current_dental_trials_s/50.htm.

33. Hanson C, Anderson-Berry A, Lyden E, et al: Intake of key pregnancy nutrients in Midwest adolescents of childbearing potential. *ICAN: Infant, Child, & Adolescent nutrition* 4(6):355–360, 2012.

34. Blumfield ML, Hure AJ, Macdonald-Wicks L, et al: A systematic review and meta-analysis of micronutrient intakes during pregnancy in developed countries. *Nutr Rev* 71(2):118–132, 2012.

35. Thangaratinam S, Rogozinska E, Jolly K, et al: Effects of interventions in pregnancy on maternal weight and obstetric outcomes: meta-analysis of randomized evidence. *BMJ* 344:e2088, 2012.

36. Ferland-McCollough D, Fernandez-Twinn DS, Cannell IG, et al: Programming of adipose tissue miR-483-3p and GDF-3 expression by maternal diet in type 2 diabetes. *Cell Death Differ* 19(6):1003–1012, 2012.

37. Carlson SE, Colombo J, Gajewski BJ, et al: DHA supplementation and pregnancy outcomes. *Am J Clin Nutr* 97(4):808–815, 2013.

38. Gould JF, Smithers, LG, Makrides M: The effect of maternal omega-3 (n-3) LCPUFA supplementation during pregnancy on early childhood cognitive and visual development: a systematic review and meta-analysis of randomized controlled trials. *Am J Clin NUtr* 97(3):531–544, 2013.

39. ACOG Committee on Obstetric Practice: ACOG Committee Opinion No. 495: Vitamin D: Screening and supplementation during pregnancy. *Obstet Gynecol* 118(1):197–198, 2011.

40. Urrutia RP, Thorp JM: Vitamin D in pregnancy: current concepts. *Curr Opin Obstet Gynecol* 24(2):57–64, 2012.

41. Ross AC, Manson JE, Abrams SA, et al: The 2011 Dietary Reference Intakes for calcium and vitamin D: What dietetics

practitioners need to know. *J Am Diet Assoc* 111(4):524–527, 2011.

42. Institute of Medicine, Food and Nutrition Board: *Dietary reference intakes for calcium and vitamin D.* Washington, DC, 2011, National Academies Press.

43. McNulty B, McNulty H, Marshall, B, et al: Impact of continuing folic acid after the first trimester of pregnancy: findings of a randomized trial of Folic Acid Supplementation in the Second and Third Trimesters. *Am J Clin Nutr* 98(1):92–98, 2013.

44. Blencowe H, Cousens S, Modell B, et al: Folic acid to reduce neonatal mortality from neural tube disorders. *Int J Epidemiol* 39(Suppl 1):i110–i121, 2010.

45. Branum AM, Bailey R, Singer BJ: Dietary supplement use and folate status during pregnancy in the United States. *J Nutr* 143(4):486–492, 2013.

46. Cao C, O'Brien KO: Pregnancy and iron homeostasis: an update. *Nutr Rev* 71(1):35–51, 2013.

47. Peña-Rosas JP, De-Regil LM, Dowswell T, et al: Intermittent oral iron supplementation during pregnancy. *Cochrane Database Syst Rev* 7:CD009997, 2012.

48. Bougma K, Aboud FE, Harding KB, et al: Iodine and mental development of children 5 years old and under: a systematic review and meta-analysis. *Nutrients* 5(4):1384–1416, 2013.

49. Pearce EN: Effects of iodine deficiency in pregnancy. *J Trace Elem Med Biol* 26(2-3)131–133, 2012.

50. Stagnaro-Green A, Sullivan S, Pearce EN: Iodine supplementation during pregnancy and lactation. *JAMA* 308(23):2463–2464, 2012.

51. Leung AM, Pearce EN, Braverman LE: Iodine content of prenatal multivitamins in the United States. *N Engl J Med* 360(9):939–940, 2009.

52. Connelly KJ, Boston BA, Pearce EN, et al. Congenital hypothyroidism caused by excess prenatal maternal iodine ingestion. *J Pediatr* 161(4):760–762, 2012.

53. U.S. Department of Health and Human Services: *Healthy People 2020: Reduce iron deficiency among pregnant females, NWS-22.* Accessed August 27, 2013. http://healthypeople.gov/2020/topicsobjectives2020/objectiveslist.aspx?topicId=29.

54. Institute of Medicine (IOM), Subcommittee on Nutritional Status and Weight Gain During Pregnancy: *Nutrition During Pregnancy.* Washington, DC, 1990, National Academy Press.

55. American Dietetic Association: Position of the American Dietetic Association and American Society for Nutrition: Obesity, reproduction, and pregnancy outcomes. *J Am Diet Assoc* 109(5):918–926, 2009.

56. Centers for Disease Control and Prevention: *Breastfeeding among U.S. children born 2000-2010, CDC Nation Immunization Survey.* Accessed August 27, 2013: http://www.cdc.gov/breastfeeding/data/NIS_data/index.htm.

57. Center for Disease Control and Prevention (CDC): *Breastfeeding Report Card—United States, 2013.* Accessed on August 27, 2013. Available at: http://www.cdc.gov/breastfeeding/data/reportcard.htm.

58. Centers for Disease Control and Prevention (CDC): Racial and ethnic differences in breastfeeding initiation and duration, by State—National Immunization Survey, United States, 2004-2008. *MMWR Morb Mortal Wkly Rep* 59(11);327–334, 2010.

59. Lumbiganon P, Martis R, Laopaiboon M, et al: Antenatal breastfeeding education for increasing breastfeeding duration. *Cochrane Database Syst Rev* (11):CD006425, 2011.

60. Institute of Medicine (IOM), Subcommittee on Nutritional Status and Weight Gain during Pregnancy: *Nutrition during Lactation.* Washington, DC, 1991, National Academy Press.

61. Guxens M, Mendez MA, Moltó-Puigmartí C, et al: Breastfeeding, long-chain polyunsaturated fatty acids in colostrum, and infant mental development. *Pediatrics* 128(4):e880–e889, 2011.

62. DiFilippo C: Exclusively breast-fed infants and vitamin D supplementation. *Top Clin Nutr* 26(1):78–89, 2011.

63. Wagner CL, Greer FR, and the Section on Breastfeeding and Committee on Nutrition: Prevention of rickets and vitamin D deficiency in infants, children, and adolescents. *Pediatrics* 122(5):1142–1152, 2008.

64. Colleran HL, Lovelady CA: Use of MyPyramid menu planner for moms in a weight-loss intervention during lactation. *J Acad Nutr Diet* 112(4):553–558, 2012.

65. Sakakeeny L, Roubenoff R, Obin M, et al: Plasma pyridoxal-5-phosphate is inversely associated with systemic markers of inflammation in a population of U.S. adults. *J Nutr* 142(7):1280–1285, 2012.

66. Stewart S, Hanning R: Building osteoporosis prevention into dental practice. *J Can Dent Assoc* 78:c29, 2012.

67. Davis SR, Castelo-Branco C, Chedraui P, et al: Understanding weight gain at menopause. *Climacteric* 15(5):419–429, 2012.

68. Lethaby AE, Brown J, Marjoribanks J, et al: Phytoestrogens for vasomotor menopausal symptoms. *Cochrane Database Syst Rev* (4):CD001395, 2007.

69. Take K, Melby MK, Kronenberg F, et al: Extracted or synthesized soybean isoflavones reduce menopausal hot flash frequency and severity: systematic review and meta-analysis of randomized controlled trials. *Menopause* 19(7):776–790, 2012.

70. Lewis SJ, Zuccolo L, Davey Smith G, et al: Fetal alcohol exposure and IQ at age 8: evidence from a population-based birth-cohort study. *PLoS ONE* 7(11):e49407, 2012.

71. Centers for Disease Control and Prevention (CDC): *Fetal Alcohol Spectrum Disorders (FASDs), Tracking fetal alcohol syndrome (FAS).* Assessed August 27, 2013: http://www.cdc.gov/ncbddd/fasd/research-tracking.html.

72. May PA, Gossage JP, Kalberg WO, et al: Prevalence and epidemiologic characteristics of FASD from various research methods with an emphasis on recent in-school studies. *Dev Disabil Res Rev* 15(3):176–192, 2009.

ⓔ EVOLVE RESOURCES

Please visit http://evolve.elsevier.com/Stegeman/nutritional for additional practice and study support tools.

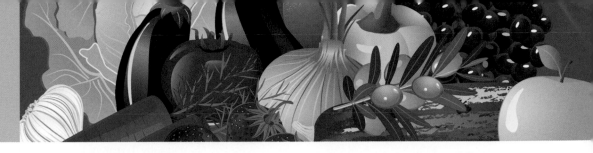

Chapter 14

Nutritional Requirements During Growth and Development and Eating Habits Affecting Oral Health

Student Learning Outcomes

Upon completion of the chapter, the student will be able to achieve the following student learning outcomes:

- Describe the procedure for introducing solid foods after the initial stage of feeding by bottle or breast.
- Discuss ways to handle typical nutritional problems that occur in infants, young children, school-age children, and adolescents.
- Apply dental aspects related to nutritional needs during infancy, early childhood, elementary school years, and adolescence to patient care.

- Assess nutrition education needs for patients during infancy, early childhood, elementary school years, and adolescence.
- Discuss physiological changes that alter the nutritional status of infants and adolescents.

Key Terms

Bruxism
Cleft lip
Cleft palate
Early childhood caries (ECC)
Food jags
Hydrolyzed protein

Innate
Necrotizing enterocolitis
Nonnutritive sucking
Sealants
Suckling

Test Your NQ

1. **T/F** Commercial infant formulas are standard in their nutrient content.
2. **T/F** Fluoride should be provided to all infants from birth if the water supply is not fluoridated.
3. **T/F** Solid foods should be introduced at 6 weeks of age.
4. **T/F** Orange juice is the first fruit juice to offer an infant.
5. **T/F** More nutrients are required during adolescence than during any other stage of life.
6. **T/F** Toddlers may refuse to eat anything except one food for several days.

7. **T/F** Breastfed infants do not need any supplements during the first 4 months.
8. **T/F** Bottle-fed infants are less likely to develop malocclusion.
9. **T/F** Energy needs of children and adolescents are high to support growth and development and physical activity level.
10. **T/F** To reduce risk of plaque biofilm, toddlers and children should not be given snacks.

Achievement of goals established in *Healthy People 2020* will improve the health of infants and children, affecting their long-term health status and life span.

INFANTS

An infant's health status, beginning at conception and affecting lifelong well-being, depends on feeding and nurturing the newborn by the mother or caretaker. Infancy is a time of rapid transition from virtually nothing but milk to a varied diet consisting of some selections from each food group being consumed on a daily basis. The infant is normally able to thrive on human milk or commercially available, artificial infant milk, but many of the physiological systems are immature at birth. Because of limited stomach capacity, frequent feedings are needed.

Pregnant patients expect the dental hygienist to provide information concerning infant feeding methods affecting the oral cavity. The practitioner should be prepared to address these issues and base their advice on scientific evidence. Feeding patterns present during the child's first 2 years create an environment for optimal development of genetically determined factors contributing to orofacial development and swallowing patterns.

Growth

Growth is the definitive test of health and is used as the most sensitive and specific indicator of nutritional status. Increased size results in greater nutritional requirements, but the need for kilocalories per kilogram decreases as one grows. Dental hygienists working with new parents, infants, and children should be familiar with normal growth and developmental patterns that reflect adequacy of nutritional intake. The birth weight of an infant doubles in 4 months (from 7.5 to 15 lb), and usually triples by 1 year of age. Length or height increases 50% by 1 year of age. The Centers for Disease Control and Prevention (CDC) growth charts for determining appropriate growth rates are available on the Evolve website.

Nutritional Requirements

Adequate nutrition is more important during infancy and childhood than during any other stage of the life cycle. As might be expected from the rapid growth rate, energy requirements are much higher per pound or kilogram of weight than for an adult: 95 to 83 kcal/kg/day between 3 and 12 months of age (energy needs per kg decrease from birth to 12 months) versus 29 to 37 kcal/kg/day for adults. Infants have a higher resting metabolic rate, and intestinal absorption is relatively inefficient.

Adequate intake (AI) for protein is 1.52 g/kg daily from birth to 6 months of age, and the RDA for older infants is 1.2 g/kg; this translates to about 9.1 to 13 g/day (Table 14-1). Recommended protein intakes are based on mean protein intake of breastfed infants. As a result of immature renal function, total protein should not exceed 20% of the kilocalories. Breast milk and artificial breast milk (commercial formula) provide approximately 50% of kilocalories from fat to supply the high energy needs.

Breast Milk

Human milk is the optimal source of nutrients for infants and contains all the right nutrients to help infants reach their

Table 14-1	**Dietary reference intakes for infants compared with nutrient content of human breast milk, cow's milk, and artificial breast milk**				
	Dietary Reference Intake[a]		Human Breast Milk (per Liter)	Cow's Milk[b] (per Liter)	Average Artificial Breast Milk (per Liter)
Nutrient	0-6 Months Old	7-12 Months Old			
Kilocalorie	95 kcal/kg (3 months)*[c] 85 kcal/kg (6 months)*[c]	83 kcal/kg[c]	650 kcal	670 kcal	680 kcal
Protein	9.1 g/day*	**13.5 g/day**	11 g	20 g	15 g
Fat	31 g/day*	30 g/day*	40-45 g	36 g	36 g
Cholesterol	ND	ND	100-200 mg	119 mg	10-30 mg
Calcium	200 mg/day*	260 mg/day*	264-210 mg	1220 mg	500 mg
Phosphorus	100 mg/day*	275 mg/day*	121-158 mg	935 mg	300 mg
Iron	0.27 mg/day*	**11 mg/day**	0.35 mg	0.5 mg	12 mg[d]
Sodium	120 mg/day*	370 mg/day*	6.6 mg	21 mg	10 mg
Potassium	400 mg/day*	700 mg/day*	13 mg	11 mg	20 mg
Renal solute load (mOsm/L)	N/A	N/A	79	221	150

Note: Recommended dietary allowances (RDAs) are presented in **bold type** and adequate intakes (AIs) are followed by an asterisk (*).
N/A, Not applicable; *ND,* not determined.
[a]Data from National Research Council: *The guide to nutrient requirements,* Washington, DC, 2006, National Academies Press; and National Research Council: *Dietary reference intakes for calcium and vitamin D,* Washington, DC, 2011, National Academies Press. Available at http://www.nap.edu
[b]Whole milk (3.5% fat content).
[c]Total energy expenditure.
[d]Iron fortified.

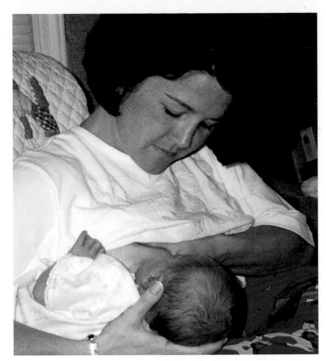

FIGURE 14-1 Breastfeeding promotes a special bonding between mother and infant. (From Lowdermilk DL, Perry SE: *Maternity nursing*, ed 8, St Louis, 2011, Mosby Elsevier.)

Table 14-2	Fluoride supplementation*		
	Parts per Million (ppm) of Fluoride in Water Supply†		
Age of Child	<0.3	0.3-0.6	>0.6
Birth–6 months	0	0	0
6 mo–3 years	0.25	0	0
3-6 years	0.50	0.25	0
6-16 years	1.00	0.50	0

From American Academy of Pediatric Dentistry Reference Manual: Guideline on fluoride therapy, revised 2013. Accessed August 30, 2013: http://www.aapd.org/media/Policies_Guidelines/G_FluorideTherapy.pdf
*Approved by the American Dental Association, American Academy of Pediatrics, and American Academy of Pediatric Dentistry.
†0.1 parts per million (ppm) = 1 mg/L.

maximum potential (Fig. 14-1). Human milk is very complex, and its exact chemical makeup is unknown. It contains living cells, hormones, active enzymes, and antibodies. Specific protein fractions synthesized in breast tissue promote colonies of healthy bacteria in the gastrointestinal tract that aid nutrient absorption and help protect infants from infections and illness. Because the infant's immune system is not fully developed, human milk provides distinct advantages over formula. Numerous organizations in the United States and worldwide strongly recommend exclusive breast-feeding for at least 4 months to reduce the incidence of atopic dermatitis, early onset wheezing, and incidence of cow's milk allergy.[1] Regardless of the nutritional status of the mother, overall composition of breast milk is constant, yet changing to meet the infant's nutritional needs.

Breast milk is normally thin with a slightly bluish color. Compared with cow's milk, human milk is high in lactose and relatively low in protein. Breast milk contains substantial amounts of long-chain fatty acids. Arachidonic acid and docosahexaenoic acid (DHA) are important in development of brain and retinal tissue. Human milk is relatively high in cholesterol. Lipase enzyme inherent in breast milk improves fat digestion. The low mineral content of human milk is ideal for the infant's immature kidneys. Although iron content is low, inherent compounds in human milk promote efficient iron utilization. Iron deficiency in exclusively breastfed infants is rare, but longer breastfeeding durations are associated with lower iron stores.[2] Because of the high bioavailability of iron, additional sources of iron are unnecessary during the first 4 to 6 months for breastfed infants. Supplemental foods during that time may reduce iron absorption.

Iron-rich foods or a daily low-dose oral iron supplement should be initiated at 4 to 6 months.

Breast milk provides approximately 0.01 mg/day of fluoride, regardless of drinking water and maternal plasma levels. Despite the low levels of fluoride breastfed infants receive during this period, risk of dental caries does not seem to increase. As shown in Table 14-2, the American Dental Association and American Academy of Pediatric Dentistry (AAPD) recommend delaying fluoride supplements for all infants until 6 months of age.

Artificial Infant Milk

Although nutrients differ slightly for various brands, all commercial formulas comply with standards set by the Infant Formula Act established in 1980 (see Table 14-1). The U.S. Food and Drug Administration (FDA) requires that these products meet strict standards. Artificial infant milk formulas duplicate breast milk as closely as technology allows, but the exact composition of breast milk cannot be duplicated. No artificial infant milk can match the benefits of breast milk. Artificial infant formulas are continually being modified to more closely duplicate components of human milk and to meet nutrient needs of various groups of infants. Nonfat cow's milk is the basis for most artificial infant formulas, modified to ensure that performance of formula-fed infants (i.e., growth, absorption of nutrients, gastrointestinal tolerance, and reactions in blood) matches that of breastfed infants. Infants given artificial infant milk tend to weigh more than breastfed infants, a negative factor that may put them at greater risk for obesity as adults; however, more research is needed to confirm this association. Breast-fed infants develop better control of their milk intake than bottle-fed infants, who have less ability to self-regulate milk intake.[3]

Almost all commercial formulas have been modified to contain DHA, which is a natural ingredient of breast milk. Brain growth relative to body weight is highest during the last trimester of a pregnancy. Decreased accumulation of DHA during brain and retinal development results in a variety of behavioral, cognitive, and visual delays, so a formula with DHA is more important for infants born during the last trimester (premature), but breast milk is still superior to all artificial infant formulas.

Adequate nutrients are provided in an appropriate caloric concentration (about 20 kcal/oz) for full-term infants. As established by the guidelines of the American Academy of Pediatrics (AAP), electrolyte, mineral, and vitamin contents are similar (see Table 14-1). Adequate amounts of these nutrients (except for fluoride and iron) are furnished if the infant receives 150 to 180 mL/kg/day of a commercial formula with iron.

Fluorosis has been associated with fluoride intake during enamel development; the severity is dependent on dose, duration, and timing of intake. Because of increasing cases of fluorosis reported, no fluoride is added to artificial infant milk; they contain a small amount of inherent fluoride as a result of some of the ingredients and processing. After 6 months of age, all infants need fluoride supplementation if local drinking water or bottled water contains less than 0.3 parts per million (ppm) of fluoride. Most bottled water does not contain fluoride. If bottled water is used, water specially marketed for babies (sometimes called "nursery water") contains appropriate amounts of fluoride. If local water contains too much fluoride, waters that contain no or minimal amounts of fluoride—purified, demineralized, deionized, distilled, or reverse osmosis filtered water—can be regionally produced and are readily available in local stores.

Infant formulas containing probiotics and prebiotics have been developed, which should be beneficial for gastrointestinal health. Infants receiving these formulas tolerate them well and show a similar rate of weight gain compared with infants fed a conventional formula. Some evidence indicates a prebiotic may help prevent food-related allergies, especially eczema.[4] Well-conducted controlled trials support the therapeutic role for probiotics toward preventing necrotizing enterocolitis in preterm infants.[5] Necrotizing enterocolitis is a condition that occurs in neonates with development of cellular dead patches in the intestines interfering with digestion and absorption. The risk of providing probiotics in artificial infant milk is minimal. Despite exhaustive research, further studies are needed before routinely recommending prebiotics for prevention of allergy in formula-fed infants.[6,7]

Commercial artificial infant milk is more appropriate for infants than cow's or goat's milk. Malnutrition has been reported in infants fed home-recipe formulas. This may be related to variations in nutrient composition or unsanitary handling practices that may result in frequent infections or gastrointestinal disorders. In other countries, infants become malnourished and die when food manufacturers fail to include required nutrients or prevent contaminants, or when water mixed with the formula is dirty or contaminated.

Many different formulas are available to substitute when an infant does not tolerate a cow's milk protein–based formula. Cow's milk allergy, the most common allergy, affects 2% to 3% of infants and young children. The American Academy of Allergy, Asthma, and Immunology (AAAAI) recommends hydrolyzed protein (protein broken down into amino acids) formula for infants at increased risk of allergic disease (family history) who are not exclusively breastfed to reduce risk of allergic disease and cow's milk allergy. Soy protein–based formulas are the most commonly used substitute, accounting for nearly 25% of the formula market. Studies using soy formulas raise no clinical concerns with respect to nutritional adequacy, sexual development, thyroid disease, immune function, or neurodevelopment, but research does not indicate that soy formula prevents atopic disease.[7,8] These formulas are not recommended for preterm infants, however, because of their different nutritional requirements.

The most common reason for using soy-based formulas is for relief of perceived formula intolerance (spitting, vomiting, fussiness) or symptoms of colic. The effects of cow's milk protein–based formulas and soy protein–based formulas on infantile colic, fussiness, or prevention of atopic disease in healthy or high-risk infants are similar. Testing of cognitive development (mental, motor, and language development) of infants fed soy formula, milk-based formula or breast milk indicate breastfed infants have a slight advantage over all other types of artificial infant formulas.[9] Soy protein–based formulas are appropriate for infants with galactosemia and hereditary lactase deficiency and for accommodating a vegetarian diet.

Lactose-free and reduced lactose cow's milk formulas are also available and are appropriate for circumstances in which elimination or a reduction in lactose is required. For infants with cow's milk protein allergy, hydrolyzed protein formula should be considered, but these more expensive formulas have not shown any benefits over intact cow protein formulas for healthy, term infants.[10] Numerous specialized formulas are available for infants with special metabolic problems, such as Phenyl-Free® (Mead Johnson Nutrition) for phenylketonuria.

Infant formulas should be discontinued by 12- to 14-months of age, and vitamin D–fortified whole milk should be provided until age 2 years. Low-fat milk is not recommended for children younger than 2 years. Special toddler formulas are nutritionally safe and do not need refrigeration, but they are unnecessary.

Feeding Practices

Although rigid feeding schedules were used in the past, infants today are generally fed on demand (when they are hungry). A pattern usually develops within about 2 weeks, with the infant eating six times daily at 4-hour intervals. This feeding pattern gradually evolves, eventually allowing the infant and parents to sleep through the night. Touching helps to strengthen feelings of love, security, and trust, and is as important as nutrients in the formula. An infant should never be left alone with a bottle propped during feedings.

Oral and Neuromuscular Development

Sucking is more difficult from the breast than from a bottle. Breastfeeding requires the infant to open the mouth wide, move the jaws back and forth, and squeeze with the gingiva to extract the milk, a process called suckling. Suckling encourages mandibular development by strengthening the jaw muscle, thus promoting maximum development of the genetically defined jaw and chin.[12] Breastfed infants are less likely to develop malocclusion—high premaxilla, abnormal alveolar ridges, and palate and posterior crossbite. Early weaning may interrupt oral motor development leading to malocclusion and oral breathing, and negatively affect swallowing, breathing and speaking.[13-15] Infants breastfed for 1 year require 40% less orthodontia than bottle-fed infants. The fatty acid profile of human milk may confer a measure of protection against persistent stuttering.[16] Sucking from a bottle or on a pacifier, thumb, or fingers may result in narrower upper and lower dental arches. When the bottle presses against the soft bones of the palate, narrow or V-shaped palates may occur; this may be predictive of snoring and sleep apnea.[17]

Nonnutritive sucking (sucking on thumb, fingers, or a pacifier), which begins in utero, is normal. Use of a pacifier does not seem to interfere with successful breastfeeding if introduced after breastfeeding is established. Nonnutritive sucking is important in development of self-regulation and ability to control emotions. However, if it continues too long, problems with tooth alignment and jaw development may occur; infants should be weaned from the pacifier between 6 months and 1 year of age, before malocclusion or skeletal dysplasias occur.[18]

Eating is not instinctive but a combination of instinctive behaviors during the first month, followed by primitive motor reflexes and learned behaviors. Eating is the most complex physical task humans do—using all the body's organ systems and requiring simultaneous coordination of all the sensory systems.

A successful feeding regimen is based on developmental stage of the infant or child. Nutrition is related to neuromuscular maturation, especially for infants. Suckling is replaced with sucking by 4 months of age, when orofacial muscles are used with the mouth more pursed, and the tongue moving back and forth. This backward movement of the tongue makes the smacking noises that occur. A forward motion of the tongue and dropping the mandible is typical during the first 3 months. If semisolid foods are offered at this time, the tongue may force food out; no discriminating taste is occurring, just reflex action.

The sucking motion becomes developed enough for the infant to eat and handle semisolid foods from a spoon around 4 to 6 months of age. Development of fine, gross, and oral motor skills to consume foods correlates with demands for additional kilocalories and nutrients. If foods are not added by 6 months of age, growth may decline below normal growth curves.

At about 6 to 8 months old, infants develop the ability to receive food and pass it to the gingiva in a chewing motion. Eight teeth normally erupt between 6 and 12 months of age. When the infant can chew, pureed foods are not required; some variety of texture is mandatory if infants are going to accept unfamiliar foods later in life. Unless textured foods are offered, the development of oral musculature may be slow or delayed, affecting the child's speech.

Introduction of Foods

Good nutrition is essential for rapid growth and development that occurs during an infant's first year. As foods are added to the infant's selections to include most food groups, timing of the transition, how the infant is fed, and quality of foods offered can have important health implications.

An infant's developmental readiness determines which foods should be fed and the texture of foods to be fed. Infants are mature enough to begin eating from a spoon when they are able to hold their necks steady and sit with support, draw in their lower lip as a spoon is removed from the mouth, and retain and swallow food. At 4 to 6 months of age, infants are usually developmentally ready to eat solid foods.

Numerous false assumptions are associated with introduction of solid foods. Despite the fact many parents introduce solid foods, especially cereals, during the first month, no nutritional advantage is associated with this practice. The most common reason for early feeding is to help the infant sleep through the night. This naturally occurs between 1 and 3 months of age, with girls typically sleeping through the night earlier than boys. This developmental milestone is not related to what is fed.

Foods should be presented to the infant with a spoon, never in a bottle. Disadvantages in starting semisolid foods too early are (a) unnecessary costs, (b) high probability of overfeeding, (c) effects on the immature digestive system, (d) increased risk of food allergies, (e) reduction of milk intake in lieu of a less nutritionally complete food, and (f) decreased iron absorption. After introduction of foods at 4 to 6 months, formula intake should remain around 32 oz daily.

Fruit juice provides no nutritional benefit for infants younger than 6 months old. To decrease risk of dental caries, fruit juice should not be given in bottles or sippy cups because these allow babies to drink easily throughout the day. Too much fruit juice, including apple, pear, and prune, can cause diarrhea, and decreases intake of other foods containing essential nutrients for infants and toddlers. Infants receiving breast milk or formula do not need additional water.

As noted in Chapter 13, breastfeeding for at least 4 months helps prevent allergies in infants.[19] Infants are at high risk of developing allergies if they have at least one first-degree relative (parent or sibling) with allergies and are not exclusively breastfed for 4 to 6 months. According to the Food Allergy Research and Education (FARE), 8% of children have a documented food allergy with young children affected most frequently. The rate of food allergy has increased among all children over the past 10 years.[20] Less than half of infants have clinically confirmed food hypersensitivity; parents report more infant adverse reactions to food than are confirmed clinically.

When the infant is 6 months old, 4 to 6 oz of fruit juice diluted with equal portions of water can be introduced in a cup. Solid foods should not be introduced before 4 to 6 months of age. Because of the possibility of a food allergy, only one new food should be introduced at a time.

Iron-fortified infant cereal, such as rice, oat, or barley cereal mixed with breast milk or artificial formula, may be introduced at 4 months without increasing the risk of developing an allergy to wheat. After introducing a new food, a waiting period of 2 to 3 days is recommended before introducing another new food to observe for allergic reactions.

Foods most commonly causing allergies include cow's milk (including ice cream), eggs, peanuts, tree nuts (e.g., walnuts, almonds, cashews, pistachios, pecans), wheat, soy, fish, and shellfish. Previously, the recommendation was to wait until after 12 months of age to introduce these foods, but the AAAAI does not find that postponing introduction of highly allergenic foods prevents allergies; in fact they suggested that early introduction of highly allergenic foods may actually reduce the risk of food allergies. Introduction of these foods should be initiated at home rather than at a restaurant or day care center.[21]

The recommended order of introduction for vegetables, meats, and fruits varies among pediatricians. Some advise the introduction of vegetables after cereals, then meats followed by fruits. Meats should be introduced early, especially for breastfed infants to provide essential nutrients, such as iron and zinc. Preference for sweet foods is an **innate** (inborn) desire. Because sweet flavors are well accepted, other foods (meats, vegetables) are offered first.

Flavors from the mother's diet are transmitted through amniotic fluid and mother's milk. So a mother's food choices, particularly for fruit and vegetables, influence later preferences and food behaviors.[22] An infant's grimace when offered a new food is innate, not a sign of dislike. When the spoon is offered again, it is very likely to be accepted.

Gradually, junior-type foods with a few lumps are introduced to initiate some chewing. The presence of a few teeth does not mean the infant is ready to masticate foods. Certain vegetables—cucumbers, onions, cabbage, and broccoli—are more difficult to digest and are introduced after 1 year of age. Commercial infant food may be used, but foods from the family menu can be pureed for use. The addition of sugar, salt, and other spices to infant foods is not recommended.

When semisolid foods are introduced, the goal should be to include all food groups as soon as possible to ensure a well-balanced diet. Guidelines for feeding infants to provide a balance of nutrients are similar to the *Dietary Guidelines* except fat and cholesterol content are not limited.

Supplements

The AAP and Health Canada recommend that exclusively breastfed infants receive 400 IU (10 μg) vitamin D supplementation beginning during the first 2 months to prevent rickets and continuing until infants are weaned and are consuming 1000 mL/day or more of vitamin D–fortified formula or whole milk.[23,24] Several cases of vitamin D deficiency have occurred in the United States in exclusively breastfed infants. In addition, all non-breastfed infants consuming less than 1000 mL/day of vitamin D–fortified formula or milk should receive a vitamin D supplement of 400 IU daily. Artificial formulas marketed in the United States provide 400 IU or more of vitamin D per 1000 mL. Vitamin D supplements on the market supply 400 IU/day. Despite these recommendations, most American and Canadian infants are not consuming the recommended amounts of vitamin D.[25,26]

Healthy, full-term infants require minimal amounts of iron during the first 6 months and more significant amounts after 6 months of age. If iron-fortified formula is not used, iron supplementation is recommended for formula-fed infants after 4 months of age, for breastfed infants at 4 to 6 months of age, and for preterm infants after 2 months of age. Iron supplementation (usually ferrous sulfate or ferric ammonium citrate) is ordinarily given as liquid drops. These drops can cause staining on erupting teeth; this can be reduced by putting the drops in water.

Fluoride supplementation is recommended for infants older than 6 months and children to increase the strength and acid resistance of developing tooth enamel. Before fluoride supplementation is prescribed, however, the AAPD recommends a caries risk assessment along with an evaluation of dietary sources of fluoride (e.g., fluoridated water).[27] Vitamin supplements containing fluoride may be prescribed by a healthcare provider or dentist (see Table 14-2).

 Dental Considerations

Assessment
- *Physical:* infant's developmental stage, neuromuscular development, age, lip biting, thumb sucking, tongue thrusting, pacifier use.
- *Dietary:* parent's knowledge of bottle-feeding, feeding of solid foods, necessity of providing oral care for the infant, source of iron, fluoride (drinking water from home, day care, and school; beverages such as soda, juice, and artificial infant milk; prepared food, and toothpaste), and use of other supplements.

Interventions
- Avoid recommending sugar-free foods, especially those containing sorbitol. This sugar substitute is a known cause of diarrhea in infants and children.
- Inform parents that supplements containing fluoride should never be added to milk; fluoride binds with milk and soy proteins, decreasing availability of fluoride significantly.
- Exposure to too much fluoride before enamel maturation may change the structure and cause fluorosis.
- Nonfluoridated or minimally fluoridated water is recommended for reconstituting powdered formulas to reduce risk of fluorosis.

 Nutritional Directions

- The AAP Committee on Nutrition recommends all water (tap or bottled, mixed with artificial infant or given plain) given to infants younger than 3 months old first be boiled for 1 to 2 minutes.
- For the first 4 months of life, 32 oz/day of formula satisfies and provides all the nutrients needed for full-term infants.
- The rate of growth is faster during infancy than at any other stage of life. Fats, a concentrated source of energy, are needed to support this rapid growth (40% to 50% of the total kilocalories

Nutritional Directions—cont'd

are recommended). Reduced-fat milk is inappropriate for children younger than 2 years.

- Despite growing concerns over CHD, cholesterol intake is important during early developmental stages of infancy. Recommending changes in fat intake before age 2 years is unnecessary.
- Store all vitamin-mineral supplements in a place that is protected from children; many children die each year from accidental iron overdose.
- Honey is inappropriate for children younger than 1 year of age because botulism may occur.
- Toddlers learn about food by touching and playing with it. Encourage this by offering finger foods when the child can sit alone and pick up items.
- During the first year, habits and preferences are beginning to form; it is important to foster healthy eating habits early.
- After solid foods are introduced, the goal is to gradually include a variety of vegetables and fruits on a daily basis. Offer dark green, leafy, and deep yellow vegetables and colorful fruits frequently.
- Nutritious foods give children a healthy head start.

Oral Health Concerns In Early Childhood

Tooth formation begins before birth and is not completed until about 12 years of age; the structure of the tooth is affected by food intake during this time. A clear relationship has been shown between nutritional deficiency during tooth development and tooth size, tooth formation, time of tooth eruption, and susceptibility to caries. One occurrence of mild to moderate malnutrition during the first year of life is associated with increased caries in primary and permanent teeth later in life. Calcium and vitamin D must be present for proper calcification of dentin and normal enamel. Vitamin D is crucial to tooth development; later deficiency may promote tooth decay.[28]

Dental caries are largely preventable, but they remain the most common chronic disease of children and adolescents. Tooth decay affects more than 25% of U.S. children ages 2 to 5 years and 50% of adolescents between 12 and 15 years of age. Children of some racial and ethnic groups and those from lower-income families have more untreated tooth decay. For example, 40% of Mexican American children ages 6 to 8 years have untreated decay, compared with 25% of non-Hispanic whites.[29] Dental caries in young children are significantly associated with lower parental education level, living at the poverty level, no breastfeeding, skipping breakfast, low fruit and vegetable intake, no annual dental visit, and amount and frequency of sugar-sweetened beverages.[30]

Infant Oral Care

Dental problems can begin early. Children who have caries as infants or toddlers have a much greater probability of subsequent caries in primary and permanent dentitions.

Good dental care starts in infancy, before the first tooth emerges. Decay and early loss can damage permanent teeth before they erupt. The infant's gingiva should be cleaned daily with gauze, or a soft infant toothbrush and water, or with an infant tooth cleaner to remove plaque biofilm.

When teeth begin erupting, parents should continue brushing the teeth with a soft infant toothbrush using a fluoride-free toothpaste. The AAPD recommends the first dental visit to occur when the first tooth erupts, typically around 6 months of age, but no later than 1 year. The earlier the dental visit, the better the chances of preventing dental problems. When the child is able to expectorate (usually around 2 to 3 years old), a pea-sized amount of fluoride toothpaste can be used. Because the child does not have the dexterity to thoroughly brush the teeth, the parent should continue brushing the child's teeth.

After the first baby teeth begin to erupt, at-will nighttime feedings should be avoided. Infants and toddlers should never be given a bottle or sippy cup of milk or juice in bed. If the infant is given a bottle in bed, it should contain only water. Children should be weaned from the bottle by 14 months of age. When children are allowed to take the bottle longer, numerous problems can develop, including speech problems, tooth erosion and deformation, and more difficulty in weaning.

Children should be offered a cup as soon as they can hold it in their hands. Between meals, the sippy cup should contain only water. Prolonged use of sugary drinks in sippy cups is a leading cause of pediatric tooth decay.

Early Childhood Caries

Early childhood caries (ECC) is the presence of one or more decayed, missing (as a result of caries), or filled tooth surfaces in any primary tooth in a child younger than 6 years old. ECC is a leading oral health problem among children younger than age 3 years. ECC, the term currently used, replaces the terms severe early childhood caries, nursing bottle caries, baby bottle tooth decay, and is characterized by early rampant decay associated with inappropriate feeding practices (Fig. 14-2). Any sign of smooth surface caries in

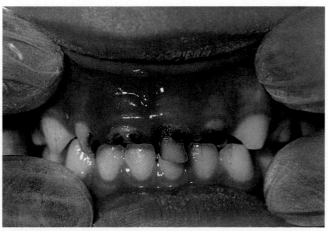

FIGURE 14-2 Early childhood caries. (From Swartz MH: *Textbook of physical diagnosis, history, and examination*, ed 7, St Louis, 2014, Saunders Elsevier.)

children younger than age 3 years is indicative of ECC, which is a serious public health problem, especially prevalent in lower socioeconomic groups. Growth of infants with ECC may be inhibited because of pain associated with eating. Baby teeth are the pattern for the bite for permanent teeth.

Treatment of ECC is costly, requiring extensive extractions or restorations or both, and causing serious future oral health problems and unnecessary suffering. Severe cases are treated under general anesthesia in a hospital. Because it is preventable, healthcare professionals and caregivers need to watch for early warning signs to detect the disease.

Contributing Factors

The primary contributing factor to ECC is infection with *Streptococcus mutans* (cariogenic bacterium). Colonization of *S. mutans* occurs only after the infant's teeth erupt. Infection with the pathogen *S. mutans* is transmitted from the caregiver to the infant. Kissing and sharing utensils or other objects contaminated with saliva are contributing factors. The infant is more likely to be infected if the caregiver has a high level of *S. mutans*. The addition of frequent or prolonged exposure to a fermentable carbohydrate feeds *S. mutans*, allowing it to proliferate and produce cariogenic acid. Destruction of the tooth surface begins and can ultimately progress to rampant caries and abscesses.

Dental caries occur when a sweet liquid (e.g., juice or milk) pools around the lingual surfaces of the teeth for extended periods in the presence of caries-producing bacteria within plaque biofilm (Box 14-1). Acid produced by bacteria leads to demineralization of enamel. Allowing an infant to go to bed at night or at naptime with a bottle, frequent daytime bottles, and habitual use of a no-spill training cup are risk factors for ECC. Breast milk and artificial infant milk are equally cariogenic.

As the child sleeps, cleansing action of saliva is diminished because of reduced salivary flow. The ultimate effect is poor clearance of the drink that has pooled in the mouth. Also, the natural or artificial nipple rests on the palate during sucking, allowing the liquid to pool around the maxillary incisors. The position of the tongue covers and protects the mandibular incisors. Because the disease state follows the eruption pattern, maxillary incisors are affected, followed by first molars, and then canines.

Nutritional Advice

Parents must understand their role in preventing childhood dental disease. Begin dietary advice as soon as the dental team is apprised of the pregnancy. During the initial visit with the child, an assessment can be made to determine the level of fluoride intake and risk of oral problems. Recommendations to parents about controlling oral bacteria and appropriate infant and preschool feeding practices are important. Obtain diet histories of both parents, especially focusing on the primary caregiver to reveal cariogenic eating patterns that may be transferred to the infant. It is critical to analyze the frequency of fermentable carbohydrate intake and oral hygiene habits in order to alert parents to potential problems (see Chapter 18). Intercepting and modifying damaging health practices before birth can prevent ECC and decrease the likelihood of rampant caries in the future.

> ### BOX 14-1   Sources of Fermentable Carbohydrates for Infants
>
> **Liquids**
> - Cow's milk, plain and flavored
> - Breast milk
> - Artificial infant milk
> - Unsweetened fruit juice
> - Sweetened fruit juice and fruit drinks
> - Syrup added to water
> - Sweetened soft drinks
> - Any sugar-sweetened beverages
>
> **Other Sources**
> - Some infant foods
> - Medication
> - Use of sweets to comfort or reward infant, or relieve constipation such as a pacifier dipped in honey or corn syrup
> - Infant cereals, teething biscuits, crackers
> - Dry cereals
> - Arrowroot biscuits and other cookies, pretzels
> - Fruits

Dental Considerations

Assessment
- *Physical:* cursory oral examination to detect decalcification or carious lesions in teeth; frequency of daily cleaning; destructive habits such as lip biting, thumb sucking, tongue thrusting, or pacifier use.
- *Dietary:* parental knowledge of ECC and what causes it; parental preferences for sweets; sharing of utensils contaminated with saliva; use of bottle propping, especially at night, or continual availability of a sippy cup throughout the day; use of corn syrup in the bottle; dipping the bottle nipple or pacifier in honey or molasses; continued use of the bottle after age 1 year; and appropriate fluoride consumption.

Interventions
- Recommend routine dental visits, and provide guidance to parents on feeding practices and nutritional needs.
- Teach parents to clean the infant's gingiva after feedings with a clean cloth. A soft infant toothbrush and water can be used when the infant has several teeth.
- If the water supply is optimally fluoridated, encourage using a pea-sized amount of toothpaste and avoidance of fluoride-containing dentifrices until the child learns to expectorate.
- If a fluoride supplement is recommended, tablets should be thoroughly chewed and swished between the teeth before swallowing. The child should not eat or drink for 30 minutes after taking the supplement and should avoid milk products for 1 hour because calcium may interfere with bioavailability of fluoride.
- Wean the child from the bottle at about 12 months of age or fill the bottle with water.

Dental Considerations—cont'd

- Educate all expectant parents and parents of infants about techniques for avoiding ECC: when feeding an infant, hold the infant and bottle; avoid bottle propping or using the bottle or sippy cup as a pacifier at bedtime or throughout the day. Use other methods instead of a bottle at bedtime and naptime to quiet and relax the child, such as rubbing the child's back, rocking in a chair, singing to the child, or providing a stuffed toy.
- Parents should be advised to avoid saliva-sharing practices, such as sharing a spoon when tasting food, to prevent transmission of caries-causing bacteria (*S. mutans*) to the infant.
- Educate parents about ECC when (a) carious lesions are initially noted in a young child, (b) either parent has active caries or dentures, or (c) sweets are used to comfort or reward the infant.
- Explain the importance of primary teeth (appearance, speech, ability to eat). Patients may be under the false impression that because primary teeth fall out anyway, they serve no purpose.
- Discuss the role of carbohydrates (including those present in fruit juice and milk) in the decay process.
- Utilize *MySmileBuddy*, an internet-based application that helps dental professionals assess a child's risk for ECC and counsel the family on preventive lifestyle changes to prevent ECC.

Nutritional Directions

- Do not let the infant suck the bottle unattended.
- Do not put fruit juice or other carbohydrate-containing beverages in a bottle. Offer juice in a cup.
- Describe disadvantages of rampant decay in an infant (discomfort, future dental phobia, infection, cost, tongue-thrust habit).
- Limit the child's access to a sippy cup containing milk or juice.
- Home filtration systems may remove fluoride, so tests should be conducted to measure fluoride content of filtered and treated water. Most state health departments assess the fluoride content of water for a minimal fee.
- During the first year, foods that require chewing should be added based on the number of erupted teeth.
- Wean infants from the bottle soon after the first birthday.

Cleft Palate and Cleft Lip

One of the most common birth defects in the United States is **cleft lip** or **cleft palate**, or cleft lip/palate, a malformation in which parts of the upper lip or palate fail to grow together. Approximately 1 of 1000 infants is born with cleft lip with or without cleft palate.[31] Scientists believe numerous factors, including drugs, heredity, and folic acid deficiency, may cause this malformation.

The main priority is to ensure adequate nutrition. Feeding the infant with a cleft palate, with or without a cleft lip, presents unique problems. Length of time needed for feedings to provide adequate nutrients can be exhaustive for both mother and infant. Because of the opening between the roof of the mouth and floor of the nasal cavity, negative pressure needed for sucking cannot be created (see Figs. 14-3 and 14-4, *A*). However, breastfeeding sometimes can be successful; the infant adapts by squeezing or chewing the nipple.

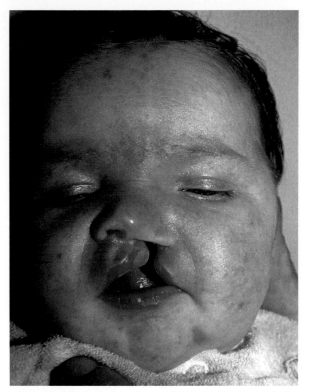

FIGURE 14-3 Cleft lip/palate. (From Kaban L, Troulis M: *Pediatric oral and maxillofacial surgery*, Philadelphia, 2004, Saunders Elsevier.)

Special feeding devices are available if necessary. These are recommended when more than one hour is required per feeding. The infant is held in a sitting position to prevent formula from entering the nose. Other feeding difficulties include nasal regurgitation, excessive air intake, and frequent burping. As soon as possible, spoon feeding is introduced. In severe cases, a prosthesis is made when the child is older (see Fig. 14-4, *B*). Patience is required, and extra time for feeding must be allowed to provide needed nutrients (see guidelines in Box 14-2).

Infants born with cleft palates are at high risk of developmental delays, including motor skill delays. They also have increased rates of dental abnormalities, including supernumerary, missing, or malformed teeth.

Dental Considerations

Assessment
- *Physical:* cleft palate/lip, aspiration.
- *Dietary:* feeding technique and past experiences in feeding infants.

Interventions
- Explain the principal problem is a lack of normal suction, and by modifying feeding techniques, the infant can obtain adequate nutrients.
- Feed the infant slowly at a 60- to 80-degree angle to provide nutrients while minimizing risks.

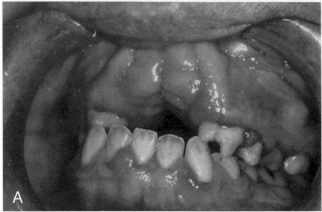

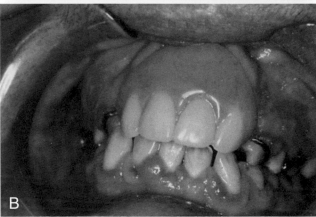

FIGURE 14-4 A, Cleft palate. **B,** Cleft palate with removable prosthesis. (Courtesy of Kathleen B. Muzzin, The Texas A&M University System, Baylor College of Dentistry, Dallas, TX.)

Nutritional Directions

- Introduce spoon feeding as soon as possible.
- Oral skills develop after surgery to correct the problem.
- Acidic and spicy foods may irritate delicate tissue in the cleft area.
- Young children with cleft palate are at increased risk for choking on foods that may slip into the trachea.
- Because of increased incidence of enamel hypoplasia, encourage meticulous oral hygiene practices and limited cariogenic food or liquids to avoid carious lesions at these sites.
- Refer parents to local support groups and to the American Cleft Palate Association for literature.

DIETARY RECOMMENDATIONS AND GUIDELINES FOR GROWTH (CHILDREN OLDER THAN 2 YEARS OF AGE)

The general consensus is that most children's diets "need improvement" or are "poor." Nutrient intakes below the RDA include vitamins C (87%), A (71.6%), and E (11.4%); calcium (78.9%); phosphorus (80.6%); magnesium (62.2%); and fiber (48.2%).[32] Intake of many of these nutrients decreases with age; intake of teenagers, especially girls, is notably lower than intake of younger children. Also of concern are the excessive amounts of several nutrients compared to their Tolerable Upper Intake Levels (UL): sodium intake is more than

double the Adequate Intake (AI), and saturated fat intake of 85% of children is above the Acceptable Macronutrient Distribution Range (AMDR) (Box 14-3). Kilocalories from fats and added sugars account for 39% of total caloric intake. Nutrient inadequacies and excesses are more prevalent in children from households with lower incomes.

Children's diets containing adequate energy and 25% to 35% of total energy from fat have positive effects on health later in life. Omega-3 fatty acids in childhood contribute to ongoing cognitive development.[33] Dietary patterns with high fat, sugar, and processed food content in early childhood may be associated with small reductions in IQ in later childhood as compared with a healthy diet containing principally nutrient-rich foods that may slightly increase IQ.[34]

The *MyPlate* website (http://www.ChooseMyPlate.gov) for preschoolers (ages 2 to 5 years) and children (ages 6 to 11 years) provides guidance for healthy food choices and an active, healthy lifestyle. The website is designed for parents, providing the information they need to help their children make wise food choices. As discussed in Chapter 1, and depicted in Fig. 1-3, the plate divides foods into five major food groups: grains, vegetables, fruits, dairy, and proteins. As children grow, needs may differ from those in the *MyPlate* guide. A doctor, nurse, or RDN should be consulted about a child's nutritional needs and how to best meet them.

The most powerful predictor for how much children eat is how much food is put on their plate. The sections on the plate for kids are the same as for adults, but serving sizes differ, so smaller sized plates are encouraged. One of the keys to the cause and prevention of overweight is knowledge of the caregiver. When parents assume control of food portions or coerce children to eat rather than allowing them to focus

BOX 14-3	Acceptable Macronutrient Distribution Ranges for Children and Adolescents

Acceptable macronutrient distribution ranges (AMDRs) as a percent of energy intake for carbohydrates, fat, and protein are as follows:

- Carbohydrates—45% to 65% of total kilocalories for ages 1 to 18 years
- Fat—30% to 40% of kilocalories for ages 1 to 3 years, and 25% to 35% of kilocalories for ages 4 to 18 years
- Protein—5% to 20% for ages 1 to 3 years, and 10% to 30% for ages 4 to 18 years

Added sugars should not exceed 25% of total calories (to ensure sufficient intake of essential micronutrients). This is a maximum suggested intake and not the amount recommended for achieving a healthful diet.

Consumption of saturated fat, trans fatty acids, and cholesterol should be as low as possible, while maintaining a nutritionally adequate diet.

Adequate intake (AI) for total fiber is as follows:

- Children ages 1 to 3 years: 19 g/day
- Children ages 4 to 8 years: 25 g/day
- Boys ages 9 to 13 years: 31 g/day
- Girls ages 9 to 13 years: 26 g/day

Data adapted from A Report of the Panel on Macronutrients, Subcommittees on Upper Reference Levels of Nutrients and Interpretation and Uses of Dietary Reference Intakes, Standing Committee on the Scientific Evaluation of Dietary Reference Intakes. *Dietary reference intakes for energy, carbohydrate, fiber, fat, fatty acids, cholesterol, protein, and amino acids (macronutrients)*, Washington, DC, 2005, National Academies Press; and U.S. Department of Agriculture and U.S. Department of Health and Human Services: *Dietary guidelines for Americans*, ed 7, Washington, DC, December 2010, U.S. Government Printing Office.

on internal cues of hunger, children's ability to regulate their own meal size is diminished. Large portion sizes of snacks and fast foods parallel dramatic increases in childhood obesity. Portion sizes and numbers of servings increase when children reach puberty, and needs are greater because of accelerated growth rate and increased size, but one of the principal concerns is an inappropriate increase in portion sizes contributing to the prevalence of overweight. Family mealtime is essential for children's nutrition, health, and overall well-being.

"Health and Nutrition Information" (http://www.choosemyplate.gov/preschoolers.html and http://www.choosemyplate.gov/children-over-five.html) provides guidelines, tips, and encouragement for mothers to help children (a) grow up healthy, (b) develop positive eating habits, (c) try new foods, (d) play actively every day, and (e) follow food safety rules. This website provides information about appropriate foods and portion sizes and suggestions for meal patterns or snacks. After creating a profile in *SuperTracker*, menus can be analyzed for adequacy, and *Food-A-Pedia* can help determine nutritional information for specific foods. Additionally, kitchen activities with preschoolers are suggested. Being healthy role models for their children is the most important step for parents to take.

"Health & Nutrition Information for Children Over Five" provides an interactive computer-based game called "Blast Off," which helps children become more aware of the connection between their food choices and physical activities. Concrete examples are provided on how to choose the right foods from each food group for "lift off." It is a fun way for children to learn about their nutritional needs, and the child must stay engaged in the activity for at least one hour to provide the space shuttle with adequate battery power for launching. The website also has links to coloring pages, worksheets, and classroom materials for teachers.

MyPlateKidsPlace (http://www.choosemyplate.gov/kids/), designed for children 8 to 12 years old, also helps parents and healthcare educators encourage healthier food choices. This webpage includes games, activity sheets, recipes, and tips.

The key message of *Dietary Guidelines* (variety, moderation, and balance in food choices) applies to childhood nutrition. Physical activity is also important. The main concern with providing dietary recommendations and guidelines for children older than 2 years is to (a) provide adequate kilocalories and nutrients to support growth and development, and (b) reduce risk of diet-related chronic diseases later in life (see Box 14-3). Children's diets need improvement, especially increasing consumption of whole fruit, whole grains, dark green and orange vegetables, and legumes. On the other hand, they usually consume too much saturated fat, sodium, and added sugars and fats.

After many studies and much deliberation, the AAP Committee on Nutrition recommends that between ages 2 and 5 years, children should gradually adopt a diet consistent with the *Dietary Guidelines* in regard to fats and cholesterol. The basic reasoning for implementing the fat and cholesterol guideline is based on the fact that childhood obesity and cholesterol levels usually continue into adulthood. Fat intake in children should be maintained at a moderate level (25% to 35% of kilocalories) to ensure their genetic growth potential. By using fat-free or low-fat or equivalent milk products instead of reduced-fat or whole milk (for children older than age 2 years), lean meats in place of higher fat meats, or lower fat products rather than high-fat products, energy and nutrient requirements can be achieved. Though the average percentage of energy from total fat and saturated fat in 2000 had decreased from 1971, still only 38% of the population 2 years and older met the guideline of less than 30% of energy from total fat, and 41% met the guideline of 10% or less of energy from saturated fat.[35] Serum lipids have improved in recent decades, but almost 1 in 10 youth have an elevated total cholesterol level.[36]

A BMI above the normal range significantly increases the risks for CHD in school aged children.[37] The AAP and American Medical Association recommend screening children 2 to 10 years old who have a genetic predisposition for CHD, or who have other risk factors for cardiovascular disease, such as obesity, hypertension, and diabetes.[38,39] The

Expert Panel recommends that all children older than 2 years should follow the *Dietary Guidelines* and make lifestyle changes, such as increasing physical activity and making dietary changes. Most children with abnormal cholesterol levels should be treated with diet and physical activity; a few with very high levels of low-density lipoproteins, the "bad" cholesterol, should consider drug treatment, especially if other risk factors are present. Although there are no studies showing long-term safety or effectiveness of nutritional modifications, lifestyle changes, or medications to prevent development of CHD, the safety and efficacy of these modifications appear to be similar to effects in adults.

Dietary modifications are similar to those recommended for adults (see Chapter 6). However, these dietary adjustments may require involvement of a RDN to help families make appropriate changes without compromising good nutrition. Children can learn how to read food labels and determine which foods are healthier selections. The entire family usually benefits from implementing these guidelines.

Energy needs of children and adolescents are high to support growth and development, and energy intake must balance with the child's physical activity level and/or other genetic and environmental factors (Table 14-3). Prepubescent children burn more fat per kilocalorie of energy expended than adults and need fat to fuel growth.

Physical activity is important for bone mineralization, growth, and cardiovascular health. Parents should encourage individual physical activities and model them for the children (Fig. 14-5).[39] Children should be given the opportunity to participate in a variety of activities, from walking to jumping rope to competitive sports. In reality, children will not be physically active unless they are having fun. Activity is important in helping control weight and reducing the risk for heart attack, colon cancer, diabetes, and high blood pressure.

The *Physical Activity* links on the *MyPlate* website and the *Let's Move!* (http://www.letsmove.gov) website provide information and encourage physical activities to help balance energy intake for a healthy lifestyle. The Institute of Medicine (IOM) recommends that childcare providers provide toddlers and preschool children with "opportunities for light, moderate, and vigorous physical activity for at least 15 minutes per hour while children are in care."[40] This translates to 3 hours daily for children who are in daycare for 12 hours; Australia and Great Britain have made similar

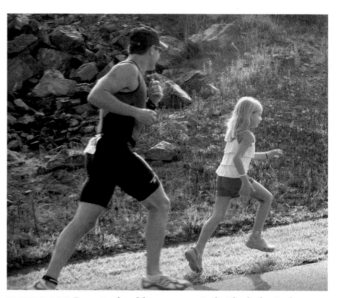

FIGURE 14-5 Parents should encourage individual physical activities and model these behaviors. (Photo courtesy of Sara Birkemeier, Raleigh, NC.)

Table 14-3	Daily estimated calories and recommended servings for children, by age and sex						
Nutrient/Food Group		**Girls**			**Boys**		
	2-3 Years Old	4-8 Years Old	9-13 Years Old	14-18 Years Old	4-8 Years Old	9-13 Years Old	14-18 Years Old
Calories*	1000-1400	1400-1600	1600-2000	2000	1400-1600	1800-2200	2400-2800
Protein foods (lean meat/beans) (oz equivalents)	2	4	5	5	4	5	6½
Dairy (cup)	2	2½	3	3	2½	3	3
Fruits (cup)	1	1½	1½	1½	1½	1½	2
Vegetables (cup)	1	1½	2	2½	1½	2½	3
Grains (oz equivalents)†	3	5	5	6	5	6	8
Oils (tsp)	3	4	5	5	4	5	6

From U.S. Department of Agriculture and U.S. Department of Health and Human Services. *Dietary guidelines for Americans*, ed 7, Washington, DC, December 2010, U.S. Government Printing Office.
*Calorie estimates are based on a moderately active lifestyle. Physical activity requires up to 200 kcal/day increase for physically active lifestyle or a decrease of up to 200 kcal/day for a sedentary lifestyle.
†Half of all grains should be whole grains.

recommendations. The Physical Activity Guidelines for Americans recommended by the U.S. Department of Health and Human Services advocates one hour or more of physical activity for children 6 to 17 years old. Most of the 60 or more minutes should be either moderate- or vigorous-intensity aerobic physical activity and should include vigorous-intensity physical activity at least three days a week; part of the 60 or more minutes of daily physical activity should include muscle-strengthening physical activity at least three days a week; part of the 60 or more minutes of daily physical activity should include bone-strengthening physical activities at least three days a week.[41] *SuperTracker* (http://www.choosemyplate.gov/supertracker-tools.html) can be used to record time spent in various activities to determine kilocalories expended.

Several organizations have endorsed the recommendation that a reasonable goal for dietary fiber intake during childhood and adolescence is approximately equivalent to the age of the child plus 5 g/day. This formula (age >5) represents a level that would provide health benefits, such as normal laxation, without compromising mineral balance or caloric intake in children older than 2 years of age. Based on this formula, the daily minimal dietary fiber intake would be 8 g/day for a 3-year-old, and would gradually increase to 20 g for a 15-year-old. The gradual increases are consistent with current guidelines for adult dietary fiber intake (25 to 35 g/day). Average dietary fiber intake among children 2 to 11 years old is 6.68 g/100 kcal; it is 6.15 g/1000 kcal for children 12 to 18 years old.[42] This is more than 60% lower than the recommendation. By using whole-grain breads and cereals, as recommended in the *Dietary Guidelines*, fiber and other nutrient guidelines can be met. At least half of the grain servings should be whole grains. The *Dietary Guidelines* and *MyPlate* promote increasing fruit and vegetable consumption to five or more servings daily. To increase fiber intake, fresh fruits are recommended over fruit juice. Unfortunately, fruit juice consumption has increased significantly over the years.[43]

Because of the high calcium requirement to increase bone mineral density in children, milk and dairy products are an essential part of the child's diet. Calcium levels were established for achievement of optimal bone mineral health to decrease the risk of osteoporosis later in life. Inadequate amounts of calcium and vitamin D during the toddler years, however, could cause rickets when infants are weaned to diets with minimal dairy content. Adolescents (12 to 19 years old) typically consume about 1 cup of milk daily and children (2 to 11 years old) consume about $1\frac{1}{3}$ cup.[44] Calcium intake can be favorably increased by using calcium-fortified beverages, such as orange juice with calcium or milk products such as low fat yogurt. Milk is also the primary contributor of phosphorus, magnesium, and potassium in children's diets. The percentage of preschool children that consume milk decreased from 85% in 1976 to 77% in 1994.[45]

TODDLER AND PRESCHOOL CHILDREN

Growth

After the child reaches 1 year of age, the growth spurt slows down. A toddler gains approximately 4 to 6 lb until 2 years old, and height doubles by age 4 years. In a normally growing child, height increases parallel that of weight. Children grow approximately 2 to 3 inches a year and gain around 5 lb a year. One-half of adult height is achieved by $2\frac{1}{2}$ to 3 years of age.

Nutrient Requirements

During the past 30 years, the nutritional status of children in the United States has improved, with few nutrient deficiencies being observed. Iron, zinc, calcium, and vitamin D are frequently deficient in the diet. Poor nutritional status of children (as measured by growth rate and biochemical indices) is generally more prevalent in lower socioeconomic groups, in which the amounts and variety of foods may be limited. Although most children fail to meet recommendations in *MyPlate* (especially in fruits, vegetables, whole grains, and dairy groups), average intake of most vitamins and minerals in 2- to 11-year-olds is adequate.

Anemia remains a public health concern among young (less than 2 years old) low-income children. Approximately 10% of all children, regardless of socioeconomic background, may be iron deficient. The incidence of anemia usually declines with age and is observed consistently more often in African American children than in white, Asian, Native American, or Hispanic children. Iron-rich foods, such as meat, and fresh fruits and vegetables that contain vitamin C, which enhance iron absorption, are expensive compared with calorically-dense foods such as chips or candy. Milk is a poor source of iron, and large amounts of milk deter absorption of iron. Iron deficiency during infancy results in lower cognitive abilities and motor skills that continue throughout childhood and adolescence.

As mentioned earlier, research studies note that ensuring vitamin D sufficiency throughout childhood and during the time of maximal bone mineral accrual seems particularly warranted. Depending on vitamin D intake, a supplement may be needed.

Because of high activity level, basal metabolic rate, and growth, the caloric requirement is relatively high, roughly 1000 kcal plus 100 kcal per year of life. Younger children need to eat foods with high nutrient and energy density because they are unable to eat large quantities of food at any particular time. Healthy snacks can contribute vital nutrients. The extra nutrient needs for growth and development result in dietary deficiencies occurring more quickly and with more severe consequences than in adults. Table 14-4 lists the dietary reference intakes (DRIs) for major nutrients. However, overweight is pandemic (see *Health Application 14*). By striving toward healthy eating and physically active habits, children may achieve healthful weights, which may prevent lifetime risks of chronic health problems.

Table 14-4   Dietary reference intakes for selected nutrients for children through adolescence

Nutrients	Children 1-3 Years Old	Children 4-8 Years Old	9-13 Years Old		14-18 Years Old	
			Boys	Girls	Boys	Girls
Protein (g)	**13**	**19**	**34**	**34**	**52**	**46**
Vitamin C (mg)	**15**	**25**	**45**	**45**	**75**	**65**
Calcium (mg)	**700**	**1,000**	**1,300**	**1,300**	**1,300**	**1,300**
Iron (mg)	**7**	**10**	**8**	**8**	**11**	**15**
Total fiber (g)	19*	25*	31*	26*	38*	26*

Data from National Research Council: *The guide to nutrient requirements*, Washington, DC, 2006, National Academies Press);and National Research Council: *Dietary reference intakes for calcium and vitamin D*, Washington, DC, 2011, National Academies Press. Available at www.nap.edu.
Note: Recommended dietary allowances (RDAs) are presented in **bold type** and adequate intakes (AIs) are followed by an asterisk (*).

Food-Related Behaviors

Lifelong habits and food attitudes are formed during pre-school years that to some extent affect health throughout life. A variety of foods should be available providing the needed nutrients. Basic understanding of nutrient content of foods, the role of foods in health, and food-related behaviors for these age groups is important for parents to promote food habits conducive to adequate nutrient intake (Box 14-4). Healthful eating produces benefits in cognitive and physical performance, fitness, psychological well-being, and energy level.

Parental attitudes and food preferences, eating habits, and food choices are influential factors in the child's food preferences. Foods disliked by one or both parents are not served often or may not be served at all. The key influence on the quality of children's diet is the quality of the primary caregiver's diet. Children model their parents and tend to enjoy foods preferred by their parents. Providing fruits for snacks and serving vegetables at mealtime affect a preschooler's eating patterns for life.

When planning menus, parents must consider the child's food preferences, but parents should control the options. Without appropriate guidance, young children do not independently make healthy food choices; the parents' role is to offer nutritious foods. Children can choose how much or even whether they will eat the food provided. Feeding problems can result when either the parent or child crosses this line of responsibility. More food is eaten by the child when the family eats together, rather than just offering food for the child to eat alone.

Toddlers (1 to 3 Years Old)

During the second year of life, development of fine motor skills results in toddlers learning to feed themselves, but skills and capabilities do not occur at exactly the same time for every child. Although this is a messy learning process, this transitional period stabilizes by age 2 years. Finger feeding may be preferred to spoon feeding; some finger foods should be provided at every meal. A toddler can manipulate a cup by about 18 months of age. Rotary chewing skills develop in the second year. Until then, finely chopped meats are accepted better and minimize the risk of choking.

BOX 14-4   Healthy Snack Choices

- Cut-up fresh vegetables with low-fat dip or salad dressing
- Air-popped popcorn with a sprinkle of parmesan cheese
- Fresh fruit*
- Frozen fruit (grapes, bananas)*
- Nuts
- Low-fat cheese (sticks, strings, cubes, or slices)
- Low-fat cottage cheese or yogurt
- Peanut butter on apple slices* or celery sticks
- Pretzels*
- Baked chips*
- Hard-boiled eggs
- Animal crackers*
- Graham crackers*
- Sliced turkey or chicken
- Dry, low-sugar cereal*
- Rice cakes*
- Low-fat pudding*
- Sugar-free gelatin with fruit
- Mini bagels*
- Pickles
- Frozen juice bars*

*Cariogenic potential. Encourage tooth-brushing after snacks.

Toddlers prefer regularity, so eating at the same time is desirable and helps control appetite. Regular meals also help to avoid fatigue, which can lead to an overly emotional situation that interferes with appetite. Tired children eat poorly. If the child has been very active, a short rest period before the meal improves intake.

Small amounts of food should be offered several times a day. Serving sizes should be based on appetite, but initially about 1 Tbsp can be offered for each year of age. Studies show that providing larger than age-appropriate portion sizes may result in children consuming more food and kilocalories. They do not compensate for this by adjusting the amount they eat in response to how much they ate at the previous meal or in the past 24 hours, or the caloric density of their meal. When children serve themselves from family size bowls, they choose smaller portions and are less likely to overeat. The amount of liquids consumed can affect the child's appetite. Either the child has a poor appetite for foods or consumes more food in addition to the kilocalories provided in liquid form, which can increase the risk of obesity.

Brightly colored foods are especially appealing to children. Children older than 1½ years of age who are still taking a bottle containing milk or sweetened liquids are more likely to be overweight and to develop anemia because of low iron intake, in addition to increased risk of tooth decay.

Food jags—refusing to eat anything except one food for several days—in toddlers and children are common and are a way to assert independence. This typical developmental stage is temporary. The food obsession may cause parental concern, but overreaction may prolong rather than correct such behaviors. Refusing to eat is a way to attract attention. Appetites, which are erratic and unpredictable, are a strong reflection of the current growth rate. Parents should not force children to eat when they are not hungry. When well-balanced meals are provided, caloric intake at any given meal varies greatly, but compensation at subsequent meals results in little variability in total energy intake. If sufficient amounts are not eaten at the meal, parents may limit snacking or provide nutrient-dense snacks. Snacks can contribute significantly to adequate nutrient intake (see Box 14-4).

Until age 4 years, children are at risk for choking on food that gets caught in the airway. Food is not chewed thoroughly until the molars erupt. To prevent choking, closely supervise children while eating, and do not allow walking, playing, talking, laughing, crying, or lying down while they are eating. Additionally, avoid foods most likely to cause choking: (a) small nuts and seeds; (b) round, firm, smooth foods such as grapes, hard candy, hot dogs, and round candies; (c) dry or hard foods such as raw carrots, cookies, pieces of pretzels, potato chips, and popcorn; and (d) sticky or tough foods such as peanut butter, raisins, tough meat, and caramel candy.

Preschool Children (4 to 6 Years Old)

Preschoolers are relatively independent at the table and can feed themselves. Certain factors need to be considered to make the mealtime pleasant rather than an ordeal. By allowing children to eat with adults, they imitate adults in manners and food habits. Parental insistence on proper utensil usage, manners, and other demands is inappropriate for this age group and may result in less food intake. Parents need to ignore some inappropriate mealtime behaviors and focus on positive non-mealtime activities. Conversation and role modeling can reinforce appropriate eating behavior and promote food intake.

Few children eat the recommended five servings of fruits and vegetables daily. Strong-flavored vegetables (overcooked cabbage and onions) are generally disliked, but are more popular if served raw. Crisp, raw vegetables are well accepted. Tough stringy fibers, such as those in celery or string beans, should be removed. Because preschool children still enjoy eating with their fingers, cutting fruits and vegetables into small pieces increases their acceptance.

Preschoolers generally prefer their foods separate; casseroles and stews may not be well accepted. Foods that can be easily chewed are more readily accepted. Snacks are still important for adequate nutrient intake (see Box 14-4). The body uses food more effectively and energy levels are more consistent when children "refuel" every 2 to 4 hours. The number of snacks varies, depending on the family schedule and the child's activity and hunger levels. Parents should lead by example. When parents eat more fruits and vegetables, so do their children.

Preschoolers are likely to be suspicious of any new foods introduced. Eight to 15 exposures to a new food may be needed to achieve acceptance. Even after they have accepted a food, preschool children may not eat it every time it is served. Rather than bargaining with a child who does not want what is on the menu or become a short-order cook, it is better to give the child the option to eat or not. Children eventually eat more of what they should eat if they are not forced to eat it.

Dental Considerations

Assessment

- *Physical:* socioeconomic level, child's age, and child's developmental level.
- *Dietary:* eating environment, frequency of meals and snacks, quantity of foods consumed, adequacy of intake, parental beliefs and food preferences.

Interventions

- Encourage eating meals at regular times. Serve food shortly after being seated to avoid restless behavior.
- Evaluate and assess children's diets at regular intervals.
- Growth charts are available on the *MyPlate* and Evolve websites for children that can be used by parents to instill healthy eating habits during the most influential time for determining a child's future food choices.
- Stress the importance of providing adequate amounts of protein; vitamins A, C, and D; calcium; phosphorus; and fluoride during formation and calcification of teeth.
- If sufficient amounts are not eaten, limit snacking or provide nutrient-dense snacks; offer cheese cubes, fresh fruit, raw vegetable sticks, low-fat milk or yogurt, fruit juices, whole-grain cereals, and bread.
- Consider the parents' attitudes, cultures, beliefs, fears, and educational levels when developing and providing oral health education.
- Help parents clarify any misconceptions interfering with a child's ability to consume foods to meet their nutrient needs for growth and development, such as "healthy foods do not taste good" or "healthful eating means eliminating all high-fat foods."
- Recommendations for fluoride usage should be determined by need, based on risk indicators.
- Encourage the use of fluoridated toothpastes for children older than 2 to 3 years.
- Encourage parents to assume responsibility for the child's oral healthcare and model good oral health behaviors.
- Refer low-income patients to any government or local social programs (WIC, food stamp program) for which they may be eligible.

Nutritional Directions

- The goal for parents is to prevent caries and plaque biofilm formation.
- The child is expected to taste each new food that is prepared and served, but the taste may be very small.
- Atherosclerosis probably begins in childhood; a reduction of dietary fats (especially saturated) and cholesterol after the second birthday most likely decreases the risk of this disease. However, undue restriction of fat intake could compromise a child's growth and development, and potentially lead to eating disorders or unhealthy attitudes about food.
- Until age 6 years, a good rule of thumb is 1 Tbsp of vegetables, fruit, or meat per year of life.
- Food, especially sweet foods, should not be used as a bribe or reward.
- Teach children to recognize and honor their hunger and satiety cues rather than cleaning their plates.
- Children who are told to "clean your plate" may have a more negative response and consume less food.
- Caregivers must understand that diet and lifestyle choices during early childhood affect lifelong eating patterns and have an impact on later disease risk. Accelerated weight and fat mass gain seem to predict adult disease conditions.
- Present disliked foods in a matter-of-fact manner, serving small portions (1 to 2 Tbsp); discard without comment if the child does not eat them.
- Successful childhood feeding may be best accomplished by providing a variety of healthful foods and allowing children to eat without coercion.
- Provide healthy snacks, but prevent the child from grazing throughout the day to ensure a good appetite at meal time (see Box 14-4).
- Children who avoid drinking milk are at increased risk for prepubertal fractures.
- Children generally eat better when the family or at least one adult sits at the table and eats with them.
- Offer a wide variety of vegetables and fruits daily, especially dark green, leafy, and deep yellow vegetables and colorful fruits.
- Water is the ideal beverage between meals; omitting sugar-sweetened beverages (sodas and fruit juice) helps prevent risks of excess weight gain (by limiting extra kilocalories) and dental caries (by lowering the frequency of tooth exposure to sugar).
- If a wide variety of foods is offered to toddlers who are healthy and growing appropriately, parents need not be overly concerned about risk of nutrient deficiency.
- Teach the child to use a pea-size amount of toothpaste to limit the amount accidentally swallowed.
- A dental examination is recommended every 6 to 12 months; topical fluoride may be applied if the water supply is not fluoridated. The dental team determines the appropriate fluoride regimen for each child.
- Encourage children to eat whole fruits rather than drink fruit juices and beverages.
- Good oral health is directly correlated to good dietary habits that promote daily breakfast consumption and fruit and vegetable intake in conjunction with fluoridation.

ATTENTION-DEFICIT/HYPERACTIVITY DISORDER

Attention-deficit/hyperactivity disorder (ADHD) is the most common developmental disorder of childhood. Despite the fact that parents report that between 5.6% and 15.6% of children 4 to 17 years of age have ADHD, only approximately 3% to 7% of these children are diagnosed with ADHD.[46] Hyperactivity is characterized by chronic age-inappropriate behaviors, including inattention, impulsiveness, hyperactivity, or restlessness. For a diagnosis of ADHD, the child must exhibit specific symptoms before age 7 years. Many theories have been proposed on the causes of hyperactivity, but none has been proven conclusively. Inherited genetic factors affecting the function of chemicals in the brain that help regulate attention and activity may be responsible. The National Institute of Mental Health indicates that certain parts of the brains of children with ADHD develop about 3 years later than children without ADHD.[47]

Many parents and teachers believe sugar causes hyperactivity, or ADHD, in children. Two theories have been proposed for sugar affecting behavior: (a) an allergic response to sugar and (b) a hypoglycemic response. A meta-analysis of scientific studies indicated that sugar does not affect behavior or cognitive performance of children.[48] The origin of the idea that sugar is responsible for hyperactivity seems to be purely based on the fact that sugar is a source of energy, as are other carbohydrates. External cues, such as parties or celebrations, possibly associated with a higher sugar intake, may cause hyperactivity, not the increased sugar intake.

Some studies suggest several food additives (e.g., colorings, flavorings, and preservatives) may increase hyperactivity in children with behavior problems. Restriction of synthetic food color additives for children with ADHD has been identified to be beneficial for some children, but appears to be more effective in individuals with food sensitivities.[49,50] Some children with ADHD and a personal or family history of food allergies show slight improvement of ADHD by eliminating the allergic foods. Researchers found only small benefits associated with supplementation of omega-3 and omega-6 fatty acids.

For children exhibiting behavior problems such as hyperactivity, the use of dietary manipulation tends to be a more acceptable approach to treatment than use of drugs, but evidence of an association between diet and behaviors is considered weak and limited. The use of dietary treatments alone is unlikely to be sufficient treatment for many children with ADHD. Many experts agree and recommend a nutritionally well-balanced, high-protein diet that limits added sugars and more complex carbohydrates, and ensures sufficient amounts of omega-3 fatty acids. Inappropriate dietary treatment without scientific support could (a) detract from efforts to identify effective treatment and prevention of delinquent behavior; (b) lead to nutritional deficiencies or excesses; and (c) provide offenders with a dietary excuse for their behavior, rather than assuming responsibility for their own behavior. Data supporting new treatments for ADHD should be scrutinized for scientific study design, clinical safety, and scientific validity before recommending them as modes of therapy.

CHILDREN WITH SPECIAL NEEDS

Health conditions, such as mental retardation of unknown origin, cerebral palsy, Down syndrome, infantile autism, and muscular dystrophy, have significant oral health and oral hygiene implications. Gum disease is frequently observed in children with Down syndrome. Mastication and swallowing problems occur in all these conditions except Down syndrome. Some children with oral–motor problems can improve; others cannot.

Children with cerebral palsy and Down syndrome may practice bruxism. Bruxism is involuntary grinding or clenching of teeth, which results in abnormal wear patterns on teeth and joint or neuromuscular problems. Loosened teeth interfere with the child eating chewy foods such as meats. Children with cerebral palsy, Down syndrome, and intellectual disabilities are likely to have abnormal sensory input and muscle tone. Difficulties with sucking, swallowing, spoon-feeding skills with semisolid or solid foods, chewing development, and independent feeding are common. Tongue thrust associated with many of these conditions results in significant food waste and may jeopardize nutritional status. Dental problems may become exaggerated in these children as a result of difficulty in maintaining good oral hygiene, the child's unique dietary habits and patterns, and the effect of their prescribed medications. Such problems include oral infections, dental caries, and periodontal disease.

The dental hygienist may become involved in team treatment of these children. Treatment is individualized, depending on potential capabilities and skills of the child. Nutritional intervention for feeding skill difficulties is assistance in planning a diet that is easiest for the child to eat and still meets nutritional needs.

Dental Considerations

Assessment
- *Physical:* condition of the oral cavity, presence of dental caries, plaque biofilm, abnormal oral-motor habits, such as tongue thrust, bruxism, oral–motor development, medications.
- *Dietary:* intake of fermentable carbohydrates, frequency of snacking, calcium and vitamin D intake, source of fluoride, pica.

Interventions
- Behaviors that are rewarded will increase in frequency. Provide reinforcement throughout the dental procedure by verbally praising desirable behavior, tangible rewards (stickers, tattoos, baseball cards) or a behavioral contract. Provide appropriate recommendations or referrals.
- Because these children are less likely to maintain good oral hygiene, recare appointments should be scheduled more frequently.

Nutritional Directions

- Provide nutritious snacks such as cheese cubes or raw vegetables. Fibrous foods promote salivary flow, increasing the buffering capacity of saliva.
- Vitamin D–fortified milk and cheeses not only provide nutrients needed for healthy teeth, but also are cariostatic.
- Provide an opportunity to brush the teeth after eating; if brushing is impossible, rinse mouth with water.
- Inappropriate dietary habits and unhealthy food preferences developed during childhood have lifelong implications.
- Limit sticky carbohydrate foods, such as candies, cookies, crackers, pastries, and raisins, between meals. If these foods are frequently consumed as snacks, the carbohydrate content and physical properties of these foods may contribute to dental caries risk.

SCHOOL-AGE CHILDREN (7 TO 12 YEARS OLD)

Middle childhood years are the result of early growth and development; reserves provide stores for upcoming rapid adolescent growth. New activities and new friends begin to influence choices and broaden the child's horizon. Students who choose an adequate amount of fruit, vegetables, protein, fiber, and other components of a healthy diet are more likely to perform better in school.[51] The child is exposed to different foods and food patterns and usually begins to accept more foods. These new ideas may affect food choices at home.

Almost all foods are liked. Vegetables are the least favorite, with only 22% of all children consuming three servings daily. Planning menus around food groups is important to include all the necessary nutrients. Foods containing mostly sugars or fats need not be eliminated, but they should not replace recommended amounts from the food groups. The appetite is usually good; but food habits and intake may suffer because children do not take time for meals (15 to 20 minutes). Enforcement of a specific amount of time to eat may prevent the child from forming the habit of eating too fast. Poor appetite may be caused by stresses, such as schoolwork and emotional difficulties.

Students are ravenous after school. Although bakery products, soft drinks, candy, and chips are favorites, nutritious snacks are preferable. More access to money and the influence of peers and mass media may result in expenditures at fast food restaurants and from vending machines. These foods are usually high in fat, salt, and sugar.

Children may continue to have problems with allergies to milk and eggs. Children with allergies to milk, egg, wheat, and soy may outgrow their allergy by age 5 years, but allergies to peanuts, tree nuts, fish, or shellfish are generally lifelong allergies.[52]

Dental Caries in School-Age Children

According to the CDC, trends in oral health prevalence of untreated tooth caries in the permanent teeth of children 6 to 19 years old decreased from approximately 23.6% in

1988-1994 to 16.2% in 2005-2008. Although strides are being made in prevention of tooth decay, this disease remains a problem for some racial, ethnic, and lower socioeconomic groups who continue to have more treated and untreated tooth decay compared with other groups. In children from families at less than 200% of the poverty level, only 26.7% of children have had a dental visit in the past year.[53] Children with untreated dental disease miss more days from school, may be unable to concentrate in school, and have poorer academic performance in addition to having feelings of embarrassment, withdrawal and anxiety.[54]

This age range also generally marks exfoliation of all or most of the primary teeth and the eruption of most permanent teeth. This is significant because application of topical fluoride (professionally applied and self-applied) now becomes as effective as systemic fluoride administration. Topical administration of fluoride can help in reduction of tooth decay. Topical fluoride sources include dentifrices, rinses, gels, fluoride supplements, varnishes, and fluoridated water. Systemic fluoride is effective before eruption and during the mineralization phase of erupting teeth. When 1 ppm of fluoride in drinking water is present during tooth formation, caries rate is reduced 60% along with reduction in prevalence of plaque biofilm and remineralization of teeth. To provide maximum protection, systemic fluoride is recommended through age 16 years for children in nonfluoridated or inadequately fluoridated areas.

Application of sealants (a clear or shaded plastic material applied to occlusal surfaces of permanent teeth) acts as a barrier protecting decay-prone areas of teeth from plaque biofilm and acid. Approximately 25.5% of children 6 to 9 years old and 19% of teens 12 to 19 years old have had sealants applied.[55] However, even the combined use of a toothbrush, dental floss, fluoride toothpaste, and sealants cannot completely control caries formation.

Another factor in caries formation is food selection and patterns of consumption. Cariogenicity of food is influenced by the presence of fermentable carbohydrates, physical properties, and frequency of consumption (see Chapter 18). The use of products (e.g., chewing gum, candy, topical oral syrup) containing xylitol can be effective in preventing tooth decay by reducing levels of harmful *S. mutans* bacteria in plaque biofilm.[56]

Dental Considerations

Assessment
- *Physical:* schoolwork or emotional difficulties, activity level, sports interests.
- *Dietary:* nutrient and fluid intake, appetite, food preferences and eating patterns, child's and parent's beliefs about nutrition.

Interventions
- Recommend nutritious snacks be readily available (see Box 14-4). Cutting foods into shapes often creates interest in the snack, such as cheese sandwiches cut into stars.

- Evaluate sources of fluoride to ensure optimal intake to protect erupting and newly erupted teeth, while minimizing excessive intake and risk for fluorosis.
- Antimicrobial agents, such as chlorhexidine, can be used to control existing plaque biofilm and formation of new plaque biofilm by controlling bacteria and limiting acid production.
- Ask low-income patients about the child's participation in governmental child nutrition programs (National School Lunch, School Breakfast, Summer Food Service, and Special Milk).

Nutritional Directions

- Children involved in meal preparation are more likely to eat the food they prepare and to be aware of what is in the food.
- Have nutritious foods available for snacks, such as sliced apples, yogurt, popcorn, low-fat cheese, or dry roasted seeds or nuts.
- As children grow older, they consume larger quantities of food, but food choices deviate more from the *Dietary Guidelines*.
- Encourage appropriate oral hygiene techniques.

ADOLESCENTS
Growth and Nutrient Requirements

Major biological, social, psychological, and cognitive changes occur during adolescence. Because of these changes and rapid growth rates, 17% of U.S. teenagers are considered to be at nutritional risk, consuming inadequate amounts of nutrients. Healthy eating helps reduce one's risk for becoming obese, or developing osteoporosis, iron-deficiency anemia, and dental caries. Poor dietary habits result in inadequate intake of folate; vitamins A, B_1, B_6, C, and D; iron; and calcium. Many adolescent eating practices place them at risk for developing chronic diseases later in life.

Poor food choices result in poor compliance with *MyPlate* and the *Dietary Guidelines*. The caloric percentage of dietary fat intake for adolescent boys and girls in 2002-2004 was approximately 33%, with approximately 21% of the kilocalories from solid fats.[57] Declining fitness levels are another contributing factor for weight gain. The American Heart Association is concerned that poor cardiovascular health behaviors, especially physical activity and dietary intake, will contribute to a worsening prevalence of obesity, hypertension, hypercholesterolemia, and diabetes as current adolescents reach adulthood.[58]

Fiber intake is about one-half the recommended amount. The lack of dietary fiber and excessive amounts of fat could be corrected by increasing fruit and vegetable consumption and choosing more whole-grain products. Researchers found that high school students consume fruits and vegetables 1.2 times per day. Overall, 28.5% of these students consumed one fruit or less daily and 33.2% consumed vegetables less than once a day.[59]

The slow childhood growth rate accelerates with pubescence until the rate is as rapid as that of early infancy. Growth of long bones, secondary sexual maturation, and fat and muscle deposition create increased nutrient requirements. The end of this adolescent growth spurt is signaled by a deceleration of growth, completion of sexual maturation, and closure of the epiphyses of long bones.

Although the DRIs provide nutrient recommendations based on chronological age, nutrient needs closely parallel physical development. Adolescent girls need to increase their energy intake sooner and decrease it more quickly than boys because of earlier onset of puberty and lower total body weight after adulthood is reached. Adolescent boys have greater nutritional needs than adolescent girls because of growth rates and body composition changes (see Table 14-4). A very active 18-year-old boy requires approximately 3800 kcal compared with almost 2900 kcal for an 18-year-old girl. Most adolescents need and are able to eat large quantities of food many times a day. However, teens need to be careful of amounts and frequency of eating when their rapid growth rate levels off.

Average protein intake is well above recommendations (see Table 14-4). However, if for any reason, such as weight-loss diets or chronic illness, overall intake becomes insufficient, dietary protein may be used to meet energy needs and would not be available for needed growth and repair.

The need for calcium, vitamin D, and iron is of particular importance throughout childhood. Adolescents are particularly vulnerable to an insult to their bones. A lack of calcium or vitamin D can have profound implications for their future skeletal health because mild deficiency of either can be unrecognized until severe skeletal damage has occurred. During adolescence, 45% of adult skeletal mass is formed; calcium needs are greater than at any other time of life. Building good bone mass during adolescence is thought to be the best way to prevent osteoporosis in old age. Physicians and healthcare educators should talk with teenagers about the importance of bone health, achieving maximum bone density, and maintaining strong bones. Boys and girls ages 9 to 13 years, and girls between the ages of 14 and 18 years are getting less than 50% of their respective DRIs from foods and supplements.[60] Daily calcium intake of 1300 mg in addition to exercise during adolescence promotes calcium retention and bone mineral density. Studies suggest the possibility of a relationship between vitamin D levels and bone mineral density in adolescents. Vitamin D deficiency in adolescents may possibly place them at risk for later osteoporosis.[61-62]

Increased iron is required because of the expansion of blood volume; increase in red blood cell mass and muscle mass, especially in boys; and the need to replace iron losses associated with menstruation in girls. Participation in sports activities leads to red blood cell destruction.

Influential Factors on Eating Habits

Eating is an important part of socialization and exerting one's independence. Food choices are influenced by complex external factors, such as family, peers, mass media, economic and sociocultural factors, and internal factors, such as physiological needs, body image, self-concept, food preferences, and personal values and beliefs about health and nutrition. Probably the strongest influential factor among teenagers is peer pressure.

Most adolescents are stressed because of continual changes. Sexuality, body image, scholastic and athletic pressures, relationships with friends and relatives, finances, career plans, and ideological beliefs may cause conflicts as adolescents try to establish and understand their identity. The presence of stress can decrease utilization of several nutrients, particularly vitamin C and calcium.

Increasing numbers of children and adolescents are overweight (see *Health Application 14*). Adolescents, especially girls, are often obsessed about their body image and a desire to be thin. They are eager to try fad diets and other unsafe weight-loss methods, which may be inadequate in nutrients. Dieting is not recommended for adolescents because nutrients during this period are necessary to build and strengthen their bodies to last a lifetime. Obesity, anorexia nervosa, and bulimia are serious health concerns amenable to early treatment. Extreme weight control behaviors during adolescence increase the risk for anorexia and bulimia 10 years later. Intervention for individuals in preadolescence and adolescence is most appropriate to prevent weight concerns from becoming life-threatening conditions as experienced with anorexia nervosa.[63] A discussion of oral problems associated with eating disorders is presented in Chapter 17. Prevention is the most successful treatment.

Favorite food choices among adolescents are carbonated beverages, sports and energy drinks, flavored milk, steak, hamburgers, tacos, chips, pizza, spaghetti, chicken, french fries, ice cream, oranges, orange and apple juice, apples, bread, candy (sour, hard, or chewy), and snack cakes. Vegetables are unpopular.

Adolescents have increased their snacking in recent years, consuming an average of more than 500 kcal which may cause excessive caloric intake. Actually the more snacks in a day, the more kilocalories are consumed, but snacking frequency is not associated with higher body mass index (BMI).[64]

The total amount of added sugars consumed by children decreased significantly; adolescents consume more added sugars than younger children. Surprisingly, 59% of the added sugar came from foods and 41% from beverages. More added sugars were consumed at home than away from home. The average intake for boys was 16.3% of their kilocalories from added sugars and 15.5% for girls. Most of this decrease was attributed to decreased soda consumption, but energy drink consumption increased.[65]

Not surprisingly, adolescents consume more carbonated beverages than adults. Numerous organizations have recommended elimination of the sale of soft drinks, sports drinks, and energy drinks in schools to prevent health problems. Potential health problems are likely to occur as a result of high intake of sweetened drinks: (a) overweight attributable to additional caloric intake; (b) displacement of milk consumption, resulting in calcium deficiency with an attendant risk of osteoporosis and fractures; and (c) dental caries and potential enamel erosion. Healthcare providers and parents are urged to monitor inappropriate use of these beverages because of the caloric contribution, and because large amounts of caffeine and other stimulant substances in energy drinks are not advisable for children and adolescents. Current data indicate that the percentage of children age 6 to 17 years who drink sugar-sweetened sodas is significantly less now than it was from 2001-2006.[66]

An increase in soda consumption may replace more nutritious beverages such as 100% fruit juice and milk. Numerous studies support this, citing lower dietary intake of vitamins A and C, calcium, magnesium, and riboflavin in children and adolescents.[67] However, a study following children and adolescents for 4 years found that average milk consumption was not related to changes in sweetened-beverage consumption, but caloric beverages generally were complementary with each other: as children increased their intake of one caloric beverage, they also increased intake of others.[68] Water, milk, and 100% fruit juices are consumed on a daily basis, whereas 24.5% of high school students drank a serving of regular soda, 16.1% drank a serving of a sports drink, and 16.9% drank a serving of another sugar-sweetened beverage one or more times daily.[69] Most studies indicate sugar-sweetened beverages promote weight gain.[70]

Artificially sweetened beverages have gained popularity among children and adolescents, the amount of low-calorie sweetened beverage consumption doubling from 1999-2000 to 2007-2008.[71] Avoidance of sugar is usually recommended; however, changing to artificially sweetened sodas is not especially helpful in regards to oral health because the phosphoric and citrus acids in all soft drinks can cause tooth enamel erosion.[72]

Approximately 25% of an adolescent's kilocalories come from high-calorie, low-nutrient-dense foods, making overeating easy. Adolescents have more access to food outside the home and experiment more with food selections than younger children. Foods chosen away from home most likely come from fast food outlets, restaurants, and schools. Fast food restaurants, vending machines, and convenience stores fit adolescents' busy, active lifestyles. These foods can increase daily caloric intake by 145 kilocalories and lower diet quality because of increased amounts of fat, saturated fat, and sodium compared with food prepared at home.[73] This results in such problems as excessive intake of sodium, sugar, and fat.

Fast foods are acceptable nutritionally when consumed in moderation as a part of a well-balanced diet. During the transition from middle adolescence to young adulthood, the proportion of boys who reported frequent fast food intake (three or more times weekly) increased from 23.6% to 33%. Lower-calorie items and a wider variety of menu selections, such as salads and low-fat milkshakes, can contribute to nutrient requirements without providing excessive kilocalories.

Adolescents 15 to 18 years old are notorious for skipping breakfast—25% of boys and 35% of girls. Omission of breakfast is more prevalent with children from lower socioeconomic levels, who also have higher rates of overweight and obesity. Many studies show positive short-term effects of breakfast on cognitive functioning and alertness; implications of the effect of skipping breakfast on mental stability and academic performance are stronger for boys than girls.

Nutritional Advice

Despite adolescents being knowledgeable about healthy eating and wise choices, they frequently choose foods they perceive are unhealthy. Promoting change is more important than providing information. Factors negatively affecting food choices are time, availability of healthy foods, and lack of concern about healthy eating. Listening to adolescents' feelings followed by sound advice works well for those who are willing to listen and make changes. Adolescents can frequently be motivated by responsibility, collaboration, fear of failure, and respect for the healthcare provider. Techniques such as negotiation and reflective listening can enhance their critical thinking skills (see Chapter 21).

Effective tactics for providing nutritional advice to adolescents are to appeal to their physical image or their muscular development and competitiveness for sports, and to praise better food choices, ignore choices that are neutral, and discourage harmful choices. By presenting nutrition and health information in terms relevant to adolescent lifestyles and personal interests, dental professionals can help teenagers understand how current eating and exercise habits affect their current and future health.

Dental Considerations

Assessment
- *Physical:* activity level, growth spurt, use of illicit drugs, use of tobacco products, body image, self-efficacy, influence of peer pressure, stress level.
- *Dietary:* adequacy of nutrient intake based on *MyPlate;* amount and frequency of carbonated beverages, and sports and energy drinks; use of fast foods, convenience foods, or vending machine foods; food preferences and personal values and beliefs about health and nutrition; dietary and nutritional supplements; breakfast; and alcohol intake.

Interventions
- Encourage use of calcium-rich and vitamin D–rich foods.
- Praise good eating patterns; collaboratively work with adolescents to modify food choices and suggest substitutions.
- Determine the frequency, quantity, and form of cariogenic foods.
- Encourage a smoking cessation program for adolescents who smoke (see Chapter 19, *Health Application 19*).
- Provide knowledge to teens regarding risks of using smokeless tobacco and other tobacco products.
- Encourage parents to promote healthy dietary behavior and provide healthy choices that can contribute to oral health and appropriate weight gain.

Nutritional Directions

- Teenagers should be aware of long-term risks and benefits of good nutrition, but the best approach is to focus on short-term benefits of eating well.
- Restriction of kilocalorie intake during rapid growth periods compromises lean body mass accumulation despite a seemingly adequate protein intake.
- Intense physical activity can cause increased urinary loss of calcium and red blood cell destruction. Referral to a RDN may be needed to ensure adequate nutritional intake.
- Snacking can have a positive influence on overall nutritional and health status of the teenager. Kitchens should be stocked with nutritious snack foods, such as cooked meats, raw vegetables, milk, cheese, fresh and dried fruit, nuts and seeds, peanut butter, pretzels, and popcorn to encourage good eating habits.
- Water and low-fat or fat-free milk are the most healthful beverages, and moderate use of 100% fruit juice has health benefits.

- Routine ingestion of sports drinks and soda (with sugar or artificially sweetened) can lead to weight gain and dental caries.
- Use of dietary supplements by most adolescents is not needed.
- An inadequate intake of calcium and vitamin D during childhood or adolescence may result in the child not reaching the genetically predetermined peak height and bone mass.
- Children and adolescents who skip breakfast miss the opportunity to consume a nutrient-rich meal; unhealthful dietary behaviors may have an adverse effect on body weight.
- An adolescent with light skin needs to spend about 5 to 10 minutes in the sun with only part of the body exposed (arms or legs) two or three times a week to produce enough vitamin D; an African American needs to spend 15 to 30 minutes. Additionally, calcium intake should be adequate (3 cups of milk or equivalent milk products).

HEALTH APPLICATION 14   Childhood and Adolescent Obesity

Childhood obesity is the greatest challenge to child health in the 21st century, and children born since 1980 may be the first generation in America to live shorter life expectancy than their parents as a direct consequence of the obesity epidemic.[74] Childhood obesity, similar to adult obesity, is a complex disease caused by an imbalance between kilocalorie intake and output. The rate of childhood obesity tripled in the 1980s, yet that there were no significant changes between 1999-2000 and 2007-2008 is encouraging. In 2009-2010, the prevalence of obesity in children and adolescents was 16.9%.[75] A growing number (about 5%) of U.S. children and teenagers are severely obese.[76] The prevalence of obesity is about the same in both boys and girls. Childhood obesity is more prevalent in families with lower socioeconomic groups. This is probably related to a number of factors: prepregnancy and current maternal weight, lower household education, lack of knowledge for choosing nutrient dense foods, and low nutrient density of snacks and other food selections.

The CDC recommends that World Health Organization growth standards be used to monitor growth for infants and children from birth to age 2 years. The BMI charts are appropriate for boys and girls older than 2 years of age (see Evolve website). BMI is a screening tool, not a diagnostic tool, used to detect weight problems. CDC defines overweight as a BMI at or between the 85th and 95th percentiles and obesity at or above the 95th percentile.[77] Because children grow in spurts and frequently grow in height for a while, followed by an increase in muscle mass and adiposity before growing taller again, these charts are not to be used as diagnostic tools, but to help form an overall clinical impression of trends for the individual. Children with a high BMI do not necessarily manifest clinical complications or health risks related to increased body fat. A high BMI is a clue necessitating more in-depth assessment of the individual child to ascertain health status.

It remains very difficult for overweight children and adolescents to lose weight and even more tedious to sustain that weight loss. The ultimate goal is prevention of overweight in children and adolescents. Experts agree it is much easier to keep weight off a child than to deal with it as an adult.

Obesity in children can potentially cause significant physiologic and psychosocial complications that can lead to negative health consequences as adults. Many diagnosable and treatable conditions arise from childhood obesity. The increasing prevalence of type 2 diabetes mellitus reflects the toll of obesity in children. Type 2 diabetes was formerly diagnosed only in adults. The CDC predicts American children born in 2000 face a 1 in 3 chance of developing diabetes. Other health problems associated with obesity in children include high cholesterol and blood pressure levels, which are risk factors for heart disease; sleep apnea (interrupted breathing while sleeping); orthopedic problems; liver disease; and asthma. Sixty percent of overweight children 5 to 10 years old have at least one risk factor for heart disease. The existence of any of these conditions should be used to motivate lifestyle changes.

Obesity is a systemic problem, not isolated from oral health.[78,79] Obesity is an important issue for all healthcare professionals to discuss with their patients. The topic is a difficult subject to discuss even in a clinical setting because of current societal culture and values. To many mothers, a little "fluff" on their child looks healthy, and they do not recognize and accept the fact that their child is overweight. They may become defensive when the issue is mentioned or take offense at comments. Individuals from low-income groups frequently possess different perceptions of weight than the healthcare provider and may be unconcerned about the child's weight. Furthermore, they lack the skills and knowledge to change behaviors. Treatment of obesity for any child or adolescent requires the expertise of many healthcare disciplines.

Perhaps more devastating to an overweight child is social discrimination. Overweight children often experience psychological stress, poor body image, low self-esteem, and depression. Despite these distressing effects on American youth, the consensus seems to be that the environment, especially the sedentary lifestyle, supports a genetic predisposition to gain excessive weight. Children are more concerned about their current appearance and athletic performance than the long-term effects of weight on their mental and physical capacities and shortened life span.

Continued

The cycle of obesity and disease seems to begin before birth: women who are overweight are more likely to give birth to larger infants, who are more likely to become obese adults.[80] At-risk children begin gaining inordinate amounts during preschool years.[81] Preschool children who are modestly overweight often continue to gain weight during their school years, making later weight loss even tougher. Assisting an overweight toddler or school-age child is easier than assisting a teenager because parents have a greater control over food choices inside and outside the home.

Although the cause of the childhood obesity epidemic is multifaceted, factors driving this phenomenon include rapid changes in modern food selections and activity levels of children superimposed onto genetic and metabolic predispositions for weight gain. The problems of American children eating too many high-kilocalorie fast foods and snacks along with being inactive are well recognized as contributing factors to this problem. The problem will not be resolved by any single action, but concerted action across many disciplines, sectors, and settings such as childcare facilities, communities, healthcare professionals, and schools.

Weight loss or gain reflects inadequate or excessive intake, which should be balanced with an appropriate amount of physical activity. This simple equation is confounded by complex social factors influencing children's eating habits, exercise, and play.

Prevention is important for numerous reasons: (a) obesity is very expensive to treat; (b) an older child regains most of the weight after an obesity management program; (c) success rates for long-term treatment of morbidly overweight teens is extremely low; and (d) access to any effective weight-loss program is limited for high-risk children. Treatment requires a motivated child and parent, and indeed the whole family.

The goal for obese children has been weight maintenance or reduction in the rate of weight gain while height increases. By "growing into their weight," body fat decreases without compromising lean body mass and growth. Many experts believe overweight children should not be put on a diet because of the importance of providing adequate nutrients to promote optimal linear growth. Although the goal for all children and adolescents who are overweight or at risk for being overweight is a BMI for age less than the 85th percentile, this goal should be secondary to healthy eating and activity.

Beneficial effects of child obesity prevention programs on BMI exist, especially if the target audience is between 6 and 12 years of age.[82] Favorable outcomes are more likely to occur when these components are included: (a) school curriculum that includes healthy eating, physical activity, and body image; (b) increased sessions for physical activity and the development of fundamental movement skills throughout the school week; (c) improvements in nutritional quality of the food supply in schools; (d) environments and cultural practices that support children eating healthier foods and being active throughout each day; (e) support for teachers and other staff to implement health promotion strategies and activities (e.g. professional development, capacity building activities); and (f) parental support and home activities that encourage children to be more active, eat more nutritious foods, and spend less time in screen-based activities. A key parenting practice is to create a protective home environment, substituting nutritious foods for unhealthful ones and facilitating physical activities instead of sedentary pursuits.

Interventions to reduce BMI are aimed at changing lifestyle behaviors—including increased physical activity, decreased sedentary activity, increased healthy dietary habits, and decreased unhealthy dietary habits to prevent pediatric obesity. The multifaceted topic of food consumption includes types of food consumed, location, food preparation, and eating habits of other household members. Food choices of children and adolescents are usually dictated by the mother (or other primary caregiver) which is influenced by her heritage and level of education. The first step in addressing this epidemic is to teach parents of young children how to make healthy choices. Nutritional imprinting starts early, so early childhood is the ideal time to start discussing proper feeding practices.

Nutrition education for the child and family is needed to provide a well-balanced diet with some caloric restriction. Many experts believe children should not be required to eat food that is different than the rest of the family; only food portions should be different. Drinks with kilocalories, including fruit juices, should be limited to less than 12 oz daily. Even though juice is natural and healthy, fresh fruits are preferable. When parents change how the whole family eats, and offer children wholesome rewards for not being couch potatoes, obese children begin to shed pounds. Instead of rewarding children with snacks, alternative ways of spending quality time with them is recommended. Environmental change is fostered by restructuring family mealtimes and leisure-time activities, and reinforcing appropriate eating cues (Box 14-5).

Technology has increased the use of media devices such as televisions, iPods, video game devices, and interactive portable devices. These electronic advancements expose children to advertisements that may use toys, cartoon characters, video games, professional athletes, or pop stars. In addition to children watching 3 to 5 hours of television daily, they spend more hours in front of a computer screen. "Inactive entertainment" has paralleled the disturbing increase in obese and overweight children.

Necessary lifestyle changes, although challenging to the child and family are effective in improving weight. Physical activity and healthy eating habits are two lifestyle practices that children need to learn to prevent obesity. Physical activity should be encouraged with consideration of the child's interests and preferences. The whole family should engage in some form of physical activity on a routine basis.

Behavioral treatment of obesity may be more effective for children than adults. A family-based, multifactor intervention can be implemented by a multidisciplinary team after a comprehensive, in-depth assessment when obesity is diagnosed. The whole family should be involved in development of a behavior modification program for maximum success. Effective behavioral programs are labor-intensive and require intensive parental involvement. Changes such as taking time to chew food, minimizing sugar-laden beverages, eating more vegetables, and walking for exercise can be effective in gaining control of the weight problem.

The goal is to establish an environment that supports behavior changes, while minimizing any perceptions of restrictions or limitations on the child. Successful programs focus on encouragement and "small victories" to sustain involvement in improving fitness levels. Parents need help in

HEALTH APPLICATION 14   Childhood and Adolescent Obesity—cont'd

communicating about eating and exercise habits with their children in positive and encouraging ways and to learn how to help children improve their fitness levels.

Because of the lack of success in weight loss and maintenance programs for severely obese children and adolescents, even with intensive behavioral treatment, clinicians have begun resorting to medication therapy and bariatric surgery to ameliorate pediatric obesity. Comprehensive weight-management programs that incorporate counseling and behavioral management techniques targeting diet and physical activity are the most effective. These guidelines stress that medication or surgical treatment should not be offered to overweight or obese children until more modest measures, including intensive dietary, behavioral, and activity-related lifestyle changes, are attempted.[83,84] Only adolescents who have not lost weight through lifestyle modifications should be considered for medication or gastric surgery and even then only when other comorbidities exist, and the individual continues to adhere to previously implemented diet and exercise interventions.

BOX 14-5   Help Children Maintain a Healthy Body Weight

- Be supportive. Children know if they are overweight, and do not need to be reminded or singled out. They need acceptance, encouragement, and love.
- Be a positive role model. Note lifestyle habits contributing to overeating and inactivity, and help them avoid the situation.
- Start the day off on the right foot. Breakfast helps spread the kilocalories throughout the day and helps avoid mid-morning unhealthy snacks.
- Set guidelines for the amount of time children spend watching television, playing video games, or playing on the computer.
- Set goals for physical activity; plan family activities involving physical activity. Instead of watching TV, go hiking or biking, wash the car, or walk around a mall. Offer choices, and let children decide.
- Be sensitive. Find activities children will enjoy that are not difficult or could cause embarrassment.
- Eat meals together as a family, and eat at the table, not in front of a television. Eat slowly and enjoy the food. Eating at home with family often translates into a healthier diet.
- Avoid using food as a reward or punishment. Spend some quality time together; take a walk or go on a long bike ride.
- Focus on positive goals. Allow children to determine goals they want to achieve, such as being able to swim five laps in a specified time. Focusing on positive goals is better than focusing on weight loss.

- Do not be too restrictive; focus on moderation. Children should not be placed on restrictive diets, unless ordered by a pediatrician (for medical reasons). Encourage kid-sized portions. Sweets and fast foods should be curtailed, but they can be used sparingly.
- Children need food for growth, development, and energy, but if they are forced to clean their plates, they are doing their bodies a disservice.
- Make eating a family activity. Involve children in meal planning, grocery shopping, and meal preparation. This helps them learn and gives them a role in decision making.
- Keep healthy snacks on hand. Good options include fresh, frozen, or canned fruits and vegetables; low-fat cheese, yogurt, or ice cream; frozen fruit juice bars; and cookies, such as fig bars, graham crackers, gingersnaps, and vanilla wafers.
- Watch what children drink. High-energy drinks provide a lot of sugar with little health benefit.
- Make small changes as a family. Menu changes should be implemented for all family members. Begin parking the car a little farther away or eating fast food less often.
- Focus on small, gradual changes in eating and activity patterns. This helps form habits that can last a lifetime.
- Get active. Plan activities involving the whole family, such as skating, hiking, or biking. Make an after-dinner walk a regular part of the family's evening.

Case Application for the Dental Hygienist

A mother brings her 3-year-old son in because of the need for a routine oral examination required by the Head Start program he is attending. She knows he has some white spots on his front teeth, but he will not allow her to brush his teeth, and she does not routinely ensure he brushes his teeth. He is still using a sippy cup, but gave up the bottle at age 18 months.

Nutritional Assessment
- Willingness to seek nutritional information
- Desire for increased knowledge of nutritional health habits
- Knowledge of community resources
- Cultural or religious influences
- Knowledge regarding the *Dietary Guidelines*, Nutrient Facts, and *MyPlate*

Nutritional Diagnosis
Health-seeking behaviors related to lack of knowledge concerning optimal nutrition practices in relation to dental health.

Nutritional Goals
The parent verbalizes correct information concerning the importance of oral hygiene and foods and beverages affecting the oral cavity; is aware of snacks that do not promote dental caries; is able to read food labels; and can name the food groups in *MyPlate*, the number of servings needed for the child, and portion sizes from each group.

Continued

Case Application for the Dental Hygienist—cont'd

Nutritional Implementation

Intervention: Ask the parent to write down everything the child ate yesterday and from the time he got up this morning until the office visit. Also ask the parent to document everything she ate.

Rationale: This will help tailor the information provided to the needs of the patient. You especially need to know the child's access to the sippy cup during the day, what beverage is in the cup, and whether he goes to bed with it. The parent's diet recall reflects the primary caregiver's preferences and habits. Any changes in her diet ultimately help the child.

Intervention: (a) Encourage variety of food intake, using *MyPlate.* Review the number of servings needed and what consists of a serving size. (b) Recommend substituting fresh fruit for juices and limiting fruit juice to 4 to 6 oz daily. (c) Instruct her to avoid products that contain fermentable carbohydrates, such as cookies, crackers, or cereal, between meals.

Rationale: It is the total balance of diet that matters, and the best balance incorporates variety to promote optimal nutrition. Providing the minimal number of servings prevents nutritional deficiencies in healthy individuals. Certain foods, although they may be wholesome and nutritious, may not be advisable for oral health.

Intervention: (a) Explain how to read labels for carbohydrate content. The name of most sugars ends in *"-ose."* (b) Emphasize moderation of sugar intake. (c) Explain that "dietetic" and "sugar-free" do not mean that the product is low in kilocalories or low in cariogenic potential. (d) Explain the relationship between carbohydrate and the caries process; emphasize the importance of proper oral hygiene after its use.

Rationale: Refined sugar contains kilocalories and no other nutrients, but is acceptable when used in items that contain appreciable amounts of other nutrients (e.g., a pudding would provide more nutrients than a gelatin dessert or carbonated beverage).

Intervention: (a) Review an entire label with the mother to help her understand how to use it, (b) determine a serving size, and (c) explain the types of carbohydrates.

Rationale: Knowledge increases compliance and allows the mom to make informed choices regarding food selections.

Intervention: Discuss the importance of three regular mealtimes and three healthy snacks and avoidance of grazing.

Rationale: Adequate nutrients are important for growth and health of the child; snacking is needed for a 3-year-old to obtain adequate nutrients. Assist the child in tooth brushing after meals and snacks.

Intervention: Ask the mother how she feels about being able to implement the changes.

Rationale: This will give you the opportunity to empathize with her about the difficulties of changing food habits and perhaps make further suggestions for implementing changes.

Intervention: Refer the patient to governmental programs for which she may be eligible—WIC, food stamps, or expanded nutrition programs.

Rationale: These agencies may help in providing healthy foods and provide practical guidelines via newsletters, workshops, and written materials to improve health.

Evaluation

To determine effectiveness of care, have the parent read labels; have the parent state the number of servings and portion sizes needed for her son. Additionally, the parent should be able to plan a menu using foods recommended, and to state how to obtain or use community information and support. The parent should be able to indicate how changes in food choices will not only improve overall health, but also maintain health of the oral cavity and ensure optimal growth of her son with minimal or no problems in the oral cavity.

STUDENT READINESS

1. Plan meals for 1 day for a family with a 2-year-old toddler, a 10-year-old boy, and a 15-year-old girl.
2. Discuss feeding an infant from birth to 12 months.
3. What is considered normal weight for a newborn?
4. Create an outline for discussing ECC with an expectant parent.
5. A mother wants to know why snacks are needed and which ones to give her preschooler to lessen the risk of developing dental cavities. What would you tell her? Provide a list of specific suggestions and food choices for the mother.
6. A mother states that because her child is hyperactive, she is going to eliminate all sugar. What is a good response to this statement?
7. List barriers for not being able to decrease use of fast food restaurants. List healthier choices available at favorite fast food restaurants.

CASE STUDY

Mrs. C. is at her 6-month recall visit and talks about her 6-month-old daughter, Jennifer. Jennifer weighed 7 lb at birth and now weighs 15 lb. She was bottle-fed from birth. At 3 months, Mrs. C. introduced cereals, but Jennifer has resisted all attempts to increase her solid food intake. She is allowed to go to sleep with a bottle propped in her crib at the daycare center.

1. What additional assessment data do you need?
2. Is Jennifer's weight gain within the expected range?
3. How much should she gain in the next 6 months?
4. What tentative dental diagnosis could you derive?
5. The dental hygienist encourages Jennifer's mother to discontinue the habit of putting her in bed with a bottle and to request that the daycare center do the same. Why?
6. The healthcare provider recommends solid foods be introduced gradually to Jennifer. What foods should be introduced first?
7. When will Jennifer be old enough for finger foods?
8. Why should honey be withheld until 1 year of age?
9. Why would the dental hygienist want to assess Mrs. C's dietary intake?

CASE STUDY

R.J. is a large 16-year-old boy (6 feet, 4 inches, 190 lb) who has complained to you about pain from dental caries. He is active in athletics in school and has a part-time job. You determine from his dietary history that his appetite is very good, and his nutrient intake is adequate except for vegetables. Snacking, principally soft drinks, candy, and cookies, constitutes almost 50% of his total caloric intake.

1. How would you advise R.J.? What motivational factors would you consider for him?
2. What are some dental nutritional diagnoses and goals and interventions for Raymond?
3. What further data are needed for a complete assessment?
4. When having R.J. choose better snack options, what are some that you would recommend?
5. How do you think R.J. will feel about your suggestions?

CASE STUDY

Norma returns for a 6-month recall visit. Since her last checkup, this 17-year-old girl has developed 12 new dental caries in the mandibular anterior teeth. Norma's parents are in their 50s. Her father has lost numerous teeth as a result of periodontal disease, and her mother is completely edentulous. Norma has no medical problems other than rhinitis (inflammation of the nasal mucous membranes secondary to allergies), which causes her to breathe through her mouth much of the time. The oral examination showed normal color and tone of the oral mucosa, tongue, and gingiva. Her decayed, missing, filled rate was 17. She reports eating a varied, well-balanced diet, except for fruit and vegetable intake. Because of the dryness in her mouth, she relies heavily on cough drops and chewing gum.

1. What is a possible cause of these new dental caries?
2. What suggestions would you give her to relieve mouth dryness?
3. Based on her dietary habits, what nutrient(s) may be inadequate?

References

1. Fleischer DM, Spergel JM, Assa'ad AH, et al: Primary prevention of allergic disease through nutritional interventions. *J Allergy Clin Immunol* 1(1):29–36, 2013.
2. Maguire JL, Salehi L, Birken CS, et al: Association between total duration of breastfeeding and iron deficiency. *Pediatr* 131(5): 31530–31537, 2013.
3. Li R, Fein SB, Grummer-Strawn LM: Do infants fed from bottles lack self-regulation of milk intake compared with directly breastfed infants? *Pediatrics* 125(6):e1386–e1393, 2010.
4. Deshpande G, Rao S, Patole S, et al: Updated meta-analysis of probiotics for preventing necrotizing enterocolitis in preterm neonates. *Pediatrics* 125(5):921–930, 2010.
5. Osborn DA, Sinn JK: Prebiotics in infants for prevention of allergy. *Cochrane Database Syst Rev* 3:CD006474, 2013.
6. Sinn J: Probiotics in infants for prevention of allergic disease and food hypersensitivity. *World Allergy Organ J* 6(Suppl 1):72, 2013.
7. Vandenplas, Y, DeGreef E, Devreker T, et al: Probiotics and previotics in infants and children *Curr Infect Dis Rep* 15(3):251–262, 2013.
8. Ibid, Fleischer, 2013.
9. Andres A, Casey PH, Clever MA, et al: Body fat and bone mineral content of infants fed breast milk, cow's milk formula, or soy formula during the first year of life. *J Pediatr* 163(1):49–54, 2013.
10. Ibid.
11. Berseth CL, Mitmesser SH, Ziegler EE, et al: Tolerance of a standard intact protein formula versus a partially hydrolyzed formula in healthy, term infants. *Nutr J* 8:27, 2009.
12. Picard PJ: Bottle feeding a preventive orthodontic. *J Calif State Dent Assoc* 35:90–95, 1959.
13. Salone LR, Vann WF, Dee DL: Breastfeeding: an overview of oral and general health benefits. *JADA* 144(2):143–151, 2013.
14. Davis D, Bell PA: Infant feeding practices and occlusal outcomes: a longitudinal study. *J Can Dent Assoc* 57(7):593–594, 1991.
15. Palmer B: The influence of breastfeeding on the development of the oral cavity: a commentary. *J Hum Lact* 14(2):93–98, 1998.
16. Mahunn-Smith J, Abrose NG: Breastfeeding may protect against persistent stuttering. *J Commun Disord* 2013. Accessed September 2, 2013: http://pediatrics.aappublications.org/content/131/4/e1101.short.
17. Palmer B: Breastfeeding: reducing the risk for obstructive sleep apnea. *Breastfeed Abstr* 18(3)19–20, 1999.
18. Sexton S, Natale R: Risks and benefits of pacifiers. *Am Fam Physician* 79(8):681–685, 2009.
19. Greer FR, Sicherer SH, Burks AW: American Academy of Pediatrics Committee on Nutrition; American Academy of Pediatrics Section on Allergy and Immunology: Effects of early nutritional interventions on the development of atopic disease in infants and children: the role of maternal dietary restriction, breastfeeding, timing of introduction of complementary foods, and hydrolyzed formulas. *Pediatrics* 121(1):183–191, 2008.
20. The Food Allergy Research & Education (FARE): *Facts and statistics.* Accessed August 30, 2013: http://www.foodallergy.org/facts-and-stats.
21. Ibid, Fleischer 2013.
22. Mennella JA, Lukasewycz LD, Castor SM, et al: The timing and duration of a sensitive period in human flavor learning: a randomized trial. *Am J Clin Nutr* 95(5):1019–1024, 2011.
23. Pettifor JM: Nutritional rickets: pathogenesis and prevention. *Pediatr Endocrinol Rev* 10(Suppl2):347–353, 2013.
24. Health Canada: *Vitamin D supplementation for breastfed infants—Questions and answers for professionals.* Accessed August 30, 2013: http://www.hc-sc.gc.ca/fn-an/surveill/nutrition/commun/prenatal/vit_d_sup-eng.php.
25. Perrine CG, Sharma AJ, Jefferds ME, et al: Adherence to vitamin D recommendations among US infants. *Pediatrics* 125(4):627–632, 2010.
26. Gallo S, Jean-Philippe S, Rodd C, et al: Vitamin D supplementation of Canadian infants: practices of Montreal mothers. *Appl Physiol Nutr Metab* 35(3):303–309, 2010.
27. American Academy of Pediatric Dentistry (AAPD): *Guideline on Fluoride Therapy.* Revised, 2012. Accessed August 30, 2013: http://www.aapd.org/media/Policies_Guidelines/G_FluorideTherapy.pdf.
28. Pacey A, Nancarrow T, Egeland GM: Prevalence and risk factors for parental reported oral health of Inuit preschoolers: Nunavut Inuit Child Health Survey, 2007-2008. *Rural Remote Health* 10(2):1368, 2010.
29. Centers for Disease Control and Prevention (CDC): *Oral Health-Preventing cavities, gum disease, tooth loss, and oral cancers at a glance 2011.* Accessed August 30, 2013: http://www.cdc.gov/chronicdisease/resources/publications/AAG/doh.htm.

30. Evans EW, Hayes C, Palmer CA, et al: Dietary intake and severe early childhood caries in low-income, young children. *J Acad Nutr Diet* 113:1057–1061, 2013.

31. National Institute of Dental and Craniofacial Research (NIDCR): *Prevalence (number of cases of cleft lip and cleft palate).* Accessed August 30, 2013t: http://www.nidcr.nih.gov/DataStatistics/FindDataByTopic/CraniofacialBirthDefects/PrevalenceCleft+LipCleftPalate.htm.

32. U.S. Department of Agriculture, Food and Nutrition Service, Office of Research, Nutrition and Analysis: *Diet quality of American school-age children by school lunch participation status: Data from the National Health and Nutrition Examination Survey, 1999-2004, 2008.* Accessed on August 30, 2013: http://www.fns.usda.gov/ora/MENU/Published/CNP/FILES/NHANES-NSLP.pdf.

33. Carlson SJ, Fallon EM, Kalish BT, et al: The role of the omega-3 fatty acid DHA in the human life cycle. *JPEN J Parenter Enteral Nutr* 37(1):15–22, 2013.

34. Northstone K, Joinson C, Emmett P, et al: Are dietary patterns in childhood associated with IQ at 8 years of age? A population-based cohort study. *J Epidemiol Community Health* 66(7):624–628, 2010.

35. Position of the American Dietetic Association: Nutrition guidance for healthy children ages 2 to 11 years. *J Am Diet Assoc* 108(6):1038–1047, 2008.

36. Kit BK, Carroll MD, Lacher DA, et al: Trends in serum lipids among US youths aged 6 to 19 years, 1988-2010. *JAMA* 308(6): 591–600, 2012.

37. Friedemann C, Heneghan C, Mahtani K, et al: Cardiovascular disease risk in healthy children and its association with body mass index: systematic review and meta-analysis. *BMJ* 345:e4759, 2012.

38. Psaty BM, Rivara FP: Universal screening and drug treatments of dyslipidemia in children and adolescents. *JAMA* 307(3):257–258, 2012.

39. Expert Panel on Integrated Guidelines for Cardiovascular Health and Risk Reduction in Children and Adolescents: Expert panel on integrated guidelines for cardiovascular health and risk reduction in children and adolescents: summary report. *Pediatrics* 128(Suppl 5):S213–S256, 2011.

40. Pate RR, O'Neill JR: Physical activity guidelines for young children: an emerging consensus. *Arch Pediatr Adolesc Med* 166(12):1095–1096, 2012.

41. U.S. Department of Health and Human Services (USHHS): *2008 Physical activity guidelines for Americans.* Accessed August 30, 2013: http://www.health.gov/paguidelines/.

42. Brauchla M, Juan W, Story J, et al: Sources of dietary fiber and the association of fiber intake with childhood obesity risk (in 2-18 year olds) and diabetes risk of adolescents 12-18 year olds: NHANES 2003-2006. *J Nutr Metab* 2012:736258, 2012.

43. Fulgoni VL, 3rd, Quann EE: National trends in beverage consumption in children from birth to 5 years: analysis of NHANES across three decades. *Nutr J* 11:92, 2012.

44. Sebastian RS, Goldman JD, Enns CW, et al: *Fluid milk consumption in the United States: what we eat in America, NHANES 2005-2006. Food Surveys Research Group Dietary Data, Brief No. 3.* September 2010. Accessed August 30, 2013: http://ars.usda.gov/Services/docs.htm?docid=19476.

45. Ibid., Fulgoni VL 3rd, 2012.

46. CDC Data & Statistics: *Attention-deficit/hyperactivity disorder.* Accessed August 30, 2013: http://www.cdc.gov/NCBDDD/adhd/data.html.

47. Shaw P, Eckstrand K, Sharp W, et al: Attention-deficit/hyperactivity disorder is characterized by a delay in cortical maturation. *Proc Natl Acad Sci U S A* 104(49):19649–19654, 2007.

48. Wolraich ML, Wilson DB, White JW: The effects of sugar on behavior or cognition in children. a meta-analysis. *JAMA* 274(20):1617–1621, 1995.

49. Nigg JT, Lewis K, Edinger T, et al: Meta-analysis of attention-deficit/hyperactivity disorder or attention-deficit/hyperactivity disorder symptoms, restriction diet, and synthetic food color additives. *J Am Acad Child Adolesc Psychiatry* 51(1):86–97, 2012.

50. Sonuga-Barke EJ, Brandeis D, Cortese S, et al: Nonpharmacological interventions for ADHD: systematic review and meta-analyses of randomized controlled trials of dietary and psychological treatments. *Am J Psychiatry* 170(3):275–289, 2013.

51. Florence MD, Asbridge M, Veugelers PJ: Diet quality and academic performance. *J Sch Health* 78(4):209–215, 2008.

52. Ibid, Food Allergy Research & Education (FARE).

53. Centers for Disease Control and Prevention (CDC), National Center for Health Statistics: *Health, United States, 2011: Access to preventive services (OH-8). Hyattsville, Maryland. 2012, Table 76.* Accessed September 2, 2013. Available at: http://www.healthypeople.gov/2020/topicsobjectives2020/objectiveslist.aspx?topicId=32#186.

54. Seiraway H, Faust SH, Mulligan R: The impact of oral health on the academic performance of disadvantaged children. *Am J Public Health* 102(9):1729–1734, 2012.

55. Ibid., Centers for Disease Control and Prevention (CDC).

56. Milgrom P, Ly KA, Tut OK, et al: Xylitol pediatric topical oral syrup to prevent dental caries: a double-blind randomized clinical trial of efficacy. *Arch Pediatr Adolesc Med* 163(7):601–607, 2009.

57. Reedy J, Krebs-Smith SM: Dietary sources of energy, solid fats, and added sugars among children and adolescents in the United States. *J Acad Nutr Diet* 110(10):1477–1484, 2010.

58. Shay CM, Ning H, Daniels SR, et al: Status of cardiovascular health in US adolescents: prevalence estimates from the National Health and Nutrition Examination Surveys (NHANES) 2005-2010. *Circulation* 127(13):1369–1376, 2013.

59. Centers for Disease Control and Prevention (CDC): Fruit and vegetable consumption among high school students—United States, 2010. *MMWR Morb Mortal Wkly Rep* 60(46):1583–1586, 2011.

60. Bailey RL, Dodd KW, Goldman JA, et al: Estimation of total usual calcium and vitamin D intakes in the United States. *J Nutr* 140(4):817–822, 2010.

61. Donaldson AA, Gordon CM: Bone health in adolescents. *Contemporary Pediatr* Apr 2013; Accessed September 2, 2013: http://contemporarypediatrics.modernmedicine.com/contemporary-pediatrics/news/modernmedicine/welcome-modernmedicine/bone-health-adolescents?page=0,4&contextCategoryId=8.

62. Nestle M, Nesheim MC: To supplement or not to supplement: The U.S. preventive services task force recommendations on calcium and vitamin D. *Ann Intern Med* 158(9):701–702, 2013.

63. Neumark-Sztainer, D, Wall M, Larson NI, et al: Dieting and disordered eating behaviors from adolescence to young adulthood: findings from a 10-year longitudinal study. *J Am Diet Assoc* 111(7):1004–1011, 2011.

64. Sebastian RS, Goldman JD, Enns CW: *Snacking patterns of U.S. adolescents: what we eat in America, NHANES 2005-2006. Food Surveys Research Group. Dietary Data Brief No. 2.* September 2010. Accessed on August 30, 2013: www.ars.usda.gov/research/publications/publications.htm?seq_no_115=255987.

65. Ervin RB, Kit BK, Carroll MD, Ogden CL: Consumption of added sugar among U.S. children and adolescents, 2005-2008. *NCHS Data Brief* (87):1–8, 2012.

66. Quann E: *National Health and Nutrition Examination Surveys (NHANES) data.* Presented at the 2012 Academy of Nutrition and Dietetics Food & Nutrition Conference & Expo, October 6-9, 2012, Philadelphia, PA.

67. Fiorito LM, Marini M, Mitchell DC, et al: Girls' early sweetened carbonated intake predicts different patterns of beverage and

nutrient intake across childhood and adolescence. *J Am Diet Assoc* 110(4):543–550, 2010.

68. Oza-Frank R, Zavodny M, Cunningham SA: Beverage displacement between elementary and middle school 2004-2007. *J Acad Nutr Diet* 112(9):1390–1396, 2012.

69. Centers for Disease Control and Prevention (CDC): Beverage consumption among high school students—United States, 2010. *MMWR Morb Mortal Wkly Rep* 60(23):778–780, 2011.

70. Malik VS, Pan AA, Willet WC, et al: Sugar-sweetened beverages and weight gain in children and adults: a systematic review and meta-analysis. *Am J Clin Nutr* 98(4):1084–1102, 2013.

71. Sylvetsky AC, Welsh JA, Brown RJ, et al: Low-calorie sweetener consumption is increasing in the United States. *Am J Clin Nutr* 96(3):640–646, 2012.

72. Bassiouny MA: Effect of sweetening agents in acidic beverages on associated erosion lesions. *Gen Dent* 60(4):322–330, 2012.

73. Mancino L, Todd J, Guthrie J, et al: *How food away from home affects children's diet quality. Economic Research Service Report No. (ERR-104), October 2010.* Accessed September 2, 2013: http://www.ers.usda.gov/publications/err-economic-research-report/err104.aspx.

74. American Heart Association: *Overweight in children,* updated April 2012. Accessed August 30, 2013: http://www.heart.org/HEARTORG/GettingHealthy/Overweight-in-Children_UCM_304054_Article.jsp.

75. Ogden CL, Carroll MD, Kit BK, et al: Prevalence of obesity and trends in body mass index among US children and adolescents, 1999-2010. *JAMA* 307(5):483–490, 2012.

76. Kelly AS, Barlow SE, Bao G, Inge T, et al: American Health Association Scientific Statement: Severe Obesity in Children and Adolescents: identification, associated health risks, and treatment approaches. *Circulation* 128(9):1689–1712. 2013.

77. Centers for Disease Control and Prevention (CDC): *Basics about childhood obesity.* Updated April 27, 2012. Accessed August 30, 2013: http://www.cdc.gov/obesity/childhood/basics.html.

78. Benguigui C, Bongard V, Ruidavets JB, et al: Evaluation of oral health related to body mass index. *Oral Dis* 18(8):748–755, 2012.

79. Must A, Phillips SM, Tybor DJ, et al: The association between childhood obesity and tooth eruption. *Obesity (Silver Spring)* 20(10):2070–2074, 2012.

80. Ludwig DS, Rouse HL: Currie. Pregnancy weight gain and childhood body weight comparison. *PLOS Medicine.* September 2, 2013. Accessed October 13, 2013: http://www.plosmedicine.org/article/info%3Adoi%2F10.1371%2Fjournal.pmed.1001521

81. Haas SA: Developmental origins of disease and health disparities: limitations and future directions. In Landale NS, McHale SM, Alan B, editors: *Families and Child Health (National Symposium on Family Issues),* New York, 2013, Springer Science.

82. Waters E, de Silva-Sanigorski A, Hall BJ, et al: Interventions for preventing obesity in children. *Cochrane Database Syst Rev* (12):CD001871, 2011.

83. Hoelscher DM, Kirk S, Ritchie L, Cunningham-Sabo L: Position of the Academy of Nutrition and Dietetics: interventions for the prevention and treatment of pediatric overweight and obesity. *J Acad Nutr Diet* 113(10):1375–1394, 2013.

84. U.S. Preventive Services Task Force: Screening for obesity in children and adolescents: U.S. Preventive Services Task Force Recommendation Statement. *Pediatrics* 125(2):361–367, 2010.

ⓔ EVOLVE RESOURCES

Please visit http://evolve.elsevier.com/Stegeman/nutritional for additional practice and study support tools.

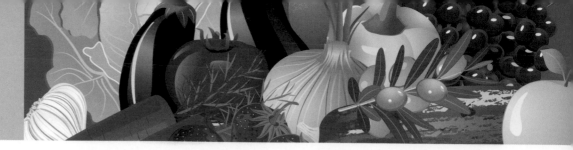

Nutritional Requirements for Older Adults and Eating Habits Affecting Oral Health

Student Learning Outcomes

Upon completion of this chapter, the student will be able to achieve the following student learning outcomes:

- Discuss ways to handle typical nutritional problems occurring in older adults.
- Examine dental considerations of nutritional needs that occur in older patients.
- Identify nutrition education needs for older patients.
- Discuss physiological changes altering an older individual's nutritional status.

- Discuss differences in amounts of nutrients needed by older patients compared with younger patients.
- Describe factors influencing food intake of older patients.
- Suggest dietary changes that could be implemented to provide optimum nutrient intake for older patients.

Key Terms

Age-related macular degeneration
Atrophic gastritis
Dysphagia
Genomics
Homeostatic mechanisms
Hypogeusia

Incontinence
Nocturia
Nutrigenomics
Nutritional genomics
Sarcopenia

Test Your NQ

1. **T/F** Normal physiological changes occurring in older adults do not affect nutritional requirements.
2. **T/F** Nutritional requirements for a 50-year-old patient are different from those for an 81-year-old patient.
3. **T/F** Food selection is highly correlated with dentition.
4. **T/F** Edentulous patients should puree their food.
5. **T/F** Dehydration is seldom observed in older adults.

6. **T/F** Older adults need more vitamins D and B$_{12}$ than individuals younger than 51 years of age.
7. **T/F** Healthy older women require increased amounts of iron.
8. **T/F** Energy requirements decrease with age.
9. **T/F** Self-medication with vitamins is a healthy practice for older adults.
10. **T/F** Exercise is of no benefit to older adults.

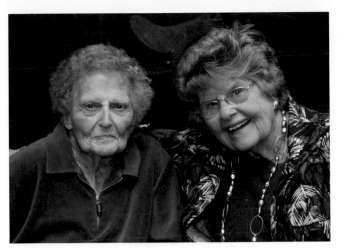

FIGURE 15-1 Relatives celebrating their 100th (*left*) and 90th (*right*) birthdays. Life expectancy is higher for baby boomers than for current older population. (Reprinted with permission of D2 Studios, www.d2studios.net.)

Major shifts in the age of the U.S. population are affecting healthcare needs. Compared with 2000, when more than 35 million people were age 65 years and older (13% of the population), this group is expected to increase to approximately 55 million by 2020 (36% increase). The 85 years and older group is the fastest growing segment of the older population (Fig. 15-1), and this group is projected to increase from 5.5 million in 2010 to 6.6 million in 2020.[1] Research indicates that genetics account for about 20% to 30% of an individual's life span, with the rest attributed to diet and lifestyle choices. Individual healthy lifestyle choices (never smoking, moderate alcohol consumption, physical activity, and eating fruits and vegetables daily) are moderately associated with successful aging; their combined impact is substantial.[2] Improved medical care since infancy has also helped increase Americans' life span, but it is important to increase the quality of that life by changing lifestyles and food choices. Quality of life is defined by the World Health Organization as an individual's perception of their position in life in the context of the culture and value systems in which they live and in relation to their goals, expectations, standards, and concerns.[3] Whereas people were once disabled by things like vision and coronary heart disease (CHD), which are now more treatable, currently degenerative conditions like Alzheimer and dementia are plaguing older individuals.

The *Dietary Guidelines* recognize that people older than 50 years of age need special consideration. Some changes in food habits are needed in later life to adjust to physical and metabolic changes that occur with aging. Dietary quality and obesity are two modifiable health risks and behaviors that can improve longevity and quality of life.[4] It is never too late to make lifestyle changes to improve one's health.

GENERAL HEALTH STATUS

The most common nutritional disorder in older individuals is obesity. The prevalence of obesity increases progressively from 20 to 60 years of age and decreases after age 60 years.

Between 1988-1994 and 2009-2010, the percentage of people older than age 65 years who were obese increased from 22% to 38%; 29% of individuals older than 75 years were obese in 2009-2010.[5] More men than women are overweight, but more women than men are obese. Obesity is more common among African Americans, and slightly higher among Mexican Americans, than among non-Hispanic whites.[6]

Obesity causes serious medical complications and impairs quality of life. Approximately 80% of older Americans have one chronic disease, and 42% have been diagnosed with two or more chronic conditions.[7] Obesity contributes to some of the chronic conditions commonly seen in older adults, including CHD, diabetes, cancer, and Alzheimer disease. Most of these conditions increase the risk of poor nutritional status. Routine nutritional care for older adults can help prevent or manage chronic diseases. Obesity can exacerbate the age-related decline in physical function and cognitive disability.[8]

Malnutrition is another nutrition-related problem diagnosed in older adults admitted to hospitals and nursing homes and in those with serious medical problems. Malnutrition is associated with impaired immune response, muscle and respiratory function; delayed wound healing; overall increased complications; longer rehabilitation; greater length of hospital stay; and increased mortality.[9] Several major identifiable biological or environmental circumstances, or events that increase risk and suggest special care and attention, have been identified as key risk factors of poor nutritional status in individuals older than age 65 years. Factors considered to be contributing causes of older individuals being at risk of malnutrition include less education and lower income; housebound, or inability to purchase food; multiple medications; physical disabilities, depression, and other mental challenges; recent drastic lifestyle changes, such as death of spouse; and lacking regularly cooked meals. Even after age 75 years, healthy lifestyle behaviors (e.g., not smoking and physical activity) are associated with longevity.[10] An example of a nutritional assessment questionnaire is available on the Evolve website. Identifying individuals at nutritional risk is critical to cost-effectiveness for the healthcare system and to assist older patients in maintaining their independence and personal well-being. Food choices are also related to oral problems, so a dental assessment should inquire about food intake and oral problems affecting intake.

Dietary restrictions associated with management of chronic diseases, such as diabetes, renal disease, or CHD, can be confusing, especially if more than one condition exists. Improper food selection or fear of choosing unhealthy foods may be a factor for inadequate nutrition. The result of certain treatments, such as with cancer, can affect eating by creating loss of appetite, nausea and vomiting, diarrhea or constipation, xerostomia, or changes in the taste of food.

A substantial number of older adults take multiple prescription drugs as well as multiple dietary supplements. Approximately 33% of older adults take three or more prescription drugs and three or more supplements; 10% combine five or more prescription drugs with as many dietary supplements.[11] Some of these drugs can interfere with appetite and nutrient absorption. Although drug-nutrient interactions can compromise anyone's nutritional status, these problems are amplified in older adults. Physiological and pathophysiological changes, such as decreased hepatic and renal clearance, result in greater variability and less predictability of a drug's effects.

PHYSIOLOGICAL FACTORS INFLUENCING NUTRITIONAL NEEDS AND STATUS

Aging significantly impacts body composition. Many organ functions decline with age, some beginning as early as age 30 years. These physiological changes may significantly influence nutritional requirements of older adults by affecting absorption, transportation, metabolism, and excretion of nutrients. With aging, the body is less able to correct nutrient imbalances, such as increasing absorption when intake is decreased; the precarious physiological balance may be upset by disease, physical and mental challenges, and environmental, economic, and social disabilities. However, chronological age and functional capacity do not always correlate. Older individuals differ from one another in physiological and health status more than any other age group, meaning that chronological status is not useful in predicting physiological abilities and health status.

Impairment of visual, auditory, and olfactory sensory organs is common. Poor vision makes food preparation difficult, even hazardous in some cases, and may be responsible for senior citizens not identifying contaminated foods, a potential cause of foodborne illness. Poor hearing increases isolation and decreases socialization.

Oral Cavity

Oral health problems (e.g., chewing, swallowing, and compromised dentition) are indicators of nutritional risk and may be primary contributors to malnutrition. Persistent oral health problems are associated with impaired intake of certain foods and nutrients. When the ability to smell declines, cariogenic food choices usually increase. A progressive decline in gustatory and olfactory sensitivity affects food choices and quantity because "nothing tastes good." Olfactory and taste receptors are affected by impaired chewing and swallowing.

Some conditions and certain medications also lead to deterioration of taste sensitivity or perception. Hypogeusia (loss of taste) may be associated with certain disorders rather than being a normal component of the aging process. Older adults may confuse taste sensations, describing sour foods as metallic and salty foods as tasteless. Many people gradually begin to lose their sense of smell around age 50 years, a condition called anosmia. As a consequence of anosmia and hypogeusia, foods may be overly seasoned with salt or sugar. Losses in salt or sugar perception make it difficult to comply with low-sodium or diabetes guidelines. Other seasonings can help replace the taste of salt or sugar.

Xerostomia, which affects half of all older adults, compromises oral processing of foods and use of nutrients. Most individuals taking five medications report problems with xerostomia. Xerostomia causes difficulties with chewing and initiating a swallow. Lack of saliva increases the risk for oral disease because saliva contains antimicrobial components and minerals that can help rebuild tooth enamel after acid-producing, decay-causing bacterial attacks. Although crunchy foods stimulate saliva flow, older patients with xerostomia are more likely to avoid crunchy foods such as raw vegetables and crispy fruits. They also tend to shun dry foods, such as bread, and sticky foods such as peanut butter. Many patients may choose hard candy or gum to stimulate saliva flow and relieve the dryness; however, this frequent exposure to fermentable carbohydrate promotes root caries and reduces intake of nutrient-dense foods (see Chapter 20 for further discussion of xerostomia).

The prevalence of root caries, further discussed in Chapter 20, is much higher in older adults than in younger adults. Less than 10% of individuals 20 to 29 years old have root caries compared with 38% of adults age 75 years and older.[12] Root caries are more prevalent in men, frequently with a history of tobacco use. Recession of gingival tissues exposes root surfaces of teeth to the oral environment; this process increases with aging. The lack of a protective enamel layer on the root, surface roughness of roots, and demineralization related to a lower pH, make the area highly susceptible to dental caries.

Periodontal disease increases the likelihood of weight loss in older adults; the more extensive and severe the disease, the greater the weight loss. Approximately 17% of individuals older than 65 years have periodontal disease and almost 11% have moderate or severe periodontal disease. This condition is partially responsible for loss of teeth. The function and position of the remaining teeth seem to indicate chewing ability more accurately than the total number of teeth present.

Edentulism is not inevitable with advancing age. Edentulism among adults older than age 50 years has decreased significantly. Native Americans and African Americans have the highest rates of edentulism.[13] Calcium is readily mobilized from trabecular bone. A negative calcium balance results in loss of calcium from the maxilla and mandible, which are primarily trabecular bone. Normally, alveolar bone is maintained in response to occlusal forces associated with chewing. Age-related bone loss affecting alveolar bone results in tooth loss and edentulism. Bone resorption accelerates causing rapidly diminishing bone height in edentulous patients. Low calcium intake is related to increased risk of tooth loss.[14]

The combination of periodontal disease and thinning bones may put postmenopausal women at particular risk of tooth loss. A primary risk factor for tooth loss is the degree of deterioration in alveolar bones supporting the teeth. Because postmenopausal women lose bone at an increased rate, control of periodontal disease can significantly reduce their tooth loss. Tooth loss and edentulism reflect differences in healthy behaviors, attitudes toward oral health, and dental care.

Many individuals in the United States older than age 60 years only have 19 teeth. More seniors with lower incomes are edentulous than those in higher income brackets. Older people who have no or few teeth at age 70 years are more likely to have mobility problems within the next 5 or 10 years, so tooth loss may be an early indicator of accelerated aging.[15]

Dental status significantly affects diet and nutrition. Loss of teeth, edentulous status, and conventional dentures increase risk of malnutrition in older adults.[16,17] When dentition status is compromised, nutrient intake decreases as the total number of teeth decreases. Periodontal conditions, edentulous areas, and/or ill-fitting appliances tend to alter their food choices to reduce chewing or because of fear of choking. Food intake is affected more if the patient feels the dentures do not fit well.[18-20] Patients who are missing a significant number of teeth generally consume fewer fruits and vegetables, especially raw carrots and tossed salads, and dietary fiber than individuals with all their teeth, and consequently have lower serum levels of beta-carotene, folate, and vitamin C.[21] Compromised dental status negatively affects animal protein intake, reducing intake of total protein, vitamins B_1 and B_6, niacin, and pantothenic acid. Individuals who have lost numerous teeth are more likely to be obese than are individuals with more teeth.[22-24]

Having fewer teeth is related to swallowing dysfunction.[25,26] Generally, patients who wear dentures have reduced masticatory efficiency—75% to 85% less than with natural teeth. After edentulous individuals fully adjust to new dentures, caloric intake increases, yet dietary intake of magnesium, folic acid, fluoride, zinc, and calcium continues to be low. Even if they own dentures, some may not wear them, or they may be unable to chew because of a periodontal condition. Treatment with mandibular implant-supported dentures may have positive effects on the clinical aspects of mastication and swallowing in older individuals.[27]

Weight changes, common among older adults, can be a reason for an ill-fitting dental appliance. Weight gain (usually secondary to edema) results in a tight-fitting denture, which may cause ulcerations; weight loss causing loose-fitting dentures also can increase risk of ulcerations. If severe mandibular resorption occurs, it is very difficult to construct a well-fitting dental prosthesis.

Nutrient intakes of patients with compromised dentition can fall below minimum requirements. Many older individuals or their families do not believe the cost of a new or replaced appliance is warranted because of the patients' perceived life expectancy.

Gastrointestinal Tract

Changes in esophageal motility and deterioration of nerve function may cause dysphagia (difficulty with swallowing). This frequently observed disorder increases risk of aspiration pneumonia and morbidity from inadequate nutrition. Individuals with swallowing problems eat slowly and may be unable to consume adequate amounts.

Atrophic gastritis, a chronic stomach inflammation with atrophy of the mucous membrane and glands and diminished hydrochloric acid production, is frequently observed in older patients. Diminished hydrochloric acid secretion may affect calcium, iron, and vitamin B_{12} absorption. Additionally, lack of acid permits overgrowth of bacteria that compromise vitamin B_{12} availability.

Constipation may be a consequence of altered gastrointestinal motility, loss of bowel muscle tone, medications, inadequate food and fluid intake, low-fiber diet, and inactivity. Additional causes include chronic laxative use and some medications, especially analgesics, antihypertensives, and narcotics. Problems with constipation may be averted by increasing fiber-containing foods, fluid intake, and activity level.

Hydration Status

Decreased thirst sensations are associated with aging; dehydration occurs more frequently in older adults. Fluid intake may not increase automatically to offset increased water losses from the compromised kidney. As a result of poor fluid intake, susceptibility to caries is increased.

Homeostatic mechanisms indicate the body's ability to correct imbalances, such as decreased nutrient intake accompanied by an increase in the nutrient's absorption or efficiency of use. Certain chronic illnesses (heart and kidney disease) lead to impairment of various homeostatic mechanisms controlling water balance. Fever, which can lead to mild dehydration in healthy individuals, may result in severe dehydration in older adults. Other seemingly mild stresses, such as the presence of infection or diarrhea, or use of diuretics, can upset the normal homeostasis of an older individual.

Dehydration is probably the primary cause of confusion in older hospitalized patients and can occur because of the kidney's inability to concentrate urine, changes in thirst sensation, changes in functional status, side effects of medications, and lack of mobility. Dehydration can lead to loose-fitting dentures. Dehydration frequently results in hospitalization as a result of fecal impaction, cognitive impairment, and overall functional decline.

Musculoskeletal System

Two nutrition-related conditions encountered by older persons involving the musculoskeletal system are osteoporosis and sarcopenia, so maintaining bone health and muscle mass are primary concerns. As discussed in Chapter 9 *Health Application 9,* osteoporosis or shortening and outward bowing of the spine may develop. Bone resorption progresses rapidly in older patients. Trabecular bone loss may be associated with physical inactivity, unavailability of calcium (inadequate dietary intake, imbalance in calcium-to-phosphorus ratio, and decreased calcium absorption), changes in hormones affecting calcium metabolism, lack of vitamin D, or altered vitamin D metabolism associated with impaired renal function. Bone loss increases susceptibility to fractures, which can result in disability.

Sarcopenia is the reduction of skeletal muscle mass and its replacement by fat that occurs in older adults. This condition affects functional capacity, leading to frailty, reduced mobility, and loss of balance. If enough muscle is lost, it can be debilitating. The prevalence of sarcopenic obesity differs substantially among studies because of the lack of a standard definition. Approximately 5% to 10% of adults older than age 60 years have sarcopenia; prevalence increases significantly in adults older than age 80 years.[28] Sarcopenia can even occur in an obese person (body mass index [BMI] >27 kg/m²) (called sarcopenic obesity).

Inactivity is responsible for loss of muscle strength and balance, which increase the likelihood of falling. Physical activity can help ameliorate some chronic health problems, yet two-thirds of people older than age 65 years do not exercise. An active lifestyle also helps to improve physiological well-being, and it relieves symptoms of depression and anxiety. Box 15-1 lists some benefits of physical activity. Many older adults can be motivated to make changes to prevent or delay a decline toward ill health and disability if information is presented with an understandable rationale. The *Physical Activity Guidelines for Americans* (see Chapter 7) issued by the U.S. Department of Health and Human Services addressing adults also apply to older adults.[29] Older adults who are unable to do 150 minutes of moderate-intensity aerobic activity a week because of health conditions should be as physically active as their abilities and conditions allow. Older adults with chronic conditions should understand whether and how their conditions affect their ability to do regular physical activity safely. Exercises that maintain or improve balance are recommended if falling is a risk.

The amount of muscle mass is determined in part by how much muscles are used. Exercising muscles to the limits of their capacity (e.g., weightlifting) results in maintaining or increasing muscle mass and strength. Women have less muscle than men but lose it more slowly during aging. Because older women do not use protein as effectively as men, muscle that has been lost is harder to replace. The older person becomes weak and frail, creating functional problems that further contribute to sarcopenia. Adequate amounts of protein are essential to replace muscle lost during the aging process.

With aging, intra-abdominal fat increases more than subcutaneous or total body fat, and peripheral muscle declines more than central muscle mass. As musculature shrinks, fat tissue accumulates. Instead of focusing on losing weight, the goal should be to increase muscle and reduce fat. A slightly higher BMI seems to be protective in maintaining immunity to diseases.

Even with no increase in weight, fat stores replace lean muscle mass. Low protein intake contributes to muscle loss and a negative nitrogen balance that causes muscle breakdown. Maintaining muscle is essential to reduce the risk of falling. Diminished sense of taste and smell, rapid satiety, poor oral health, decreased metabolism, gastrointestinal changes, and dementia—all increasingly common with aging—result in decreasing food intake and increased adiposity (caused by fatigue and lack of activity). This creates a vicious cycle that leads to more gain in fat and more muscle loss, eventually resulting in functional consequences (e.g., disability), reduced quality of life, and early death.

On the brighter side, sarcopenia is not inevitable with aging. High-protein foods stimulate muscle protein synthesis, even in older adults. Protein use may be impaired, but this can be overcome by consuming high-quality protein at each meal and doing resistance training. Resistance exercise combined with consuming proteins from animal sources elicits the greatest anabolic response and may help older individuals produce a "youthful" muscle protein synthesis response. The International Osteoporosis Foundation also recommends balancing a high-protein diet with adequate amounts of fruits and vegetables to reduce risk of sarcopenia. Maintaining appropriate blood levels of vitamin D may also aid in retaining muscle strength and physical performance.[30]

Whether benefits of weight loss outweigh risks in the older population is unknown. But in postmenopausal women who lost approximately 12% of their body weight, 84% of those who regained more than 4 lb deposited more than four times as much fat as muscle.[31] Muscle mass can be preserved by increasing physical activity. When older people diet without exercising, they lose more lean muscle mass and less fat compared to those who exercise while dieting.

Less lean body mass results in a decreased basal metabolic rate (Fig. 15-2). In older individuals, the basal metabolic rate may be 10% to 12% below the level of 20-year-olds (see Chapter 7). In other words, the body burns fewer kilocalories than during earlier years, so less food is needed to prevent weight gain. Less intake of vital proteins inhibits healing after a physiological injury or insult and also contributes to the declining function of many organ systems.

BOX 15-1	Health Benefits of Physical Activity

- Improves chances of living longer and healthier
- Decreases risk of heart disease, stroke, high blood pressure, and adverse blood lipid profile
- Helps decrease risk of developing certain cancers, including colon and breast cancer
- Helps prevent or delay the onset of type 2 diabetes and metabolic syndrome
- Prevents weight gain, promotes weight loss (if combined with reduction of caloric intake)
- Improved heart-lung and muscular fitness
- Decreases risk of falls
- Relieves symptoms of depression and anxiety and improves mood
- Improves cognitive function
- Improves sleep quality
- Increases bone density and decreases risk of hip fractures

Adapted from U.S. Department of Health and Human Services. *2008 Physical activity guidelines for Americans.* Accessed September 6, 2013: http://www.health.gov/paguidelines/.

SOCIOECONOMIC AND PSYCHOLOGICAL FACTORS

Many changes occur that may affect food intake of older adults (Fig. 15-3). Most retired people live on fixed incomes significantly lower than when they were employed. Approximately 3.4 million older adults live in poverty with approximately 9 million at risk of hunger.[32] Inflation, failing health, and medical bills (especially cost of medications) can have a devastating effect on fixed incomes. The food budget frequently is affected and is a risk factor for inadequate nutrition. Fresh fruit and vegetable choices may be curtailed because of their high cost and limited shelf life. Title III Nutrition Programs for the Elderly (congregate dining and Meals-on-Wheels) are available to improve nutritional and health status of older patients and possibly prevent or postpone more expensive services of long-term care institutions. Nutritious meals are furnished at a minimal charge to older adults or free for those who qualify. These programs have been proven to improve dietary intakes of recipients whose diets were previously below the RDA.

An inability to drive or lack of access to transportation affects use of health services and availability of food. Approximately one-third of noninstitutionalized individuals older than age 65 years live alone. Individuals who live with another person and are socially active tend to consume a larger variety of foods. An inactive person who lives alone may lack motivation to prepare well-balanced meals, especially if the appetite is poor.

Apathy and depression can predispose older individuals to decreased appetite and interest in food. Depression is difficult to distinguish from symptoms related to stresses of later life such as illness and changes in lifestyle. Some older individuals may consider depression as a natural, inevitable component of aging and may not seek treatment. Loneliness is related to dietary inadequacies.

Dental Considerations

Assessment

- *Physical:* blood pressure, diagnosis of chronic disease, dentures, swallowing process, xerostomia, condition of oral cavity and gingiva; financial status, socioeconomic status, mental status, educational level, psychological status; types of drugs taken, including over-the-counter drugs, herbal supplements, and aspirin use.
- *Dietary:* screen for nutritional health (see the assessment form available on Evolve); motivation to eat and drink; beliefs and attitudes about foods or products to delay the aging process.

Interventions

- Encourage new denture wearers to swallow liquids with the dentures first, then to chew soft foods, and, last to bite and masticate regular foods. It is easier to master complex masticatory movements in this order, and the mouth is protected from becoming sore. New denture wearers need to eat slowly, chew food longer, and cut raw fibrous foods such as apples and carrots into bite-size pieces.
- Wearing dentures may promote positive calcium balance and decrease alveolar resorption. If calcium intake is poor, supplements containing both calcium and vitamin D may help promote positive calcium balance.
- For edentulous patients, inquire about the preferred texture of food. Do not assume edentulous patients require pureed foods; because of lack of visual appeal and flavor, appetite may be affected if only pureed foods are offered.

Continued

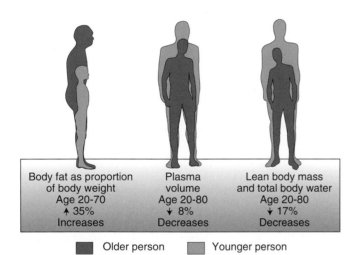

FIGURE 15-2 Changes in the body with aging. Younger person, age 20 years. Older person, age 80 years. (Redrawn from Vestal RE: *Drugs and the elderly*, NIH Publication No. 79-1449, Washington, DC, 1979, U.S. Department of Health, Education, and Welfare.)

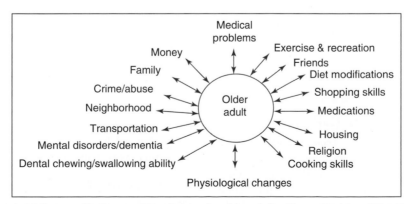

FIGURE 15-3 Multiple interrelated factors affecting nutritional status for older adults. (From American Dietetic Association: Position of the American Dietetic Association: Nutrition, aging, and the continuum of care. *J Am Diet Assoc* 2000; 100(5):580-594.)

Dental Considerations—cont'd

- Teach older patients about appropriate oral hygiene techniques to minimize recession, followed with a fluoride regimen.
- Assess the fit of a denture or any prosthesis. The dental team may need to make recommendations for adjusting the prosthesis for a better fit or refer the older patient to a healthcare provider for assessment and management of unintentional weight changes.
- Encourage older patients to eat slowly and chew their food well.
- Often healthcare providers recommend lemon glycerin swabs to moisten oral tissues in patients with xerostomia. This may be detrimental to the mouth for two reasons: (a) because lemon is an acid, it may cause decalcification of the teeth, and (b) glycerin is a form of alcohol that can further dry oral tissues. A better alternative would be to moisten a swab with water and apply it to the dry mucosa.
- Avoidance of certain food categories (fresh fruit and vegetables and meats) because of masticatory difficulties may aggravate other nutrition-related problems; these foods are major sources of vitamins and minerals.

Nutritional Directions

- Factors that slow the aging process include regular exercise, abstinence from smoking, and reduction of stress. Physical exercise and activity enhance muscle strength and preserve muscle mass.
- Effective interventions are available to prevent and control oral disease to achieve good oral health which is essential to healthy aging.
- Less muscle tissue and a lower activity level result in a reduced caloric requirement.
- If xerostomia is present, use artificial saliva products (oral moisturizers), gum, or hard, sugarless candies (preferably containing xylitol); practice frequent oral hygiene care; and drink adequate noncariogenic fluids.
- For patients with compromised natural dentition or xerostomia, suggest including fluids, sauces, or gravies with each meal to make chewing easier. However, beverage consumption should not interfere with food intake.
- Because of decreased stomach acid, older adults should take calcium citrate with vitamin D supplements between meals for optimal absorption or use calcium carbonate supplements with meals.
- Moderate exercise, such as walking, is beneficial in reducing the risk of CHD in older adults.
- By exercising 45 minutes a day, older adults can significantly improve muscle strength and slightly increase bone density.[33] The promotion of physical activity in older adults should emphasize moderate-intensity aerobic activity, muscle-strengthening activity, flexibility, and balance.

NUTRIENT REQUIREMENTS

Dietary Reference Intakes (DRIs)

The revised DRIs separated the recommendations for individuals 51 to 70 years old from those for individuals older than 70 years. Metabolism to maintain body functions requires all the same nutrients, but the requirements for most micronutrients are increased because of the effects of aging on absorption, use, and excretion. With few exceptions, the recommended amounts for most nutrients for both groups are the same. Energy needs are lower for older individuals because of declining basal metabolism and activity level. Recommendations for several nutrients differ from those for adults 31 to 50 years old, including fiber, calcium, chromium, iron (for women), and vitamins D and B$_6$ (Table 15-1).

Fluids

In normal situations, at least eight glasses of fluids per day are recommended (Fig. 15-4). Fluid intake is of particular concern because older individuals are susceptible to fluid imbalances secondary to physiological changes. An older patient may intentionally restrict fluids because of nocturia (excessive urination at night), incontinence (inability to control urinary excretion), pain associated with movement related to arthritis, or having to request assistance to go to the toilet.

Energy and Protein

Energy balance is usually recommended for older adults. Clinical recommendation of weight loss remains controversial because of the potential for loss of lean muscle and physical function. Protein intake may be compromised because of illness, debilitating injuries, depressed appetite, or difficulty eating. If intentional caloric deficit to lose weight (and consequently fatty tissue) is accompanied by routine exercise to maintain physical fitness, mobility and walking speed can improve.[34] However, weight loss, even with intentional caloric restriction and improved health indices, does not increase life span.[35]

Despite what is indicated in the RDAs, protein needs are proportional to body weight, not energy intake.[36] Essential amino acid requirement is increased for older adults to produce a positive response in muscle protein synthesis and metabolism and stimulate bone protein metabolism. Approximately 25 to 30 g (or slightly more than 3 oz of meat) of high-quality protein will maximize muscle protein synthesis, but this amount of protein is needed three times a day rather than eating most of the protein at one meal.[37,38]

Inadequate protein intake was observed in 1% to 5% of men between 51 and 71 years and 9% to 24% in women over 71 years of age. Animal sources provided more than 60% of the protein intake. The percentage of protein from animal sources predicts the probability of meeting the RDA.[39] Older persons who consume higher percentages of protein have less age-related reduction in lean tissue mass.[40] Exercise at any age increases the body's need for protein, so protein intake slightly above the RDA (1.0 g/day) may be needed for increasing bone-mineral density and muscle mass.[41] Protein also plays a pivotal role in maintenance of bone health by increasing calcium absorption and muscle strength and mass, thereby benefiting the skeleton.[42]

Vitamins and Minerals

Older patients (especially women) usually have a negative calcium balance and lose bone mass, leading to osteoporosis

Table 15-1	Dietary reference intakes (DRIs) for selected nutrients for older adults			
	Age 51-70 Years		**Age Older than 70 Years**	
Nutrients	Men	Women	Men	Women
Protein (g)	56	46	56	46
Carbohydrate (g)	130	130	130	130
Fiber (g)	30*	21*	30*	21*
Fat-Soluble Vitamins				
Vitamin A (μg)	900	700	900	700
Vitamin E (mg)	15	15	15	15
Vitamin D (μg/IU)†	15/600	15/600	20/800	20/800
Vitamin K	120*	120*	90*	90*
Water-Soluble Vitamins				
Ascorbic acid (mg)	90	75	90	75
Folate (μg)	400	400	400	400
Niacin (mg)	16	14	16	14
Riboflavin (mg)	1.3	1.1	1.3	1.1
Thiamin (mg)	1.2	1.1	1.2	1.1
Vitamin B_6 (mg)	1.7	1.5	1.7	1.5
Vitamin B_{12} (μg)†	2.4	2.4	2.4	2.4
Biotin	30*	30*	30*	30*
Choline	550*	550*	550*	550*
Minerals				
Calcium (mg)	1000	1200	1200	1200
Phosphorus (mg)	700	700	700	700
Iodine (μg)	150	150	150	150
Iron (mg)	8	8	8	8
Magnesium (mg)	420	320	420	320
Zinc (mg)	11	8	11	8
Selenium (μg)	55	55	55	55

Data from Institute of Medicine, Food and Nutrition Board: *Dietary reference intakes for: calcium and vitamin D*, Washington, DC, 2011, National Academies Press; Institute of Medicine, Food and Nutrition Board: *Dietary reference intakes for vitamin C, vitamin E, selenium, and carotenoids*, Washington, DC, 2000, National Academies Press; Institute of Medicine, Food and Nutrition Board: *Dietary reference intakes for calcium, phosphorus, magnesium, vitamin D, and fluoride*, Washington, DC, 1997, National Academies Press; Institute of Medicine, Food and Nutrition Board: *Dietary reference intakes for vitamin A, vitamin K, arsenic, boron, chromium, copper, iodine, iron, manganese, molybdenum, nickel, silicon, vanadium, and zinc*, Washington, DC, 2001, National Academies Press; and Institute of Medicine, Food and Nutrition Board: *Dietary reference intakes for carbohydrates, fats, protein, fiber, and physical activity, parts 1 and 2*, Washington, DC, 2002, National Academies Press. Available www.nap.edu.

Note: Recommended dietary allowances (RDAs) are presented in **bold type** and adequate intakes (AIs) are followed by an asterisk (*).

†1 μg cholecalciferol = 40 IU vitamin D.

and spontaneous fractures. Inadequate calcium intake is one possible reason for this, but genetic, hormonal, and environmental factors are also important. Decreased physical activity contributes to calcium loss over the years. The RDA of 1200 mg of calcium for everyone older than age 70 years is higher than for younger adults so as to maintain bone mass and reduce risk of osteoporosis. Calcium supplements are largely ineffective for remodeling bone matrix if adequate protein (at least 1.0 g/kg) is not available.[43]

The Third National Health and Nutrition Examination Survey (NHANES III) estimated 30% of individuals 60 years old and older who reside in lower latitudes have vitamin D insufficiency in the winter, and 26% residing in higher latitudes have vitamin D insufficiency in the summer.[44] Prevalence of vitamin D deficiency is even higher in homebound or institutionalized older individuals. Vitamin D insufficiency may occur in older adults because aging skin cannot synthesize vitamin D as efficiently, they are less likely to spend much time outdoors, and their vitamin D intakes may be inadequate. A deficiency may be the result of several causes that reduce production of vitamin D_3 by the skin, such as increased clothing to cover the skin and use of sunscreen. Other causes of vitamin D deficiency include dietary insufficiency, malabsorption, kidney disease, and use of glucocorticoids.

As many as half of older adults in the United States could be vitamin D deficient as evidenced by the numbers of hip fractures.[45] The RDAs may be adequate for most older individuals, but these amounts may not be adequate for high risk seniors—those who are obese, have osteoporosis, have

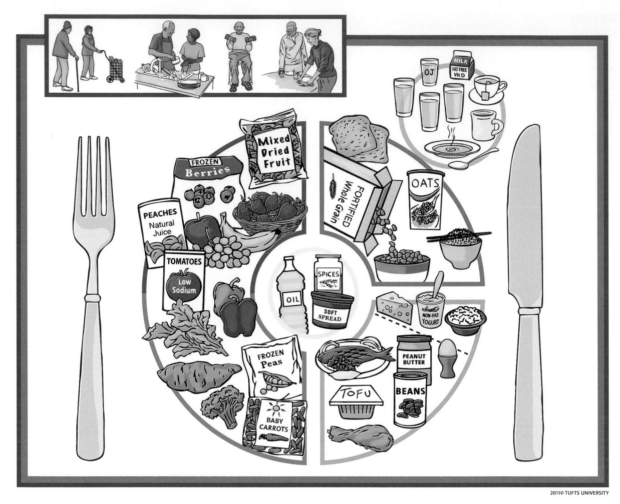

FIGURE 15-4 *MyPlate for Older Adults.* The Tufts University *MyPlate for Older Adults* icon provides food, fluid and physical activity guidance, corresponds with the federal government's 2010 Dietary Guidelines (© 2011 Tufts University. Reprinted with permission from Lichtenstein AH, et al: Available at http://nutrition.tufts.edu.)

limited sun exposure, or experience malabsorption. For these individuals, the International Osteoporosis Foundation recommends providing supplementation based on measurement of serum 25-OHD (1,25-dihydroxyvitamin D3) level.[46] Supplementation with vitamin D reduces risk of falls only in older people whose vitamin D levels are low.[47]

Vitamin D insufficiency leads to reduced active transport of calcium from the intestine. In older individuals with vitamin D insufficiency, supplementation reduces bone loss. Muscle performance also is improved, which reduces the risk of falling and fracture risk.[48-50] To prevent problems with bone mineralization, the recommendation for vitamin D intake is higher for individuals over 70 years—20 μg/day (800 IU). It is important to ensure that patients receive adequate calcium in addition to vitamin D.

Physiological requirements for vitamins B_6 and B_{12} are increased to prevent a decline in cognitive function associated with aging and to reduce risk for coronary artery disease.[51] Cobalamin (vitamin B_{12}) may be less available in

older adults because of atrophic gastritis and bacterial overgrowth. Approximately 10% to 30% of older adults have decreased absorption of vitamin B_{12} and many are at risk because of the effects of medications. Choosing foods fortified with vitamin B_{12} or taking a vitamin B_{12}-containing supplement is recommended to meet the DRIs. Symptoms such as cognitive decline, confusion, disorientation, and neurological problems may decrease in individuals treated with vitamin B_{12}.[52,53]

Economic factors and chewing problems may negatively affect meat consumption, thus negatively affecting vitamins B_6 and B_{12} intake. Edentulous men with inadequate natural masticatory function and no dentures could be at much greater risk of dementia than those with adequate natural chewing skills.[54] Neurological symptoms similar to dementia may result from deficiencies of vitamins B_6 and B_{12} when intake is reported to be marginal.

In addition to these neurological symptoms, metabolic abnormalities may occur before vitamin B_{12} levels in the blood decrease; pernicious anemia occurs only in severely vitamin B_{12}–depleted individuals. When serum levels are depressed, low oral doses of vitamin B_{12} can be used rather than the painful and more expensive injections. Oral vitamin B_{12} is effective in benefiting symptoms of depression in some older adults.[55]

High levels of folic acid intake resulting in elevated blood folate concentrations may negatively affect an older adult's health. High folate levels can cause cognitive decline and impaired cognitive performance. Whereas folic acid supplementation was encouraged in the past for CHD, further studies indicate higher folate levels may increase risk of cancer mortality.[56] Both men and women taking supplements are more likely to have elevated folate concentrations, but smoking reduces the amount of folate in the blood.[57]

Dietary mineral intake, especially sodium, may need to be adjusted based on the patient's physiological status. Excess or even normal dietary levels can have deleterious consequences in certain diseases, particularly chronic illnesses such as hypertension or congestive heart failure. Rigid and severe restrictions may seriously affect food acceptance. Individualization is crucial.

EATING PATTERNS

Deficiencies

Compared with younger age groups, the diets of Americans older than age 65 years rate better with regard to higher consumption of fruits and lower consumption of sodium and cholesterol. As with most Americans, the prevalence of low-energy-dense diets that are more likely to provide adequate amounts of nutrients is low. More than 80% of individuals older than age 71 years consumed empty kilocalories exceeding the discretionary caloric allowances.[58] Overall, most older adults are not meeting the RDA for many nutrients.[59,60] A notable deficiency was a lower proportion of older adults consuming the recommended number of servings of meat.

Dairy products, fruits, and vegetables are frequently lacking in the diet, especially for individuals living alone. Milk is important for calcium needs, but daily consumption is difficult because of frequent trips needed to purchase it. Dry milk, although less palatable than regular milk, can be incorporated into many foods without deleterious effects on taste. Additionally, lactose intolerance may contribute to inadequate calcium intake (see Chapter 2, *Health Application 2*). The choice of soft foods usually results in a decrease in protein and more simple carbohydrate intake. Inadequate monetary resources to purchase meat products may result in less protein consumption. Older individuals at highest risk of consuming minimal amounts of fruits and vegetables are those who are socially isolated, are missing pairs of posterior teeth, have poor self-reported health, and are obese. Older adults who adhere to the *Dietary Guidelines* by choosing recommended amounts of vegetables, fruit, whole grains, low-fat dairy products, poultry, and fish may have a low risk of mortality.[61]

Snacks and Nutritional Supplements

For some older adults, energy intakes decline. Snacking may ensure consumption of adequate amounts of kilocalories and protein for those who have experienced weight loss. Underweight is a recognized risk factor for disease and disability. Between-meal snacks can be used to offset some nutrient deficits.

Milk-based food supplements, such as an instant breakfast mix, are economical and can help prevent nutrient deficiencies. A tasty supplement can augment overall nutrient intake to maintain nutritional status. Commercial liquid nutrition supplements, such as Ensure (Abbott Nutrition) and Sustacal (Nestlé Lanka Group), are more convenient and may be preferred. Some of these liquid supplements are lactose-free. These supplements, when used routinely, may produce a small but consistent weight gain and may have a beneficial effect on mortality of older undernourished people.[62] Oral nutritional supplements for acutely ill patients can be used to improve nutritional status and avoid hospital admissions. Referral to the healthcare provider or registered dietitian (RDN) is recommended for these patients.

Food Safety

Foodborne illness can be very serious for older patients. Many older adults are more susceptible to foodborne illness because of a compromised immune system (placing them at risk for infections), decreased secretion of gastric hydrochloric acid, and reduced smell and taste. Food poisoning (discussed more fully in Chapter 16) is caused by food contaminated with pathogenic bacteria, toxins, viruses, or parasites.

MYPLATE FOR OLDER ADULTS

MyPlate for Older Adults focuses on the unique needs associated with the aging process (see Fig. 15-4). This updated version is based on the *Dietary Guidelines* and *MyPlate*.

MyPlate for Older Adults emphasizes nutrient-dense food choices and the importance of fluid balance, but has additional guidance about types of foods that best meet the unique needs of older adults and importance of regular physical activity. The groupings on this plate are slightly different than for *MyPlate*: (a) icons of many bright colored fruits and vegetables occupy half of the plate; (b) whole, enriched, and fortified grains cover one-fourth of the plate; (c) protein sources, including meats, dry beans and nuts, eggs, and tofu, make up the other one-fourth of the plate; and (d) a small part of the protein section contains milk and cheese icons. In the center of the plate are icons depicting liquid vegetable oils and soft spreads (to avoid foods high in animal fats that contain saturated fat and other processed foods containing *trans* fats), and spices other than salt to reduce sodium intake to below 1500 mg/day.

Icons of fruits and vegetables are presented in different forms (frozen, pre-peeled fresh, dried, and canned options). Canned low-sugar fruits and low-sodium vegetables are healthy and nutrient content is similar to fresh or frozen products; they are easier to prepare, may be less expensive, and have a longer shelf life. Above the right side of the plate are fluids such as water, tea, coffee, and fat-free milk as a reminder of the importance of drinking liquids to help avoid dehydration. *MyPlate for Older Adults* promotes regular physical activity whether it is household chores, walking, or regular exercise routines. Eating should be an enjoyable routine and, whenever possible, mealtimes should involve social interaction.

Vitamin-Mineral Supplements

Sometimes food choices of older adults are not as well balanced as they should be, or less food is consumed. Because of impaired absorption of nutrients and reduced food intake, many older individuals may benefit from a multiple vitamin-mineral supplement. Daily multivitamin-mineral supplementation at 100% of the RDI levels is helpful in protecting against a decline in immune response and preventing anemia.

For older adults, poor appetite, decreased sense of taste and smell, and denture problems all can contribute to a poor diet, as can eating alone and depression. Natural foods are the best source of vitamins and minerals, so if additional food is needed for adequacy, healthy snacks should be encouraged. However, because of increased need for calcium and vitamins D and B$_{12}$, accompanied by poor intake and decreased caloric requirements, a vitamin and/or mineral supplement may improve cognition and nutritional status.[63,64]

A discussion with the healthcare provider about the need for nutritional supplements may be in order. The following recommendations about dietary supplements should be considered in concurrence with the individual's regular food intake with a goal of ensuring nutrients in the amounts listed in Table 15-1.[65]

- Calcium—Calcium supplements should not be more than 2500 mg/day. For better absorption, calcium should be taken in two 600-mg doses. Calcium not only keeps bones healthy, but also helps muscles function properly and normalizes blood pressure.
- Vitamin D—Vitamin D supplements should be limited to less than 4000 IU each day. This should be taken in conjunction with calcium to increase calcium absorption. This amount should not be increased without a recommendation from the healthcare provider.
- Vitamin B$_{12}$—Because of poor absorption of vitamin B$_{12}$, increased amounts (above 2.4 μg) may be needed, which may help improve cognitive function and symptoms of depression and prevent pernicious anemia.

The *Dietary Guidelines* recommend eating fish twice a week. People who do not eat much fish may benefit from a fish oil supplement (300 mg of omega-3 fatty acid), which can help reduce triglyceride levels.

As many as 70% of older adults take dietary (vitamin-mineral) supplements to maintain a healthy life, or prevent a disease/medical problem, because they know their eating patterns are not ideal, or because a healthcare professional recommended them. Although it may be important to take dietary supplements, 27% exceed the upper limit for a nutrient.[66]

Age-related macular degeneration is a deterioration in the central area of the retina (back of the eye) in which lesions lead to loss of central vision. Studies have found a lower risk of macular degeneration in people who consume a diet rich in lutein and zeaxanthin (carotenoid vitamins, related to beta-carotene and vitamin A) and diets rich in fatty fish, such as salmon. Previously, antioxidant vitamins and/or minerals have been recommended for prevention of age-related macular degeneration. Researchers have reported that taking vitamin E and beta-carotene supplements are unlikely to prevent age-related macular degeneration.[67] Foods may contain something other than these nutrients that explains the lower risk of eye disease associated with eating them. Evidence is lacking with respect to any antioxidant supplements preventing or delaying the onset of age-related macular degeneration. These vitamin supplements are generally recognized as safe, but they could have harmful effects; clear evidence of benefit is needed before recommending them. Referral to the healthcare provider or a RDN is necessary to assess the need for supplements.

Dental Considerations

Assessment
- *Physical:* visual appraisal of weight status; dry mucous membranes.
- *Dietary:* adequacy of nutrients and fluid intake based on the *MyPlate for Older Adults*; multivitamin/mineral/herbal use.

Interventions
- To prevent dehydration, encourage older patients to use caffeine in moderation and to take medications with 8 oz of fluid. Encourage nutrient-dense foods, especially for older patients whose kilocalorie expenditure is low.
- Healthy snacks such as cheese, hard-boiled eggs, low-fat milk products, bananas, and canned fruit can be recommended.
- Older patients who have had an unintentional weight change of 10% (loss or gain) in 6 months should be referred to a healthcare provider.
- Absorption of vitamin B$_{12}$ from vitamin supplements or fortified foods is not affected by atrophic gastritis. Suggest enriched or fortified cereals to increase intake of iron and vitamin B$_{12}$.
- Encourage consumption of milk and dairy products or adding dry milk powder in foods.
- Encourage consumption of a vitamin C–rich food daily.
- Review economical sources of folate and cooking practices to retain folate.
- Encourage wise selections of convenience foods. Explain how to read food labels to make selections appropriate for restricted diets or to provide a well-balanced diet.

Nutritional Directions

- A well-balanced diet following the *MyPlate for Older Adults* may delay symptoms of aging.
- Consume 2 to 4 oz of meat or other protein source at each meal.
- Lack of vitamin B_{12} can cause poor memory and impaired balance.
- Nutrition counseling by a RDN can provide information on consuming adequate amounts of high-quality protein to help patients living on a limited budget and offer alternatives to eating problems.
- Nonfat or low-fat milk is the best source of calcium and vitamin D.
- Dietary intake should strive to optimize immune function and reduce risk of disease in older adults.
- Calcium supplements should also contain vitamin D to enhance calcium absorption and increase bone density.
- Discuss economical fruit, vegetable, and meat selections (see Chapter 16).
- Adequate fluid intake is beneficial in preventing and treating constipation.
- Soups, juices, milk products, decaffeinated soft drinks, and decaffeinated tea and coffee can enhance fluid intake.
- Because many older adults cannot efficiently use vitamin B_{12} found in animal foods, vitamin B_{12} present in breakfast cereals or supplements is better absorbed.

- Older adults should check with their healthcare provider or RDN to find out whether supplements are needed.
- Older patients should contact their healthcare provider when their food choices are limited over a period of time because of illness, chewing problems, lack of appetite, or inability to shop for or prepare food.
- Vitamin supplements providing more than 100% of the RDI should be taken only in cases of specific need or recommendations by a healthcare provider. Use of vitamin-mineral supplements does not eliminate the need to consume a nutritionally-balanced diet, and supplements do not protect against development of chronic diseases associated with inappropriate food intake.
- Excess supplementation of vitamins and minerals may cause more problems with hypervitaminosis and detrimental effects on other nutrients. Zinc supplements can result in copper imbalance and reduce high-density lipoprotein cholesterol levels. Refer the patient to a healthcare provider or RDN.
- Heed food safety guidelines to ensure foods do not cause illness.

HEALTH APPLICATION 15 Genomics

The word *genome* refers to the entire DNA sequence of an organism. DNA located in the nucleus contains the instruction for developing and directing the activities of nearly all living organisms. A complete set of DNA is called the organism's genome. Mutation of a cellular DNA produces an abnormal protein which can disrupt normal physiological processes and lead to a disease. Virtually every disease has some basis in the individual's genes.

In 2001, scientists associated with the Human Genome Project announced completion of the sequence mapping of the human genome.[68] Since everyone's gene pool is unique, the sequence is a generic sequence from multiple people. Genomics is the scientific discipline of mapping, sequencing, and analyzing the genome. Research related to genomics is contributing to a better understanding of cellular and molecular mechanisms underlying diet–disease relationships. This information is being used to develop more effective diagnostic tools with a future vision of using it to better understand health needs and design individualized approaches to disease prevention and treatment.

By integrating and applying genomics technology into nutrition research, current studies are aimed at prevention and control of chronic disease, such as cancer, CHD, diabetes, and obesity. The scientific study of how foods or their components interact with genes, and how individual genetic differences affect responses to nutrients (and other naturally-occurring compounds), is referred to as nutrigenomics or nutritional genomics. Nutrigenomics will eventually be able to characterize genetic susceptibility to diet-related chronic diseases and molecular responses to dietary factors. Integration of genomics and nutrition in research is needed to develop programs aimed at prevention and control of chronic disease through nutritional interventions.

Genes have a powerful influence over a person's health but are not the only determinant over destiny because nutrition, emotions, and environmental factors also influence health. These factors further complicate research by adding innumerable variables. For example, more than 25,000 bioactive (nonnutrient) food components have been identified with many unanswered questions about their modes of interaction and duration of activity.[69]

A nutritionally-related birth defect has almost been cut in half by implementation of a dietary measure. Folate is an example of a nutrient extensively studied because of its impact on DNA synthesis in the human genome. Variants (different forms) of genes that are responsible for folate-dependent enzymes can alter efficiency of DNA synthesis and provide protection from and risk for developmental conditions such as neural tube defects. Folate fortification in the food supply was targeted at a distinct group—women of childbearing age who are at genetic risk for having an infant with a neural tube defect—to prevent this birth defect. This public health measure has been successful in lowering the rate of neural tube defects. This is just one example of how a nutritional intervention might be individualized based on knowledge of nutrigenomics.

Nutritional genomics has tremendous potential to not only change the future of personal nutrition recommendations, but also dietary guidelines for the population. Health promotion advice as promoted in the *Dietary Guidelines* is based on population-based data; for example, what is statistically likely to occur with respect to risk factors and disease outcomes. On the other hand, nutrigenomics research focuses on tweaking this advice based on an individual's genetics.

The current knowledge base for nutrigenomics is in its infancy. Nutrigenomics will someday provide the basis for

Continued

HEALTH APPLICATION 15   Genomics—cont'd

personalized dietary recommendations based on the individual's genetic makeup. Chronic disease may be preventable, or delayed, by prescribing a personalized regimen of a specific nutrient based on an analysis of a person's genes.

Cutting edge research is exciting and encouraging, but nutrigenomics is not ready for clinical implementation. The Evaluation of Genomic Applications in Practice and Prevention Working Group reported in 2010 that specific genetic types affecting metabolism and nutritional factors have been identified that influence an individual's health, but existing clinical data does not show a significant clinical effect.[70]

As genetic analysis rapidly develops and becomes more cost effective, potential problems will result in exploitation of the basic hypotheses. Many scientific research studies are essential when determining whether a hypothesis is true, and many of these studies will need to be long-term. A single study claiming to show a specific effect is not considered evidence-based research, ready for implementation in a clinical setting. Unscrupulous individuals will use cutting edge research to make clinical claims that are years or decades premature by basing their work on knowledge that currently does not exist.[71] Currently, clinical claims regarding genomics and nutrition or

health conditions are premature and misleading by pretending to be knowledgeable where evidence-based studies do not exist.

Already, websites are claiming to treat autism, multiple sclerosis, Parkinson disease, and other conditions using "nutrigenomics." There is currently no evidence for any nutritional treatment to prevent or cure any of these diseases, and especially not based on genetic types. Nutrigenomics is an exciting legitimate field of research, but it is an area subject to dangerous quackery.

A symposium in 2012 considering all the research pertaining to nutrigenomics concluded[72]:

"The modulation of an individual's response is influenced by both genetic and environmental factors. Many nutrigenetics studies have attempted to explain variability in responses based on a single or a few genotypes so that a genotype may be used to define personalised dietary advice. It has, however, proven very challenging to define an individual's responsiveness to complex diets based on common genetic variation. In addition, there is a limited understanding of what constitutes an optimal response because we lack key health biomarkers and signatures."

Case Application for the Dental Hygienist

A 75-year-old edentulous patient is not eating because he states he has difficulty chewing, and food does not taste good. He reports he dislikes a lot of red meat and milk. He has lost 14 lb since his last recare appointment (usual weight 170 lb).

Nutritional Assessment
- Height; weight; appropriateness of BMI; significant weight changes, especially loss
- Nutrient and fluid intake in relation to DRIs
- Medications
- Alterations in taste, smell, or vision
- Support group, significant others, living arrangements, social support
- Psychological status

Nutritional Diagnosis
Altered nutrition: less than body requirements related to taste changes and chewing difficulty.

Nutritional Goals
The patient will consume a well-balanced diet (based on the *MyPlate for Older Adults*) and verbalize ways to increase protein and calcium intake and exercise.

Nutritional Implementation
Intervention: Encourage small, frequent meals.
Rationale: This helps the older patient consume adequate amounts of nutrients by decreasing fatigue and feelings of fullness that may occur with larger meals.
Intervention: Suggest use of spices such as pepper, thyme, and basil.
Rationale: These spices may improve the taste of foods because the older patient's ability to detect tastes is altered.
Intervention: Encourage fluids with meals.
Rationale: Drinking fluids with meals makes chewing and swallowing easier.

Intervention: Examine and question about the fit of the prosthesis. Clinically, conduct an intraoral and extraoral examination, especially noting any deviations from normal of the underlying tissue.
Rationale: The weight change may have created a loose-fitting denture and ultimately difficulty in chewing. An ill-fitting denture may also result in weight loss.
Intervention: Teach the patient to perform an oral self-examination.
Rationale: The patient also can identify oral problems earlier for more effective treatment.
Intervention: Emphasize use of eggs, turkey, chicken, fish, tenderized meat in marinades (e.g., wine or vinegar), and soy products such as tofu.
Rationale: Because he does not like red meats, the patient may obtain needed protein in a more acceptable manner.
Intervention: Emphasize the use of low-fat or nonfat dairy products, such as yogurt, cream cheese, cheese, or frozen yogurt.
Rationale: His dislike of milk lessens the likelihood of his choosing milk; these foods are alternatives to supply the needed calcium.
Intervention: Encourage adding powdered milk to soups, sauces, cereals, and casseroles.
Rationale: These are methods to increase protein and calcium consumption.
Intervention: Encourage the patient to walk outdoors for 10 to 20 minutes daily and to eat foods that require more chewing, such as lettuce salads, raw carrots, cabbage, and apples.
Rationale: Exercise is important to maintain bone density in the mandible and throughout the body. Available dietary calcium is better absorbed because it is dependent on vitamin D, which can be obtained through sunshine.
Intervention: Suggest mixing meat with vegetables.

Case Application for the Dental Hygienist—cont'd

Rationale: Because he enjoys vegetables, this form may be more palatable for him and would enhance protein intake.

Intervention: Refer the patient to Meals-on-Wheels or another federally funded program (e.g., food stamps), community meals centers, or church-sponsored centers.

Rationale: Anorexia may be a result of a lack of socialization during mealtimes.

Evaluation

The patient should be eating at least 75% of the number of food servings from *MyPlate for Older Adults* and steadily gaining weight until desired body weight is achieved. Other behaviors, such as consuming yogurt, eggs, fish, and dry milk in foods, will increase calcium and protein intake.

STUDENT READINESS

1. Plan a day's menus for an older edentulous patient.
2. What are some vitamin and mineral deficiencies that might influence mental attitudes of older patients?
3. Discuss reasons older patients might not eat adequately.
4. Visit a group meal program. Review the menu with the RDN, and discuss beneficial effects of the program's various activities.
5. List nutritional interventions to help a healthy older patient with full dentures to eat a well-balanced diet.
6. Observe the staff at an extended-care facility, and note positive activities related to maintaining good oral health and activities that can be improved.
7. Why are older individuals prone to dehydration? How can dehydration affect oral status?
8. Describe procedures for encouraging adequate food intake for new denture wearers.
9. What are some suggestions you could make for a patient experiencing xerostomia?
10. Name three differences in *MyPlate* and *MyPlate for Older Adults*.

CASE STUDY

A 75-year-old man widowed for 2 years is seen in the healthcare clinic for decreased intake and a weight loss of 6 lbs in the past year. He states nothing tastes good. He is on a limited, fixed income from Social Security. His current weight is 130 lb, and his height is 5 feet, 7 inches. He is edentulous and refuses to get dentures because he feels he is "too old."

He fixes a bologna sandwich occasionally, but mostly eats frozen food dinners. He thinks meats and fruits are too expensive to buy, and states, "They spoil before I can eat them." He eats overcooked vegetables in the summer because a neighbor shares fresh produce from his garden. He does not want to use any community resources because he objects to "a handout."

1. Explain why "food does not taste good."
2. What psychological and social factors may influence his dietary patterns?
3. What are some practical ways to increase protein and calcium in his diet?
4. How could you address his attitude of not wanting to accept "a handout"?

5. What medical and dental information should you assess on this man to determine nutritional status?
6. What are the strengths and weaknesses of his diet?
7. What behaviors would indicate this patient is meeting his nutritional needs?

References

1. Bernstein R: *Census bureau releases comprehensive analysis of fast-growing 90 and-older population.* Thursday, November 17, 2011. Accessed September 6, 2013: http://www.census.gov/newsroom/releases/archives/aging_population/.
2. Sabia S, Singh-Manoux A, Hagger-Johnson G, et al: Influence of individual and combined healthy behaviors on successful aging. *CMAJ* 184(18):1985–1992, 2012.
3. World Health Organization Quality of Life assessment (WHOQOL): Position paper from the World Health Organization. *Soc Sci Med* 41(10):1403–1409, 1995.
4. Anderson AL, Harris TB, Tylavsky FA, et al: Dietary patterns and survival of older adults. *J Acad Nutr Diet* 111(1):84–91, 2011.
5. U.S. National Institute on Aging/U.S. National Center for Health Statistics, newsroom: *Federal report details health, economic status of older Americans, August 16, 2012.* Accessed September 11, 2013: http://www.nia.nih.gov/newsroom/2012/08/federal-report-details-health-economic-status-older-americans.
6. Sommers AR: *Obesity among older Americans.* CRS Report for Congress 7-5700, February 20, 2009. Accessed September 11, 2013: http://www.aging.senate.gov/crs/aging3.pdf.
7. Freid VM, Bernstein AB, Bush MA: Multiple chronic conditions among adults aged 45 and over: trends over the past 10 years. *NCHS Data Brief* 100:1–8, 2012.
8. Houston DK, Nicklas BJ, Zizza CA: Weighty concerns: the growing prevalence of obesity among older adults. *J Am Diet Assoc* 109(11):1886–1895, 2009.
9. Milne AC, Potter J, Vivanti A, et al: Protein and energy supplementation in elderly people at risk from malnutrition. *Cochrane Database Syst Rev* (2):CD003288, 2009.
10. Rizzuto D, Orsini N, Qiu C, et al: Lifestyle, social factors, and survival after age 75: population based study. *BMJ* 345:e5568, 2012.
11. Nahin RL, Pecha M, Welmerink DB, et al: Ginkgo Evaluation of Memory Study Investigators: concomitant use of prescription drugs and dietary supplements in ambulatory elderly people. *J Am Geriatr Soc* 57(7):1197–1205, 2009.
12. U.S. Department of Health and Human Services: *Healthy People—Oral health.* Accessed September 6, 2013: http://www.healthypeople.gov/2020/topicsobjectives2020/objectiveslist.aspx?topicId=32.

13. Wu B, Liang J, Plassman BL, et al: Edentulism trends among middle-aged and older adults in the United States: comparison of five racial/ethnic groups. *Community Dent Oral Epidemiol* 40(2):145–153, 2012.

14. Adegboye AR, Fiehn NE, Twetman S, et al: Low calcium intake is related to increased risk of tooth loss in men. *J Nutr* 140(10):1864–1868, 2010.

15. Holm-Pedersen P, Schultz-Larsen K, Christiansen N, et al: Tooth loss and subsequent disability and mortality in old age. *J Am Geriatr Soc* 56(3):429–435, 2008.

16. Cousson PY, Schultz-Larsen K, Christiansen N, et al: Nutritional status, dietary intake, and oral quality of life in elderly complete denture wearers. *Gerodontology* 29(2):e66–e692, 2012.

17. Kikutani T, Yoshida M, Enoki H, et al: Relationship between nutrition status and dental occlusion in community-dwelling frail elderly people. *Geriatr Gerontol Int* 13(1):50–54, 2013.

18. Cousson PY, Bessadet M, Nicolas E, et al: Nutritional status dietary intake and oral quality of life in elderly complete denture wearers. *Gerodontology* 29(2):e685–e692, 2012.

19. Nowjack-Raymer RE, Sheiham A: Numbers of natural teeth, diet, and nutritional status in US adults. *J Dent Res* 86(12):1171–1175, 2007.

20. Wakai K, Naito M, Naito T, et al: Tooth loss and intakes of nutrients and foods: a nationwide survey of Japanese dentists. *Community Dent Oral Epidemiol* 38(1):43–49, 2010.

21. Ervin RB, Dye BA: The effect of functional dentition on Healthy Eating Index scores and nutrient intakes in a nationally representative sample of older adults. *J Public Health Dent* 69(4):207–216, 2009.

22. Benguigui C, Bongard V, Ruidavets JB, et al: Evaluation of oral health related to body mass index. *Oral Dis* 18(8):748–755, 2012.

23. De Marchi RJ, Hugo FN, Hilgert JB, et al: Number of teeth and its association with central obesity in older Southern Brazilians. *Community Dent Health* 29(1):85–89, 2012.

24. Gorman A, Kaye EK, Apovian C, et al: Overweight and obesity predict time to periodontal disease progression in men. *J Clin Periodontol* 39(2):107–114, 2012.

25. Furuta M, Komiya-Nonaka M, Akifusa S, et al: Interrelationship or oral health status, swallowing function, nutritional status, and cognitive ability with activities of daily living in Japanese elderly people receiving home care services due to physical disabilities. *Community Dent Oral Epidemiol* 41(2):173–181, 2013.

26. Okamoto N, Tomioka K, Saeki K, et al: Relationship between swallowing problems and tooth loss in community-dwelling independent elderly adults: the Fujiwara-kyo study. *J Am Geriatr Soc* 60(5):849–853, 2012.

27. Berretin-Felix G, Machado WM, Genaro KF, et al: Effects of mandibular fixed implant-supported prostheses on masticatory and swallowing functions in completely edentulous elderly individuals. *Int J Oral Maxillofac Implants* 24(1):110–117, 2009.

28. Patel HP, Syddall HE, Jameson K, et al: Prevalence of sarcopenia in community-dwelling older people in the UK using the European Working Group on Sarcopenia in Older People (EWGSOP) definition: findings from the Hertfordshire Cohort Study (HCS). *Age Ageing* 42(3):378–384, 2013.

29. U.S. Department of Health & Human Services: *2008 Physical activity guidelines for Americans,* updated 09/16/2011. Accessed September 6, 2013: http://www.health.gov/paguidelines/.

30. International Osteoporosis Foundation (IOF): *Preventing sarcopenia.* Accessed September 11, 2013: http://www.iofbonehealth.org/preventing-sarcopenia.

31. Beavers KM, Lyles MF, Davis CC, et al: Is lost lean mass from intentional weight loss recovered during weight regain in postmenopausal women? *Am J Clin Nutr* 94(3):767–774, 2011.

32. AARP foundation: *Drive to end hunger.* Accessed September 6, 2013: http://www.drivetoendhunger.org.

33. Nelson ME, Rejeski WJ, Blair SN, et al: Physical activity and public health in older adults: recommendation from the American College of Sports Medicine and the American Heart Association. *Med Sci Sports Exerc* 39(8):1435–1445, 2007.

34. Ibid, Beavers KM, et al: 2013.

35. Shea MK, Nicklas BJ, Houston DK, et al: The effect of intentional weight loss on all-cause mortality in older adults: results of a randomized controlled weight-loss trial. *Am J Clin Nutr* 94(3):839–847, 2011.

36. Layman DK: Dietary Guidelines should reflect new understandings about adult protein needs. *Nutr Metab (Lond)* 6:12, 2009.

37. Paddon-Jones D, Rasmussen BB: Dietary protein recommendations and the prevention of sarcopenia. *Curr Opin Clin Nutr Metab Care* 12(1):86–90, 2009.

38. Symons TB, Sheffield-Moore M, Wolfe RR, et al: A moderate serving of high-quality protein maximally stimulates skeletal muscle protein synthesis in young and elderly subjects. *J Am Diet Assoc* 109(9):1582–1586, 2009.

39. Berner LA, Wise GBM, Doi J: Characterization of dietary protein among older adults in the United States: amount, animal sources, and meal patterns. *J Acad Nutr Diet* 113(6):809–815, 2013.

40. Bauer J, Biolo G, Cederholm T, et al: Evidence-based recommendations for optimal dietary protein intake in older people: a position paper from the PROT-AGE Study Group. *J Am Med Dir Assoc* 14(8):542–559, 2013.

41. Valenzuela RE, Ponce JA, Morales-Figueroa GG, et al: Insufficient amounts and inadequate distribution of dietary protein intake in apparently healthy older adults in a developing country: implications for dietary strategies to prevent sarcopenia. *Clin Interv Aging* 8:1143–1148, 2013.

42. Surdykowski AK, Kenny AM, Insogna KL, et al: Optimizing bone health in older adults: the importance of dietary protein. *Aging health* 6(3):345–357, 2010.

43. Bonjour JP, Kraenzlin M, Levasseur R, et al: Dairy in adulthood: from foods to nutrient interactions on bone and skeletal muscle health. *J Am Coll Nutr* 32(4):251–263, 2013.

44. Looker AC, Dawson-Hughes B, Calvo MS, et al: Serum 2-hydroxyvitamin D status of adolescents and adults in two seasonal subpopulations from NHANES III. *Bone* 30(5):771–777, 2002.

45. Institute of Medicine, Food and Nutrition Board: *Dietary reference intakes for calcium and vitamin D.* Washington, DC, 2010, National Academy Press.

46. Dawson-Hughes B, Cooper C: IOF statement on new IOM dietary reference intakes for calcium and vitamin D. *Osteoporos Int* 21(7):1151–1154, 2010.

47. Gillespie LD, Robertson MC, Gillespie WJ, et al: Interventions for preventing falls in older people living in the community. *Cochrane Database Syst Rev* (9):CD007146, 2012.

48. Moyer VA, on behalf of the U.S. Preventive Services Task Force: Prevention of falls in community-dwelling older adults: U.S. preventive services task force recommendation statement. *Ann Intern Med* 157(3):197–204, 2012.

49. Bischoff-Ferrari HA, Willett WC, Orav EJ, et al: A pooled analysis of vitamin D dose requirements for fracture prevention. *N Engl J Med* 367(1):40–49, 2012.

50. Dawson-Hughes B: Serum 25-hydroxyvitamin D and muscle atrophy in the elderly. *Proc Nutr Soc* 71(1):46–49, 2012.

51. Harris E, Macpherson H, Vitetta L, et al: Effects of a multivitamin, mineral and herbal supplement on cognition and blood biomarkers in older men: a randomised, placebo-controlled trial. *Hum Psychopharmacol* 27(4):370–377, 2012.

52. Morris MS, Selhub J, Jacques PF: Vitamin B_{12} and folate status in relation to decline in scores on the mini-mental state

examination in the Framingham heart study. *J Am Geriatr Soc* 60(8):1457–1468, 2012.

53. Leishear K, Boudreau RM, Studenski SA, et al: Relationship between vitamin B$_{12}$ and sensory and motor peripheral nerve function in older adults. *J Am Geriatr Soc* 60(6):1057–1063, 2012.

54. Paganini-Hill A, White SC, Atchison KA: Dentition, dental health habits, and dementia: the Leisure World Cohort Study 2012. *J Am Geriatr Soc* 60(8):1556–1563, 2012.

55. Vidal-Alaball J, Butler CC, Cannings-John R, et al: Oral vitamin B$_{12}$ versus intramuscular vitamin B$_{12}$ for vitamin B$_{12}$ deficiency. *Cochrane Database Syst Rev* (3):CD004655, 2005.

56. Dietary Guidelines Advisory Committee: *Report of the Dietary Guidelines Advisory Committee on the Dietary Guidelines for Americans, 2010.* Part D. Science base. Section 2. Nutrient adequacy. Washington, DC, 2010, Agricultural Research Service.

57. Vanderwall CM, Tangney CC, Kwasny MJ, et al: Examination of circulating folate levels as a reflection of folate intakes among older adult supplement users and nonusers in the National Health and Nutrition Examination Survey 2003–2004. *J Acad Nutr Diet* 112(2):285–290, 2012.

58. Krebs-Smith SM, Guenther PM, Subar AF, et al: Americans do not meet federal dietary recommendations. *J Nutr* 140(10):1832–1838, 2010.

59. Hsiao PY, Mitchell DC, Coffman DL, et al: Dietary patterns and diet quality among diverse older adults: the University of Alabama at Birmingham Study of Aging. *J Nutr Health Aging* 17(1):19–25, 2013.

60. Schröder H, Vila J, Marrugat J, et al: Low energy density diets are associated with favorable nutrient intake profile and adequacy in free-living elderly men and women. *J Nutr* 138(8):1476–1481, 2008.

61. Anderson AL, Harris TB, Tylavsky FA, et al: Dietary patterns and survival of older adults. *J Am Diet Assoc* 111(1):84–91, 2011.

62. Milne AC, Potter J, Vivanti A, et al: Protein and energy supplementation in elderly people at risk from malnutrition. *Cochrane Database Syst Rev* (2):CD003288, 2009.

63. O'Leary F, Allman-Farinelli M, Samman S: Vitamin B$_{12}$ status, cognitive decline and dementia: a systematic review of prospective cohort studies. *Br J Nutr* 108(11):1948–1961, 2012.

64. Fabian E, Bogner M, Kickinger A, et al: Vitamin status in elderly people in relation to the use of nutritional supplements. *J Nutr Health Aging* 16(3):206–212, 2012.

65. National Institute on Aging, National Institutes of Health: *Dietary supplements.* Accessed on September 6, 2013: http://www.nia.nih.gov/health/publication/dietary-supplements.

66. Albright CL, Schembre SM, Steffen AD, et al: Differences by race/ethnicity in older adults' beliefs about the relative importance of dietary supplements vs prescription medications: results from the SURE study. *J Acad Nutr Diet* 112(8);1223–1229, 2012.

67. Evans JR, Lawrenson JG: Antioxidant vitamin and mineral supplements for preventing age-related macular degeneration. *Cochrane Database Syst Rev* (6):CD000253, 2012.

68. Institute of Medicine (IOM): *Nutrigenomics and beyond: Informing the future.* Washington, DC, 2007, National Academies Press.

69. Ibid.

70. Evaluation of Genomic Applications in Practice and Prevention (EGAPP): *Evidence reports.* Last updated April 5, 2012. Accessed September 11, 2013: http://www.egappreviews.org/.

71. Novella S: *Nutrigenomics—not ready for prime time.* Science-based Medicine. Posted January 2, 2013. Accessed September 11, 2013: http://www.sciencebasedmedicine.org/index.php/nutrigenomics-not-ready-for-prime-time/.

72. de Roos B: Personalized nutrition: ready for practice? *Proc Nutr Soc* 72(1):48–52, 2013. Accessed on September 11, 2013: http://journals.cambridge.org/action/displayAbstract?fromPage=online&aid=8822953.

ⓔ EVOLVE RESOURCES

Please visit http://evolve.elsevier.com/Stegeman/nutritional for additional practice and study support tools.

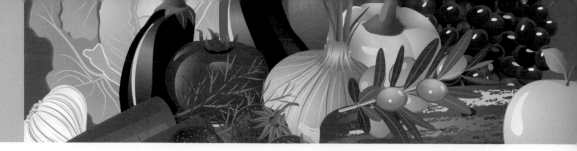

Chapter 16

Food Factors Affecting Health

Student Learning Outcomes

Upon completion of this chapter, the student will be able to achieve the following student learning outcomes:

- Explain how a patient can obtain adequate nutrients from different cultural food patterns.
- Identify reasons for food patterns.
- Respect cultural and religious food patterns while providing nutritional recommendations for patients.
- Explain to a patient how to prepare and store food to retain nutrient value.
- Provide referrals for nutritional resources.

- Inform patients of ways to make economical food purchases.
- Explain to a patient how food processing, convenience foods, and fast foods affect overall intake.
- Discuss reasons why food additives are used.
- List reasons why health quackery can be dangerous.
- Identify common themes of health quackery and why they are contrary to evidence-based research.

Key Terms

Chelation therapy
Colonics
Cortisol
Detoxification
Dietary acculturation
Evidence-based
Food deserts
Food fad
Food insecurity
Food patterns
Food quackery

Hunger
Irradiated foods
Meta-analysis
Neurotransmitters
Nutrient density
Nutritionist
Observational studies
Organic
Stable nutrients
Systematic reviews
Very low food security

◉ Test Your NQ

1. **T/F** Religion can affect food patterns.
2. **T/F** Adults usually avoid the foods they ate during childhood.
3. **T/F** The nutritional content of food is the most important determinant for food choices.
4. **T/F** Most consumers spend about 25% of their income on food.
5. **T/F** Fad diets are usually well balanced and nutritious.

6. **T/F** Organic foods are more nutritious.
7. **T/F** All food processing is detrimental to the nutritional quality of foods.
8. **T/F** Fast foods are usually a good source of protein.
9. **T/F** Food additives improve the nutritional value of foods.
10. **T/F** Individual food preferences do not ordinarily influence nutritional adequacy of the diet.

HEALTHCARE DISPARITIES

Healthcare disparities are a serious problem in the United States for the underprivileged of all ages, especially for ethnic minorities and low income groups. The Institute of Medicine reports that quality of healthcare in the United States varies according to the patient's race and ethnicity, resulting in healthcare disparities.[1] By 2060, 57% of the American population may consist of ethnic minorities in contrast to 37% in 2012.[2] Not all ethnic minorities are disadvantaged, but many come from different cultural backgrounds with dissimilar beliefs and expectations, are not cognizant of American healthcare systems and policies, and may experience communication problems as a result of language barriers. The health status of the underprivileged and many racial and ethnic minority groups is poor.

Patients who only speak, understand, or read a different language, have different levels of acculturation and socioeconomic status, understand illness uniquely, or have a different perspective on healthcare, are challenging to healthcare workers educated in the American mainstream system. Health professionals need to be able to provide healthcare to accommodate different cultural attitudes. Cultural competence of healthcare providers contributes substantively in reducing racial and ethnic disparities in health and healthcare that pervade the U.S. healthcare system. Cultural competency requires a dedication of dental professionals to understand and be responsive to a variety of attitudes, perspectives, values, verbal cues, and body language. Additionally, they should be familiar with health problems common among the ethnic groups they serve most frequently, whether they be African Americans, Asians, Hispanics/Latinos, Native American/Alaskan Natives, Pacific Islanders, or poorly educated and impoverished Americans. The Centers for Disease Control and Prevention (CDC) identified these oral health disparities in *Healthy People 2020*[3]:

- More untreated dental caries in children age 3 to 9 years.
- Fewer dental sealants in black adolescents.
- Fewer Hispanic and black adults between 45 and 64 years of age having a full set of permanent teeth (excluding third molars).
- More edentulous older adults age 65 to 74 years live below the federal poverty level.

FOOD PATTERNS

In terms of food choices, people are creatures of habit. Patterns throughout societies are quite evident; however, the term "habit" connotes inflexibility. People change their food habits for numerous reasons; hence, the term "food pattern" is more descriptive of food choices. Many factors are associated with formation of food patterns and preferences. Food patterns are generally developed during childhood and reflect the family's lifestyle and its ethnic or cultural, social, religious, geographical, economic, and psychological components. All of these influence one's attitudes, feelings, and beliefs about food. However, cultural and economic factors typically have the greatest influence on food choices.

No culture has ever been known to make food choices solely on the basis of nutritional and health values of food. Nutritional value is secondary, especially if a food has established social, religious, or economic status. For example, kale is one of the most nutritious vegetables (based on nutrient density) available in the United States but is a less-popular vegetable; whereas the tomato, the most commonly eaten vegetable, comparatively rates very low as a source of vitamins and minerals. Nutrient density is the amount of nutrients in a food relative to the number of kilocalories it provides. A raw carrot is more nutrient dense than a candy bar because the carrot contains more nutrients per kilocalorie.

Cultural Influences

The United States is more culturally diverse today than at any time in its history. The immigrant population has changed dramatically. Dietary needs unique to foreign-born immigrants have a direct impact on the national health of the United States. One of the most interesting and visible ways cultural identity is expressed is through an individual's food choices. Although milk is the only food used worldwide, many cultures consider it appropriate only for infants and children.

Children of different cultures accept as the norm what adults in their family eat. Cultural food patterns establish the foundation for a child's lifelong eating patterns regarding meal times and frequency of eating, foods acceptable for specific meals, preparation methods, likes and dislikes, foods suitable for specific members of a group or specific time of day, table manners, the social role of foods and eating, and attitudes toward eating and health (Fig. 16-1).

Many ethnic groups have brought a rich heritage of various food patterns to the United States, resulting in distinct and discrete patterns of food consumption. American diets have become more homogeneous because of transportation, advertising, mobility, new methods of production, changes in income distribution, and appreciation of one another's heritage. Food preferences are being influenced by the influx of immigrants, yet some regional food patterns are still evident—few people in northern states would routinely choose grits, and many Southerners would not recognize lentils. Individual food preferences do not influence nutritional adequacy of the diet.

Status and Symbolic Influences

Two cultures often regard a food differently. For example, beef is regarded as a high-status food among some people in the United States, but some Hindus from India consider cows sacred and do not eat beef. The choice of different foods is influenced by religious beliefs, availability, cost, cultural values, and traditions, or even the endorsement or condemnation of a highly respected person.

Because of symbolic meanings of food, eating becomes associated with sentiments and assumptions about oneself

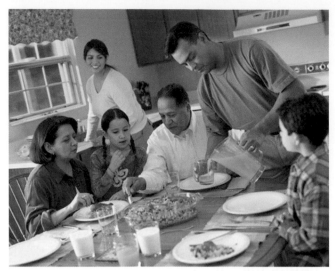

FIGURE 16-1 Eating habits are established at a very young age. (From Food and Nutrition Service, U.S. Department of Agriculture and Food and Nutrition Information Center, National Agricultural Library: SNAP-Ed Connections: photo gallery. Beltsville, MD, 2005. Retrieved September 13, 2013. http://snap.nal.usda.gov/foodstamp/photo_gallery.php?mode=mealtime)

and the world. Foods sometimes become symbolic because of religious connotations and use as rewards. After a child has fallen, a mother may give the child ice cream or candy to help forget the pain and stop crying. Food is also withheld for bad behavior.

WORKING WITH PATIENTS WITH DIFFERENT FOOD PATTERNS

Respect for Other Eating Patterns

Dental hygienists must be prepared for the unexpected. People are partial to their own food pattern; however, too many people, including dental professionals, are convinced their own beliefs, attitudes, and practices are best and assume everyone should follow them. Multicultural competence is the ability to discover each patient's cultural and ethnic preferences, and effectively adapt interventions.

Even when the facts are known, an analysis of the situation may be clouded because of unique individual habits. Information should be obtained regarding food habits using open-ended questions, rather than questions that put words into a patient's mouth. For example, "Tell me everything you had to eat this morning" might elicit a different response than the open-ended question, "What did you have for breakfast this morning?"

Effecting Change

Knowledge of food preferences and attitudes is important for recognizing and respecting differences to effect change if needed. An empathetic, observant dental hygienist understands and is aware of unique characteristics of different cultures in the area and treats each patient with respect.

Several basic facts help in approaching patients from various ethnic groups to promote sound nutritional practices.

Cultural food patterns have contributed to survival of the group in a particular environment. People have a remarkable ability to obtain a nutritious diet out of available foodstuffs. Some eating patterns that seem strange may actually be adaptive by enhancing or preserving nutritional value.

Food patterns of other countries are in some instances nutritionally superior or at least comparable to "ordinary" American traditions. When people relocate, they retain their traditional food patterns only if their native foods are available in a new location at an affordable price. Finding native foods that were the basis of their family traditional food pattern may be a challenge.

Problems arising within various cultural groups are generally economic, rather than faults of traditional food patterns. Foods from the country of origin, which were cheapest at "home," may be very expensive or possibly unavailable in the new location. Immigrants may find their culturally preferred foods easily in urban areas because many Americans are interested in exotic and ethnic cuisines, increasing availability of ethnic foods in supermarkets and ethnic restaurants. If the location is a rural, less populated area, finding native foods may be more difficult.

Each food, food-related behavior, and tradition can be categorized as beneficial, neutral, or potentially harmful. A food that is beneficial promotes health by contributing necessary nutrients. Neutral foods are not especially beneficial, but are not harmful to health. Foods are not usually harmful, but customs affecting nutritional content of the food may be potentially harmful. Efforts should be made to alter only patterns undesirably affecting nutritional value or health. For example, because many water-soluble vitamins are destroyed by heat, the practice of cooking foods (especially vegetables) for long periods is discouraged unless the liquids are consumed or iron cookware is used.

Food patterns are generally deeply ingrained, contribute to psychological stability, and are hard to change. If dietary changes are indicated for health or dental reasons, suggest minimal alterations in the patient's normal patterns and, if possible, present the information with options. Rather than indicating a patient needs to stop eating a food that is a part of the cultural heritage, talk about portion control of the food. Healthcare workers who do not address individual patient needs are ineffective, and patients feeling uncomfortable with the information will not use it.

Cultural patterns tend to be used more consistently by older family members. First-generation immigrants are still rooted in their homeland and usually have at least one native meal a day. Dental professionals should learn about ethnic foods for immigrants in the area so they can assist in suggesting alternatives or similar types of foods. Gradually, the diet conforms to food resources of the new location, a process called **dietary acculturation**. Second-generation Americans are raised without that direct native connection, and their parents, often struggling with new

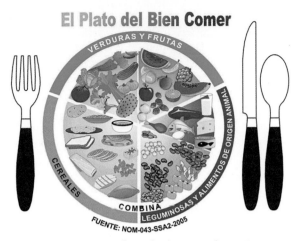

FIGURE 16-2 Mexican Food Guide. (From Mahan LK, Escott-Stump S, Raymond JL: *Krause's food and the nutrition care process*, ed 13, St Louis, 2012, Saunders.)

foods themselves, may not have the knowledge to educate their children about healthy American foods.

It is impossible to cover the dietary practices of all cultures and religions in this text. Figure 16-2 is a food guide for Mexico. The Canadian Food Guide was presented in Chapter 1 (see Fig. 1-6). Additional food guides can be found in the back of the book and on Evolve. Table 16-1 categorizes foods of different cultures and regions and includes brief descriptions that help introduce some unique and interesting foods.

Religious Food Restrictions

Religious beliefs affect eating patterns, attaching symbolic meanings to food and drink. Some examples are the bread and wine served during Christian communion service, and Hindu reverence for the cow. Many Seventh Day Adventists are vegetarians; some are vegans. These patterns do not usually result in any nutritional problems, but could affect one's food patterns and require consideration before making dietary recommendations.

- Be tactful and allow longer response times for patients from different cultures.
- Patients are more receptive to minor changes in the diet pattern. The key is to ease patients into change.
- Identify advantages and faults for each cultural food pattern in your area.
- Use an understanding of ethnic food habits to encourage or incorporate beneficial practices into the patient's diet.
- Compliance is improved when a patient has input into changes in food choices, understands why changes are indicated, and feels responsible for following the suggestions.
- Individuals from all cultures have unique tastes and preferences; stereotyping members of cultural groups should be avoided.
- In many cases, American food practices adopted by immigrants have been deleterious to their health by contributing to the same chronic diseases typical in the United States.

FOOD BUDGETS

Foods available in the home are primarily the result of food shopping behaviors. If nutrient-dense healthful foods are not purchased, they cannot be consumed; likewise, if more energy-dense foods are purchased, they compete with more healthful choices even if more nutritious foods are available. Despite increasing interest in optimal nutrition, many Americans are anxious about food prices and constantly attempt to conserve their food dollars. Food prices have been increasing annually at a rate of 2% to 3% per year since 2006 and will probably continue to increase. Fluctuating prices from year to year reflect supply and demand both within the United States and internationally, with supply being affected significantly by weather conditions. Evidence that poor or fair health status and malnutrition increase as income level decreases is discussed in *Health Application 16* in this chapter.

The average American family spends approximately 15% of its income on food; families at the poverty level may spend 33%. American families report spending anywhere from $50/week to $300/week, with an average expenditure of $151 weekly.[4] Based on U.S. Department of Agriculture (USDA) food plans for 2012, the weekly cost of food for a family of 4 ranges between $128 and $291 (based on all meals and snacks being prepared at home).[5] Purchasing the most nutritious products using available money is a common concern at most all income levels.

Table 16-1   Cultural and regional foods

Name of Food	Culture/Region	Type of Food	Description
Adobo	Filipino	Protein	Meat with soy sauce
Ajinomoto	Japanese	Grain	Wheat germ
Anadama	New England	Grain	Cornmeal-molasses yeast bread
Arroz blanco	Puerto Rican	Grain	Enriched white rice
Bacalao	Puerto Rican	Protein	Salted codfish
Bagel	Jewish	Grain	Bread dough, doughnut-shaped, boiled in water and baked
Baklava	Greek	Dessert	Layered pastry made with honey
Bok choy	Asian	Vegetable	Green leafy, stalk-like vegetable
Brioche	French	Grain	Egg-rich cake bread, used as sweet roll or shell for entrees
Bulgur	Middle Eastern	Grain	Granular wheat product with nutlike flavor
Burrito	Mexican	Combination	Tortilla filled with beef-bean mixture and fried or baked
Café con leche	Latin American	Beverage	Coffee with milk
Cape Cod turkey	New England	Protein	Codfish balls
Challah	Jewish	Grain	Sabbath or holiday twisted egg-bread
Chappati	Indian	Grain	Unleavened bread
Chayote	Mexican	Vegetable	Squash-like vegetable
Chitterlings	Southern U.S.	Protein	Intestine of young pigs, soaked, boiled, and fried
Chorizo	Mexican	Protein	Sausage
Cilantro	Mexican	Seasoning	Coriander, similar to parsley
Crackling	Southern U.S.	Fat/snack	Crispy pieces of fried pork fat
Croissants	French	Grain	Buttery, flaky, crescent-shaped rolls
Crumpets	English	Grain	Muffin-like product cooked on griddle then toasted
Cush	Montana	Grain	Cornbread mixed with butter and water and fried
Dandelion greens	Southern U.S.	Vegetable	Leaves from dandelion plant
Dhal	Indian	Vegetable protein	Thick lentil soup with onion, tomatoes, and spices
Dolmathes	Greek	Combination	Grape leaves stuffed with beef
Dosal	Indian	Combination	Pancakes with lentils
Edamame	Oriental	Vegetable	Baby soybean in the pod
Enchiladas	Mexican	Combination	Tortilla filled with meat and cheese
Escargots	French	Protein	Snails
Falafel	Middle Eastern	Vegetable protein	Vegetarian-type meatball
Fatback	Southern U.S.	Fat	Fat from loin of pig
Feijoada	Brazilian	Protein	Black beans with meat
Feta	Greek	Milk	Soft, salty white cheese from sheep or goat milk
Finnan haddie	Scottish	Milk	Salted, smoked haddock
Frijoles fritos	Mexican	Vegetable protein	Refried pinto beans
Gazpacho	Spanish	Vegetable soup	Cold soup with chopped tomatoes, green peppers, and cucumbers
Gefilte fish	Jewish	Protein	Seasoned fish ground and shaped into balls
Goulash	Hungarian	Protein	Stew seasoned with paprika
Grits	Southern U.S.	Grain	Hulled and coarsely ground corn
Guava	Cuban	Fruit	Small, yellow or red, sweet tropical fruit
Gumbo	Creole	Combination	Well-seasoned okra stew with meat or seafood
Hangtown fry	California	Protein	Fried oysters and eggs

Table 16-1   Cultural and regional foods—cont'd

Name of Food	Culture/Region	Type of Food	Description
Hoe cake	Southeast U.S.	Grain	Thin corn cake
Hog maw	Southern U.S.	Protein	Stomach of pig
Hoppin' John	Southern U.S.	Combination	Black-eyed peas and rice
Hushpuppy	Southern U.S.	Grain	Fried cornbread
Idli	Indian	Combination	Steamed dumplings with lentils
Jalapeños	Latin American	Vegetable	Hot peppers
Jambalaya	Creole	Combination	Well-seasoned combination of seafoods, tomatoes, and rice
Kale	Southern U.S.	Vegetable	Dark green leafy vegetable, similar to spinach
Kasha	Jewish	Grain	Coarsely ground buckwheat, toasted before cooking in liquid
Kelp	Asian	Vegetable	Seaweed
Kibbeh	Middle Eastern	Protein	Fresh raw lamb, ground and seasoned, similar to meat loaf
Kielbasa	Polish	Protein	Sausage
Kimchi	Korean	Vegetable	Peppery fermented combination of pickled cabbage, turnips, radishes, and other vegetables
Kuchen	German	Dessert	Yeast cake
Lard	—	Fat	Shortening-like product from pork
Latkas	Jewish	Grain	Pancakes, sometimes from potatoes
Limpa	Swedish	Grain	Rye bread
Lox	Jewish	Protein	Smoked salmon
Matzo	Jewish	Grain	Unleavened bread
Menudo	Mexican	Protein	Stew made with tripe (cow's stomach)
Minestrone	Italian	Vegetable/soup	Vegetable soup
Miso	Asian	Vegetable protein	Fermented soybean paste
Moussaka	Greek	Combination	Meat and eggplant casserole
Mush	Southwestern U.S.	Grain	Cooked cereal, usually cornmeal
Pan Dowdy	New England	Dessert	Dumplings and fruit
Pasta	Italian	Grain	Macaroni, spaghetti, and noodles in various shapes made from wheat
Pepperoni	Italian	Protein	Hot sausage
Phyllo	Greek	Grain	Paper-thin pastry for making meat, vegetables, cheese, and egg dishes and sweet pastries
Pilaf	Middle Eastern	Grain	Rice enriched with fat and sometimes vegetables, bits of meat, and spices
Poi	Polynesian	Vegetable	Root vegetable, especially taro, cooked and pounded, mixed with water, and sometimes fermented
Polenta	Italian	Grain	Cornmeal or cornmeal mush
Polk	Southern U.S.	Vegetable	Dark green leafy vegetable
Poori	Indian	Grain	Deep-fried whole-wheat bread
Potato latkes	Jewish	Vegetable	Potato pancakes
Pot liquor (likker)	Southern U.S.	Vegetable	Liquid from cooking green vegetables or bones
Prickly pear	Native American	Fruit	Fruit of cactus
Prosciutto	Italian	Protein	Ready-to-eat, cured, smoked ham
Pumpernickel	German	Grain	Yeast bread with wheat, corn, rye, and potatoes
Ratatouille	French	Vegetable	Well-seasoned casserole of eggplant, zucchini, tomato, and green pepper
Red-eye gravy	Southern U.S.	Gravy	Fried ham gravy
Sake	Asian	Beverage	Rice wine

Continued

Table 16-1   **Cultural and regional foods—cont'd**

Name of Food	Culture/Region	Type of Food	Description
Salt pork	Southern U.S.	Fat	Salted pork fat from the belly
Sancocho	Puerto Rican	Combination	Soup with meat and viandas (vegetable)
Sashimi	Japanese	Protein	Raw fish
Sauerbraten	German	Protein	Pot roast in spicy, aromatic, sweet-and-sour marinade
Scones	English	Grain	Round, flat, unleavened sweetened bread
Scrapple	Pennsylvania Dutch	Combination	Solid mush from cornmeal and by-products of hog butchering
Shoofly pie	Pennsylvania Dutch	Dessert	Molasses pie
Shoyu	Japanese	Seasoning	Soy sauce
Sofrito	Puerto Rican	Seasoning	Specially seasoned tomato sauce
Sopapillos	Mexican	Grain	Rich fried bread
Spatzle	German	Grain	Small dumplings
Spoonbread	Virginia	Grain	Baked dish with cornmeal
Spumoni	Italian	Dessert	Fruited ice cream
Stollen	German	Dessert	Christmas fruitcake
Strickle sheets	Pennsylvania Dutch	Dessert	Coffee cake
Strudel	German	Dessert	Light pastry, filled with fruit or cheese
Tacos	Mexican	Combination	Fried tortillas, filled with meat, vegetables, and hot sauce
Tamales	Mexican	Grain	Pancake-like leathery bread
Tempura	Japanese	Combination	Deep-fried seafood or vegetables
Teriyaki sauce	Hawaiian	Seasoning	Sweetened soy sauce
Tofu	Asian	Vegetable protein	Soybean curd
Trotters	Southern U.S.	Protein	Pig's feet
Viandas	Puerto Rican	Vegetable	Starchy tropical vegetables, including plantain, green bananas, and sweet potatoes

From Davis JR, Sherer K: *Applied nutrition and diet therapy for nurses*, ed 2, Philadelphia, 1994, Saunders.

Frequently, a family spends significantly more money eating in restaurants or fast food establishments than on food prepared in the home. In general, a large proportion of the food dollar is spent on processed foods. A general awareness of food costs can be used to assist patients in stretching their food dollar (Box 16-1). The amount of money a household spends on food provides insight into how adequately nutritional needs are being met. Higher-priced foods may not be the most nutritious; palatable, nutritious foods can be provided economically.

Most people believe that healthy foods (such as fruits and vegetables) are more expensive than calorie-dense foods (e.g., foods high in sodium, added sugars, or saturated fats). An extensive study determined the price of more than 4000 foods, assessing price per 100 kilocalories, price per 100 edible grams (after cooking, ready-to-eat), and price per average portion. Based on the price-per-calorie measure, some vegetables are considerably more expensive than less-healthy foods. However, the price-per-edible-gram showed that numerous nutrient-dense foods (fruits and most

vegetables) cost no more than many less-healthy foods. Both fruits and vegetables are also less expensive than less-healthy foods when measured by price per average portion. This was true for all the food groups except the protein group.[6] Households have shifted from refined grains toward more whole grains, but continue to purchase too few fruits, vegetables, and too many refined grains, fats, and added sugars. Increasingly, more processed and packaged foods are being purchased.[7] Consumers can save money and eat healthier by reducing portion sizes, especially of energy-dense foods, and buying fewer calorie-dense foods.

Based on the *Dietary Guidelines*, food choices of low-income households are generally less desirable than those of higher income households. Compliance with recommendations for fruits and vegetables is the biggest concern. Low-income households earning below 130% of the poverty line are more likely to spend less on all categories of foods except for eggs. This suggests that low-income households may consume less food, and/or lower-quality foods. A small increase in income results in increased expenditures on beef

---

BOX 16-1   **Basic Principles for Economical Food Purchases**

1. Take inventory before going to the supermarket.
2. Plan weekly menus using *MyPlate* as a guideline. Prepare a shopping list and stick to it.
3. Plan menus around seasonal foods or weekly specials.
4. Never shop when hungry.
5. Purchase the least-expensive items in each food group that you will eat.
6. Rely on minimal servings of meats. On the average, purchase 1 lb ground beef or turkey for 4 people. When purchasing steaks, check the weight; most would serve at least 2 people.
7. Use meat substitutes (e.g., legumes, nuts, peanut butter, and cheese) several times each week.
8. Serve adequate quantities of grains, cereals, and pasta products (6 to 11 servings per day), but be aware of portion sizes. For instance, one serving of pasta is one-half cup cooked, but pasta labels may identify 1 serving as 1 cup cooked.
9. Purchase smaller quantities of whole-grain products in place of a larger quantity of refined grains. The first ingredient in the bread should be 100% whole grain.
10. Prepare most foods from scratch rather than buying convenience items, such as frozen pizza.
11. Limit highly processed foods that are expensive or have low nutrient density (e.g., carbonated beverages and chips). Replace these foods with fresh fruits and vegetables.
12. Avoid impulse buying, but be prepared to make substitutions if a similar item is a better buy.
13. Purchase store brands, which are usually a wise choice. Store brands, often found on the lowest shelves, are equal in quality and taste to well-advertised national brands.
14. Read labels to determine nutritive value and compare with similar products.
15. Compare unit prices. If available, the price per unit (e.g., ounce) stated on the shelf below the grocery item facilitates comparing various sizes.
16. Buy larger sizes (which are usually cheaper per serving) if the food will be eaten before it spoils, but purchase individual serving sizes of products such as low-fat yogurt, if portion control is important.
17. Shop at large supermarkets rather than small stores or convenience stores for more economical purchases.
18. Avoid purchasing high-energy snack foods and breakfast cereals with a high sugar content.
19. Do most of your shopping around the perimeter of the store, where seasonal items and basic essentials such as fresh meat, milk, and eggs are located. Highly processed foods line the inner supermarket shelves.
20. Frozen meats are cheaper and as healthful as fresh meat.
21. Plan to use highly perishable items, such as fresh fish or strawberries, as soon as possible after purchasing.
22. Use convenience foods wisely. In general, the more someone else does in preparing food, the more the product will cost.
23. Use dating information on products to select the freshest foods. Do not let food in the pantry or refrigerator go to waste.
24. Avoid purchasing bruised, moldy, and mushy produce.
25. Pay attention at the checkout counter to be sure the advertised price or the price indicated on the shelf is what is charged.
26. Plan to use leftovers for soups, salads, and sandwiches.

---

and frozen prepared foods. Thus, a small increase in income is unlikely to induce more spending for fruits and vegetables. Households earning 10% above the 130% of the poverty line are more likely to allocate additional resources to fruits and vegetables.[8]

On the basis of nutrient density, spinach, liver, turkey, canned tuna, lentils/beans, nonfat and low-fat milk, cottage cheese, tofu, eggs, and fresh carrots are usually the most economical. Some less-expensive fruits per serving size are bananas, watermelons, raisins, apples, grapefruit, grapes, and oranges; least-expensive vegetables include potatoes, carrots, cucumbers, green beans, onions, mustard greens, kale, romaine and iceberg lettuce, bell peppers, tomatoes, and broccoli. Buying fruits and vegetables that are home-grown and in season is more economical. Generally, more of the food dollar should be spent for fruits, vegetables, grain products, milk, and dry beans; less is needed for meats and high-sugar, high-fat food items (e.g., candy, carbonated beverages, and chips).

People with limited financial resources are hampered by other constraints. **Food deserts** are located in lower-income, inner-city and rural areas with few supermarkets but numerous small stores that stock limited nutritious food items, particularly fruits and vegetables, at affordable prices. Without transportation, low-income consumers are often limited to shopping close to where they live, or they must spend money for travel or delivery services. Produce is 30% to 70% more expensive in small, independent stores.[9] Cost, lack of availability, and poor quality are deterrents to eating healthier for very-low-income consumers. Small, low-income-area grocery stores are less consistent for stocking whole grains, low-fat cheeses, lean ground beef, and larger package sizes. Changes in the Special Supplemental Nutrition Program for Women, Infants, and Children (WIC) program (see Referrals for Nutrition Resources on page 332) made in 2009 have prompted some small stores in desert areas to stock healthier foods, especially reduced fat milk and whole-grain breads.[10] One study identified another benefit from the food package changes: 1-year-olds weighed 6% less than previously, and 2- to 4-year-olds weighed 3% less.[11]

Families on food stamps or on a very low food budget need to learn skills in buying and storing food. Households with better financial management skills are better equipped to provide enough food for the household.[12] Low-income shoppers spend less on food purchases despite the fact that food prices are higher where they are compelled to shop. Low-income shoppers can buy more food with less money by purchasing lower-priced foods, by selecting less-expensive meats and fresh fruits and vegetables, and by consuming less

Table 16-2 Cost of 20 g of protein from various meats and meat alternatives*

Food	Cost ($)/Market Unit	AP† to Provide 20 g Protein	EP‡ Amount to Provide 20 g Protein	Cost ($)/20 g Protein
Turkey, ready-to-cook	1.29/lb	3½ oz	2⅓ oz	0.19
Pinto beans, dry	2.79/2 lb	¾ cup	1½ cup	0.32
Eggs (large)	1.59/dz	3	3	0.40
Chicken whole fryer	1.39/lb	5.2 oz	2.6 oz	0.49
Chicken breasts with bone and skin	2.49/lb	3¾ oz	2⅓ oz	0.50
Milk, skim	3.78/gal	2½ cup	2½ cup	0.59
Loin pork chops (rib with bone)	3.13/lb	3.3 oz	2.6 oz	0.65
Tuna, canned in water	.94/5 oz	3.5 oz	3.5 oz	0.66
Ham, boneless	2.78/lb	4 oz	3.3 oz	0.70
Peanut butter	3.79/16.3 oz	5½ Tbsp	5½ Tbsp	0.71
Bread, whole-grain (sandwich sliced)	3.39/20 oz	5½ slices	5½ slices	0.75
Beef liver	3.49/lb	3.5 oz	2.4 oz	.76
Beef, ground, regular	3.79/lb	3.5 oz	2.5 oz	0.83
Ham, cured picnic, bone-in	1.49/lb	4.3 oz	3.4 oz	0.98
Beef, chuck roast, bone-in	4.33/lb	3.7 oz	2.4 oz	1.00
Bread, white enriched (sandwich slices)	2.99/20 oz	9 slices	9 slices	1.22
Pork and beans, canned	1.39/15 oz	1⅔ cup	1⅔ cup	1.32
Beef, round steak, boneless	6.29/lb	3.5 oz	2.5 oz	1.38
Bologna, beef, sliced	3.49/lb	6.5 oz	6.5 oz	1.42
Cheese, American processed	4.29/12 oz	4 oz	4 oz	1.43
Turkey, ground	7.99/20 oz	3¾ oz	2.8 oz	1.49
Frankfurters	3.99/lb	3⅓ franks	3⅓ franks	1.66
Cod or catfish fillet, fresh	6.99/lb	4 oz	3 oz	1.75
Salmon, fresh fillets	8.99/lb	3.4 oz	2.6 oz	1.91
Chicken wings	2.29/lb	3.5 wings	3.5 wings	2.25
fish fillets, breaded, frozen	7.99/2.5 oz	12.5 sticks	12.5 sticks	3.33
Bacon, sliced	6.99/lb	10 slices	10 slices	3.50

*Prices at Randalls, Lakeway TX; October 2012.
†AP, as purchased, including weight of bone, skin, and fat.
‡EP, edible portion, cooked.

energy-dense foods. Table 16-2 shows the relative cost of 20 g of protein from various foods.

MAINTAINING OPTIMAL NUTRITION DURING FOOD PREPARATION

From the time any produce is removed from the plant or a grain product is harvested, nutrient content begins to degrade. Harvesting, processing, and cooking food means nutrient losses are occurring, but good handling processes, such as chilling or freezing, minimize losses and bacterial growth.

Methods of Preparation

In many instances, cooking enhances palatability, increases digestibility of food, and destroys pathogenic organisms. Cooking affects acceptability and nutritional value of food. Following a few guidelines can help preserve nutrients during cooking (Box 16-2).

Adding large amounts of fats during the cooking process, as in frying, is discouraged. Methods of preparing meats, such as broiling or cooking on a grill, are recommended to lessen natural fat content. Meats cooked to the well-done stage contain less fat. To remove fats during cooking, meats

---

**BOX
16-2**   **Guidelines for Preserving Nutrients During Preparation**

1. Prepare fresh produce as near to serving time as possible to prevent deterioration of many nutrients when they are exposed to air. Refrigerate within 2 hours of cutting or peeling.
2. Do not soak fruits and vegetables that have been cut to prevent loss of water-soluble vitamins and some minerals (especially potassium) into the water. If cut-up fruits and vegetables are soaked in water, use the water in food preparation.
3. Scrub fruits and vegetables rather than pare them to increase fiber and nutrient intake. When necessary, pare as thinly as possible to maintain nutrients.
4. Boil nonconsumable parings and portions of vegetables in water and incorporate in soup stock or gravies. This is a very rich source of potassium and water-soluble vitamins.
5. Leave produce whole or in large pieces so that less surface area is available for oxidation of nutrients.
6. Carotenoids, like beta-carotene, lycopene, and lutein, are more easily absorbed when vegetables are cooked than raw.
7. Store any fruits or vegetables that have been cut or otherwise processed, such as fruit juice, in airtight containers. Container size should be appropriate for the amount to be stored to prevent excessive oxidation from air inside the container.
8. Quick-cooking methods rather than extended cooking times are usually best to retain the B and C vitamins. Boiling leaches water-soluble vitamins, so quick steaming or sauteing is recommended to reduce loss into the cooking medium unless the liquid is also consumed (e.g., in soups or incorporated into a gravy).
9. A covered pan minimizes cooking time by increasing the temperature inside.
10. Use the least amount of liquid possible in cooking. Serve vegetables as soon as they are prepared.
11. Do not use baking soda when cooking vegetables.

---

can be boiled, microwaved in a colander or on paper towels, or roasted or broiled on a rack. Absorption of fat-soluble vitamins requires availability of a small amount of fat, i.e., absorption of vitamins A, D, E, and K from a vegetable salad is enhanced with a salad dressing (not fat-free) or cheese, or some other food containing fat.

Cooking increases digestibility of protein in meats. Cooking generally softens cellulose in fresh produce. Total volume and bulk of the food decrease, so a greater quantity of these low-calorie foods can be eaten. Stir frying is an old Asian technique that is a highly recommended method, which has the added benefit of being quick. Bite-sized pieces of food are cooked very briefly over high heat with or without a small amount of vegetable oil. Vegetables retain their nutrient value, color, and crispness.

A microwave oven is another timesaver because of shorter cooking times. Vitamin content of foods cooked in a home microwave oven is about the same as foods prepared conventionally, especially if a minimal amount of water is added.

Greens, such as spinach, increase in folate, lutein, beta-carotene, and vitamins E and K content during exposure to light, even with continuous exposure to grocery store lighting.[13] The only vitamin detrimentally affected is vitamin C. Apparently, as long as the plant is green, photosynthesis continues. Vitamin levels begin to degrade when wilting begins. Actually, baby greens are typically more nutritious than more mature greens—younger leaves have greater nutrient density than older leaves.[14,15]

Food Sanitation and Safety

Food carefully chosen for its nutritional value may be adversely affected by handling techniques and preparation for consumption. More than 9 million foodborne illnesses are estimated to be caused by major pathogens. The CDC attributes 46% of these illnesses to produce and found that more deaths were attributed to poultry than to any other commodity.[16] Of the 31 pathogens known to cause foodborne illness, 6 account for most of the illnesses, hospitalizations, and deaths annually—*Campylobacter, Escherichia coli (E. coli), Listeria monocytogenes, Salmonella, Vibrio,* and *Yersinia.* In recent years, progress has been made in significantly reducing foodborne infections caused by *E. coli, Listeria,* and *Campylobacter,* but infections from one of the more common germs, *Salmonella,* are still rampant.[17] Spices from other countries, especially Mexico and India, have been implicated in foodborne illness due to salmonella contamination. Symptoms include diarrhea, fever, headache, and vomiting. For most people, the illness resolves on its own, but these illnesses can be fatal for younger and older individuals and those with weakened immune systems. Illness caused by *Listeria* can result in miscarriage, fetal death, or severe illness or death of a newborn (see Chapter 13).

The CDC estimates that at least one-third of cases caused by foodborne pathogens could be prevented by following safe food-handling and preparation recommendations, and by avoiding consumption of raw or undercooked foods of animal origin such as eggs, ground beef, and poultry; unpasteurized milk, cheese, and juices; and raw or undercooked oysters.[18] Because of the prevalence of foodborne illness, the *Dietary Guidelines* address food safety in general terms. The five major control factors for pathogens are personal hygiene, adequate cooking, avoiding cross-contamination, cooking and maintaining food at safe temperatures, and avoiding foods from unsafe sources. Edibles must be handled with care to prevent contamination with foodborne organisms, and sometimes must be properly cooked to kill any organisms naturally present. Many foods, especially meat, poultry, and eggs, require sufficiently high temperatures to destroy microorganisms. Bacteria and other organisms grow at an astonishing rate between 40° F and 140° F. Box 16-3 lists some specific guidelines for handling food.

In recent years, nationwide recalls of tainted food products have included meats, peanut butter, vegetables, salad,

- Keep kitchen countertops, refrigerator, cookware, and cutlery clean. Disinfect countertops and sink with a weak chlorine (1 tsp household bleach in 1 gallon water) solution.
- Wash your hands before preparing meals and handling any foods.
- Purchase pasteurized juice to avoid harmful bacteria.
- Avoid cross-contamination by keeping fresh produce away from uncooked meats.
- Avoid washing fruits and vegetables until just before eating. Natural coatings keep moisture inside; washing makes them spoil sooner.
- Refrigerate fresh produce within 2 hours of cutting or peeling.
- Wash all prepackaged produce, even if the package says "prewashed."
- Refrigerate or freeze meat, poultry, eggs, and other perishables as soon as possible.
- Bacteria can live on the rinds or skins—clean the whole thing, even inedible parts. The knife cutting into the edible portion can transfer bacteria from the rind/peel.
- Gently rub fruits and vegetables under running water. Soaps, detergents, bleaches, or commercial sprays and washes will leave their own residue on the produce.
- Scrub firmer items such as apples and potatoes with a vegetable brush while rinsing with clean water to remove dirt and residues.
- Remove and discard the outer leaves of lettuce and cabbage heads, and thoroughly rinse the rest of the leaves.

- Rinse berries and other small fruits thoroughly and allow them to drain in a colander.
- People with a compromised immune system should consider eating only cooked produce, especially sprouts, and well-cooked meats and fish.
- Never use the same utensils or cutting surfaces for preparing meats and vegetables. Use different cutting boards for fresh produce, dairy products, poultry, fish, and meats. Wash with a weak chlorine solution after using.
- Wash the tops of all cans, including pop-top beverages, before opening.
- Use an appliance thermometer to ensure the refrigerator temperature is between 40°F and 32°F and freezer is 0°F or below. Use a food thermometer to ensure meats are cooked to appropriate temperature—beef, pork, veal, lamb, 160°F; turkey, chicken, 165°F; ham, 140°F; finfish, 145°F; leftovers, 165°F.
- Refrigerate leftovers to 40°F or below within 2 hours of serving. Seal leftovers in an airtight, clean container labeled with the expiration date.
- Discard leftovers and other refrigerated foods as soon as possible after expiration date. Leftovers should be eaten within 2 days.
- Foods left unrefrigerated for more than 2 hours should be discarded.
- Wash your reusable grocery bags.
- Defrost meats in the refrigerator or the microwave.

snacks, fast foods, and dessert items, causing thousands of illnesses and even a few deaths. Many of these foods were imported, but some were domestic products grown in areas considered to be safe. New foods have been implicated—organically grown spinach, sprouts, and peanut butter were perplexing problems. Increasing numbers of people consuming more fresh produce is good nutritionally, but harmful microbes on some fruits and vegetables have created problems. Contrary to popular opinion, pathogens that cause illness arc odorless, colorless, and invisible, so smelling, tasting, or looking at the food is not a good gauge of whether it may be contaminated. Spoilage bacteria evidenced by slimy films on lunch meat, soggy edges on vegetables, or sticky chicken are not as toxic as pathogens.

Concern has intensified over the possibility of contaminated food caused by terrorist acts. The Food and Drug Administration (FDA) is authorized in the Public Health Security and Bioterrorism Preparedness and Response Act of 2002 (Bioterrorism Act) to detain suspect food. The FDA Food Safety Modernization Act (FSMA) was signed into law in early 2010, but has not been fully implemented because funding is pending; regulations, processes, and systems are being developed. The FSMA enables the FDA to better protect public health by focusing on preventing food safety problems rather than reacting to problems after they occur. A science-based system is being developed that addresses hazards from farm to table, putting greater emphasis on

preventing foodborne illness. The FDA will be able to hold imported foods to the same standards as domestic foods. Congress established specific implementation dates in the legislation; some parts have already been implemented. The first rule focuses on keeping fresh produce safe from becoming contaminated with microorganisms (water, soil amendments, etc.). The second proposed rule requires domestic and foreign food producers to develop plans to prevent their products from becoming contaminated and to have procedures in place to correct any problems that might arise.

Processed Foods

Actually everything that is done to a food after harvesting to prepare for consumption is food processing, whether it occurs at home or is provided by the food manufacturer. Active, mobile lifestyles and an increasing number of women working full-time or part-time outside the home have led to a continued increase in consumption of processed foods. Although growing one's own food and making foods from "scratch" can give consumers control over how food is handled and what is added, this is not feasible for most Americans.

Effect of Processing on Nutrients

Many consumers have been misled in assuming that nutrient content of our food supply has deteriorated. Based on studies conducted by USDA, nutrient changes are mixed—some nutrients have gone down whereas others have improved. A significant change is that most fruits and vegetables are bred to be bigger and juicier.[19]

Nutrient content of foods can be affected by the way food is handled—that is, the type of processing to which the food is subjected (e.g., milling, cooking, freezing)—and how it is stored. In general, most minerals, carbohydrates, lipids, proteins, and vitamin K and niacin are **stable nutrients**. Nutrients are considered stable if at least 85% of the original level is retained during processing and storage. Thiamin, riboflavin, folate, and ascorbic acid are most likely to be seriously depleted by processing and storage and method of food preparation. The nutritional value of home-cooked foods is frequently about the same as processed foods.

Manufacturers involved in food processing attempt to maintain optimal qualities of taste, freshness, safety, cost, and value—five traits important in consumer choices. Not everything done to foods by food processors has been good; however, not all processing is detrimental. The milling process removes the bran coat of grains. Removal of the high lipid-containing bran produces a more stable grain, increasing its shelf life. Nutritionally, however, this results in a reduction of fiber and loss of 70% to 80% of thiamin, riboflavin, vitamin B_6, and other nutrients. Enrichment replaces some nutrients (thiamin, riboflavin, niacin, folic acid, and iron) lost in processing, but not all of them (see Chapter 1, Table 1-2). Without the enrichment and fortification processes, many American diets would be deficient in nutrient intake of vitamins A, C, and D, thiamin, iron, and folate.[20]

Fresh fruits and vegetables have a higher nutritive value and better taste immediately after harvest, but rapidly deteriorate if transported long distances or improperly stored. Frozen foods packed immediately after harvesting may be higher in nutritive value than their fresh counterparts available in the supermarket. Because canned vegetables have prolonged exposure to water, they usually lose more nutrients than frozen ones, but even canned vegetables are better than no vegetables at all. On the other hand, some canned foods, especially tomatoes, but also carrots, sweet potatoes, peaches, beans (legumes), tuna, and salmon, are cheaper and as nutritious as their counterpart fresh products.

The most negative effect of food processing has been the addition of ingredients that enhance taste and desirability of the product—sweeteners, salt, and artificial colors and flavors. Because of the way foods are processed quickly and transported rapidly, fresh produce is available year round, harmful microorganisms are reduced, maximum efficiency in production results in reduced costs, and foods are fortified or enriched with nutrients. Highly processed foods are usually less nutritious than the fresh form (i.e., potato chips are less nutritious than a baked potato). Consumers are free to choose foods that are minimally processed and thus healthier, or ready-to-eat foods that may contain less-desirable ingredients (Fig. 16-3). Reading nutrition and ingredient labels is important.

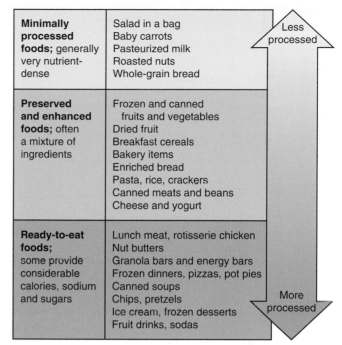

Minimally processed foods; generally very nutrient-dense	Salad in a bag Baby carrots Pasteurized milk Roasted nuts Whole-grain bread	Less processed
Preserved and enhanced foods; often a mixture of ingredients	Frozen and canned fruits and vegetables Dried fruit Breakfast cereals Bakery items Enriched bread Pasta, rice, crackers Canned meats and beans Cheese and yogurt	
Ready-to-eat foods; some provide considerable calories, sodium and sugars	Lunch meat, rotisserie chicken Nut butters Granola bars and energy bars Frozen dinners, pizzas, pot pies Canned soups Chips, pretzels Ice cream, frozen desserts Fruit drinks, sodas	More processed

FIGURE 16-3 How do I make sure that I am eating "healthy" processed foods? The chart shows the range of processed foods available. Minimally processed foods are similar to, and sometimes even more nutritious than, the same foods in their unprocessed form. Although the "ready-to-eat" category contains some foods that are high in calories and nutrient-poor, this category also includes convenient, ready-to-eat meals and snacks that provide a significant source of nutrients. (Reprinted with permission by the Dairy Council of California © 2013. Processed foods: a range, not a dichotomy. 2012. Accessed September 13, 2013: http://www.healthyeating.org/Portals/0/Documents/Health%20Wellness/White%20Papers/ProcessedFoods_72dpi.pdf)

Convenience Foods

Convenience foods are usually popular because they save time in meal preparation, planning, purchasing, and cleanup. The variety of foods available is also expanded. Convenience foods prepared by food manufacturers may cost more because of extra handling and packaging (Table 16-3). Convenience foods also require more preservatives and may contain more sodium and fat than home-cooked products.

Irradiated Foods

Foods treated with controlled amounts of ionized radiation for a prescribed period to kill spoilage-causing and disease-causing bacteria and molds in meats and produce are known as **irradiated foods**. This process has stimulated a lot of controversy, with opponents criticizing the process as being a stopgap measure that ignores the bigger problem of how food is grown, processed, and sold. This process that breaks down DNA molecules of harmful organisms, without significantly increasing the temperature of the food, is often called "cold pasteurization." Irradiation can extend the period of ripeness of fruits and vegetables, prolong the freshness of many foods, and prevent certain foodborne illnesses.

Table 16-3	Eating healthy on a budget					
Highly Processed Foods				**Minimally Processed Foods**		
Food	Serving	Price/serving*		Food	Serving	Price/serving*
Chocolate milk	1 cup	0.40		Skim milk	1 cup	0.24
Cheez Whiz	2 Tbsp	0.38		Mild cheddar cheese	1 oz	0.25
White bread	1 slice	0.15		Whole-wheat bread	1 slice	0.15
Fruit Loops	1 cup	0.29		Cheerios	1 cup	0.29
Instant packaged oatmeal	1 package (½ cup)	0.36		Old fashioned oats	½ dry	0.23
Chicken wings	¼ lb	0.69		Whole chicken	¼ lb	0.35
Frozen fish sticks	5	1.33		Chunk light tuna in water	2 oz	0.38
Refried beans	½ cup canned	0.43		Dried pinto beans	½ cup cooked	0.11
Tater tots	9 pieces	0.20		Cabbage	1 cup raw	0.11
Carrot cake	1 slice	1.25		Carrots	½ cup cooked	0.27
Orange juice, reconstituted, refrigerated	1 can	0.50		Fresh orange	1	0.14

*Price per serving October 12, 2012 at Randalls in Lakeway, TX.

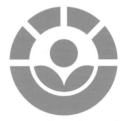

FIGURE 16-4 Official package label for irradiated foods. (From United States Department of Agriculture Food Safety and Inspection Service. Accessed September 13, 2013: http://www.epa.gov/radiation/sources/food_labeling.html.)

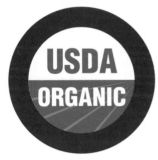

FIGURE 16-5 Official USDA organic seal. (From the National Organic Program, Agricultural Marketing Service, U.S. Department of Agriculture, Washington, D.C. Accessed September 13, 2013. http://www.ams.usda.gov/AMSv1.0/ams.fetchTemplateData.do?&template=TemplateC&navID=NationalOrganicProgram&leftNav=NationalOrganicProgram&page=NOPOrganicSeal&description=The%20Organic%20Seal&acct=nopgeninfo.)

Washing fresh fruits and vegetables can reduce risk of food contamination, but irradiation can kill bacteria that are beyond the reach of conventional chemical sanitizers, such as inside the leaves of curly spinach and lettuce. (Irradiated foods are not sterile.) At the low doses of radiation allowed, nutrient losses are either not measurable or are not significant. Foods have been safely irradiated in the United States for more than 50 years, and more than 40 other countries use the process. The process is carefully controlled and monitored by numerous government organizations; irradiated foods bear the label shown in Figure 16-4.

Organic Foods

The sharp rise in consumer demand for organic food has outpaced domestic supply. Driven by consumer choice, organic food sales experienced 9.4% growth in 2011.[21] The fastest-growing sector, the meat, fish, and poultry category, is still less than fruit and vegetable sales. This rapid growth may be driven by consumers' perception that organic foods are healthier, more nutritious, fresher, and free of pesticides.

In 2002, the USDA passed regulations defining organic food and permitting use of a seal (Fig. 16-5) for foods meeting specific standards. Organic certification regulates how these foods are grown, handled, and processed. Foods labeled organic are grown without synthetic pesticides, growth hormones, antibiotics, or genetic engineering. Organic farmers are allowed to use pesticides approved by the National Organic Standards Board that are usually naturally-occurring chemicals, principally animal and crop wastes; botanical, biological, or non-synthetic pest controls; or specific synthetic materials that quickly degrade when exposed to oxygen and sunlight.

Animals raised by organic producers cannot be given antibiotics to stimulate growth, so organic meats, poultry, milk, or eggs do not contain residues of these drugs. New standards became effective in 2011 requiring that all organic animals have year-round outdoor access; ruminant animals must graze on pastureland during the entire grazing season; and at least 30% of their dry nutrition must be from the pasture while they are grazing. Beef and lamb must come from animals that were not confined during the finishing period (when animals are usually fattened on grain).

Food manufacturers voluntarily provide information to USDA about substances and practices used in food production, including how nonorganic and organic foods are kept separate. The USDA is responsible for inspecting the site annually and certifying a producer. Products labeled "Made with Organic Ingredients" must contain at least 70% organic ingredients. A product containing more than 5% of the allowable pesticide tolerance level established by the Environmental Protection Agency cannot be labeled organic.

Whether organic foods are more nutritious than conventional foods has been a point of contention for years. Two systematic reviews, one analyzing more than 250 research studies and the other evaluating more than 160 studies published in the scientific literature over the past 50 years, found no overall difference in vitamin and mineral content between foods produced using organic and conventional methods.[22,23] After examining all available evidence, the American Association of Pediatricians concluded that organic foods (produce, meats, milk) do not have any meaningful nutritional benefits or deficits.[24] Numerous studies indicate organic produce contains more polyphenols or antioxidants having potential human health benefits.[25-27]

Nonorganic produce is 30% more likely to have pesticides than organic fruits and vegetables.[28] E. coli contamination does not differ between organic and conventional produce. Organic produce can acquire synthetic pesticides from the environment (in the air), or in packing (from water or packing materials) or storage. Congress passed the Food Quality Protection Act (1996) restricting the amount and type of chemical pesticides permitted. Pesticides currently allowed metabolize quickly and are not stored in the body; a few days after ingesting a pesticide, it is completely gone from the body. Pesticides in the U. S. food supply have decreased significantly, so approximately 80% of the risk from pesticides is from imported foods and only approximately 20% from domestically-grown food.[29]

The health risks of pesticides in humans are unclear. Although organic produce contains fewer pesticide residues than conventional ones, the difference is insignificant; actual levels of contamination in all foods grown in the United States are well below acceptable limits established by Environmental Protection Agency.[30] Food surveys of conventional foods indicate estimated exposures from 34 pesticides were less than 1% of the United Nations Food and Agriculture Organization/World Health Organization's acceptable daily intake, and four other pesticides contributed 1% to 4.8% of the acceptable daily intake. A typical human exposure at 1% of the acceptable daily intake represents an exposure 10,000 times lower than levels that do not cause toxicity in animals.

Several measures can be taken to ensure minimal intake of questionable chemicals other than purchasing only organic products, as described in Box 16-3. Blanching, boiling, canning, frying, juicing, peeling, and washing fruits and vegetables reduces pesticide residues.[31] Even after washing fruits and vegetables, some foods still contain higher levels of pesticide residue than others. These foods include apples, berries, grapes, green leafy vegetables, and potatoes, so the priority would be to choose organic for these foods. Also, buying locally produced fresh vegetables and fruits in season is helpful because fewer pesticides are used when long storage periods and long-distance shipping are not required. Eat a wide variety of fruits and vegetables to limit exposure to any one type of pesticide residue. Purchase only fruits and vegetables subject to USDA regulations. Imported produce is not grown under the same regulations as those enforced by the USDA.

Nonorganic animals do not contain antibiotic residues because FDA regulations prohibit farmers from giving feed with antibiotics to conventionally raised animals for a period of time before slaughter. This "withdrawal time" is specific to the antibiotic used to ensure the drug is at a safe level in the animal's system before the meat or milk enters the food supply. Tests rarely detect traces of antibiotics or other drugs in conventionally-produced meat, poultry, milk, or eggs.

Organic produce is no less likely than conventional choices to be contaminated by dangerous bacteria. In both methods of farming, bacterial contamination of chicken and pork is common. Bacteria resistant to three or more antibiotics was higher in conventional than in organic chicken and pork.[32] Standards for organic and conventional foods require specific procedures regarding the composting of animal manures, or the manure must be applied more than 90 days before harvest.

Organic food generally comes at a premium cost for many reasons, including higher production and labor costs, lower yields, and high demand. Also, profit margins are higher than those of conventional foods. Organic products cost approximately 10% to 50% more than conventional products. When deciding whether the additional cost for organic food is worth it, remember: eating a lot of fruits and vegetables with pesticides outweighs any possible risk from ingesting trace amounts of pesticides. Although organic foods have been on the market for many years, it is premature to say that either organic or conventional foods are superior with respect to safety or nutritional composition.

Consumers state other good reasons for choosing organic foods: (a) organic farming tends to build topsoil; (b) environmental reasons, such as less use of fertilizer; (c) better taste; (d) fresher; and (e) more humane treatment of animals and less antibiotic-resistant bacteria.

Organic farming is sustainable for a population of about 2 to 3 billion people, but not for the current worldwide population of more than 7 billion people. Available arable land is limited, prohibiting organic crop rotation to feed the world. Drastically cutting consumption of poultry and meat could make the possibility of feeding everybody organic products a possibility.

The food industry has developed many new organic products that are not wise healthy choices. For instance, a jelly bean is all sugar, and not a healthy food choice, whether it is 100% organic or not. To know whether a product is healthy, read food labels (nutrition and ingredient labels) to determine levels of kilocalories, saturated fat, sugar, sodium, as well as protein, fiber, and vitamins and minerals. Organic crackers may be made with wheat flour. If whole grain is not the first ingredient, the cracker is inconsistent with the *Dietary Guidelines.* Organic foods to be careful of include sweetened beverages, crackers, candy, energy bars, and chips. These foods are high in kilocalories and are not nutrient dense.

The term "natural" is popular on food packaging. Consumers assume a product labeled "natural" is probably healthier. "Natural" does not mean organic. The FDA has not established a standardized legal definition for this term, and no organization regulates this claim on food products. The FDA does not object to foods being labeled as "natural" if they do not contain added color, artificial flavors, or synthetic substances. "Natural" labels are meaningless and misleading for consumers.

Fast Foods and Other Food Establishments

Fast foods have become an integral part of the American fast-paced lifestyle. Spending for meals and snacks away from home has increased substantially since 1965 and accounts for more than double the amount spent on food eaten at home.

Although some people believe fast food is junk food, this is not always true. Nutritional analyses by fast food chains and independent studies reveal their menu items contain rich sources of protein (30% to 50% of the recommended dietary allowances [RDAs]). Additionally, items are available that (if selected) provide 20% to 30% of the RDAs for thiamin, riboflavin, ascorbic acid, and calcium. When a hamburger or roast beef sandwich is selected, substantial amounts of iron are supplied. Most fast food menus lack a rich source of vitamin A. Because of consumer demand, salads and other healthier items have been added to menus. This provides a source of vitamins A and C and dietary fiber; however, the cost may be two to seven times higher than the same foods purchased at supermarkets. Shortages of other nutrients—specifically biotin, folate, pantothenic acid, and copper—are also reported.

Several other problems with fast foods raise concern: (a) The kilocalorie count of a regular meal is generally 900 to 1800 kilocalories (33% to 66% of the RDA for young men or 45% to 90% for young women); (b) sodium content is very high (1000 to 2515 mg); (c) fat content of some fast food meals is 51% of kcalories consumed; and (d) mega-size portions contain a day's worth of kilocalories in one meal. The impact of fast foods on nutritional status depends on how frequently they are consumed, composition of each item selected, and other foods eaten during the day. Wise choices are possible when an individual's nutritional needs and nutrient content of menu items are known. New menu items and reduced portion sizes by several fast food chains simplify decisions to choose healthier foods. Nutritional analysis of menu items is available from most fast food chains.

Providing nutrition information at restaurants is one avenue for educating consumers about what they are eating. The Patient Protection and Affordable Care Act (2010) requires chain restaurants with 20 or more locations to post the number of kilocalories and other nutritional information in each standard menu item. The FDA was authorized to establish uniform requirements affecting many chain restaurants within a year, but this process has been slow. The FDA is writing menu labeling regulations, which should come out in the near future. Nutrition information will be displayed prominently on menus and menu boards, including drive-through locations, and next to self-service foods, such as items in a salad bar. Menu labeling will ensure that customers can process the kilocalorie information as they are deciding what to eat.

While some consumers say labeling is helpful, others find it confusing or disregard the information. A systematic review evaluating the effect of nutrition labels available in restaurants and fast food establishments indicates they may not have the intended effect of decreasing kilocalorie purchases or consumption.[33,34] Another possible advantage of labeling is that posting nutrition information may pressure chain restaurants to reformulate and make healthful changes in their products.

Food Additives

The use of food additives is regulated by law. During the 1950s, the Delaney committee investigated food additives. The Delaney clause prohibits use of any food additive that is carcinogenic in humans or animals. Additives deemed to be harmless were labeled "generally recognized as safe." These substances met certain specifications of safety under what might be called a "grandfather clause"—in other words, they are generally recognized by experts as safe, based on their use in foods for years without any known occurrence of health problems.

In 1960, similar regulations were passed for color additives. Colors currently in use were required to undergo further testing to continue being marketed. Since then, approximately 90 of the original 200 color additives have been classified as safe and continue to be added to foods.

Before a newly proposed additive can be marketed, it must undergo strict testing to establish its safety for the intended purpose. Safety levels of additives established by FDA limit the quantity and use of the additive. Currently, additives are specific, well-known substances meeting specifications for purity and have been shown as convincingly as possible to be free from harmful effects in amounts commonly used.

Almost all food additives (99%) are derived from natural sources or are synthetically produced to be identical to the natural chemical substance. In many instances, effects of chemicals naturally present in a food are observed, and this chemical is added to other foods to achieve a similar effect. For instance, calcium propionate in Swiss cheese was observed to retard mold; therefore, it was added to bread to inhibit mold growth.

Currently, additives are as safe as science can make them. "Absolute safety" cannot be guaranteed for anything in life. They are designed not to be toxic, and most of them would have to be ingested in very large amounts to produce acute symptoms. Some people experience allergic reactions to food additives, just as allergies to natural foods can occur.

One of the controversial chemicals used in food contact materials, bisphenol A (BPA) was approved by FDA in the 1960s. BPA is not a food additive, but when used in food packaging, it becomes a contaminant. For more than 40 years, BPA has been used in manufacturing many hard plastic food containers such as baby bottles, water bottles, reusable cups, hard plastic cookware, and in the lining of metal food and beverage cans. Trace amounts of BPA are found in some foods packaged in these containers. Because of scientific studies indicating subtle effects from low doses of BPA in laboratory animals, FDA responded to citizen petitions. Based on a review of BPA research studies available in 2008, FDA judged containers with BPA to be safe, but in 2012, they ordered manufacturers of infant bottles and feeding cups to stop using BPA. More research was requested to better understand health effects of human exposure to BPA. To further avoid risk of BPA contamination, choose products in materials other than metal cans, like glass containers; minimize purchasing canned goods, especially tomato products and green beans; and avoid microwaving foods in plastic containers not labeled as microwave safe.

The use of food additives makes many foods more readily available by preventing spoilage and keeping food wholesome and appealing. Complicated chemical names found on labels can be intimidating. Even names of vitamins on labels (e.g., thiamin mononitrate or cyanocobalamin) can cause apprehension for consumers unfamiliar with the terms. Food additives have the following benefits (Table 16-4):

1. They improve nutritional value. Enrichment and fortification have helped reduce malnutrition in the United States. Nutrients added help ensure adequate intake of vitamins or minerals. All added nutrients must be listed on product labels.
2. They maintain wholesomeness and palatability of foods. Bacterial contamination can cause foodborne illnesses. Preservatives retard spoilage caused by mold, air, bacteria, fungi, or yeast, and preserve natural color and flavor. Antioxidants prevent oxidation of fats and oils, fruits, and vegetables.
3. They maintain product consistency. Emulsifiers enable particles to mix and prevent separation. Stabilizers and thickeners contribute to a smooth, uniform texture.
4. They provide leavening or control pH. Leavening agents, such as yeast and baking powder, are used to make foods light in texture and to cause baked goods to rise.

5. They enhance flavor and appearance. These substances are the most widely used and the most controversial additives. Included in this category are coloring agents, natural and synthetic flavors, spices, flavor enhancers, and sweeteners. Sugar, corn syrup, and salt are used in the largest amounts. Without these additives, foods are less appealing, a factor that influences selection and nutrient intake.

Dental Considerations

- Stress following the recommendations on how to retain nutrients during preparation listed in Box 16-2.
- Clarify any misinformation about use of organic foods, but respect patients' beliefs and assist them in obtaining economical products that are acceptable to them.

Nutritional Directions

- Products that can be stored at room temperature should be kept in cool, dry areas in airtight containers.
- Regular ground beef is more economical than ground round, and total fat content can be significantly reduced by using a low-fat cooking method and by rinsing crumbled ground beef after cooking.
- Organic foods cost more but are not more nutritious or significantly different in taste. Fresh, locally grown produce is ideal.
- Organic produce may not look as attractive and unblemished as traditionally grown produce; organically processed foods have a shorter shelf life than products containing preservatives.
- The terms "natural" and "organic" were used interchangeably in the past to describe food that was minimally processed and free of artificial additives or preservatives; however, consumers should be aware that only products with an organic label have met USDA standards. Legally, use of terms such as "natural" or "all-natural" can mean anything the manufacturer wants them to mean.
- Food additives are tested before they can be used. They are considered safe, but should be consumed in moderation. Choosing fresh foods is usually the ideal situation; these foods usually have fewer additives.
- Populations consuming large amounts of fruits and vegetables, even with the use of fertilizers and pesticides, have a lower rate of cancer.
- Buying organic foods should be a personal choice, based on availability, price, appearance, and taste, as well as personal values of the consumer. The most important factor is eating a wide variety of fruits and vegetables.

FOOD FADS AND MISINFORMATION

Nutrition is a very popular subject, but even with all the current knowledge, it is no easier to understand today than it was in 1938:

> More food notions flourish in the United States than in any other civilized country on earth, and most of them are wrong. They thrive in the minds of the same people who talk about their operations; and like all

Table 16-4 | **Guide to food additives**

Type or Function	Commonly Used Additives	Food Usage
Vitamins and minerals improve nutritive value of foods	Vitamin D	Milk, margarine
	Potassium iodide (iodine)	Iodized salt
	Thiamin mononitrate (vitamin B_1), riboflavin (vitamin B_2), niacin (vitamin B_3), folate and ferrous sulfate (iron)	Enriched or fortified breakfast cereals, macaroni, pastas, breads, flour
	Ascorbic acid/sodium ascorbate (vitamin C)	Fruit juices and fruit drinks, cured meats, cereals
Preservatives maintain wholesomeness and palatability of foods	Butylated hydroxyanisole (BHA)	Cereals, chewing gum, potato chips, vegetable oil
	Tocopherols (vitamin E)	Vegetable oils
Antioxidants prevent unsaturated fats and oils, flavorings, and colorings from oxidation, which would result in rancidity, flavor changes, and loss of color	Citric acid	Instant potatoes, fruit drinks, sherbet
	Ascorbic acid (vitamin C)	Cured meats, fruit drinks
	Propyl gallate	Vegetable oils, meat products, potato sticks
	Erythorbic acid	Cured meats
Other preservatives control growth of mold, bacteria, and yeast	Sodium benzoate	Pickles, preserves, fruit juice
	Calcium (or sodium) propionate and potassium sorbate	Breads, rolls, pies, cakes
	Sulfites	Dried fruit, frozen potatoes, wines
	Sodium nitrite/nitrate	Bacon, ham, frankfurters, luncheon meats, smoked fish
	Sorbic acid, potassium sorbate	Cheese, syrup, jelly, cake, wine, dry fruits
Processing aids product consistency and texture; emulsifiers keep oil and water mixed together with uniform dispersion of tiny particles	Monoglycerides and diglycerides	Baked goods, margarine, candy, peanut butter
	Lecithin	Baked goods, chocolate ice cream
	Polysorbate 60	Frozen desserts, imitation dairy products
Stabilizers (other processing aids) help maintain smooth texture and uniform color and flavor	Alginate and propylene glycol alginate	Ice cream, cheese, yogurt
	Carrageenan	Ice cream, jelly, chocolate milk, artificial breast milk
Thickeners (more processing aids) provide desired thickness or gel	Various gums (Arabic, guar, xanthan)	Beverages, salad dressing, cottage cheese, frozen pudding
	Casein/sodium caseinate	Ice cream, sherbet, coffee creamers
	Pectin	Jelly
	Gelatin	Powdered dessert mixes, yogurt, ice cream, cheese spreads
	Starch/modified starch	Soup, gravy, baby food
Acids and bases control the pH of many foods and may act as buffers or neutralizing agents, or as leavening agents	Citric acid and sodium citrate	Frozen desserts, fruit drink, candy, instant potatoes
	Fumaric acid	Powdered drinks, pudding, pie fillings, gelatin desserts
	Lactic acid	Olives, cheese, powdered foods, cured meats, carbonated beverages
	Phosphoric acid	Breads, pastries, baked goods
	Sodium bicarbonate	
Colorings, cosmetic additives in natural and synthetic forms, enhance the appearance of foods	Beta carotene	Margarine, shortening, nondairy whiteners
	Caramel color	Carbonated beverages, candy
	Artificial colors	Beverages, candy, baked goods, cherries in fruit cocktail, sausage, gelatin desserts
	Ferrous gluconate	Black olives

Table 16-4	Guide to food additives—cont'd	
Type or Function	**Commonly Used Additives**	**Food Usage**
Flavoring agents, cosmetic additives available in natural and synthetic forms, enhance flavors	Artificial and natural flavoring	Carbonated beverages, candy, breakfast cereals, gelatin desserts
	Hydrolyzed vegetable protein (HVP)	Instant soups, frankfurters, sauce mixes, beef stew
	Vanillin (substitute for vanilla)	Ice cream, baked goods, beverages, chocolate, candy, gelatin desserts
	Monosodium glutamate (MSG)	Tonic water, bitter lemon
	Quinine	Soup, potato chips, crackers
	Salt (sodium chloride)	
Sweeteners are cosmetic additives used to increase sweetness	Dextrose (corn syrup, glucose)	Candy, toppings, syrups, snack foods, imitation dairy foods
	High-fructose corn syrup	Soft drinks, processed foods
	Invert sugar	Candy, soft drinks
	Sugar (sucrose)	Table sugar, sweetened foods
	Lactose	Whipped topping mix, breakfast pastry
Alternative sweeteners are cosmetic additives replacing sugar in products to reduce kilocalories or to reduce risk of dental decay	Acesulfame-K	Baked goods, chewing gum, gelatin desserts, soft drinks
	Aspartame	Soft drinks, drink mixes, frozen desserts, gelatin desserts
	Mannitol	Chewing gum, low-kilocalorie foods
	Saccharin	"Diet" products, soft drinks
	Sorbitol	Dietetic drinks and foods, candy, shredded coconut, chewing gum
	Sucralose	Diet foods
Other additives needed for processed foods to be prepared, stored, and shipped include anticaking agents; humectants; curing agents; sequestrants; and firming, bleaching, and maturing agents	Calcium (or sodium) stearyl lactylate	Bread dough, cake fillings, processed egg whites
	Ethylenediamine tetraacetic acid (EDTA)	Salad dressing, margarine, processed fruits and vegetables, canned shellfish
	Glycerin	Marshmallows, candy, fudge, baked goods

mythology, they are a blend of fear, coincidence, and advertising.[35]

As consumers' interest in nutrition increases, myths surrounding the subject continue to confuse. Purveyors of nutritional misinformation capitalize on fears and hopes by exaggerating and oversimplifying health virtues or curative properties of foods. Too few consumers understand the effects of various nutrients on the body and how nutrients are used, opening the door to food faddism or nutrition quackery.

Food fad is a catchall term covering all aspects of nutritional nonsense, characterized by exaggerated beliefs about the value of nutrition in health and disease. A food fad may be based on a fact or fallacy. People often begin a diet or believe claims for specific foods or supplements on the basis of something they read or hear without investigating its validity or effectiveness. Some fad diets are nutritionally inadequate and could lead to serious deficiencies. A fad is sometimes harmful because this therapy is substituted for advice of a healthcare provider and consumers delay medical treatment.

Fad diets are prevalent in the United States as Americans continue to search for a magic formula to lose weight and defy the aging process. According to promoters of weight loss diets, specific foods or food combinations facilitate weight loss, implying that a specific food or combination of foods oxidizes body fat, increases metabolic rate, or inhibits voluntary food intake. These diets are frequently deficient in essential nutrients and can be dangerous. Other benefits, such as rapid weight loss, may not be long-lasting (see Evolve website for information to evaluate popular diets).

Fad diets may promise to melt away fat with an immediate weight loss of several pounds, without exercise or limiting food intake. Miraculous promises are a good reason to run the other way. Diets that provide adequate nutrients and changes in lifestyle behaviors are desirable and more effective. Fads, whether for weight loss or other purposes, can be recognized instantly when they promise secret formulas to "cure all."

Food quackery is the promotion of nutrition-related products or services having questionable safety and/or effectiveness for claims made. These claims or promises may be due to ignorance, delusion, misconception, or deliberate deception. Americans spend more than $10 billion annually for cures scientists deem as quackery.

The unknowns of medicine and disagreement among reputable scientists regarding interpretation of research findings foster nutritional misinformation. Given the right circumstances, such as confronting a chronic or incurable disease, everyone is potentially capable of exchanging sound judgment and common sense for the promise of a miraculous cure.

Numerous unproven theories abound regarding food allergies and intolerances, ranging from illegitimate diagnostic testing to treatment with diets and supplements not proven effective in scientific studies. Unconventional procedures for nutritional assessment are numerous. Hair analysis is used to recommend vitamin and mineral supplements. Hair analysis can indicate exposure to toxic heavy metals, but vitamins are not present in hair except in roots below the skin. Hair grows very slowly and does not reflect current body status. Hair mineral content can be affected by shampoos, bleach, dye, and many other factors, including environmental and geographical factors.

Many theories have been proposed to delay the aging process and chronic diseases such as cancer, rheumatoid arthritis, multiple sclerosis, and migraine headaches. Nutritional manipulations are implemented based on these theories to extend a person's life. To date, no proven methods exist to extend the life span.

Other than lead or arsenic toxicities, medical research has no proof of toxic levels from food, so little to no scientific support is available for detoxification methods. The American Academy of Nutrition and Dietetics defines **detoxification** as the biochemical process that transforms non–water-soluble toxins and metabolites into water-soluble compounds that can be excreted in urine, sweat, bile, or stool.[36] Alternative complementary medicine has been a promoter of detoxification, a poorly defined theory. The media and popular culture advocates detoxification through diet, herbal supplements, fasts, juicing, cleanses, chelation therapy, purging products, and removal of mercury fillings. Many chemicals from food, water, and air can be deposited in fat cells. The human body is an amazing machine, cleansing itself from the inside out; cells die and are removed naturally. The intestinal wall and liver are constantly neutralizing potentially toxic substances for elimination via the kidneys, colon, gallbladder, lungs, and skin. Each chemical has a different level of toxicity. However, if one of these systems is not functioning properly, or if the systems are overloaded with excess toxins, a state of toxicity could occur.

During any of the detoxification processes, individuals may experience side effects of fatigue, malaise, aches and pains, emotional duress, headaches, and allergies. Research available on detoxification is largely testimonial—individual personal accounts of healing without controlled scientific experiments.

Detoxification diets are generally high fiber; vegetarian; low in fat, processed foods, alcohol, and caffeine; and utilize supplements with numerous vitamins, minerals, and antioxidants. A detoxification diet based on whole foods with fruits and vegetables, adequate fiber, and water may accelerate the body's detoxification pathways. Phytochemicals from numerous foods promote detoxification enzymes: cruciferous vegetables, celery, herbs (cilantro, rosemary, turmeric, milk thistle, and curry), and dark green leafy vegetables, green and herbal teas, fibrous foods, probiotics, eggs, garlic, and onion. This diet can be well balanced and consistent with the *Dietary Guidelines*. The recommendation for using foods for detoxification is not endorsed by most science-based healthcare providers; claims are based on preliminary and questionable studies.

Juicing is the extraction of juice from fresh fruits or vegetables. This juice contains most of the vitamins, minerals, and phytonutrients found in the whole fruit; however, whole fruits and vegetables contain fiber that may be lost in juicing. Whether juicing actually reduces risk of cancer, boosts the immune system, helps remove toxins, aids digestion, and helps with weight loss is unproven. Freshly squeezed juice can develop harmful bacteria unless consumed soon, and juices contain significant amounts of sugar that can actually lead to weight gain.

Herbal laxatives and high-fiber products, such as psyllium seeds, may be used to cleanse the digestive tract and promote elimination. The use of **colonics** to cleanse the lower intestines is based on the assumption that years of bad diet causes the colon to become caked with layers of accumulated toxins. This is a false assumption because colon examinations routinely performed on millions of people have not observed this even in people who routinely make poor food choices.

Chelation therapy uses specific chemicals to bind and eliminate heavy metals from the body. It has been proposed to rejuvenate the cardiovascular system, treat cancer and immune disorders, and retard aging. This treatment has caused kidney damage and may result in people not seeking competent medical treatment. Sweating therapies help release toxins stored in subcutaneous fat cells. In addition to saunas, therapeutic baths, and exercise, massage therapy and acupressure may be used.

The removal of mercury fillings is based on the concept that mercury in amalgam causes numerous health problems, so fillings are removed to prevent or treat disease. Although it is indisputable that mercury can be toxic, scientific evaluation generally indicates mercury levels in people with fillings are significantly below those necessary to cause toxic symptoms.

Because governmental organizations do not monitor the production and marketing of herbal supplements, numerous concerns are associated with their use. Herbal medicine should not be regarded as quackery, but should be approached with caution. Herbs, including herbal teas and other plant-based formulations, are marketed as being the only natural method to prevent and cure numerous conditions. A recent study indicated herbal products available may be contaminated or contain alternative plant products not listed on the label.[37] Deaths and severe health problems, including CHD, cirrhosis, and renal failure, have occurred from use of some herbal preparations in the United States.

Identifying Sources of Nutrition Misinformation

How do unscrupulous health promoters get away with their lies and fake products? Strict laws protect against false advertising and mislabeling, but health food deception and "food terrorism" thrive. The government actively pursues health swindlers, but enforcement agencies lack adequate staff and resources needed to handle all the problems reported.

The First Amendment to the United States Constitution protects free speech and free press; it also protects a person's right to dispense false, misleading, or deceptive health claims. If the label on a food product makes false or misleading claims, the FDA can take action because of mislabeling. Health-related claims are permitted on food labels if (a) it is well documented that a particular nutrient can reduce risk and (b) the benefits of this nutrient are not offset by another ingredient present. (For instance, a high-fiber cereal high in fat could not be touted as being healthful because of its fat content.)

The Federal Trade Commission can take action if false claims are made in advertising, so claims made on labels or in promotions are not usually false. However, products can be legally promoted in the media and on the Internet because of protection under the First Amendment.

Consumer interest in health and nutrition information is high as consumers are taking more responsibility for their own healthcare. The American culture is bombarded with nutrition information—television and radio talk shows, commercials, infomercials, magazines, newspapers, books, Internet, family and friends, and healthcare providers. People are frequently influenced by testimonials. Celebrities, sports figures, fitness experts, and others without nutrition expertise frequently are featured in advertisements purporting a nutritional product.

The Internet is an unregulated source of nutrition information, reaching millions of people with sales of fraudulent and illegal nutritional and medical products. The emergence of blogs and tweets on the Internet are other sources of information that need to be questioned for credibility. Information may be presented as fact, but the validity of information on websites, especially those with products to sell, should be verified before making a purchase. Therefore, the information is to be questioned regarding its scientific basis. Blogs and YouTube videos may be personal testimonials that are true, but the drawn conclusions may not be related to any purported cause; that is, what works for one person may not work on anyone else.

A popular tactic is to discredit the interpretation of scientific research by the medical community and governmental agencies. Inaccurate information is based on misunderstanding and misrepresentation. Evaluating nutritional information for its legitimacy and validity can be tedious. Healthcare professionals, regardless of where the nutrition information is presented—on the Internet, on television, or in print—should evaluate the findings in light of well-established nutrition principles.

BOX 16-4   Scrutinizing for Fraudulent Information

1. Under the Food, Drug, and Cosmetic Act, a product is a drug if medical claims are made or if it affects body functions. All medical manufacturers who market products interstate must register and list the products with the FDA. The FDA prohibits introduction of any food, drug, device, or cosmetic not labeled correctly. (a) Even though the FDA must approve products before they are marketed, the term *FDA* is not permitted in any claim suggesting approval. (b) Ask to see the firm's FDA registration letter, product's listing letter, or FDA marketing approval letter.

2. Look for use of superlative terms, such as "amazing," "exclusive," "miracle," or "breakthrough," or extravagant terms, such as "cure" or "long life," or emotionally appealing terms, such as promises of "youth," "beauty," or "glamour." Scientific literature does not use these terms. Serious medical problems cannot be cured with remedies marketed mail order, door to door, or on the Internet.

3. Study the label on the product. (a) The instructions on the label should clarify the benefits for the user. (b) Information in the advertisement or promotional material should agree with the product label. Most false claims do not appear on the label because of FDA regulations. Unsubstantiated false claims are usually found in books, television, brochures, infomercials, and promotional materials. Because of the First Amendment, which allows free speech and press, these types of materials are not regulated.

4. Insist on full identification of the institution or researcher promoting the product. Determine whether this information is from a credible source, or if credentials of the promoter are from an accredited college or university. Medical clinics or medical personnel willingly provide full names, addresses, and phone numbers.

5. Beware of "cures" for serious diseases and of products that claim to cure multiple health problems.

6. Be careful of self-diagnosis based on a person's symptoms. Symptoms of many illnesses are similar, and a misdiagnosis can be hazardous if the condition is not being treated appropriately. A proper diagnosis requires an assessment, including a physical examination, by a health professional. Delaying treatment may allow progression of the disease beyond help.

7. Investigate information based on testimonials or case histories or promoted by movie stars, sports figures, or any "big name" person. This is not scientific evidence. The FDA cannot regulate a testimonial about a product.

8. Be cautious of recommendations for vitamin or mineral doses more than the RDAs or over the tolerable upper intake levels for the nutrient. Reliable sources recommend only vitamin and mineral doses in line with the RDAs. Nutrients in amounts greater than the RDA or tolerable upper intake level may be used as medications, as is done when niacin is used to reduce blood cholesterol levels. Only certain conditions require doses beyond the RDAs, and a legitimate medical source should monitor the effects.

9. If it sounds too good to be true, it probably is.

Probably the best way to begin a search on the Internet is to go to credible websites of trusted health organizations with names you recognize, universities, and state and national government agencies and offices, and click on links provided on these websites. Reliable nutrition websites are given throughout this text and on the Evolve website. The information provided in Box 16-4 is helpful for evaluating oral or written claims.

The news media often have a poor understanding of research methods and statistics, and seldom report the extent and limitations of information or important nuances of a research study. Frequently, reporters are anxious to publish before the competition and may "jump the gun" to get "to press" without fully checking out the story. They generally report medical findings as "facts." Consumers are confused by listening to journalists presenting research studies that provide conflicting information. Two physicians developed four valuable guidelines published in the *New England Journal of Medicine* to help prevent misinterpretation of scientific studies[38]: (a) an association between two events is not the same as a cause and effect; (b) demonstrating one link in a postulated chain of events does not mean that the whole chain has been proven; (c) probabilities are not the same as certainties; and (d) the way a scientific result is framed can greatly affect its impact.

Dental professionals and consumers can begin by checking credentials of the person making a questionable claim. Most articles appearing in established medical and scientific journals were submitted to a board of peer scientists for

evaluation before publication. If peer reviewers consider conclusions to be well supported by the research, it is published for others to read. A single study never proves a theory; it may provide conclusive information, but provoke more questions for further studies. A single study usually serves as another piece of the puzzle if it can be replicated.

When evaluating individual studies, consideration must be given to the number of participants and length of the study and other pertinent information as described in Box 16-5. For instance, the Nurses' Health Study that began in 1976, has involved almost 122,000 women ages 30 to 55 years, and is still ongoing. This National Institutes of Health-funded study to investigate potential long-term consequences of oral contraceptives has limitations in its credibility because professionally trained healthcare workers may have different values and practices than a cross-cultural sample of women.

Many types of studies—epidemiological, case-control, placebo-controlled, randomized, crossover-design, double-blind, clinical trials or interventions—together help provide conclusive information. The gold standard for research studies is "evidence-based," a term used for medical practices that have been thoroughly evaluated using scientific methods. Interventions used in the studies are evaluated based on risks and benefits revealed during clinical trials that are randomized and placebo-controlled. Experts review data from numerous studies to determine whether or not treatment can be recognized as safe or effective. The Cochrane Collaboration is dedicated to creating systematic reviews of

---

BOX 16-5   How to Determine Whether a Claim or a Source Is Legitimate

Consider the Source: Is the source recognized as creditable by your industry or profession? Does it have a history of imparting information that is balanced and unbiased? Is it potentially biased due to stated or inherent political, social, or professional affiliations? Is the source externally or internally monitored to ensure the information it imparts is fair and unbiased? Is it a primary or secondary source of information?

Check Reviews of Sources: Some common sources of reviews include *Book Review Index* and *Periodical Abstracts*. Sources dedicated to vetting online information include Factcheck.org, prwatch.org, and http://www.imediaethics.org/.

Determine Whether the Source Is a Member of or Governed by Reputable Industry Organizations: Some leading organizations, such as the American Business Media, an umbrella group for business-to-business publications, require members to maintain strict standards of journalistic ethics, regardless of whether the information is imparted in print or on websites, social networks, e-newsletters, directories, search engines, blogs, digital editions, videos, podcasts, or webcasts.

Look for a Corroborating Source: Does an equally creditable source support the information imparted by the initial source? If not, does the difference lie in the manner in which facts are stated or in the manner they are interpreted? Either way, proceed with caution.

Identify the Intended Audience: Is the source imparting information to a general audience or to an audience allied with your profession? If the information is directed to a general audience, is it thoroughly presented? Does it identify professional sources?

Identify Potential Conflicts of Interest: Is the source supported by advertising? If so, is the information imparted "advertiser friendly?"

Research the Author: Does the author have a degree or other credentials pertaining to the subject of interest? If the author or the author's professional affiliation isn't identified, what makes the author a creditable source?

Evaluate the Source's/Author's Sources: Does the author cite sources to support the author's statement? Do the sources have a degree or credentials pertaining to the statement? Is there any potential bias as a result of political, social, or professional affiliations?

Look for Peer Reviews: Assuming the information derives from a journal, determine whether it has been peer reviewed, meaning evaluated by qualified individuals in a related field.

Check the Date: Information gathered by online search engines frequently isn't dated. As a result, the information may be out dated.

From Gregerson J: Truth, lies, and rumors in the media: consider the source. *J Acad Nutr Diet* 2012;112(5):602-609.

peer-reviewed studies. The Academy of Nutrition and Dietetics also maintains an evidenced-based library of nutrition-related studies. Meta-analysis combines all relevant studies from independent sources using a statistical technique, most often used to assess clinical effectiveness of healthcare interventions. A meta-analysis provides a precise estimate of treatment effect. Systematic reviews also provide reliable information based on all relevant published and unpublished evidence, selecting studies for inclusion, assessing the quality of each study, then compiling the findings, and interpreting them to present a balanced and impartial summary while defining limitations of the evidence. Observational studies are epidemiological research studies with no type of intervention or experiment. These may be used to discover possible relationships between lifestyle and diseases. For instance, "people who love ice cream are obese" may survey thousands of participants, but does not clearly determine a cause.

Dental Considerations

- Assess patients' use of food fads, economic level, educational level, and the nutrient adequacy of any fad diet undertaken.
- If a patient restricts food choices because of a food fad or belief, ensuring nutrient adequacy is more difficult. A thorough assessment and evaluation by the dental hygienist may indicate risk for a nutritional insufficiency or deficiency. Referral to a registered dietitian nutritionist (RDN) may be needed.
- Help patients choose a variety of foods to ensure a balanced intake and decrease amounts consumed of any particular food to minimize risk of excessive contaminants from any one source. For instance, consumption of fish is encouraged because of beneficial substances to prevent CHD. However, fish, especially large fish such as swordfish, shark, mackerel, tilefish, and tuna, contain methylmercury so that eating too much fish has the potential to cause neurological problems.
- Provide patients with positive advice based on a broad knowledge base and understanding nutritional concepts and current research findings.
- Answer any questions about therapies, products, or treatments a patient may be contemplating, or refer the patient to a reliable source.
- Speak out to protect the public from misinformation.
- Do not offer remedies unless they have been proven to be safe and effective.
- If a patient is using or contemplating using a food fad or diet you are unfamiliar with, do not hesitate to consult an RDN, home economist, or nutrition professor.

Nutritional Directions

- Although some fads are physically harmless, they may create an economic hardship for individuals with limited income because the foods or supplements may be expensive.
- Results of fad diets can be devastating and have even led to death.
- The mainline medical community is divided on whether detoxification has any benefits.

REFERRALS FOR NUTRITIONAL RESOURCES

Frequently, patients need special assistance for nutritional problems. At some point during 2012, approximately 25% of Americans participated in at least one of the USDA's 15 domestic food and nutrition assistance programs.[39] A variety of governmental programs are available to help financially, assist with food budgeting, teach basic nutrition and meal planning, or help clarify nutrition misconceptions. Local chapters of many health-related organizations, listed in the telephone directory, furnish free or inexpensive literature, audiovisual material, and health-oriented programs on various topics.

Dental hygienists can identify patients or families with nutritional needs, provide appropriate referrals, and help them participate in applicable programs (Table 16-5). RDNs and many nutritionists are trained to assist with nutritional or dietary problems. A nutritionist may have at least a 4-year degree in foods and nutrition, and may work in a public health setting assisting people in the community.

One of the best sources is the city or county health department. State and local health departments usually have various programs to provide nutrition services, such as well-baby clinics and family health centers. Health departments and county hospitals are excellent resources for information about various programs available. The federal government administers several nutrition programs through the USDA and the U.S. Department of Health and Human Services.

The Area Information Center (2-1-1) maintains comprehensive databases of resources, including federal, state, and local government agencies, and community-based and private nonprofit organizations. Information and referral services is a national dialing code to link people in need of assistance with appropriate providers of services in their community.

The Supplemental Nutrition Assistance Program (SNAP) (formerly the Food Stamp Program) is the cornerstone for nutrition safety in the United States. This federal assistance program is available to individuals with incomes up to 130% of the poverty level. The program was renamed because benefits are provided through an Electronic Benefit Card (EBT) to low-income households that meet certain requirements, rather than food stamp coupons. The program, designed to help low-income households purchase nutritious food, is based on family income and household size. Local offices that administer the program are widely distributed throughout the United States. The program was initially designed to boost food consumption and energy intake.

Food stamp usage has hit a new high. The declining and persistently weak economy, and high rates of unemployment or underemployment in the American workforce are attributed to increasing numbers of people having to rely on federal programs. The number of people on SNAP has more than doubled from 23 million in 2004 to more than 47 million in May 2013.[40] Currently more than 1 in 7 Americans

Table 16-5 | **Referral chart for community nutrition resources**

Population Group	Risk Factor	Referral Source*	Contact†
Pregnant and lactating women	Low income	Supplemental Nutrition Assistance Program (SNAP)	State food stamp hotline number available at http://www.fns.usda.gov/snap/contact_info/hotlines.htm
	Anemia, inadequate weight gain, age-related risk factor, inadequate healthcare, or lack of food and nutrition information	WIC Program	City, county, or state health department
		Maternity and Infant Care Project	State health department
		Expanded Food and Nutrition Education Program (EFNEP)	Land-grant universities
			Prenatal clinic or private healthcare team
Infants	Low-birth-weight, failure to thrive, or poor growth patterns	Prenatal education	City, county, or state health department
	Inadequate healthcare	WIC Program	State health department
Children	Poor growth patterns or overweight, inadequate diet, or anemia	WIC Program (up to 5 years old)	City, county, or state health department
	Low income	Children and Youth Project (up to 18 years old)	State health department
		Head Start (preschool)	Local community action project
		School lunch	Board of education
		School breakfast	Local school district
Older adult	Low income	Supplemental Nutrition Assistance Program (SNAP)	State food stamp hotline number available at http://www.fns.usda.gov/snap/contact_info/hotlines.htm
		Congregate meal sites	State and local agencies on aging
	Homebound	Meals on Wheels	Locations available at www.mealcall.org/meals-on-wheels/index.htm
General adult	Obesity	Weight Watchers International, Thin Within, Dieters workshop, TOPS, and other weight reduction groups	Local chapters
	Hyperlipidemia, cardiovascular disease, or hypertension	American Heart Association	Local chapter
	Diabetes	American Diabetes Association	Local chapter
	Low income	Supplemental Nutrition Assistance Program (SNAP)	State food stamp hotline number available at http://www.fns.usda.gov/snap/contact_info/hotlines.htm
	Reliable food and nutrition information	EFNEP	Land-grant universities
	General consumer information for all populations	Community nutrition groups and community cooperatives	Local groups
		Academy of Nutrition and Dietetics	Available at www.eatright.org/Public/
		Center for Science in the Public Interest	Available at http://www.cspinet.org/about/index.html
		U.S. Department of Health and Human Services	Available at dhhs.gov/
		Healthfinder	Available at healthfinder.gov
		WebMD	Available at http://www.webmd.com/a-to-z-guides/common-topics/default.htm

*This is only a partial listing. Programs may vary in different parts of the United States.
†Call 2-1-1 for free access to health and human services information and referrals in local communities.

receives SNAP. Adjusting for inflation in food prices, the maximum SNAP benefit declined by about 7% from 2009 to 2011.[41]

SNAP program benefits are critically important to help feed families in need. For October 2012 through September 2013, the maximum monthly allotment for a family of 4 was $668 per person, $367 for a family of 2.[42] Without good money management skills, the monthly food allowance may run out mid-month. The program is meant to supplement a household's food budget; it is not intended to be the total food budget. Although it took careful planning and shopping, two chefs and a magazine food editor planned seven days of meals for a family of four using the SNAP budget, and were either within the budget of $68.88 per person (the maximum benefit for 2010), or very close to that amount.[43] Eating healthy on the SNAP program is challenging but doable—a back-to-basics style of eating.

Because poor diets exert heavy costs in medical expenditures and lost productivity, measures for promoting healthful food choices could yield considerable benefits. State governments and health advocates recognize that additional modifications to reinforce nutrition education, restrict foods allowed with food stamp benefits, and expand benefits to encourage purchases of more healthful foods, such as fruit and vegetables, are needed.

While the program is intended to improve the nutritional and health status of families needing help, consumers frequently do not use the funds to purchase foods wisely. Recipients can use the Electronic Benefit Card to buy any foods sold in participating grocery stores, with the exception of prepared hot foods. Billions of SNAP dollars purchase products inconsistent with the goal of helping improve health. A study conducted by Yale University's Rudd Center for Food Policy and Obesity estimated that the SNAP benefits pay at least $1.7 to $2.1 billion annually for sugar-sweetened beverages purchased in grocery stores.[44]

The Special Supplemental Food Program for Women, Infants, and Children (WIC) is designed to prevent nutritional problems in this high-risk, low-income group. The WIC program is available to pregnant and lactating women, infants, and children up to 5 years old who are considered to be at nutritional risk. Some of the criteria for nutritional risk are evidence of iron deficiency, inadequate weight gain during pregnancy, teenage pregnancy, failure to thrive, poor growth patterns, and inadequate dietary patterns. In addition to supplemental foods, nutrition education and referrals to healthcare sources are provided. Studies of the WIC program have shown positive effects on iron status and growth and development of infants and children. The program also saves millions of dollars by decreasing the rate of low-birth-weight infants, so funding has remained relatively stable.

In 2009, significant, nutritionally beneficial changes were made in the food packages. The goals for changes were to better support breastfeeding and provide healthier foods more consistent with the *Dietary Guidelines*. Food packages for mothers and infants are financially equivalent in the costs of food provided, whether the mother is breastfeeding or not. For instance, since formula feeding is more expensive, breastfeeding mothers are allowed more foods equivalent to the cost received by the formula-fed infant. The full formula package provides less food for the mother, and all food benefits for the mother stop when the formula-fed infant is 6 months old. Fresh fruits and vegetables are permitted, and only low-fat or skim milk is allowed for children older than 2 years of age and mothers. Foods provided must meet strict nutritional standards by providing a specific amount of fiber, vitamin C, or vitamin D.

School breakfast and lunch programs provide nutritious meals for children at school. Nutritional standards for school lunch require lunch provide at least one-third, and breakfast at least one-fourth, of the RDAs for children. Free and reduced-price meals are provided based on household income and size. New guidelines for overhauling the school food program were written in 2010, with initial implementation by Fall 2012.[45] These new requirements are more consistent with the *Dietary Guidelines*, significantly changing the maximum amount of allowable kilocalories, sodium, saturated and *trans* fats. Because of difficulties in meeting the lower sodium requirement, some of the targets will be gradually decreased through 2022. The standards for age-grade groups include more food groups and limiting kilocalories. Milk must be fat-free (plain or flavored) or plain low-fat (1% milk fat). More whole fruit is required at both meals. Dark green vegetables, red/orange vegetables, beans/peas (legumes), and starchy vegetables ($\frac{1}{2}$ cup equivalent) must be offered at least weekly. Fruits and vegetables are not interchangeable. At least half of the bread/grain offerings must meet the criterion for a whole-grain–rich food; by 2014, all grains must be whole-grain rich. Many students claimed the school lunch that met the guidelines did not provide enough kilocalories and protein. Because of protests of parents and students, the requirements were liberalized somewhat in 2013.

The Nutrition Program for the Elderly (Title III) provides group and home-delivered meals. The purpose of this program is to improve nutritional and health status of older adults and offer participants opportunities to form new friendships and create informal support networks. The Elderly Nutrition Program provides a range of services (including social services) through approximately 4000 nutrition service providers. Of the participants served, 73% are at high nutritional risk, 25% at moderate risk.[46] More than 3 million elderly participants receive an estimated 40% to 50% of required nutrients from meals provided by this program. Many of the participants report they do not always have enough money or food stamps to buy food.

The Expanded Food and Nutrition Education Program is designed to help lower socioeconomic groups with all aspects of nutrition. The Expanded Food and Nutrition Education Program is available through county extension services of land-grant universities and assists with meal planning, budgeting, cooking, and other food-related and nutrition-related problems. Nutrition aides are low-income homemakers who are trained to visit homes of low-income families to assist in providing well-balanced meals.

Head Start is a preschool educational program for low-income families. Breakfast, lunch, and snacks are furnished for the children, and nutrition education is available for parents.

Locally-funded food agencies providing assistance through food banks and food pantries have increased substantially. Food pantries, which usually do not base eligibility for benefits on income status, currently serve millions of Americans. Foods available at food pantries provide inadequate amounts of calcium and vitamins A and C, but many of these facilities are trying to improve the quality of foods they provide. Emergency food providers serve a diverse population with different reasons for needing the assistance. These providers are especially helpful for people during a short-term setback, such as an unexpected emergency medical bill; others need emergency kitchens to receive a hot meal or supplement food stamps. On the dismal side, in many cases, emergency food pantries are not being used just to meet temporary, acute food needs. Almost 75% of participants at a food pantry in Connecticut were black, 59% female, and 75% of participants had an income level of less than $1,000/month.[47] More than half of the clients consistently or frequently receiving food from the food pantry are SNAP recipients, or are older than 65 years of age.[48]

ROLE OF DENTAL HYGIENISTS

What role can the dental hygienist play in combating nutrition fads and misinformation? Natalie Van Cleve stated in 1938, when times were different but widespread misinformation on diet was just as prevalent as today[49]:

> It is the duty of all professions active in the field of food and nutrition to cooperate in clarifying any misconceptions of the laity. If the [healthcare providers] do not know their vitamins, the patients will find a radio announcer who does.

Healthcare providers, dental hygienists, and even RDNs have sometimes promoted nutritional misinformation by failing to apply their knowledge, misunderstanding how nutrients are used, or searching for fame and fortune. The dental professional is in a unique position to understand the causes of food fads and to recognize their dangers. First, understanding patients and their love of "miracle" answers should help in recognizing the appeal of such misinformation. Second, a scientific background permits assessment of potential effects or uselessness of food fads. Dental hygienists can help patients understand the true essence of nutritional science—the process of nourishing or being nourished—rather than the polypharmacy of supernutrition. Many legitimate resources include governmental and professional organizations; these are referenced on the Evolve website to help evaluate the legitimacy of nutritional claims. Many legitimate medical journals are also available on the Internet, as listed on the Evolve website.

The dental professional can help by referring patients to appropriate resources and agencies or to a social worker for assistance in filling out forms. These embarrassing issues should be discussed in a matter-of-fact manner. Patients may benefit by ventilating feelings and beliefs about food "handouts." Information should be presented in a positive manner, stating how it would benefit the patient and family. Most parents desire the best for their children; it is important to stress benefits children would receive (e.g., increased growth, learning, productivity) by participating. Help patients recognize that having inadequate funds for food is not a sign of failure, and that asking for help shows strength, courage, and wisdom. In due time, they may be able to help someone else. Dental professionals can also help by serving at community food resource centers or food donation drives. Some centers offer dental care using volunteer dental hygienists and dentists.

Dental Considerations

- Identify patients needing food assistance, and refer them to appropriate sources.
- If kilocalories, sodium, and fat should be restricted, discourage patronage of fast food establishments or provide suggestions for appropriate fast food selections (e.g., salads or baked chicken).
- Low-income households must allocate a higher proportion of both their income and time to planning, purchasing, and preparing food if they wish to consume nutritious meals.
- When recommending foods to patients, consider the income level. Suggesting steak or lobster as a protein source for low-income patients is inappropriate.
- In addition to government health agencies already mentioned, numerous health and professional organizations listed on the Evolve website provide health information. Other organizations, such as the Better Business Bureau, may also be helpful.

Nutritional Directions

- Protein sources are generally the most expensive budget items; however, it is unnecessary to buy choice quality grades of meat for good nutrition. ("Select" and "standard" are more economical grades of meat.)
- Discuss guidelines for economical food purchases (see Box 16-1) to help low-income patients modify food purchases.

HEALTH APPLICATION 16   Food Insecurity in the United States

Food security, or access to enough food for an active, healthy life by all family members at all times, is a universal dimension of household and personal well-being and considered a fundamental requirement for a healthy, well-nourished population. However, food insecurity and hunger continue to exist in the United States. Hunger, or an uneasy or painful sensation caused by lack of food, typically precedes food insecurity. Food insecurity refers to the lack of access to enough food to meet basic needs fully at some time during the year because of insufficient funds or resources for food. Food insecurity means having to decide which bills to pay—food, housing, heat, electricity, water, transportation, childcare, or healthcare. Food insecurity is usually recurrent or transient, but not chronic, and may involve a low-quality diet that is monotonous and lacking in nutrients. Approximately 14.9% of U.S. households were food insecure sometime during 2011 (Fig. 16-6). Prevalence of food insecurity in America has increased significantly since 2007 (Fig. 16-7).

Food-secure households typically spend more on food than food-insecure households, but low-income households spend a larger proportion (33%) of total income on food.[50] Hunger rates decrease as income increases, but food insecurity is not exclusive to very-low-income families. The Food Research and Action Center indicated the food hardship rate was 18.2% during the first 6 months of 2012.[51] Approximately 5.7% of households (7 million) experienced very low food security (at times during the year, food intake of household members was reduced and normal eating patterns disrupted because of insufficient funds or other resources to obtain food) in 2012 (see Fig. 16-6).[52]

Rates of food insecurity are substantially higher than the national average for households with children headed by a single woman and in households with children (Fig. 16-8). Black and Hispanic households had rates of food insecurity more than twice those of white non-Hispanic households.[52] Nearly half of American children live in homes that at some point receive governmental nutrition programs.[53]

A work-limiting disability substantially increases the risk of food insecurity for low-income families. In addition to the disabled individual being unable to work and incurring burdensome medical costs and other expenses, an adult caretaker may be restricted in work opportunities and hours. The homeless make up a large percentage of the hungry. Millions of people in the United States maintain a home and may even work full-time but live below the poverty level. (In 2012, poverty was defined as an annual income less than $29,960 for a family of 4 in the 48 contiguous states.)

Several factors may account for the increase in food insecurity—the state of the American economy; unemployment rate; and the changing composition of the United States population, particularly households headed by single women. People who are unemployed for a long period deplete their assets, exhaust unemployment insurance, and turn to SNAP for help. Households attempt to avoid hunger by using various strategies, such as eating less-varied diets, skipping meals, participating in federal food assistance programs (57%), and/or getting emergency food from community food pantries. Emergency food from pantries is being used to regularly supplement monthly shortfalls in contrast to earlier usage of food pantries for temporary acute food needs. Emergency food assistance remains at unprecedented levels, yet sources for approximately 25% of the food available from food pantries has declined significantly, limiting their ability to meet the communities' needs. Two groups of low-income Americans are facing problems, requiring more reliance on food banks—seniors and people enrolled in the SNAP program.[54]

Food insecurity may cause a variety of negative health outcomes for everyone affected, but younger populations are most at risk. In most households, older family members protect children, especially younger ones, from substantial reductions in food intake and ensuing hunger. Effects on health and behavior have been observed, especially with persistent or chronic food shortages. Insufficient food intake affects mental and physical health, having both acute and chronic effects. Food-insecure children younger than 3 years old were nearly twice as likely to be in "fair or poor" health, and a larger percentage of children were more likely to have been hospitalized since birth than were food-secure children. Ensuring food security may reduce health problems and hospitalizations in children. Growth stunting without muscle wasting is

Continued

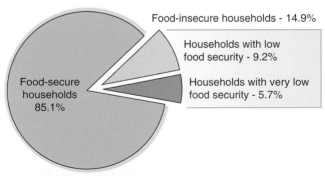

FIGURE 16-6 U.S. households by food security status, 2011. (Calculated by USDA, Economic Research Service based on Current Population Survey Food Security Supplement data. Coleman-Jensen A, Nord M, Andrews M, Carlson S: *Household food security in the United States in 2012,* ERR-155, U.S. Department of Agriculture, Economic Research Service, September 2013. Accessed September 14, 2013. Available at: http://www.ers.usda.gov/media/884525/err141.pdf.)

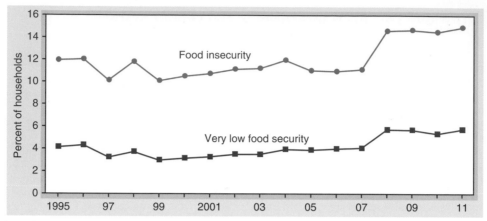

FIGURE 16-7 Trends in the prevalence of food insecurity and very low food security in U.S. households, 1995-2011. Prevalence rates for 1996 and 1997 were adjusted for the estimated effects of differences in data collection screening protocols used in those years. (Calculated by USDA, Economic Research Service based on Current Population Survey Food Security Supplement data. Coleman-Jensen A, Nord M, Andrews M, Carlson S: *Household food security in the United States in 2012,* ERR-155, U.S. Department of Agriculture, Economic Research Service, September 2013. Accessed September 13, 2013. Available at: http://www.ers.usda.gov/publications/err-economic-research-report/err141.aspx.)

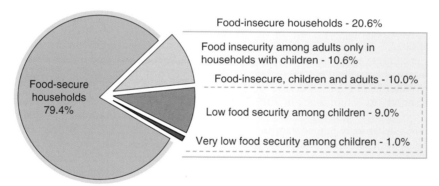

FIGURE 16-8 U.S. households with children by food security status of adults and children, 2011. (Calculated by USDA, Economic Research Service based on Current Population Survey Food Security Supplement data. Coleman-Jensen A, Nord M, Andrews M, Carlson S, et al: *Household food security in the United States in 2012,* ERR-155, U.S. Department of Agriculture, Economic Research Service, September 2013. Accessed September 13, 2013. Available at: http://www.ers.usda.gov/media/884525/err141.pdf.)

HEALTH APPLICATION 16   **Food Insecurity in the United States—cont'd**

characteristic of homeless children who experience moderate chronic nutritional stress. Hungry children are more likely to experience undesired weight loss, fatigue, irritability, concentration problems, and dizziness, frequent headaches, ear infections, and colds.

Cognitive and academic performance are also detrimentally affected. Missing a meal, particularly breakfast, can reduce a child's ability to respond to the environment, negatively affecting learning. Apathy, disinterest, irritability, and a low tolerance for frustration are common behaviors in hungry children. Hungry children are unable to concentrate in school and are less likely to reach their potential to become fully-productive adults. Additionally, psychosocial problems are observed more often: difficulty getting along with peers, suspension from school, and adolescent suicide. **Neurotransmitters,** such as serotonin, acetylcholine, and norepinephrine, relay chemical messages to the brain to increase function, and

each chemical has a different role in maximizing capabilities. Proteins, fats, some minerals and vitamins are necessary for production of neurotransmitters. Having a healthy, balanced diet improves brain capacity, minimizes cognitive capabilities, and improves academic performance.[55]

Paradoxically, low income individuals, especially women, with food insecurity have disproportionately higher rates of obesity than those with food security. A consensus of research indicates participation in the program does not increase likelihood of being overweight or obese for men or children, but hunger along with food insecurity is related to greater body mass indexes.

Low-income people are subject to the same influences and problems as other Americans (e.g., more sedentary lifestyles, increased portion sizes), but they also face unique challenges in adopting healthful behaviors. Individuals who skip meals or postpone mealtimes are more likely to consume more kilocalories when food is available. When adequate food supplies are not always available, people find themselves in a cycle of overeating and then hunger when money or food stamps run out. Mothers, usually the food managers in the household, may take several actions to protect their children from hunger, including skipping meals and eating cheaper, less nutritious foods. Irregular eating can cause a metabolic response that supports fat deposition.[56] Persistent household food insecurity without hunger is related to child obesity, but these associations depend on maternal weight status.[57]

Overconsumption is even easier with more readily available cheap, energy-dense foods. In low-income neighborhoods, full-service grocery stores and farmers' markets are lacking, healthy food is more expensive or may not be available, and fast food establishments are plentiful. Lower-income neighborhoods provide fewer opportunities for physical activity (fewer parks, bike paths, and recreational facilities, unsafe playground equipment, more problems with crime and traffic, and less participation in organized sports).

Nutritionally, adults and children from food-insufficient households are more likely to consume substantially less than recommended dietary allowances (RDA) for certain food groups and nutrients. Unfortunately, SNAP participants have lower quality diets than income-eligible non-participants.[58] The first food group eliminated from an impoverished person's diet is produce. Over the long-term, these deficits increase the risk of developing chronic diseases, cardiovascular disease and diabetes, more frequent and severe disease complications, and increased demands and costs for healthcare services.[59]

Food insecurity represents a major public health and public policy challenge by causing health problems, increasing education costs, and less than optimal productivity. Yet this serious health problem is treatable with a simple inexpensive cure: providing food. Proper nutrition can decrease money spent on health problems. SNAP participants choose how to spend their benefits. However, many lack money management skills, creating problems at the end of the month when benefits are depleted. They have no clue about the healthiest foods to purchase with their limited allotment. Educational efforts are needed to focus on supporting resource-limited SNAP participants in making healthful selections that will help with weight management while providing adequate nutrients. The American Academy of Nutrition and Dietetics advocates "systematic and sustained interventions to achieve food and nutrition security for everyone in the United States," recommending adequate funding for and increased use of food and assistance programs and innovative programs to promote and support economic self-sufficiency.[60]

Use of dietary supplements containing the recommended amounts of vitamins and minerals has been proposed because the average cost of one tablet is less than a dime. However, dietary supplements do not provide energy, which is especially important for children and older adults.

The goal of *Healthy People 2020* is to increase quality and years of healthy life and to eliminate health disparities; this requires improved food and nutrition security. By increasing food security among American households to 94% (from the baseline of 89%), hunger would also be reduced. U.S. federal assistance programs discussed earlier in this chapter are available to address hunger. Full use of these programs, with increased availability and benefits, and increased awareness of programs are a good place to start.

Case Application for the Dental Hygienist

A patient reports he has found a miracle cure for his advanced periodontal disease. He plans to follow a diet and take recommended supplements "to strengthen my gums." This diet eliminates all foods from two food groups on *MyPlate*.

Nutritional Assessment
- Dietary intake, especially which of the food groups are omitted; nutrients most likely to be lacking
- Nutrition knowledge
- Supplements used and dosage
- Economic status
- Where most meals taken; food preparation

Nutritional Diagnosis
Knowledge deficit related to nutritional requirements.

Nutritional Goals
The patient will receive adequate nutrients to maintain oral health status by consuming a well-balanced diet.

Nutritional Implementation
Intervention: Discuss *MyPlate*—different groups, numbers of servings needed from each group, portion sizes, and nutrients provided from each group.
Rationale: Healthy oral structures depend on a variety of nutrients that can be obtained by following this guideline.

Intervention: Discuss nutrients that are deficient in his proposed diet and why those nutrients are important.
Rationale: When essential nutrients are omitted, the body cannot function effectively, and its immune response is compromised.
Intervention: Discuss the importance of obtaining nutrients from foods rather than supplements.
Rationale: Foods are the natural way of obtaining nutrients; when supplements are used, many times they are in proportions that cannot be absorbed, or they may interfere with absorption of other nutrients. Other components of food may affect use of the nutrient. In general, most supplements are not as effective as the food itself (see *Health Application 11* in Chapter 11).
Intervention: Discuss specific foods and oral care that would be helpful in preventing further deterioration.
Rationale: Adequate nutrition and oral self-care promote healing and repair of disease tissue. Maintaining a well-balanced diet provides the nutrients needed to support a healthy periodontium and resist disease activity.

Evaluation
The patient will practice effective oral care and consume a well-balanced diet; as a consequence, his periodontal health will improve.

STUDENT READINESS

1. Which ethnic group is most prevalent in your area?
   - Identify at least one thing good about this ethnic group's food pattern.
   - List at least one potential dietary problem of this ethnic group, and provide some suggestions for altering the diet.
   - Plan a 2-day menu that would fulfill the RDAs using many favorite foods or habits.
   - Would a patient have any problem following that menu, such as economic hardship or the local availability of special foods?
   - Does that ethnic group have any predominant dental problems?
2. Think of two general statements that apply to all of your family/roommates (e.g., always eat breakfast, never drink milk, etc.). Discuss these statements with a group of your fellow students and see how many actually conform to your statement. Other than good foods to eat, what other lifelong eating customs are learned as a child?
3. State some reasons why people in the United States do not have similar eating patterns.
4. Plan an inexpensive menu for one day using low-cost foods.
5. A patient wants to know about convenience and fast foods. What would you tell the patient?
6. Study the meats at a grocery store. Categorize the types of meats that contain nitrate preservatives. Look at your own daily intake for three days, and evaluate how frequently you are consuming nitrate-containing foods.
7. Americans are dependent on commercially prepared frozen foods or purchased foods outside the home. Look at the caloric density of foods consumed in commercial restaurants and the nature of the diseases that relate to obesity and cardiovascular health. What has consumer demand done to change selections offered in commercial food service establishments?
8. Prepare a rough budget showing how your personal funds are expended on a month-to-month basis. Evaluate the percentage of your own personal income that is earmarked for food prepared at home versus food prepared commercially in a restaurant or convenience items purchased in a grocery store. How well do you spend your own food dollar? Make some conclusions about how you could better use your dollar to provide nutrient-dense foods for you and your family.
9. Compare the cost of three foods from a health food store or health food section of a supermarket with the cost of similar items in a supermarket. Can you think of any reasons to justify the more expensive product?
10. Locate an advertisement in a popular magazine or newspaper for a health food product, and list merits of the product stated in the ad. List information about the product that might have been omitted or should be questioned.
11. Compare the cost of three organic foods with the same foods that are not labeled organic. Which would you choose to purchase and why?
12. Why are food faddism and quackery problems for the medical profession?
13. Discuss current food fads and how they may have adverse effects.
14. How can one spot a food quack?
15. Discuss the pros and cons of allowing nutritional claims on products.
16. A patient states, "I want to follow the _____ diet because my favorite actor is advertising it." How would you respond?
17. Read a nutrition research article from a reputable journal. Using information provided in this chapter, point out some problems with the validity and applicability of the research. Does the article identify these as problem areas? Summarize the article in one page or less as if presenting to a patient.

CASE STUDY

A young couple with 3 children, ages 3, 5, and 7 years, has been living on unemployment insurance payments for 9 months. The mother expresses concerns because of inadequate funds to feed the children. She is worried about their dental health.

1. Prepare a list of social services or federal service agencies in the community that should be contacted to determine potential sources of assistance to support recovery of this couple.
2. What are some nutritional concerns the dental hygienist could address with the patient?
3. What are some foods that are nutrient-dense and economical purchases?
4. List some snack foods for the children that are nutritious, economical, and noncariogenic.
5. What methods of food preparation could be suggested to the mother that would preserve the nutritional quality of the food?

References

1. Centers for Disease Control and Prevention (CDC): *Health disparities and inequalities report—United States*, 2011. Accessed September 13, 2013: http://www.cdc.gov/minorityhealth/reports/CHDIR11/ExecutiveSummary.pdf.
2. U.S. Census Bureau: *U.S. interim projections by age, sex, race, and Hispanic origin*, 2004. Accessed September 13, 2013: http://www.census.gov/newsroom/releases/archives/population/cb12-243.html.
3. Dye BA, Li X, Thornton-Evans G: Oral health disparities as determined by selected *Healthy People 2020* oral health objectives for the United States, 2009–2010. *NCHS Data Brief* 104:1–8, 2012. Accessed September 13, 2013: http://www.cdc.gov/nchs/data/databriefs/db104.htm.
4. Mendez E: *Americans spend $151 a week on food; the high-income, $180.* August 2, 2012. Accessed September 13, 2013: http//www.gallup.com/poll/156416/Americans-Spend-151-Week-Food-High-Income-180.aspx.

5. U.S. Department of Agriculture, Center for Nutrition Policy and Promotion: *Official USDA food plans: cost of food at home at four levels, U.S. average, modified January 2013.* Accessed September 13, 2013: http://www.cnpp.usda.gov/Publications/FoodPlans/2013/CostofFoodJan2013.pdf.

6. Carlson A, Frazão E: *Are healthy foods really more expensive? It depends on how you measure the price.* EIB-96, U.S. Department of Agriculture, Economic Research Service, May 2012. Accessed September 13, 2013: http://www.ers.usda.gov/media/600474/eib96_1_.pdf.

7. Guthrie J, Lin BH, Okrent A, et al: *Americans' food choices at home and away: how do they compare with recommendations?* Amber Waves 2013 Feb 21. Accessed September 12, 2013: http://www.ers.usda.gov/amber-waves/2013-february/americans-food-choices-at-home-and-away.aspx.

8. Stewart H, Blisard N: *Are lower income households willing and able to budget for fruits and vegetables?* U.S. Department of Agriculture, Economic Research Service, ERR-54, January 2008. Accessed September 12, 2013: http://www.ers.usda.gov/publications/err-economic-research-report/err54.aspx.

9. Leibtag E: *Tracking purchase behavior of low-income households: assessment of data needs.* Presented at the IOM Workshop: Defining the Adequacy of SNAP Allotments, March 28, 2012. Accessed September 12, 2013: http://www.iom.edu/~/media/Files/Activity%20Files/Nutrition/SNAP%20adequacy/05_Leibtag.pdf.

10. Hillier A, McLaughlin J, Cannuscio CC, et al: The impact of WIC food package changes on access to healthful food in 2 low-income urban neighborhoods. *J Nutr Educ Behav* 44(3):210–216, 2012.

11. Columbia University's Mailman School of Public Health: *Changes to WIC nutrition program likely had a positive impact on weight and healthy diet.* Medical News Today. MediLexicon, Intl, 2013 Jan 10. Accessed September 13, 2013: http://www.medicalnewstoday.com/releases/254729.php.

12. Gundersen CG, Garasky SB: Financial management skills are associated with food insecurity in a sample of households with children in the United States. *J Nutr* 142(10):1865–1870, 2012.

13. Lester GE, Hallman GJ, Perez JA: Gamma irradiation dose: Effects on spinach baby-leaf ascorbic acid, carotenoids, folate, alpha-tocopherol, and phylloquinone concentrations. *J Agric Food Chem* 58(8):4901–4906, 2010.

14. Farnham MW, Lester GE, Hassell R: Collard, mustard and turnip greens: effects of varieties and leaf position on concentrations of ascorbic acid, folate, B-carotene, lutein and phylloquinone. *J Food Comp Anal* 27(1):1–7, 2012.

15. Xiao Z, Lester GE, Luo Y, Wang Q: Assessment of vitamin and carotenoid concentrations of emerging food products: edible microgreens. *J Agric Food Chem* 60(31):7644–7651, 2012.

16. Painter JA, Hoekstra RM, Ayers T, et al: Attribution of foodborne illnesses, hospitalizations, and deaths to food commodities by using Outbreak Data, United States, 1998–2008. *Emerg Infect Dis* 19(3):407–415, 2013.

17. Centers for Disease Control and Prevention (CDC): *CDC Estimates of Foodborne Illness in the United States. CDC 2011 estimates: findings.* Updated October 10, 2012. Accessed September 13, 2013: http://www.cdc.gov/foodborneburden/2011-foodborne-estimates.html.

18. Centers for Disease Control and Prevention (CDC): *Trends in foodborne illness in the United States, 2012.* Updated April 18, 2013. Accessed September 13, 2013. http://www.medicalnewstoday.com/releases/254729.php.

19. Grossman J: *Nutrient decline fallacy.* The Nutrition Post. Accessed September 13, 2013. http://www.thenutritionpost.com/frontpage/nutrient-decline-fallacy.html.

20. Fulgoni VL, 3rd, Keast DR, Bailey RL, et al: Foods, fortificants, and supplements: where do Americans get their nutrients? *J Nutr* 141(10):1847–1854, 2011.

21. *U.S. organic market surpasses $31B.* Progressive Grocer, April 23, 2012. Accessed September 13, 2013. http://www.progressivegrocer.com/top-stories/headlines/consumer-insights/id35248/u-s-organic-market-surpasses-31b/.

22. Smith-Spangler C, Brandeau ML, Hunter GE, et al: Are organic foods safer or healthier than conventional alternatives? A systematic review. *Ann Intern Med* 157(5):348–366, 2012.

23. Dangour AD, Lock K, Hayter A, et al: Nutrition-related health effects of organic foods: a systematic review. *Am J Clin Nutr* 92(1):203–210, 2010.

24. Forman J, Silverstein J: Committee on nutrition, Council on Environmental Health: Organic foods: health and environmental advantages and disadvantages. *Pediatrics* 130(5):e1406–e1415, 2012.

25. Smith-Spangler C, Brandeau ML, Hunter GE, et al: Are organic foods safer or healthier than conventional alternatives? A systematic review. *Ann Intern Med* 157(5):348–366, 2012.

26. Reganold JP, Andrews PK, Reeve JR, et al: Fruit and soil quality of organic and conventional strawberry agroecosystems. *PLoS ONE* 5(9):e12346, 2010.

27. Dangour AD, Lock K, Hayter A, et al: Nutrition-related health effects of organic foods: a systematic review. *Am J Clin Nutr* 92(1):203–210, 2010.

28. Ibid., Smith-Spangler C, et al: 2012.

29. Benbrook C: Going organic: what's the payoff? *Nutr Action Health Lett* 39(8);1:3–7, 2012. Accessed September 12, 2013: http://www.cspinet.org/nah/articles/going-organic.html.

30. Magkos F, Arvaniti F, Zampelas A: Organic food: buying more safety or just peace of mind? A critical review of the literature. *Crit Rev Food Sci Nutr* 46(1):23–56, 2006.

31. Keikotlhaile, BM, Spanoghe P, Steurbaut W: Effects of food processing on pesticide residues in fruits and vegetables: a meta-analysis approach. *Food Chem Toxicol* 48(1):1–6, 2010.

32. Smith-Spangler C, Brandeau ML, Hunter GE, et al: Are organic foods safer or healthier than conventional alternatives? A systematic review. *Ann Intern Med* 157(5):348–366, 2012.

33. Ellison B, Lusk JL, Davis, D: Looking at the label and beyond: the effects of calorie labels, health consciousness, and demographics on caloric intake in restaurants. *Int J Behav Nutr Phys Act* 10:21, 2013.

34. Swartz JJ, Braxton D, Viera AJ: Calorie menu labeling on quick-service restaurant menus: an updated systematic review of the literature. *Int J Behav Nutr Phys Act* 8:135, 2011.

35. Anonymous, cited by Wilder RM: Fads, fancies, and fallacies in adult diets. *Sigma Xi Q* 26:73, 1938.

36. Foroutan R: Defining detox. *Food Nutr* 1(3):13–15, 2012.

37. Newmaster ST, Grguric M, Shanmughanandhan D, et al: DNA barcoding detects contamination and substitution in North Americal herbal products. *BMC Medicine* 11(1):222, 2013.

38. Angel M, Kassuer JP: Clinical research—what should the public believe? *N Engl J Med* 331(3):189–190, 1994.

39. Oliveira V: *Food assistance landscape: FY 2012 annual report.* United States Department of Agriculture, Economic Research Service. Economic Information Bulletin No 109, March 2013. Accessed September 13, 2013. Available at: http://www.ers.usda.gov/publications/eib-economic-information-bulletin/eib109.aspx#.UU3SGFfB98E.

40. Food Research and Action Center (FRAC): *SNAP/Food stamp participation*, 2012. Accessed September 13, 2013: http://frac.org/reports-and-resources/snapfood-stamp-monthly-participation-data/.

41. Nord M: *Effects of the Decline in the Real Value of SNAP Benefits From 2009 to 2011*, ERR-151. 2013. U.S. Department of Agriculture, Economic Research Service.

42. U.S. Department of Agriculture, Food and Nutrition Service: *Supplemental Nutrition Assistance Program.* Modified July 25, 2013. Accessed September 13, 2013: http://www.fns.usda.gov/snap/applicant_recipients/fs_Res_Ben_Elig.htm.

43. Shallwani P: *Eating well on $68.88 a week.* Updated April 2010. Accessed September 13, 2013: http://www.msnbc.msn.com/id/36507576/ns/health-diet_and_nutrition/#.UHmZ3oagFe4.

44. Andreyeva T, Luedicke J, Henderson KE, et al: Grocery store beverage choices by participants in federal food assistance and nutrition programs. *Am J Prev Med* 43(4):411–418, 2012.

45. Committee on Nutrition Standards for National School Lunch and Breakfast Programs, Institute of Medicine: *"Front Matter." School Meals: Building Blocks for Healthy Children.* Washington, DC, 2010, National Academies Press.

46. U.S. Department of Health and Human Services, Administration on Aging: *Fact sheet: elderly nutrition program.* June 16, 2009. Accessed September 13, 2013: fs_nutrition.doc.

47. Robaina KA, Martin KS: Food insecurity, poor diet quality, and obesity among food pantry participants in Hartford, CT. *J Nutr Behav Educ* 45(2):159–164, 2013.

48. Echevarria S, Santos R, Waxman E, et al: *Food Banks: Hunger's New Staple,* September 27, 2011. Accessed September 13, 2013. Available at: http://feedingamerica.org/hunger-in-america/hunger-studies/~/media/Files/research/HungerNewStaple FullReport_FINAL.ashx?pdf.

49. Van Cleve N: Food: Facts, fad, and fancy. *Am J Nurs* 38(3):285, 1988.

50. Coleman-Jensen A, Nord M, Singh A: *Household food security in the United States in 2012.* ERR-155, U.S. Department of Agriculture, Economic Research Service, September 2013. Accessed September 13, 2013: http://www.ers.usda.gov/publications/err-economic-research-report/err155.aspx.

51. Food Research and Action Center (FRAC): *Nearly one in five American households report inability to afford enough in food during first six months of 2012.* Accessed September 13, 2013: http://frac.org/nearly-one-in-five-americans-report-inability-to-afford-enough-food/.

52. Ibid., Coleman-Jensen A, et al: 2013.

53. Rank M, Hirschl T: Estimating the risk of food stamp use and impoverishment during childhood. *Arch Pediatr Adolesc Med* 163(11):994–999, 2009.

54. Fraser R: *Study: food assistance shifts from "emergency" to "chronic." Feeding America,* September 28, 2011. Accessed September 13, 2013: http://feedingamerica.org/press-room/press-releases/hungers-new-staple.aspx.

55. Rausch R: Nutrition and academic performance in school-age children: the relation to obesity and food insufficiency. *Nutr & Food Sci* 3(2):190–192, 2013.

56. Martin MA, Lippert AM: Feeding her children, but risking her health: the intersection of gender, household food insecurity and obesity. *Soc Sci Med* 74(11):1754–1764, 2012.

57. Metallinos-Katsaras E, Must A, Gorman K: A longitudinal study of food insecurity on obesity in preschool children. *J Acad Nutr Diet* 112(120):1949–1958, 2012.

58. Leung CW, Ding EL, Catalano PJ, et al: Dietary intake and dietary quality of low-income adults in the Supplemental Nutrition Assistance Program. *Am J Clin Nutr* 96(5):977–988, 2012.

59. Seligman HK, Laraia BA, Kushel MB: Food insecurity is associated with chronic disease among low-income NHANES participants. *J Nutr* 140(2):304–310, 2010.

60. American Dietetic Association: Position paper: food insecurity in the United States. *J Am Diet Assoc* 110(9):1368–1377, 2010.

ⓔ EVOLVE RESOURCES

Please visit http://evolve.elsevier.com/Stegeman/nutritional for additional practice and study support tools.

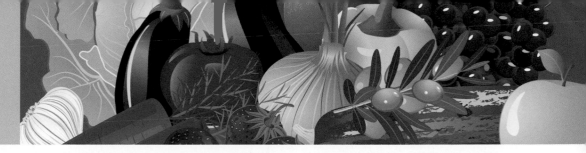

Chapter 17

Effects of Systemic Disease on Nutritional Status and Oral Health

Student Learning Outcomes

Upon completion of this chapter, the student will be able to achieve the following student learning outcomes:

- Discuss the various diseases, conditions, and treatments that commonly have oral signs and symptoms.
- Discuss disease states, conditions, and accompanying treatments likely to affect nutritional intake.

- Critically assess the implications of a patient's systemic diseases or conditions for optimal oral health.
- Plan appropriate dental interventions for patients with systemic diseases or conditions with oral manifestations based on dietary guidelines.

Key Terms

Aneurysm
Anticholinergic
Atherosclerosis
Atrophic glossitis
Binges
Bisphosphonates
Bradykinesia
Brown tumors
Chemotherapy
Dialysate
Epilepsy
Esophagitis
Gastroesophageal reflux disease
Gastrostomy
Glossodynia
Gluten
Goitrogens
Herpetic ulcerations
Hiatal hernia
Hirsutism
Ischemia
Kaposi sarcoma

Leukemia
Leukoplakia
Lipodystrophy
Macroglossia
Materia alba
Micrognathia
Mucositis
Necrotizing ulcerative periodontitis
Neoplasia
Neutropenia
Odynophagia
Osteonecrosis
Osteosclerosis
Parkinson disease
Periapices
Phantom taste
Pocketed foods
Purging
Renal osteodystrophy
Stomatitis
Syrup of ipecac
Thrombus

1. **T/F** Anorexia, associated with a chronic disease, can result in an increased susceptibility to infection.
2. **T/F** Antihypertensive, anticholinergic, and antidepressant drugs often cause a decrease in salivary flow.
3. **T/F** Iron supplements should be recommended to a patient who has anemia.
4. **T/F** It is within the scope of practice for a dental hygienist to provide nutritional advice to a patient recently diagnosed with diabetes.
5. **T/F** A patient with a hiatal hernia should be cautioned against eating before a dental appointment to prevent regurgitation while lying in a supine position.

6. **T/F** The healthcare provider should monitor protein intake closely in a patient with chronic renal failure.
7. **T/F** Kaposi sarcoma is a tumor that occurs frequently in patients with epilepsy.
8. **T/F** Phenytoin (Dilantin) can cause gingival hyperplasia and vitamin deficiencies.
9. **T/F** A dental hygienist should not confront a patient suspected to have an eating disorder, but should casually refer the patient to a healthcare provider.
10. **T/F** Patients with bulimia generally have low body weight.

As you have already learned, nutritional deficiencies frequently are manifested in the oral and head and neck areas. Oral lesions can be a reflection of or a marker for disease elsewhere. The oral cavity cannot be isolated from, and is not immune to what is occurring physiologically because oral tissues are nourished by the same blood supply providing oxygen and nutrients to cells throughout the entire body. Oral tissues may reflect changes in nutrient supply or other metabolic alterations. Oral manifestations are just a single part of the total systemic state.

Oral problems may develop as a result of disease processes or therapies, or by nutritional deficiencies. Subsequent oral issues can cause inadequate intake. Systemic diseases or medications usually prescribed for these conditions may cause alterations in the oral cavity, such as oral lesions, xerostomia, or muscular weakness (Table 17-1). These oral alterations may lead to changes in eating patterns, which frequently have a general debilitating effect on the entire body. For example, food preferences are affected by an individual's ability to chew. Patients with reduced masticatory efficiency usually choose soft foods, which may not provide adequate amounts of essential nutrients. Numerous studies have indicated that dentate status, malocclusion, and ill-fitting dentures or partials increase risk of inadequate nutrient intake. The nutrients most frequently cited include protein, fiber, some B vitamins, vitamin D, iron, magnesium, and phosphorus. The body depends on nutrients from foods eaten to regenerate and repair diseased tissues; provisions must be made to provide these nutrients in adequate amounts on a regular basis.

All disease processes result from a combination of factors: the presence of an etiologic agent (e.g., plaque biofilm), the susceptibility or resistance of the host (or activation of immune response), and environmental factors. One of the most important factors in one's ability to combat hostile agents is availability of nutrients acquired from food. Infections can spread rapidly when the immune response is depressed.

Ramifications of a patient's systemic health are important to the dental hygienist because they provide cues to possible oral problems; may change treatment goals, priorities, or scheduling; or may influence dietary recommendations provided to the patient. The dental hygienist's dietary recommendations should take into consideration the systemic health of a patient and should not contradict dietary instructions provided by the patient's other healthcare providers. In other words, nutritional advice regarding oral health problems must be done in the context of the whole patient.

More than one-third of the patients seen in a dental office do not frequently interact with a general healthcare provider.[1] Especially for these individuals, but often for other patients who visit their healthcare provider less frequently than they visit the dental office, dental hygienists are in a key position to assess and detect oral signs and symptoms of systemic health disorders. Clinical observations, radiographic findings, diet screening, and inquiries made while obtaining or updating the health history are used to detect signs and symptoms, and should be the basis for motivating the patient to visit a healthcare provider or registered dietitian (RDN). This can potentially reduce healthcare costs.

This chapter presents oral problems frequently caused by systemic health conditions or their treatment because these problems typically affect eating patterns. No attempt is made to cover pathophysiology, and the information given should not be used to diagnose conditions. If the cause of oral signs and symptoms is unknown, refer the patient to a healthcare provider, who can perform a thorough assessment, including diagnostic laboratory evaluation, for accurate diagnosis and treatment.

EFFECTS OF CHRONIC DISEASE ON INTAKE

Anorexia and Appetite

The term anorexia nervosa refers to a disease associated with a distorted body image, but anorexia may also refer to a

Table 17-1   Oral problems associated with systemic diseases

Condition	Xerostomia	Taste Alterations	Oral Lesions	Immune Response	Masticatory Efficiency	Delayed Wound Healing	Dysphagia	Sore Tongue	Risk of Bleeding	Dental Caries
Anemias										
Iron-deficiency	X	X	X	X		X		X		
Plummer-Vinson	X	X	X	X		X	X	X		
Megaloblastic		X	X	X				X		
Thalassemia					X					
Aplastic			X						X	
Other Hematological Diseases										
Polycythemia									X	
Neutropenia			X	X						
Gastrointestinal Problems										
Medications for reflux	X							X		
Malabsorptive conditions		X	X			X				
Cardiovascular Conditions										
Cardiovascular accidents							X			
Antihypertensive medications	X									
Lipid-lowering medications		X							X	
Skeletal Anomalies										
Systemic bone disturbances					X					
Metabolic Problems										
Diabetes mellitus	X	X		X		X				X
Acromegaly					X					
Hypopituitarism					X					
Cushing syndrome					X			X		
Hypothyroidism					X					X
Hyperparathyroidism					X					
Renal Disease										
Diminished kidney function			X		X	X			X	
Neuromuscular Problems										
Parkinson disease	X				X		X			
Developmental disabilities					X		X			
Epilepsy	X									
Neoplasia										
Cancer		X								
Kaposi sarcoma			X							
Leukemia				X						
Acquired Immunodeficiency Syndrome										
AIDS	X		X	X						
Mental Health Problems										
Anorexia nervosa/bulimia			X							X
Medications for mental illness	X									

condition in which a patient has a poor appetite for a variety of reasons (e.g., cancer treatment). Appetite is associated with enjoyment of food. Most healthy individuals have a good appetite with no problems eating adequate amounts. However, during illness, appetite may decrease because of pain, apathy, anorexia, drugs, inactivity, or many other reasons. Individuals may become depressed after the diagnosis of a chronic illness, causing mental stress about problems related to living with, or dying because of, the condition. A modified diet may be prescribed for a patient with a chronic illness, which may adversely affect intake. Poor food intake may further lessen the desire to eat. In some situations it may be unknown whether anorexia is a cause of the illness or an effect of the illness. Malnutrition and other stresses such as infection, surgery, and injuries resulting in anorexia deplete body stores of kilocalories, macronutrients (e.g., protein), and micronutrients (e.g., vitamin C) needed to regenerate and repair cells; the body is more susceptible to bacterial or viral invasion.

Taste and Smell Disorders

The foods people choose to eat are modulated by taste, smell, and oral textural perception. Taste and smell dramatically affect appetite and food intake. Various conditions (e.g., respiratory diseases and cancer), medications, and treatment for the conditions may result in chemosensory disorders (e.g., disorders of taste and smell). Taste perception declines during the normal aging process, except intensity of sweet taste does not diminish with age.[2] Reactions to loss of taste and smell vary. Patients with loss of smell eat less, use more spices, and eat and drink fewer sweets. Loss of saliva in disease and drug-induced xerostomia reduce solubility of flavors and the ability to taste. Many patients experiencing taste changes tend to have inadequate food intake and weight loss resulting in malnutrition.[3]

Numerous drugs may adversely influence taste perception, either by decreasing function or producing perceptual distortions or phantom taste (lingering unpleasant taste even though nothing is in the mouth). Individuals taking three or more medications are likely to have less taste sensitivity, requiring greater amounts of sodium and sugar to perceive these tastes.

Xerostomia

Saliva protects hard and soft oral tissues from mechanical, thermal, and chemical irritants in addition to its roles in buffering acids, antimicrobial activity, and remineralization. Medications (e.g., antidepressants, antihistamines, antihypertensives, diuretics, and gastrointestinal drugs), diseases or conditions (e.g., Sjögren disease), and therapies (e.g., radiation) may cause xerostomia. More than one-third of older adults experience xerostomia primarily as a result of anticholinergic (blockage of impulses through the parasympathetic nerves) medications.[4,5] Older individuals taking more than one medication are more likely to have xerostomia, but it is not caused by the aging process.[6] Hyposalivation is a known risk factor for dental caries and periodontal

disease, but may also cause taste disturbances, swallowing problems, poor chewing ability, and malnutrition.[7]

Xerostomia can affect nutritional status in several ways, as follows: (a) chewing is difficult because a bolus cannot be formed without additional moisture; (b) chewing is painful because the mouth is sore; (c) swallowing is difficult because of loss of lubrication from saliva; and (d) food intake may decrease because of changes in taste perception. Individuals with xerostomia tend to avoid dry, crunchy foods and sticky foods, which may result in malnutrition secondary to lower intake of kilocalories and other essential nutrients.[8]

ANEMIAS

Typical symptoms of all the anemias are pallor of the skin, oral mucosa, and conjunctival tissues, along with overall weakness as a result of inadequate oxygen-carrying power of the blood. The occurrence and severity of clinical symptoms depend on the degree of anemia and speed of onset. The type of anemia can be determined only after evaluation of blood tests.

Iron-Deficiency Anemia

Iron-deficiency anemia can be caused by a deficiency of dietary iron or by excessive bleeding, and is likely to occur during periods in which iron requirements are high, such as during infancy or pregnancy. Gradual depletion of iron stores may progress to iron-deficiency anemia in which iron levels are inadequate for maintaining hemoglobin levels to provide cellular oxygen. Lethargy and fatigue in addition to glossitis, aphthous ulcers, and xerostomia associated with iron-deficiency anemia can lead to changes in appetite and food intake. Clinical symptoms in the oral cavity include gingival and mucosal pallor (Fig. 17-1), angular cheilosis, and atrophic glossitis. Atrophic glossitis is described as

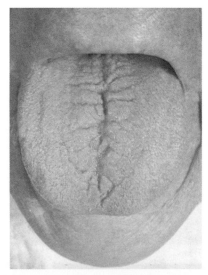

FIGURE 17-1 Clinical symptoms of iron-deficiency anemia include pallor of the gingiva, mucosa, and tongue. (Courtesy DW Beaven and SE Brooks. From McLaren DS: *A colour atlas and text of diet-related disorders*, ed 2, London, 1992, Mosby-Yearbook.)

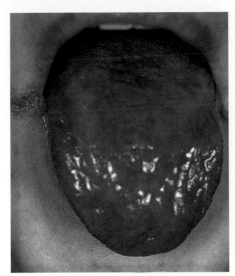

FIGURE 17-2 Iron-deficiency anemia. (From Cawson RA, Odell EW: *Cawson's essentials of oral pathology and oral medicine*, ed 8, Edinburgh, 2008, Churchill Livingstone.)

atrophy of the filiform and fungiform papillae beginning at the tip and lateral borders of the tongue and gradually spreading to the entire dorsum of the tongue. As the papillae gradually shrink in size, bald spots appear, and the tongue becomes smooth, shiny, and red (Fig. 17-2).

Iron-deficiency anemia affects the immune response and places a patient at increased risk for fungal infections, such as candidiasis. After iron supplementation is initiated, oral symptoms begin to resolve in 48 hours, and filiform papillae regenerate in 3 to 4 weeks. Depending on the severity of iron-deficiency anemia, wound healing may be impaired in response to invasive dental treatments, such as tooth extraction, nonsurgical periodontal therapy, and periodontal surgery.

Dental Considerations

Assessment
- *Physical*: burning sensation of the tongue, xerostomia, gingival and mucosal pallor, atrophy of the filiform and fungiform papillae, atrophic glossitis, angular cheilosis, dysphagia, candidiasis.
- *Dietary*: adequacy of dietary intake, especially red meats, dark green vegetables, enriched cereals and bread; use of vitamin-mineral supplements.

Interventions
- Encourage iron-rich foods (see Table 12-9); if principally nonheme sources are consumed at a meal, a source of vitamin C enhances absorption of nonheme iron.
- If the iron supplement causes nausea, suggest the patient take the supplement with food, or discuss the problem with the healthcare provider, rather than discontinue the supplement.

Evaluation
- Successful outcomes include the patient's consuming iron-rich foods and taking the ordered supplement.

Nutritional Directions

- If the iron supplement is liquid, dilute with water or juice, and drink with a straw to minimize tooth staining.
- Iron stores are replenished very slowly; therapy should be continued for at least 1 year.

Megaloblastic (Pernicious) Anemia

Vitamin B_{12} deficiency can result in a megaloblastic anemia (a small number of large red blood cells) also called pernicious anemia. This condition occurs when vitamin B_{12} is deficient in the diet, absorption is inadequate, or requirements are increased. With vitamin B_{12} malabsorption or no dietary source, normal body stores are usually sufficient for 3 to 4 years. Vitamin B_{12} deficiency is most common among vegans who consume no animal products.

Oral changes of vitamin B_{12} deficiency may be the only clinical evidence of the disease preceding significant anemia. Patients with pernicious anemia may initially present with angular cheilosis, recurrent aphthous ulcers (and erythematous **mucositis** [inflamed, flat lesions with red borders on the mucous membrane, Fig. 17-3]), and pale or yellowish oral mucosa (Fig. 17-4). Patients may also complain of a painful, sore, burning tongue with signs of atrophic glossitis associated with a beefy red color. Replacement therapy with vitamin B_{12} supplements or injections relieves symptoms within 36 to 48 hours with evidence of regeneration of tongue papillae within 4 to 7 days, and the tongue may be normal in 3 to 4 weeks.

Another type of megaloblastic anemia, caused by folic acid deficiency, is frequently associated with poor diets or medications that interfere with folate absorption or metabolism, such as phenytoin (Dilantin) or methotrexate. Oral manifestations are similar to symptoms present in pernicious anemia: glossitis, atrophy of the papillae, ulcerations, and **glossodynia** (pain in the tongue). Angular cheilitis and fungal infections in the perioral area may also be observed.

Folate replacement is necessary because diet alone is inadequate to replace lost stores. Iron supplements also may be ordered because when folate is deficient, iron is usually low as well. Folate supplementation in a patient deficient in vitamin B_{12} may produce hematological improvement, whereas neurological damage from vitamin B_{12} deficiency continues to progress.

Dental Considerations

Assessment
- *Physical*: sex; age; glazed, red, sore or painful tongue; pale skin and oral mucous membranes; shortness of breath; malabsorption, previous gastrointestinal surgeries.
- *Dietary*: dietary intake, especially dark green leafy vegetables, animal products, whole-grain breads, and fortified foods; alcohol intake.

Continued

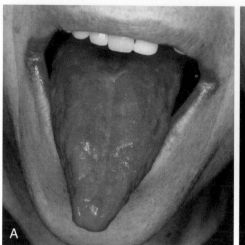
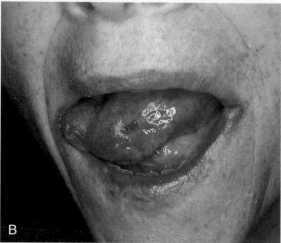

FIGURE 17-3 **A** and **B,** Pernicious anemia. (From Ibsen OAC, Phelan JA: *Oral pathology for the dental hygienist,* ed 6, St Louis, 2014, Saunders.)

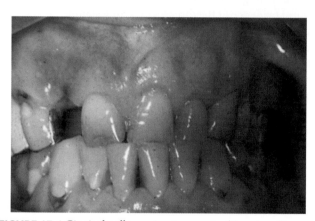

FIGURE 17-4 Gingival pallor owing to anemia. (Courtesy Dr. Edward V. Zegarelli. From Ibsen OAC, Phelan JA: *Oral pathology for the dental hygienist,* ed 2, Philadelphia, 1996, Saunders.)

Nutritional Directions

- Raw vegetables are a better source of folate than cooked vegetables; heat destroys folate.
- Daily intake of dietary folate is necessary.
- Patients with permanent gastric or ileal damage need monthly intramuscular or oral vitamin B_{12} supplementation for life.
- Vitamin B_{12} shots are not always indicated for "tired blood."
- When oral vitamin B_{12} or iron supplements are ordered, take with vitamin C–rich foods to enhance absorption.
- Large doses of folate can negate therapeutic effects of anticonvulsants, so consultation with the healthcare provider is recommended.

Dental Considerations—cont'd

Interventions

- If the patient has megaloblastic anemia caused by folate deficiency, encourage rich sources of folate (especially grains fortified with folic acid) along with a supplement meeting the RDA for folate (400 μg) (see Table 11-12).
- If the patient is not a vegan, encourage intake of foods from animal sources high in vitamin B_{12} for pernicious anemia (see Table 11-14). If the patient is a vegan, encourage fortified foods or supplementation. Dietary intake helps reestablish depleted stores.
- Refer the patient to an RDN; patients with megaloblastic anemia especially need nutritional counseling because of undesirable eating habits.

Evaluation

- Desired outcomes include the patient's consuming a well-balanced diet and foods high in folate or vitamin B_{12} (as appropriate) and taking supplements to enhance the formation of red blood cells or erythropoiesis.

OTHER HEMATOLOGICAL DISORDERS

Neutropenia

Neutropenia is a diminished number of neutrophils, the most abundant type of white blood cells (WBCs) in the blood and may predispose an immunocompromised patient to life-threatening infections. The risk of infection is directly proportional to duration and severity of neutropenia. Neutropenia results from dysfunctional bone marrow: cancer (e.g., leukemia), drugs (e.g., chemotherapeutic agents or antibiotics), radiation therapy, autoimmune disease (e.g., rheumatoid arthritis or systemic lupus erythematosus), bone marrow transplant, nutritional deficiencies (e.g., severe vitamin B_{12} or folate deficiency), or certain bacterial or viral infections (e.g., HIV, malaria, tuberculosis, or Epstein-Barr virus).

Mucositis and viral and fungal infections (e.g., candidiasis) are frequently occurring complications as a result of neutropenia. As the neutrophil count falls, incidence and severity of infection rise. Oral organisms from the dentition, periapical (area around the root apex), and periodontium can disseminate systemically, causing bacteremias and systemic infection. Mucositis may result in large ulcerative and necrotic lesions with extensive tissue destruction. Ideally, this condition is treated and managed before initiation of treatment that may result in neutropenia.[9,10] Meticulous oral hygiene is essential to prevent the progression of periodontal disease. When neutropenia is present, invasive dental treatment is usually contraindicated until WBC counts increase. If treatment is indicated, a consultation with the healthcare provider is necessary to determine if antibiotic prophylaxis is needed.

Dental Considerations

Assessment
- *Physical:* painful oral mucosal ulcerations (mucositis), candidiasis.
- *Dietary:* folate and vitamin B$_{12}$ intake.

Interventions
- For neutropenia, encourage foods high in folate (see Table 11-12) and vitamin B$_{12}$ (see Table 11-14) if the patient's intake is questionable.
- Stress the importance of frequent oral prophylaxis and meticulous oral self-care.
- Refer the patient to an RDN for nutritional counseling if eating habits are poor.

Evaluation
- Successful outcomes include patient adherence to a diet encompassing a variety of foods, concentrating on iron, vitamin B$_{12}$, or folate; use of supplementation as recommended by a healthcare provider or RDN; and frequent dental recare appointments and maintenance of good periodontal health.

Nutritional Directions

- To ensure adequate iron intake, choose meat, fish, or poultry regularly.
- To enhance iron absorption, choose a vitamin C–rich food with a meal or eat a small amount of meat with each meal.

GASTROINTESTINAL PROBLEMS

Gastroesophageal Reflux, Hiatal Hernia, and Esophagitis

Heartburn 30 minutes to 1 hour after eating is the most common symptom of **gastroesophageal reflux disease**, a return of gastric contents into the esophagus. This condition is commonly associated with **hiatal hernia** (partial protrusion of the stomach through the esophageal opening into the chest cavity), pregnancy, and obesity. Normally, the lower esophageal sphincter prevents caustic gastric acid from refluxing into the esophagus. Acidity from the stomach, alkalinity, pepsin, or bile may damage the esophageal mucosa, and esophagitis may result if left untreated. **Esophagitis** is an inflammation of the lower esophagus and may cause discomfort when swallowing.

Patients are normally advised to decrease their intake of foods that may precipitate reflux, such as fatty foods (e.g., gravy, pastries, chocolate, fatty meats, cheese, nuts, chips, salad dressing, and mayonnaise), peppermint, caffeinated foods (e.g., coffee, tea, chocolate, and some carbonated beverages), alcohol, and onions. Other foods to avoid are those directly irritating to the esophagus, such as citrus juices, tomato products, and red peppers. If appropriate, weight loss is recommended. Other suggestions to help reduce pain include eating small, frequent meals; using antacids to buffer gastric juices; wearing loose-fitting clothing; eating at least 2 to 3 hours before lying down; and sleeping with head and shoulders elevated.

Anticholinergic medications prescribed for gastroesophageal reflux disease may interfere with absorption of vitamin B$_{12}$ and folic acid. Observation for oral signs of vitamin deficiency is appropriate for patients taking these medications. Anticholinergic medications may also cause xerostomia.

Dental Considerations

Assessment
- *Physical:* type of medications used; heartburn; bitter taste; visual appraisal of weight; enamel erosion; sensitivity of the dentin.
- *Diet:* adequacy and frequency of intake; caffeine, fat, and alcohol intake; knowledge of foods that increase reflux or irritate the esophagus.

Interventions
- If weight loss is needed, refer to an RDN or a nationally-recognized weight loss program, such as Weight Watchers or TOPS (Take Off Pounds Sensibly), for a nutritionally sound reduction program.
- To reduce risk of regurgitation during dental treatment, the patient's head and neck should be positioned above the stomach in the operatory chair; encourage the patient not to eat for 2 hours before the appointment; omit the use of nitrous oxide because it may relax the lower esophageal sphincter.

Evaluation
- The patient plans frequent well-balanced meals, avoiding foods that cause reflux and irritate the esophagus.

Nutritional Directions

- The effectiveness of avoiding or limiting foods that increase likelihood of reflux to avoid irritation of esophageal tissue varies among patients and is based on individual tolerances. General recommendations include limiting caffeine, chocolate, alcohol, mint, and carbonated beverages. However, evidence-based research does not support the modifications.
- If citrus fruits and tomato products are avoided, other sources of vitamin C should be selected, including cantaloupe, potatoes, and strawberries.
- Heartburn is not caused by inadequate digestion; digestive enzyme tablets are inappropriate.
- Eat small meals, evenly distributed throughout the day.
- Reduce or eliminate cigarette smoking, which stimulates gastric acid secretion.

Malabsorptive Conditions

Many chronic diseases are associated with poor nutrient absorption, including Crohn disease, ulcerative colitis, cystic fibrosis, gluten-sensitive enteropathy (sprue or celiac disease), and AIDS. Gluten is a protein found mainly in wheat and to a lesser degree in rye, oat, and barley. Different parts of the gastrointestinal tract are affected in these disorders, and manifestations differ from one individual to another with the same condition (see Chapter 3, *Health Application 3*). Malabsorption may occur, affecting many macronutrients (e.g., gluten [protein], fat, and carbohydrates) and micronutrients (e.g., vitamin B$_{12}$).

Oral problems associated with Crohn disease and ulcerative colitis include swollen, bleeding, erythematous gingiva; diffuse pustular eruptions on the buccal gingiva; oral ulcerations (Fig. 17-5); swelling of the lips, and cobblestone-like, raised hypertrophic lesions. Additionally, taste alterations (metallic dysgeusia) and reduction in taste acuity may develop. Enamel defects and deep aphthous ulcerations may be a marker of Crohn disease, ulcerative colitis, or celiac disease, and precede gastrointestinal symptoms. These clinical signs appear when the disease is in the acute stage and disappear when it is inactive.

Diarrhea and malabsorption associated with these disease states create deficiencies of nutrients and trace elements. Nutritional requirements of these patients are usually increased; however, abdominal cramping precipitated by food intake, and anorexia and intolerance to many different food components (gluten, fat, lactose, and fiber) inhibit intake. As a result, patients are finicky and apprehensive about eating; they may present with anemia, protein and energy malnutrition, poor wound healing, and suppressed immune response.

Different nutritional modalities are used with these conditions. A diet high in kilocalories and protein with limited fat and fiber, and possible lactose or gluten restriction may be recommended for patients by their healthcare provider or RDN. Small, frequent feedings are better tolerated and increase adequacy of intake. Irritating foods are excluded. Extremely hot and cold foods and high-fiber foods are avoided because they increase peristalsis.

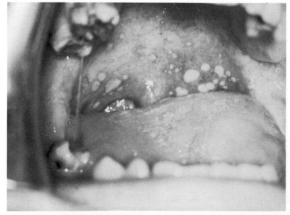

FIGURE 17-5 Oral ulcers (ulcerative colitis). (From Ibsen OAC, Phelan JA: *Oral pathology for the dental hygienist*, ed 6, St Louis, 2014, Saunders.)

Dental Considerations

Assessment
- *Physical:* edema, anemia, weight loss, abdominal pain, diarrhea, fatigue, swollen bleeding gingiva, enamel defects, aphthous ulcers (canker sores), and emotional stress.
- *Dietary:* iron, folate, vitamin B$_{12}$, and adequate protein and kilocalories.

Interventions
- Encourage the patient to eat a nutrient-rich, well-balanced diet. Reassess the diet frequently to monitor nutrient adequacy.
- The use of stress management techniques during the appointment can prevent aggravating symptoms associated with the disease.
- Consult with the healthcare provider about the need for supplemental steroids and prophylactic antibiotics before the dental appointment. The healthcare provider or RDN may also recommend vitamin and mineral supplementation.

Evaluation
- Successful outcomes include the patient's choosing foods that are well tolerated and promote weight gain or stability (as needed) and physical strength; and minimal oral problems do not affect eating.

Nutritional Directions

- Adequate rest and a relaxed, calm day before the prophylaxis help to avoid aggravating symptoms.
- Multiple nutrient deficiencies are common and can interfere with effectiveness of the prescribed medication, compromising immune function.

CARDIOVASCULAR CONDITIONS

Cardiovascular disease (CVD) encompasses numerous prevalent chronic heart problems, including hypertension, congestive heart failure, myocardial infarction, cerebrovascular accident, and arteriosclerosis. There may be a risk of CVD resulting from systemic exposure to periodontal pathogens (as measured by antibodies to *Actinobacillus actinomycetemcomitans* and *Porphyromonas gingivalis*).[11] Periodontal interventions may reduce systemic inflammation and risk of CVD; however, meta-analyses and evidence-based research have revealed conflicting results regarding the association between periodontal disease and interventions to prevent or modify the outcomes of CVD.[12]

In contrast to its many ill effects in other sites of the body, CVD produces few oral effects and usually does not have any oral manifestations that affect food intake. However, medications prescribed for cardiovascular conditions may have oral effects. Dietary adjustments recommended for these patients affect information the dental hygienist provides.

Cerebrovascular Accident

A cerebrovascular accident (also known as a stroke) results if occlusion, or ischemia, occurs in an artery supplying the brain, or if hemorrhaging in the brain occurs. Ischemia (inadequate blood flow and lack of oxygen because of constriction or obstruction of arteries) is caused by blockage of one of the arteries in a part of the body (cardiac ischemia, heart muscle). Most strokes are caused by ischemia. An artery may become blocked from atherosclerosis or a **thrombus** (blood clot). **Atherosclerosis** is caused by an accumulation of fatty materials (such as cholesterol) on smooth inner walls of arteries. As this plaque thickens, arteries become progressively narrow and rough, and blood flow carrying oxygen and nutrients may be disrupted. Hemorrhagic strokes may occur as a result of a bleeding **aneurysm** (weak or thin spot in an arterial wall). Occasionally, patients who have ministrokes do not seek medical care even though dysphagia can result. The patient may realize that things are not normal but may attribute these deficits to the aging process. A dental hygienist may suspect dysphagia in a patient who has facial muscle weakness (drooping mouth) or slurred speech; in a patient with weak oral, neck, or tongue muscles; or in a patient who coughs or chokes frequently on foods, drinks, and secretions (e.g., saliva and mucus). Neurologically-impaired patients may deny having swallowing problems. Patients suspected to have dysphagia should be referred to a healthcare provider. Normally, a speech-language pathologist and RDN work closely with these patients to ensure adequate fluid and nutrient intake. Severely-impaired patients may receive their nutrition via **gastrostomy** (a tube that provides the feeding directly into the stomach) until the swallowing reflex improves.

Liquids are very difficult to control in the mouth, especially in the oral stage of the swallow. Because of this issue, use of water for rinsing or ultrasonic instrumentation may be contraindicated during dental care. The patient may be unable to lie in a supine position for fear of choking on saliva. Water should be used sparingly, and use of high-speed evacuation may be necessary to prevent aspiration.

Neurological deficits may cause some patients to be unaware of the presence of food in the mouth. After meals, the mouth should be checked for any **pocketed foods** (foods retained in the mouth, especially in the vestibule) that should be removed to decrease risk of aspirating the food and developing dental caries.

Dental Considerations

Assessment
- *Physical:* slurred speech and inability to communicate effectively; unilateral weakness or paralysis; difficulty chewing and swallowing; loss of oral sensations; lack of tongue control (weak, flabby, and deviates to one side).
- *Dietary:* chewing and swallowing difficulties, dietary inadequacies.

Interventions
- Monitor the patient's blood pressure at each dental visit.
- Refer to the RDN when dysphagia exists.
- Consult the healthcare provider before treatment to determine the need for antibiotic prophylaxis to prevent infective

endocarditis and whether the medications will have an anticoagulant effect.

Evaluation
- Desired outcomes include adequate nourishment using modifications according to the patient's disability, maintenance of good oral hygiene with formation of no new caries, and control of the periodontal condition.

Nutritional Directions

- Encourage the patient or caregiver to maintain adequate oral hygiene, particularly because of limited self-cleansing action on the affected side of the oral cavity.

Hypertension

Blood pressure consistently 140/90 mm Hg or higher is known as stage 1 hypertension. Patients with diagnosed hypertension or congestive heart failure may have been told to increase fruits and vegetables, use more low-fat or nonfat dairy products, limit sodium, limit intake of alcohol and caffeine, quit smoking, exercise, lose weight, and reduce stress (see Chapter 12, *Health Application 12*). When many older adults are told to limit salt in their diet because of high blood pressure, they may consume less food because it does not taste good, and they may not adhere to the recommendations because of limited food choices and lack of palatability.

Diuretics are frequently prescribed for patients with congestive heart failure or hypertension to help eliminate excess fluid. These medications also negatively affect salivary flow, which causes xerostomia.

Hyperlipidemia

Patients with other types of heart disease involving elevated cholesterol levels or increased risk of atherosclerosis normally have a saturated, *trans* and total fat, and cholesterol restriction (discussed in Chapter 6, *Health Application 6*). Low-fat diets can result in weight loss, which is beneficial to many. However, for patients who are trying to maintain their weight, snacks may be needed. Dental hygienists should consider recommending noncariogenic snacks relatively low in fat, such as low-fat or nonfat cheese or skim milk.

Long-term use of bile acid sequestrants (e.g., cholestyramine and colestipol), prescribed to reduce serum lipids, may cause malabsorption of fat-soluble vitamins and folic acid. Several bile acid sequestrants may cause gastrointestinal disturbances and affect overall food intake. Patients with heart disease may also be taking anticoagulants, such as warfarin (Coumadin), which may increase risk of bleeding and affect dietary intake because foods with vitamin K are limited.

Dental Considerations

Assessment
- *Physical:* medications prescribed, xerostomia, blood pressure.
- *Dietary:* dietary recommendations, adequacy of food intake.

Interventions
- Because stress is a negative risk factor for most patients with hypertension or heart conditions, minimize stress and consider effects of the disease on the proposed dental treatment. A shortened appointment and use of nitrous oxide may need to be considered.
- Generally, hypertension has no typical physiological symptoms; monitoring blood pressure at each appointment is necessary.
- Refer the patient to the RDN for medical nutrition therapy.

Evaluation
- The patient's blood pressure is within a normal range; the patient takes prescribed medications and follows *MyPlate* guidelines.

Nutritional Directions

- Most salt substitutes contain potassium and chloride. Remind patients to check with the healthcare provider or RDN for advice on the use of salt substitutes to minimize the intake of excessive dietary potassium.
- Help the patient determine low-sodium, low-fat, and low-cholesterol foods feasible for individual lifestyle and food preferences.
- Antihypertensive drugs may be responsible for reduced salivary flow. Fluoride therapy may be necessary. Xylitol gum or mints also may be used to promote salivation and remineralization of early carious lesions.
- Calcium channel blockers can cause gingival hyperplasia. Encourage optimal oral hygiene.

SKELETAL SYSTEM

Systemic bone disturbances initially may be detected by the following changes in the maxilla or mandible during an oral examination: (a) significant increase in size or alteration in contour of the maxilla or mandible, (b) alteration in radiographic pattern, (c) mobility of individual teeth without significant periodontal disease, (d) pain or discomfort in the jaw without obvious dental pathology, (e) increased sensitivity of the teeth without obvious dental or periodontal disease, (f) changes in occlusion of the teeth, or (g) abnormal sequence of deciduous tooth loss or eruption of permanent molars in young patients. These changes may be caused by osteoporosis, metabolic disturbances such as hyperparathyroidism, or other conditions such as Paget disease or fibrous dysplasia. For denture-wearing patients with osteoporosis, rapid resorption of the alveolar ridges may lead to continuous loosening of the dentures with resultant oral lesions or the inability to consume foods that require chewing.

In addition to referring the patient to a healthcare provider for correct diagnosis and treatment, the dental hygienist needs to provide guidance to ensure adequate calcium and vitamin D for patients with missing teeth, sensitivity to hot or cold foods, or pain when eating hard foods.

Bisphosphonates are medications primarily prescribed for postmenopausal and glucocorticoid-induced osteoporosis, multiple myeloma, and intravenous use is sometimes prescribed during chemotherapy for cancer. These drugs decrease bone turnover and inhibit the bone's reparative ability. A growing concern for patients receiving bisphosphonates is the risk for osteonecrosis (bone death of the jaw) after invasive dental procedures (Fig. 17-6). Patients at risk for osteonecrosis have a history of large doses of intravenous bisphosphonates (although patients taking oral bisphosphonates for long periods may also be at risk) with poor oral health requiring invasive dental procedures (e.g., extractions or dental surgery) or mechanical trauma.[13,14]

Dental Considerations

Assessment
- *Physical:* postmenopausal changes involving bone; osteoporosis/osteopenia.
- *Dietary:* variety and a well-balanced meal plan.

Interventions
- Encourage consultation with a healthcare provider to evaluate bone mineral density, possibly with dual-energy x-ray absorptiometry.
- As a part of the healthcare team, the dental professional can explain oral concerns related to bisphosphonate use and risk of osteonecrosis of the jaw.
- Physicians have prescribed bisphosphonates for millions of people, very few of whom developed a major side effect. Osteonecrosis occurs in approximately 1 of every 1000 women taking bisphosphonates.[15] Bisphosphonates are more likely to help prevent fractures, as intended, than to cause jaw problems, especially in women with postmenopausal osteoporosis.
- Resorption of the edentulous alveolar ridge requires frequent relining of the mandibular denture to avoid oral lesions and ensure the ability to masticate food.
- Provide counseling for tobacco cessation, if necessary (see Chapter 19, *Health Application 19*).

Evaluation
- The patient seeks medical guidance and adheres to prescribed recommendations.

Nutritional Directions

- Dietary supplementation of calcium and vitamin D may slow bone loss or increase bone mass.
- Avoid excessive alcohol consumption.

METABOLIC PROBLEMS
Diabetes Mellitus

Current evidence supports an interrelationship between diabetes and oral health problems. Type 2 diabetes and risk of periodontitis are correlated.[16] Periodontal disease is considered another long-term complication associated with diabetes, along with neuropathy or nephropathy. Studies are inconsistent in regard to the impact of periodontal treatment

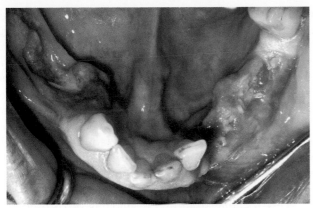

FIGURE 17-6 Bisphosphonate-associated osteonecrosis of mandibular arch. (From Damm DD, Bouquot JE, Neville BW, et al: *Oral and maxillofacial pathology*, ed 3, St Louis, 2009, Saunders.)

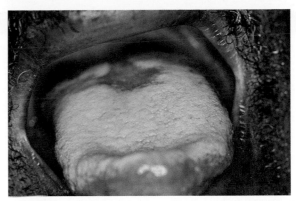

FIGURE 17-8 Oral candidiasis. (From Swartz MH: *Textbook of physical diagnosis: history and examination*, ed 7, Philadelphia, 2014, Saunders.)

Resistance to infections in these patients is lowered, and the normal healing process is slow. In poorly controlled diabetes, minor trauma to the gingiva may result in extensive tissue necrosis with eventual denudation of the underlying bone and the possibility of osteonecrosis. Treatment of oral problems should be reserved until the diabetes is under good control.

Xerostomia is also prevalent and is partially responsible for altered taste, general tenderness or burning of the mucosa, and carious lesions, all of which may affect nutrient intake. Patients with longstanding, poorly controlled diabetes are at risk of developing oral candidiasis (Fig. 17-8), partly due to increased glucose levels in saliva, which provide a substrate for fungal growth.[19]

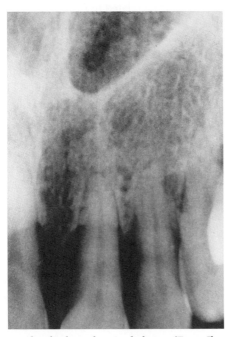

FIGURE 17-7 Alveolar bone loss in diabetes. (From Ibsen OAC, Phelan JA: *Oral pathology for the dental hygienist*, ed 6, St Louis, 2014, Saunders.)

on improving glycemic control, but because periodontal disease is an infection, evidence indicates periodontitis may be a risk factor for poor glycemic control.[17,18] Poorly controlled diabetes results in more severe periodontal disease and alveolar bone loss even in children and adolescents and may contribute to the progression of diabetes (Fig. 17-7).

Patients with uncontrolled or undiagnosed diabetes may have a characteristic fruity-smelling breath (more prevalent in type 1 diabetes), increased thirst, unexplained weight loss, or frequent urination. These symptoms are associated with elevated blood glucose levels. However, patients may be asymptomatic. Diabetes mellitus and nutrition recommendations are discussed in Chapter 7, *Health Application 7*.

Dental Considerations

Assessment

- *Physical:* polyuria, polydipsia, xerostomia, weight loss, weakness, ketosis, or asymptomatic.
- *Dietary:* polyphagia (increased hunger); adherence to prescribed lifestyle modifications, particularly fruit and vegetable intake.

Interventions

- Dental professionals can have a significant, positive effect on the oral and general health of patients with diabetes mellitus.
- Educate patients with diabetes about oral manifestations (e.g., xerostomia) and complications (e.g., periodontitis and oral candidiasis) to promote proper oral health behaviors. Few dental and periodontal changes and no oral mucosal changes are observed in individuals with well-controlled diabetes.
- Lack of fruit and vegetable intake by individuals with diabetes is associated with periodontitis.[20]
- To prevent hypoglycemia during dental treatment, the patient must eat at the usual time and take prescribed medications.
- Patients taking insulin or an oral diabetes medication in which hypoglycemia can occur may require at least 15 g of a carbohydrate source to bring blood glucose levels to a normal range.
- Some oral diabetes medications (e.g., α-glucosidase inhibitor) do not cause hypoglycemia by themselves; however, they are often combined with an oral agent that does. In this scenario, the

Continued

Dental Considerations—cont'd

patient may require a glucose source. Have 3 to 4 glucose tablets available for such events.

- When working with individuals who have diabetes, watch for the following warning signs:
  - gingival bleeding when brushing or flossing
  - red, swollen, or tender gingiva
  - suppuration
  - halitosis
  - recession
  - mobile teeth
  - malocclusion
  - changes in the fit of partial dentures or bridges
  - white or red patches on gingiva, tongue, cheeks or roof of mouth
  - pain when chewing
  - sensitivity to cold, hot or sweet
  - demineralized areas
- Periodontal infections may need to be managed with systemic antibiotic therapy and topical antimicrobials.
- Request that the patient bring the blood glucose monitor to each appointment to check the blood glucose level. Before a dental procedure begins, the patient's blood glucose level should be between 70 and 200 mg/dL. Long and stressful appointments may require testing during the appointment. Testing at the end of the appointment is also suggested; individuals with blood glucose values of less than 70 mg/dL should be treated before leaving the dental office.

Evaluation
- The patient's fasting blood glucose levels are normal, and the glycated hemoglobin A1c is less than 6.5%, indicating the diabetes is well controlled.

Nutritional Directions

- Read labels carefully for sources of carbohydrates, and choose predominantly complex carbohydrates. Foods labeled "sugar-free" may contain carbohydrates other than sucrose.
- Because of the risk of periodontal disease, meticulous daily oral self-care is imperative in conjunction with regular supportive peri-odontal therapy.

Hypopituitarism

The pituitary gland releases seven different hormones, including antidiuretic hormone, growth hormone, thyroid-stimulating hormone, and the sex hormones. Hypopituitarism may occur congenitally. In childhood hypopituitarism, decreased skeletal growth results in disproportionate retardation of mandibular growth. Prepubertal hypopituitarism, or decreased production of growth hormone, is usually caused by pressure from a cyst or tumor. Because of normal size teeth erupting into the small mandible and maxilla, proper alignment is impossible. In addition to delayed eruption, malocclusion is the principal oral problem.

Hypopituitarism may also occur secondarily to a tumor, head trauma, stroke, radiation, or infections of the brain. Symptoms of hypopituitarism in adults include poor appetite, weight loss, low blood pressure, fatigue, headache, and visual disturbances.

Cushing Syndrome

Pharmacological use of corticosteroids, and endogenous secretion of excess cortisol, as seen in Cushing syndrome, results in a state of hypercortisolism. Physical signs of Cushing syndrome include upper body obesity; round face; increased neck size; relatively slender arms and legs; high blood pressure; glucose intolerance or diabetes; muscle weakness; thin, fragile skin that bruises easily; hirsutism (excessive hair growth); osteoporosis; and depression. Muscle weakness resulting from excess amounts of cortisol may affect muscles used for mastication and the tongue. The presence of diabetes and osteoporosis may affect management of periodontal disease and associated bone loss.

Hypothyroidism

Hypothyroidism may be related to (a) inadequate consumption of iodine, (b) an inborn error of metabolism, (c) high intake of goitrogens, (d) treatment of hyperthyroidism (surgical excision, irradiation, antithyroid drugs), (e) thyroid gland disorder, or (f) deficient secretion of thyrotropin (thyroid-stimulating hormone) by the pituitary gland. Goitrogens are chemicals present in broccoli, kale, kohlrabi, cabbage, rutabagas, turnips, cauliflower, Brussels sprouts, horseradish, and soybeans that inhibit thyroid uptake of iodine. When hypothyroidism occurs at birth or in young children, the child is short in stature and has intellectual disabilities. Poor muscle tone results in a macroglossia (large, protruding) tongue, showing indentations on the lateral borders caused by pressure from the teeth (Fig. 17-9), and a tendency to choke. Eruption of the teeth is delayed, causing severe malocclusion, which makes proper oral hygiene difficult. Additionally, it places the patient at increased risk of dental caries and periodontal disease.

When hypothyroidism occurs in an adult, the tongue becomes enlarged and has decreased flexibility. Gingivitis

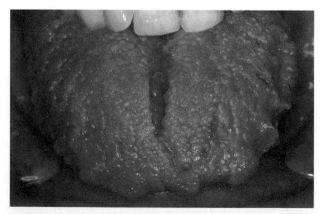

FIGURE 17-9 In hypothyroidism, the large tongue often protrudes from the mouth, showing indentation on the lateral borders caused by pressure from the teeth. (From Damm DD, Bouquot JE, Neville BW, et al: *Oral and maxillofacial pathology*, ed 3, St Louis, 2009, Saunders.)

and chronic periodontal disease may be a result of the patient's lack of interest in maintaining normal oral hygiene.

Hyperparathyroidism

Hyperparathyroidism results from hypersecretion of the parathyroid hormone, leading to alterations in calcium, phosphorus, and bone metabolism. Primary hyperthyroidism is seen more often in women older than 50 years of age. As a result of improved screening of serum calcium levels with routine laboratory tests, most cases of hyperparathyroidism are identified and treated before severe skeletal disease occurs. Clinical manifestations result from increased osteoclastic bone resorption, decreasing bone integrity. Systemic bone disturbances are reflected in the mouth by jaw enlargement and reduced bone density. In the terminal stage of the bone remodeling process, brown tumors (giant cell tumor replacement of bone as evidenced radiologically) may occur on the maxilla, palate, and mandible in addition to femur fractures.[21] These brown tumors may cause discomfort and may affect the patient's ability to consume an adequate diet but are normalized following treatment.

Renal Disease

The kidney is the primary organ that eliminates significant amounts of waste products; metabolic and endocrine functions are also affected by kidney disease. Progressive loss of nephrons in the kidney leads to chronic failure. When kidney function diminishes, complications arise as by-products accumulate from protein metabolism, and alterations occur in electrolyte levels and acid–base balance. Patients with renal disease may be on dialysis while awaiting a kidney transplant.

Because of calcium-phosphorus imbalances, various changes in bones are observed—a syndrome called renal osteodystrophy. This term describes various changes in bones associated with renal failure, such as classic hyperparathyroidism, osteomalacia, osteoporosis, and sometimes osteosclerosis (hardening or abnormal density of bone). Patients with chronically high urea levels may exhibit facial changes. Changes in facial dimensions increase in terms of width (skull base, mandible, and nose), length (mandible and nose), and depth of the mandible. Facial changes may result in a larger maxilla with a tendency toward more prominent lips.[22]

Manifestations that may be seen in the teeth and periodontium include delayed eruption, enamel hypoplasia, loss of the lamina dura, widening of the periodontal ligament, severe periodontal destruction, tooth mobility, drifting, and pulp calcifications. Numerous manifestations are seen in the bone, such as bone radiolucent fibrocystic lesions, metastatic soft tissue calcifications, decreased trabeculation and thickness of cortical bone, jaw fracture after trauma or surgery, brown tumors, and abnormal bone healing after extraction.[23,24]

Nutritional care for these individuals is extremely complex. Anorexia is often present because of dietary restrictions, uremia, and bad taste that many patients with chronic renal disease experience. High-quality protein intake is recommended to reduce nitrogen waste products (urea) and to minimize accumulation in the blood between dialysis treatments. In addition to protein, intake of minerals and electrolytes (e.g., sodium, potassium, and phosphorus) must be adjusted; adequate energy intake must be maintained; and potentially harmful intake of phosphorus, magnesium, aluminum, and some vitamins must be avoided. Fluid intake must be carefully monitored to prevent excess fluid buildup, which has a negative impact on blood pressure. For this reason, nutritional counseling should be left to an RDN who specializes in renal care.

The oral cavity reflects many signs of systemic involvement. Platelet abnormalities may result in gingival bleeding and bruising. Anemia is common, so gingival tissues may be pale in color. Other oral manifestations of chronic renal failure include complaints of a bad taste; malodor from urea buildup; xerostomia from fluid restriction; a variety of oral mucosal lesions (e.g., stomatitis [inflammation of the mouth], lichen planus, oral hairy leukoplakia [an asymptomatic white, yellow, or gray patch or plaque on the oral mucosa that cannot be removed by scraping or rubbing Fig. 17-10]; black hairy tongue, pyogenic granuloma, and nonspecific ulcerations); oral infection (e.g., candidiasis and viral infections); and Brown tumors.[25] Periodontal disease is observed frequently in patients with poor oral hygiene habits that may lead to systemic problems (pneumonia) because of

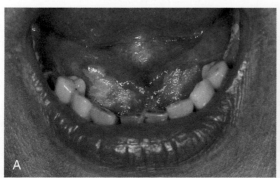 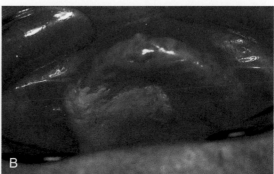

FIGURE 17-10 A, Leukoplakia on the floor of the mouth. **B,** Leukoplakia on the maxillary alveolar mucosa and palate. (From Ibsen OAC, Phelan JA: *Oral pathology for the dental hygienist*, ed 6, St Louis, 2014, Saunders.)

compromised immune status. Wound healing is slow because of general loss of tissue resistance and an inability to withstand normal traumatic insults. Evidence does not suggest an increased caries risk.

Many vitamin and mineral imbalances can develop in patients with renal disease, especially those on dialysis: poor appetite, depression, gastrointestinal symptoms, difficulty chewing and/or swallowing, and difficulty with grocery shopping and cooking, or, due to the dialysis process, dietary restrictions, excretion alterations to maintain homeostasis, and dialysate (material that passes through the membrane during dialysis) contamination. Patients on dialysis are more likely to be deficient in water-soluble vitamins (B and C) and the minerals iron and zinc.

Dental Considerations

Assessment
- *Physical:* oral manifestations and deteriorating physical status.
- *Dietary:* appetite, prescribed diet, adequacy of oral intake.

Interventions
- Consult the healthcare provider before treatment because of the bleeding tendency as a result of platelet dysfunction and anticoagulant medication and to determine the need for antibiotic prophylaxis to prevent infective endocarditis or infection of the vascular access site for dialysis or both.
- Emphasize the importance of good oral hygiene and consequences of poor oral hygiene.
- Because of the increased occurrence of oral complications, perform a careful and thorough oral examination to detect problems early.
- Medical care becomes more complicated when systemic conditions (e.g., pneumonia and diabetes) occur secondary to oral infections.
- Because of fluid restrictions for patients on dialysis, minimize water used during treatment. Because of the amount of water generated when using ultrasonic and sonic instrumentation, it is essential to use high speed evacuation.
- Transplantation patients normally require oral prophylaxis prior to being placed on the transplant waiting list.
- Consult with and refer to an RDN as needed.
- Schedule the dental appointment for a patient who is receiving dialysis the day after dialysis treatment.

Evaluation
- The patient is able to describe the relationship between the condition and effects of dietary intake on oral health.

Nutritional Directions

- Meticulous oral hygiene and frequent recare appointments prevent or reduce oral infections commonly associated with metabolic problems that can lead to difficulties in eating certain foods.
- Antimicrobial mouth rinses are helpful to minimize possible bacterial and fungal infections.

NEUROMUSCULAR PROBLEMS
Parkinson Disease

Parkinson disease is a progressive neurological condition characterized by involuntary muscle tremors, **bradykinesia** (slowness of movement), muscular weakness, rigidity, stooped posture, decreased fine motor coordination, masklike expression with absence of blinking, orthostatic hypotension, and a peculiar gait. It affects the oral cavity by causing an abnormal swallow pattern, with frequent drooling and tremor of the mandible, lips, and tongue. Decreased voluntary muscle movement affects muscles used to masticate food. Patients with Parkinson disease may have many problems associated with feeding and receiving adequate nourishment: (a) mechanical difficulties may interfere with the transfer of food from the plate to the mouth, and (b) oral disturbances may alter normal chewing and swallowing mechanisms. These problems may necessitate a change in the form or consistency of food, or special eating utensils, or both.

Poor oral health of patients with Parkinson disease may be related to lack of muscular control both orally (affecting chewing and swallowing) and hand control (affecting use of toothbrush, toothpaste, and dental floss).

Dysphagia may affect the oral phase of swallow or the pharyngeal stage of swallow. This can lead to problems such as pneumonia, dehydration, and malnutrition. The results include drooling of saliva, holding food in the mouth for extended periods, inability to tear food apart and mix it with saliva, food or liquid leaking from the nose, regurgitation, a gurgly voice, and food coating the tongue and palate after swallowing. Because of poor tongue control, a flowing, noncohesive bolus could spill over the base of the tongue before a swallow reflex is initiated, increasing risk for aspiration.

Other oral implications of Parkinson disease include salivary dysfunction (xerostomia and drooling), dysphagia, burning mouth, changes in taste and smell, root caries, and increased plaque accumulation related to challenges with oral self-care.[26,27]

The Parkinson's Disease Foundation recommends eating a balanced diet to maintain a healthy weight, maintaining bone health, bowel regularity, and balancing medications and food. Frequently, patients with Parkinson disease lose weight during early stages of the disease related to avoidance of solid foods and a decrease in food intake because of eating difficulties. Attention to subtle cues can ensure the patient does not lose a significant amount of weight and muscle mass. Nutritional supplements and high kilocalorie foods can be encouraged.

Medications are usually initiated when symptoms affect quality of life or affect work performance and disrupt an individual's daily activities. Recent research is working to find neuroprotective therapies to prevent the progression of disease since current medications only control symptoms.

The principle medication used for Parkinson disease is levodopa, which has drug-nutrient interactions with protein reducing effectiveness of the drug. Despite these interactions, adequate protein intake is crucial. Nausea and poor appetite resulting from medications can also negatively affect dietary intake. Challenges in maintaining body weight and health may necessitate consultation with an RDN to tailor a diet meeting the patient's needs.

Parkinson disease cannot be prevented. However, epidemiologic data suggest dietary patterns with high intake of fruits, vegetables, legumes, whole grains, nuts, fish, and poultry; low intake of saturated fat; and moderate intake of alcohol may protect against Parkinson disease. This is one more reason why dental hygienists need to encourage healthy eating.

Developmental Disabilities

Many disabilities may impair development of normal feeding reflexes (discussed in Chapter 14) and coordination of these reflexes with respiration. These feeding reflexes may be absent or weak and difficult to elicit. Abnormal oral-motor patterns and difficulties associated with feeding may result when structural malformations such as cleft palate, macroglossia, and micrognathia (abnormally small jaw) are present. Neuromuscular diseases, such as cerebral palsy, muscular dystrophy, and Down syndrome, may be associated with abnormal oral-motor development. The feeding experience, which is normally pleasurable, becomes a frustrating, time-consuming situation for everyone involved in the patient's care.

Oral-motor impairment may become evident during the spoon-feeding phase of feeding development. Tongue retraction, tonic bite reflex, tongue thrust, and persistence of a suckling pattern interfere with placing a spoon in the mouth and result in loss of food from the mouth (Table 17-2). A patient with tonic bite reflex may clamp down on a spoon inserted in the mouth and be unable to release the bite.

Table 17-2	Feeding problems
Condition	**Description**
Tonic bite reflex	Strong jaw closure when teeth or gingiva are stimulated
Tongue thrust	Forceful and often repetitive protrusion of an often bunched or thick tongue in response to oral stimulation
Jaw thrust	Forceful opening of the jaw to its maximal extent during eating, drinking, attempts to speak, or general excitement
Tongue retraction	Pulling back the tongue within the oral cavity at presentation of food, spoon, or cup
Lip retraction	Pulling back the lips in a very tight, smile-like pattern at the approach of food, spoon, or cup toward the face
Sensory defensiveness	A strong adverse reaction to sensory input (touch, sound, light)

Attempting to free the spoon by pulling is ineffective and may cause continued biting.

With tongue thrusting and tongue retraction, the tongue is unable to form a bolus and move it to the back of the mouth. Placing food in the mouth can be difficult with a severe tongue thrust, which also may affect the individual's ability to suck, chew, and swallow.

With lip retraction, lips may be unable to remove food from the spoon, and drinking or sucking may be impossible. Sensory defensiveness is associated with a strong emotional reaction to the unwanted tactile stimuli and can result in a severe food intake problem.

Inadequate chewing skills are associated with jaw and tongue thrusting, hyperactive or hypoactive gag reflex, abnormal intraoral sensation, and poor tongue lateralization. Oral-motor impairments make providing optimal nutritional care very difficult. Whenever intake of food is limited, because of an oral-motor problem or an inability to self-feed, these patients are at nutritional risk.

When oral-motor impairment is extremely severe, adequate nutrition cannot be provided with oral feedings, and nutrition is provided via gastrostomy feedings. Treatment is facilitated using an interdisciplinary team to determine the best treatment promoting development of feeding skills and providing foods in a form that can be handled safely.

Epilepsy

Epilepsy, or psychomotor seizures, in itself does not usually result in any specific oral or feeding problems. However, a popular drug used for seizure control, phenytoin, can significantly cause bone loss within a year. Gingival hyperplasia is noted with long-term phenytoin use (Fig. 17-11). When good oral self-care techniques are routinely practiced, inflammation and gingival overgrowth are reduced.

Phenytoin increases metabolism of vitamins D and K and folate, which may increase risk for loss of bone mineral density. Research suggests that phenytoin resulted in significant bone loss even though the participants consumed 1000 mg of calcium and were physically active.[28] This research raises concerns about long-term bone health for these

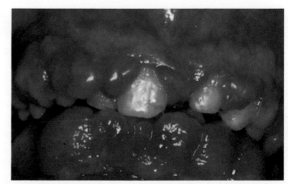

FIGURE 17-11 Hyperplasia associated with phenytoin use. (Courtesy of Barbara D. Altshuler, BSDH, MS, Clinical Assistant Professor, Caruth School of Dental Hygiene, The Texas A&M University System, Baylor College of Dentistry, Dallas, TX.)

patients. Phenobarbital, which is also used to manage convulsions in epilepsy, may also affect bone health by increasing turnover of vitamins D and K. Despite increased need for these nutrients, supplementation of folate or vitamin B₆ may decrease bioavailability of phenytoin and must be carefully monitored by a healthcare provider.

Dental Considerations

Assessment
- *Physical:* oral complications related to neuromuscular disorders; medications prescribed; nutrient supplements; orthostatic hypotension.
- *Dietary:* adequacy of intake, signs of malnutrition.

Interventions
- Carefully assess oral status of patients taking anticonvulsants.
- To reduce stress and anxiety, keep appointments brief and relaxing.
- Assess saliva flow and provide tips for preventing xerostomia associated oral problems (see Chapter 20).
- After supine positioning, have the patient with Parkinson disease sit upright for at least 2 minutes before standing to avoid orthostatic hypotension.
- Coping strategies for dysphagia, such as massaging the throat before beginning the feeding and reminding the patient to tilt the head forward before swallowing, aid swallowing problems, but become tedious and taxing for healthcare providers.
- For patients experiencing xerostomia, advise avoidance of alcohol, smoking, and caffeine.
- Instigate a rigorous preventive oral health regime tailored to the needs of individuals with neuromuscular problems.
- Schedule appointments at the individual's best time of day.
- Suggest dental gels, such as fluoride, and dentifrices for individuals with dysphagia rather than mouthrinses that may increase risk of aspiration. Refer the patient to the healthcare provider or RDN if nutrient supplementation is reported. Some nutrients may interfere with absorption of the prescribed medication.
- Suggest adaptations so the patient can maintain independence for teeth or denture cleaning (e.g., an electric toothbrush or toothbrush handle adaptations).

Evaluation
- The patient's dental health is maintained, and prescribed medications are taken.

Nutritional Directions

- Check the fit of a dental prosthesis. An improper fit may impact nutritional status.
- Encourage small, frequent nutrient-dense meals and snacks for patients experiencing anorexia and weight loss. Refer to an RDN.
- Salivary substitutions and topical fluoride treatments may be recommended for patients experiencing xerostomia.
- Antimicrobial rinses are helpful to decrease the chance of bacterial and fungal infections.
- Patients with Parkinson disease are often at risk for osteoporosis. Foods high in or fortified with calcium, magnesium, and vitamins D and K may be suggested.
- Patients taking levodopa or carbidopa should avoid eating foods high in vitamin B₆ (e.g., dry skim milk, peas, beans, sweet

potatoes, avocados, fortified cereal, oatmeal, wheat germ, yeast, pork and beef organs, tuna, and fresh salmon) when they take the medication.
- Calcium supplements are not recommended for patients taking phenytoin and phenobarbital unless closely monitored by the healthcare provider because large amounts of calcium decrease bioavailability of the drug and the mineral.
- Pyridoxine and folate supplements may alter response of phenytoin and result in increased seizure activity.
- Carbamazepine (Tegretol), another popular anticonvulsant, causes xerostomia, altered taste, and oral sensitivity.

NEOPLASIA

Neoplasia (abnormal mass of tissue), more frequently referred to as tumors, causes problems not only in the primary site, but also in regional and remote areas. The manifestations at secondary sites away from the primary lesion may be the presenting feature in some cases. The mouth and jaw may be involved in generalized malignant disease.

Nutritional requirements for patients with neoplasms are generally increased to maintain lean body mass and immune responses. Anorexia is an important symptom of an underlying neoplasm. Oral symptoms or signs may be secondary to malnutrition or nutrient deficiencies. Abnormalities in taste perception have been noted in some patients with cancer, such as an elevated threshold for sweets and a reduced threshold for bitter flavors. Altered taste sensations may be secondary to a deficiency of zinc. Hormonal factors affect the hypothalamic feeding center to reduce oral intake. Early satiety may be related to minimal digestive secretions or impaired gastric emptying.

The location of the tumor itself also may be a factor in reduced food intake, especially when the alimentary tract is affected. Intake is reduced in patients with cancer of the oral cavity, pharynx, or esophagus because of odynophagia (pain on swallowing) or dysphagia. Gastric cancer may lead to reduced gastric capacity or partial gastric outlet obstruction, resulting in early satiety, nausea, and vomiting.

Psychological factors undoubtedly affect appetite. Depression, grief, or anxiety resulting from the disease or its treatment may lead to poor appetite and abnormal eating behaviors.

Kaposi Sarcoma

Kaposi sarcoma is a highly malignant tumor of blood vessel origin that occurs on the skin and oral mucosa (Fig. 17-12). It is characterized by bluish red cutaneous nodules, usually on the lower extremities, and occurs frequently in immunocompromised individuals. These lesions appear in many HIV-positive patients. Red-purple macular lesions in the mouth may progress to raised, indurated lesions with central areas of necrosis and ulceration. Lesions can cause obstruction of the esophagus, compromising food intake.

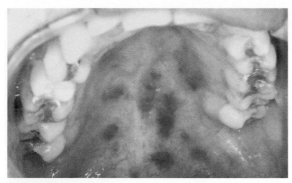

FIGURE 17-12 Kaposi sarcoma lesions on the hard palate. (From Silverman S Jr: *Color atlas of oral manifestations of AIDS*, ed 5, St Louis, 1996, Mosby.)

Leukemia

Several types of leukemia are classified according to how quickly they progress (acute or chronic). Leukemia is a generalized malignant disease characterized by distorted proliferation and development of WBCs. It is another neoplastic process with many oral manifestations that detrimentally affect food intake. Gingival tissues are especially susceptible to gingivitis because of an exaggerated inflammatory response to local etiologic factors (e.g., calculus, plaque biofilm, and materia alba [soft white deposit around the necks of teeth]). Rather than the normal response of chronic marginal gingivitis, the gingiva may become severely inflamed with tissue hyperplasia, areas of ulcerations, necrosis, and spontaneous bleeding. This is believed to be caused by the body's depressed immune response. Susceptibility to infection is increased, and healing responses are delayed.

Cancer Treatments

Cancer treatment may include surgery, radiation therapy, chemotherapy, biological therapy, or combinations of these modalities. Tumors involving the gastrointestinal tract affect the ability to ingest foods orally or digest and absorb nutrients adequately. Radical surgery in the oropharyngeal area may present problems in chewing and swallowing, and alterations in taste sensations.

Radiation therapy significantly affects the alimentary tract. Early transient effects include general loss of appetite, nausea and vomiting, and diarrhea caused by malabsorption secondary to mucosal damage in the gastrointestinal tract. Food intake is affected because of loss of taste sensation, xerostomia, difficulty in swallowing, and a burning sensation in the mouth when the larynx or pharynx area is irradiated. When a patient is exposed to a food or beverage before radiation treatment or chemotherapy, the item may become associated with the therapy, causing the patient to develop an aversion to that particular food. Rampant caries and loss of teeth may complicate adequate dietary intake further.

Chemotherapeutic drugs are used to destroy malignant cells without loss of an excessive number of normal cells. Chemotherapy has more widespread effects on the body than either radiation or surgical treatment. Rapid cell turnover rate in the alimentary tract leads to stomatitis or mucositis, oral ulcerations, and decreased absorptive capacity. As a result, changes in taste sensation and learned food aversions occur.

 Dental Considerations

Assessment
- *Physical:* fatigue, caries, adequate weight, weight loss, oral ulcerations, medications.
- *Dietary:* maintaining caloric intake, adequate fluids, food aversions (especially food groups), alterations in taste.

Interventions
- Use of an antimicrobial mouth rinse (i.e., alcohol-free chlorhexidine) may be indicated to reduce inflammation associated with cancer treatment.
- A soft or bland diet (refer to diet in Chapter 19, Box 19-4) may be recommended as deemed necessary by oral conditions.
- Discuss the relationship between fermentable carbohydrate intake, effects of xerostomia, plaque biofilm formation, and caries. Caution against eating hard candy containing fermentable carbohydrates to relieve xerostomia.

Evaluation
- A dietary recall reveals adequate nutrients and kilocalories with a minimum of fermentable carbohydrates.

 Nutritional Directions

- Small, frequent meals are appropriate to provide additional kilocalories and to counteract nausea and vomiting.
- Meticulous oral hygiene, frequent recare appointments, and fluoride therapy are essential.
- Adequate food and fluid intake not only improve the physical response to cancer treatment, but also create a more positive psychological outlook.
- Avoid foods that are hot, spicy, or acidic (e.g., citrus fruit and juices).
- Avoid alcohol-containing beverages and mouth rinses.
- Commonly used chemotherapeutic agents (bleomycin, cyclophosphamide, and methotrexate) generally cause complications such as stomatitis, nausea, vomiting, diarrhea, and anorexia.

ACQUIRED IMMUNODEFICIENCY DISEASE

HIV debilitates the body's immune system. Following identification of HIV antibodies in the blood, a positive diagnosis of HIV is made. This retrovirus causes a dysfunction in the genetic core of T lymphocytes or WBCs that normally function to resist infection. Retroviruses are characterized by the presence of reverse transcriptase, which interferes with production of DNA from RNA. Susceptibility to various opportunistic infections (especially *Pneumocystis carinii, Cryptosporidium, Candida, Mycobacterium,* and herpes simplex) and certain neoplasms (Kaposi sarcoma, non-Hodgkin lymphoma, and oral warts) is increased. These infections can appear in virtually every organ system.

Because of the body's inability to fight infections, AIDS develops.

With the advent of highly active antiretroviral therapy (HAART), HIV-positive individuals no longer exhibit the classic gaunt appearance typical of wasting. Patients receiving HAART may still lose lean body mass, but because of a dramatic increase in fat cells and lipodystrophy (rearrangement of fat deposits that can be extremely disfiguring), it may be harder to diagnose. The course of HIV/AIDS is often complicated by weight loss, wasting of lean body mass, cachexia, opportunistic infections, malignancies, diarrhea, multiple nutrient deficiencies, and particularly protein-energy malnutrition. The cause of malnutrition is multifactorial and may involve inadequate intake, malabsorption, or hypermetabolism.

At present, nutritional status is not known to affect the length of time for HIV infections to progress to AIDS. Good nutrition does not cure AIDS, but malnutrition may hasten progression of the disease and affect outcome. Many oral problems in HIV-positive patients have predictive value for development of AIDS because of their effect on appetite and food intake. Adequate dietary intake can help maintain strength, comfort, and level of functioning. Providing optimal nutrition improves resistance to opportunistic infections. Good oral hygiene improves nutritional status by promoting a desirable environment that enhances food intake.

More than 30 different oral manifestations of HIV disease have been reported since the AIDS epidemic began. However, treatment of oral problems should not be avoided when a person is HIV-positive. Individuals with a compromised immune system should practice preventive measures to avoid bacterial infections evidenced in dental caries and periodontal disease. A routine plan of care to prevent development of oral health problems is particularly important.

Anorexia may be attributed to respiratory and other infections, fever, dysgeusia, gastrointestinal complications, adverse effects of drugs, and depression. Specific nutritional deficiencies may depress appetite and exacerbate anorectic behavior. Oral and esophageal pain during eating also may decrease intake.

Several varieties of oral candidiasis are prevalent in HIV-positive individuals; *Candida* infection is a sign of immune dysfunction and should be reported to the healthcare provider. Oral candidiasis produces pain and inhibits production of saliva. Pharyngeal or esophageal lesions of Kaposi sarcoma may cause obstruction, whereas herpetic ulcerations or other ulcerations on the tongue or esophagus can cause difficulty in swallowing. Herpetic ulcerations are painful ulcerations of the oral mucosa with a red center and yellow border. The development of thrush may be attributed to herpes virus, candidiasis, chemotherapy, or drugs such as interferon.

Oral hairy leukoplakia (Fig. 17-13) is found predominantly on the lateral borders of the tongue or occasionally on the buccal or labial mucosa in patients who are HIV-positive. The white lesions or filamentous growth do not rub off. HIV-infected patients frequently have ulcerations that

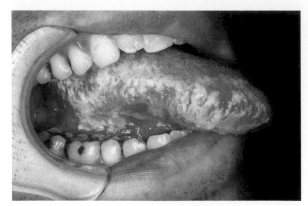

FIGURE 17-13 Hairy leukoplakia. (From Silverman S Jr: *Color atlas of oral manifestations of AIDS*, ed 5, St Louis, 1996, Mosby.)

resemble aphthous ulcers which appear as well-circumscribed ulcers with an erythematous margin. These painful ulcers may become extremely large and necrotic; they may persist for several weeks.

The level of HIV control by HAART determines how the patient responds to periodontal therapy. Patients who are not well controlled may not respond normally to standard periodontal therapy; a mild case of gingivitis can progress to severe periodontitis in a few months, resulting in the need for extraction of affected teeth. Untreated periodontal disease can lead to necrotizing ulcerative periodontitis because of the compromised immune system. Necrotizing ulcerative periodontitis is a severe form of periodontal disease with rapid loss of soft tissue and bone, (including exposure of the bone), and by rapid deterioration of tooth attachment and loss of surrounding teeth (see Chapter 19).

HIV-positive patients may have parotid gland swelling accompanied by xerostomia. Spontaneous oral bleeding may be associated with small purpuric lesions or ecchymoses or gingivitis.

Dental Considerations

Assessment
- *Physical*: weight change, oral infections and malignancies, candidiasis, periodontitis, viral load.
- *Dietary*: oral sensitivity, adequate levels of all nutrients.

Interventions
- Perform a careful oral examination to identify signs of HIV-infected patients so they can be treated appropriately.
- Individualize the care plan and treatment for each AIDS patient related to special needs.
- Systemic antibiotic therapy may be indicated for infections.
- Oral lesions will affect nutritional status because of discomfort in the mouth. Offer suggestions for palliative care (antimicrobial mouth rinse, antifungal lozenge or mouthwash; pain medication; and non-acidic foods) that will not exacerbate lesions.

Dental Considerations—cont'd

- Consultation with the healthcare provider is necessary to gather information about laboratory values (e.g., platelet count, WBC count, and viral load), medications, and history of opportunistic infections, and to determine if antibiotic prophylaxis is needed.
- The patient should use a non-alcoholic antimicrobial rinse and antifungal and antiviral agents as prescribed by the dentist or healthcare provider.
- Encourage and try to motivate the patient to maintain the highest possible level of oral self-care and regular preventive dental care.
- Refer the patient to an RDN for medical nutrition therapy.
- Side effects of HAART include diarrhea, nausea, and vomiting. Frequent vomiting can cause enamel erosion. Preventive dental care and use of topical fluoride therapy at home is essential.

Evaluation

- The patient exhibits increased attention to oral hygiene care and is maintaining current weight.

Nutritional Directions

- To promote healing and maintenance of oral tissues, encourage attention to nutrient intake. The *Dietary Guidelines* recommendation to decrease fat intake may be inappropriate for patients with HIV/AIDS.
- To add kilocalories and protein, add nuts and dried fruits to hot and cold cereals; use cream instead of milk; add ground meat or poultry or grated cheese to soups, sauces, casseroles, and vegetable dishes; use peanut butter on fruit or crackers; dip vegetables in sour cream mixes; use nutritional supplements or instant breakfast drinks as snacks.
- Limit caffeine-containing and alcohol-containing beverages if xerostomia is present.

MENTAL HEALTH PROBLEMS

Anorexia Nervosa, Bulimia Nervosa

More than 10 million Americans are affected by serious eating disorders. Although anorexia nervosa, bulimia nervosa are two different conditions, they are symptomatically related (Fig. 17-14). Anorexia nervosa is a disease primarily affecting adolescent girls and young women who have an exaggerated, intense fear of becoming fat. Zealous self-imposed restriction leads to extreme weight loss.

Individuals with anorexia nervosa may be described as achievement-oriented perfectionists who seek to rule their lives by refusing to eat in an effort to control their bodies. These young individuals are generally surrounded with all the evidences of success. Individuals with anorexia nervosa may become excellent gourmet cooks, spending hours planning menus, finding special recipes, and shopping for exotic ingredients. In-depth knowledge of nutritional and caloric value of foods is commonly exhibited by individuals with anorexia.

Diagnosis of anorexia nervosa includes weight loss equal to or exceeding 15% below expected or original body weight, rigid dieting, amenorrhea (for women), and an excessive

desire for slimness with a distorted body image. Dental complications in advanced stages of malnutrition are generally observed in patients with anorexia nervosa.

Bulimia nervosa occurs more frequently than anorexia nervosa. Bulimia is an eating disorder that is not associated with significant weight loss. An individual with bulimia might even be normal weight or slightly overweight and appear healthy. Bulimia is characterized by intentional, although not necessarily controllable, secret binges (periods of overeating) usually followed by purging (a means of counteracting the effects of overindulgence).

Typically, bulimia and anorexia nervosa occur for the same reason: fear of becoming fat. However, individuals with bulimia try to control this fear by repeatedly restraining eating, but this backfires and leads to bingeing and purging. Individuals with bulimia exhibit many of the same characteristics as individuals with anorexia, but those with bulimia are more sociable, while underneath they feel profoundly separated from other people. Usually they appear very mature, but this is a defense mechanism to hide insecurities. Appearance is extremely important to them.

Individuals with bulimia acknowledge their eating behaviors are not normal. They have strong appetites and may binge several times a day, with intakes of 1200 kcal or more per episode. Binges may last minutes to several hours and may be planned or spontaneous, but ordinarily are related to stress. Compulsive stealing of food and money to buy food is another common characteristic. Individuals binge on mainly high-carbohydrate, easily digested food.

These binges occur most often in the late afternoon or evening and end with purging. Self-induced vomiting is the main method of purging. Vomiting may be induced by sticking a finger or other object down the throat, applying external pressure to the neck, or drinking syrup of ipecac (emetic drug). Eventually, some individuals with bulimia can vomit by merely contracting their abdominal muscles.

In addition to poor overall health status, nutritional effects of bulimia stem from purging and the method employed for purging. Frequent episodes of self-induced vomiting can cause oral cavity trauma; bruises and irritations in the oral cavity may be observed. Frequent vomiting causes erosion of tooth enamel (predominantly on the lingual surfaces of the maxillary teeth) (Fig. 17-15), dentin hypersensitivity, and enlargement of the parotid glands. Lips are often red, dry and cracked and lesions on oral soft tissue bleed easily. Erosion can occur in as short as 6 months after continued regurgitation (Fig. 17-16). Teeth may be sensitive to extreme temperatures. Signs of malnutrition may also be present and observed during an oral examination (e.g., dry brittle hair, spoon-shaped nails, and cheilosis). Dental hygienists should not falsely assume oral problems result from poor dental hygiene practices; rather, these oral problems develop secondary to frequent vomiting. Another classic sign of bulimia associated with self-induced vomiting is the presence of abrasions and calluses on dorsal surfaces of fingers and hands secondary to friction of the teeth.

PRE-DISEASE/		
Anorexia	EARLY SYMPTOMS	Bulimia

Anorexia

*Low self-esteem
*Misperception of hunger, satiety, and other bodily sensations
*Feelings of lack of control in life
*Distorted body image
*Overachiever
*Compliant
*Anxiety
*Menstrual cycle stops (amenorrhea)
*Progressive preoccupation with food and eating
*Isolates self from family and friends
*Perfectionistic behavior
*Compulsive exercise
*Eats alone
*Fights with family about eating (may begin to cook and control family's eating)
*Fatigue
*Increased facial and body hair (lanugo)
*Decreased scalp hair
*Thin, dry scalp
*Emaciated appearance (at least 25% loss of total body weight)
*Feelings of control over body
*Rigid
*Depression
*Apathy
*Fear of food and gaining weight
*Malnutrition
*Mood swings (tyranical)
*Diminished capacity to think
*Sensitivity to cold
*Electrolyte imbalance (weakness)
*Lassitude cardiac arrest
*Denial of problem (see self as fat)
*Joint pain (difficulty walking and sitting)
*Sleep disturbance

EARLY SYMPTOMS / MIDDLE STAGE SYMPTOMS / CRUCIAL STAGE SYMPTOMS

Bulimia

*Low self-esteem
*Feel that self-worth is dependent on low weight
*Dependent on opposite sex for approval
*Normal weight
*Constant concern with weight and body image
*Experimentation with vomiting, laxatives, and diuretics
*Poor impulse control
*Fear of binging/eating getting out of control
*Embarrassment
*Anxiety
*Depression
*Self-indulgent behavior
*Eats alone
*Preoccupation with eating and food
*Tiredness, apathy, irritability
*Gastrointestinal disorders
*Elimination of normal activities
*Anemia
*Social isolation, distancing friends and family
*Dishonesty, lying
*Stealing food/money
*Tooth damage (gingivitis)
*Binging/high carbohydrate foods
*Drug and alcohol abuse
*Laxative and diuretic abuse
*Mood swings
*Chronic sore throat
*Difficulties in breathing/swallowing
*Hypokalemia (abnormally low potassium concentration)
*Electrolyte imbalance
*General ill health/constant physical problems
*Possible rupture of heart or esophagus/peritonitis
*Dehydration
*Irregular heart rhythms
*Suicidal tendencies/attempts

RECOVERY / REHABILITATION

Ongoing Support

*Trust/openness
*Understanding of personal needs
*Honesty
*Increased assertiveness
*Improved self-image
*Developing optimism
*Respect of family and friends
*More understanding of family
*Fully aware of and at ease with life
*Appreciation of spiritual values
*Enjoyment of eating food without guilt
*Acceptance of personal limitations
*Return of regular menstrual cycles
*New interest
*New friends
*Achievement of personal goals in a wide range of activities
*Self-approval (not dependent on weight)
*Relief from guilt and depression
*Diminished fears
*Resumption of normal eating
*Resumption of normal self-control
*Begin to relax
*Acceptance of illness
*Participation in a treatment program
*Acceptance of a psychiatric treatment plan

RECOGNITION OF NEED FOR HELP

The progressions of symptoms and recovery signs are based on the most repeated experiences of those with Anorexia and Bulimia. When a patient with Anorexia becomes Bulimic, she will experience symptoms characteristic of both eating disorders. Although every symptom in the chart does not occur in every case or in any specific sequence, it does portray an average progression pattern. The goals and resultant behavior changes in the recovery process are similar for both eating disorders.

FIGURE 17-14 Anorexia nervosa and bulimia: a multidimensional profile.

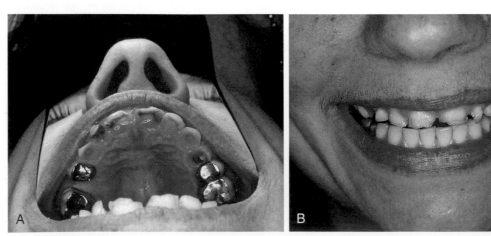

FIGURE 17-15 A and **B,** Enamel erosion caused by bulimia nervosa. (From Ibsen OAC, Phelan JA: *Oral pathology for the dental hygienist,* ed 6, St Louis, 2014, Saunders.)

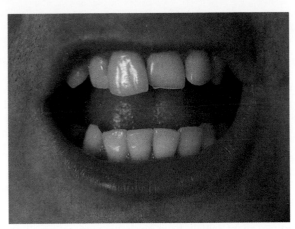

FIGURE 17-16 Bulimia nervosa. Incisor was capped because of dental caries. Continued vomiting has diminished the size of the surrounding teeth, while prosthesis remains unchanged. (Courtesy Dr. J. Treasure. From McLaren DS: *A colour atlas and text of diet-related disorders*, ed 2, London, 1992, Mosby-Yearbook.)

A third category of eating disorders is binge-eating disorder. It is defined as frequent episodes of eating significant quantities of food, even when not hungry. Accompanying feelings include lack of control, guilt, embarrassment or disgust.[29]

Successful outcomes require comprehensive treatment by a multidisciplinary team that addresses individual psychosocial, nutritional, and medical problems. The team usually comprises a psychotherapist or psychiatrist, RDN, nurse, social worker, and healthcare provider. This pooling of specialties provides effective treatment for the patient and a support system for team members when difficult decisions are necessary or progress seems slow.

Mental Illness

A few of the many different mental illnesses that occur include schizophrenia, depression, and bipolar disorder or mania. These disorders do not usually display any oral manifestations; however, drugs frequently prescribed to treat the conditions may have side effects that affect oral status. Antipsychotics (e.g., haloperidol, thioridazine, fluoxetine, and thiothixene) used to treat schizophrenia frequently cause xerostomia. Anticholinergic properties of tricyclic antidepressants, monoamine oxidase inhibitors, and trazodone used to treat depression also cause xerostomia, dental caries, ulcerations, and periodontal disease. Trazodone can also cause an unpleasant taste in the mouth.

 Dental Considerations

Assessment

- *Physical:* signs of malnutrition (e.g., thinning hair, always cold, facial hair), fatigue, dehydration, trauma to the soft palate from fingernails or objects used to induce vomiting, location of enamel erosion, parotid enlargement, weight changes.
- *Dietary:* high-carbohydrate diet, very-low-caloric intake or other unusual dietary habits, obsession with diet or weight.

Interventions

- An increased caries rate can be indicative of high-carbohydrate bingeing, low pH of saliva from vomiting, and xerostomia. Office and home fluoride therapy should be recommended.
- Discuss specific characteristics observed in the dental assessment with the patient.
- Treatment of an eating disorder involves a multidisciplinary team of healthcare professionals, including the dental professional. It is

the responsibility of the dental hygienist to be able to recognize the signs and symptoms of a suspected eating disorder, refer patients to a healthcare provider or a local hospital or eating disorder facility for assessment and treatment, and document the findings and recommendations.
- Chronic use of syrup of ipecac can affect skeletal muscle and cardiac action, which can result in congestive heart failure, arrhythmia, and sudden death.
- Encourage meticulous oral hygiene.

Evaluation

- The patient is making realistic changes by protecting the hard and soft tissues, being plaque-free, and being treated by a multidisciplinary healthcare team.

 Nutritional Directions

- To prevent further damage to teeth, caution the patient against brushing immediately after vomiting; avoid use of hard toothbrushes, abrasive toothpaste, and a "scrubbing" toothbrush method; avoid rinsing with tap water because it reduces the protective effects of saliva; encourage use of a mouth guard during vomiting episodes; rinse with sodium bicarbonate to neutralize the

oral environment; and encourage use of daily fluoride and dentinal hypersensitivity products.
- Inform the patient about various ways to relieve xerostomia and the effect of lack of saliva on hard and soft tissues.
- Nutritional advice provided should encourage health-centered behaviors rather than discussing caloric values or intake.

HEALTH APPLICATION 17 Human Papillomavirus

April is Oral Cancer Awareness Month. The American Dental Association recommends performing an oral cancer visual and tactile screening on a routine basis for early detection.[30] Several oral cancer screening technologies exist that may aid visual and tactile screening. More than 42,000 people in the United States will be diagnosed with oral or oropharyngeal cancer this year; 640,000 people worldwide. More disturbing is the fact that the survival rate after 5 years of diagnosis is only 57%.[31] Overall, cancer death rates are declining. However, oral cancer is on the rise. Dental professionals are well positioned to refer patients with lesions identified during an intra- and extra-oral examination to the healthcare provider.

Human papillomavirus (HPV) is a risk factor for oral cancer (Box 17-1). HPV is a common sexually transmitted infection that can also occur in the oral cavity, esophagus, and larynx. These lesions can be recognized during an intraoral examination; however, HPV lesions vary in form (Fig. 17-17). More than 100 different types of HPV have been identified. Low-risk HPV strains can lead to the growth of a papilloma or wart. However, some high-risk strains have shown a strong association with cancer.[32] HPV strains are numbered; HPV-16 and HPV-18 have been identified as subtypes associated with

risk factors for oral squamous cell carcinomas. Squamous cell carcinoma manifests as cancer in the head and neck area. Currently, two HPV vaccines, a series of three shots over 6 months, have received FDA approval for protection against HPV-16 and HPV-18.

HPV can be present and communicable even when lesions are not present. Salivary diagnostic testing is available to detect the presence of HPV.

Treatment regimens for cancer (surgery, chemotherapy and/or radiation) vary according to the cancer site and stage. The treatments cause or exacerbate symptoms such as anorexia, alterations or loss of taste, xerostomia, mucositis, nausea, and vomiting, all of which have an impact on eating. Before, during, and after treatment, patients with oral cancer often experience complications related to these symptoms. Malnutrition, a frequent complication, has serious implications on the outcome and response to treatment.[33,34]

As the association between HPV and oral cancer strengthens, early detection and education is the emerging responsibility of dental professionals. Communicating the message on this sensitive topic may require additional training.

BOX 17-1	Risk Factors for Oral Cancer

- HPV
- Tobacco use
- Heavy alcohol use
- Age
- Gender
- Family history
- Lichen planus
- Excessive exposure to sunlight
- Poor nutrition
- Weakened immune system
- Mouthwash*
- Irritation from dentures*

*Controversial

Data from American Cancer Society: *What are the risk factors for oral cavity and oropharyngeal cancers?* 2013. Accessed September 6, 2013: http://www.cancer.org/cancer/oralcavityandoropharyngealcancer/detailedguide/oral-cavity-and-oropharyngeal-cancer-risk-factors.

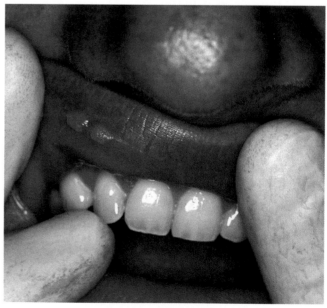

FIGURE 17-17 Papillary lesion of the upper lip caused by human papilloma virus in a patient with human immunodeficiency virus infection. (From Ibsen OAC, Phelan JA: *Oral pathology for the dental hygienist,* ed 6, St Louis, 2014, Saunders).

Case Application for the Dental Hygienist

Janie, a 17-year-old cheerleader in high school, came in for her 6-month recare appointment. She complained that "my teeth seem to be wearing down," and "I'm getting holes in my front teeth." Further questioning indicated frequent vomiting to control her weight because "everyone does it."

Nutritional Assessment
- Weight changes
- Oral assessment
- Food, nutrient, and kilocalorie intake
- Awareness of the relationship between health and nutritional intake
- Dietary habits

Nutritional Diagnosis
Consumption of large amounts of high-carbohydrate, low-nutrient foods in a short time, several times a week, followed by regurgitation.

Nutritional Goals
Patient will limit fermentable carbohydrates to reduce the incidence of decay.

Nutritional Implementation
Intervention: Conduct an oral examination to note if any of the following complications are present: trauma to the soft palate, erythematous pharyngeal area, enamel erosion, angular cheilosis, salivary gland enlargement, and xerostomia.
Rationale: These self-inflicted oral complications can indicate to the dental professional the need to investigate further the possibility of an eating disorder in a patient who denies the problem.

Intervention: Discuss effects of frequent vomiting on the oral cavity and appropriate methods to prevent further damage.
Rationale: Not brushing immediately after purging, use of mouth guards during purging, and use of daily fluoride and desensitizing agents are practices Janie is encouraged to adopt to decrease further problems in the oral cavity. Providing such information may be a factor in reducing Janie's vomiting episodes.
Intervention: Become the dental liaison in the medical/psychological healthcare team for this patient.
Rationale: Because of complicated issues involved with an eating disorder, several health disciplines are required to treat patients. The dental hygienist plays a crucial role in overall care of these patients.
Intervention: Discuss specific foods that help to prevent further deterioration of the teeth.
Rationale: Adequate nutrition is essential to support a healthy periodontium and prevents destructive dental activities. Frequent intake of simple carbohydrate foods is a factor in the high caries rate.

Evaluation
The patient is actively seeking treatment for her eating disorder. She plans to achieve small goals as she works toward improving intake of all nutrients and decreasing episodes of bingeing and purging to improve her oral hygiene status.

STUDENT READINESS

1. List ways to make a low-fat diet more appealing. Using favorite foods, create a low-fat diet for yourself for one day.
2. Describe several oral manifestations seen in various systemic diseases that create a painful mouth, making eating difficult and less enjoyable.
3. Identify strategies for a patient who is experiencing (a) nausea and vomiting, (b) bitter or metallic taste in the mouth, (c) chewing and swallowing difficulties, (d) stomatitis, and (e) xerostomia.
4. What factors contribute to anorexia in a patient with HIV/AIDS?
5. What are some cancer treatments, and what oral problems can result from these therapies?

2. Would this patient benefit from nutrition information by the dental hygienist? If so, on what areas should the dental hygienist concentrate?
3. What dietary modifications and dental care instructions would you provide this patient?
4. Create a list of helpful additional resources or agencies to refer this patient.

CASE STUDY

A new patient is seen in the office with complaints of recurrent aphthous ulcers. These ulcers make it very difficult for him to eat, and he has lost about 8 lb. During an oral examination, candidiasis, hairy leukoplakia, and a flat, bluish, nonsymptomatic lesion on the palate, indicative of Kaposi's sarcoma, are noted. HIV/AIDS may be a possible diagnosis.
1. What additional information would you like to obtain from this patient?

References

1. Strauss S, Alfano MC, Shelley D, et al: Identifying unaddressed systemic health conditions at dental visits: patients who visited dental practices but not general health care providers in 2008. *Am J Pub Health* 102(2):253–254, 2012.
2. Methven L, Allen VJ, Withers CA, et al: Ageing and taste. *Proc Nutr Soc* 71(4):556–565, 2012.
3. Solemdal K, Sandvik L, Willumsen T, et al: The impact of oral health on taste ability in acutely hospitalized elderly. *PLoS One* 7(5):e36557, 2012.
4. Desoutter A, Soudain-Pineau M, Munsch F, et al: Xerostomia and medication: a cross-sectional study in long-term geriatric wards. *J Nutr Health Aging* 16(6):575–579, 2012.
5. Shetty SR, Bhowmick S, Castelino R, et al: Drug induced xerostomia in elderly individuals: an institutional study. *Contemp Clin Dent* 3(2):173–175, 2012.
6. Villa A, Abati S: Risk factors and symptoms associated with xerostomia: a cross-sectional study. *Aust Dent J* 56(3):290–295, 2011.
7. Samnieng P, Ueno M, Shinada K, et al: Association of hyposalivation with oral function, nutrition and oral health in

community-dwelling elderly Thai. *Community Dent Health* 29(1):117–123, 2012.

8. Nykänen I, Lönnroos E, Kautiainen H, et al: Nutritional screening in a population-based cohort of community-dwelling older people. *Eur J Public Health* 23(3):405–409, 2013.

9. Soga Y, Yamasuji Y, Kudo C, et al: Febrile neutropenia and periodontitis: lessons from a case periodontal treatment in the intervals between chemotherapy cycles for leukemia reduced febrile neutropenia. *Support Care Cancer* 17(5):581–587, 2009.

10. National Cancer Institute, National Institutes of Health: *Infection.* Last modified October 23, 2012. Accessed September 6, 2013:http://www.cancer.gov/cancertopics/pdq/supportivecare/oralcomplications/HealthProfessional/page7.

11. Mustapha IZ, Debrey S, Oladubu M, et al: Markers of systemic bacterial exposure in periodontal disease and cardiovascular disease risk: a systematic review and meta-analysis. *J Periodontol* 78(12):2289–2302, 2007.

12. Lockhart PB, Bolger AF, Papapanou PN, et al: Periodontal disease and atherosclerotic vascular disease: does the evidence support an independent association?: a scientific statement from the American Heart Association. *Circulation* 125(20):2520–2544, 2012.

13. Otto S, Abu-Id MH, Fedele S, et al: Osteoporosis and bisphosphonates-related osteonecrosis of the jaw: not just a sporadic coincidence—a multi-centre study. *J Craniomaxillofac Surg* 39(4):272–277, 2011.

14. Chustecka Z: *New details on osteonecrosis risk with bisphosphonates: cancer patients using IV forms at greatest risk.* Medscape Medical News, February 24, 2011. Accessed September 6, 2013. http://www.medscape.com/viewarticle/737939.

15. Ibid.

16. Jimenez M, Hu FB, Marino M, et al: Type 2 diabetes mellitus and 20 year incidence of periodontitis and tooth loss. *Diabetes Res Clin Pract* 98(3):494–500, 2012.

17. Haseeb M, Khawaja KI, Ataullah K, et al: Periodontal disease in type 2 diabetes mellitus. *J Coll Physicians Surg Pak* 22(8):514–518, 2012.

18. Lamster IB, Lalla E, Borgnakke WS, et al: The relationship between oral health and diabetes mellitus. *J Am Dental Asssoc* 139(suppl 5):S19–S24, 2008.

19. Ibid.

20. Ibid., Jimenez M, Hu FB, Marino M, et al: 2012.

21. Sutbeyaz Y, Yoruk O, Bilen H, et al: Primary hyperparathyroidism presenting as a palatal and mandibular brown tumor. *J Craniofac Surg* 20(6):2101–2104, 2009.

22. Ferrario VJ, Sforza C, Dellavia C, et al: Facial changes in adult uremic patients on chronic dialysis: possible role of hyperparathyroidism. *Int J Artif Organs* 28(8):797–802, 2005.

23. Dentistry iQ: *Oral health and chronic kidney disease: building a bridge between the dental and renal communities.* Accessed September 6, 2013. http://www.dentistryiq.com/articles/gr/print/volume-2/issue-3/original-article/oral-health-and-chronic-kidney-disease-building-a-bridge-between-the-dental-and-renal-communities.html.

24. Proctor R, Kumar N, Stein A, et al: Oral and dental aspects of chronic renal failure. *J Dent Res* 84(3):199–208, 2005.

25. Ibid.

26. Grover S, Rhodus NL: Dental management of Parkinson's disease. *Northwest Dent* 90(6):13–19, 2011.

27. Dougall A, Fiske J: Access to special care dentistry, part l. Special care dentistry services for older people. *Br Dent J* 205(8):421–424, 2008.

28. Pack AM, Morrell MJ, Randall A, et al: Bone health in young women with epilepsy after one year of antiepileptic drug monotherapy. *Neurology* 70(18):1586–1593, 2008.

29. American Psychiatric Association: *Feeding and eating disorders.* Accessed September 6, 2013: http://www.dsm5.org/Documents/Eating%20Disorders%20Fact%20Sheet.pdf.

30. American Dental Association: *American Dental Association encourages public to get 9screened for oral cancer.* Accessed September 6, 2013: http://www.ada.org/5735.aspx.

31. Oral Cancer Foundation: *Oral cancer facts.* Accessed September 6, 2013. http://oralcancerfoundation.org/facts/index.htm.

32. Li X, Gao L, Li H, et al: Human papillomavirus infection and laryngeal cancer risk: a systematic review and meta-analysis. *J Infect Diseases* 207(3):479–488, 2013.

33. Valentini V, Marazzi F, Bossola M, et al: Nutritional counseling and oral nutritional supplements in head and neck cancer patients undergoing chemoradiotherapy. *J Hum Nutr Diet* 25(3):201–208, 2012.

34. Kiss NK, Krishnasamy M, Loeliger J, et al: A dietitian-led clinic for patients receiving (chemo)radiotherapy for head and neck cancer. *Support Care Cancer* 20(9):2111–2120, 2012.

ⓔ EVOLVE RESOURCES

Please visit http://evolve.elsevier.com/Stegeman/nutritional for additional practice and study support tools.

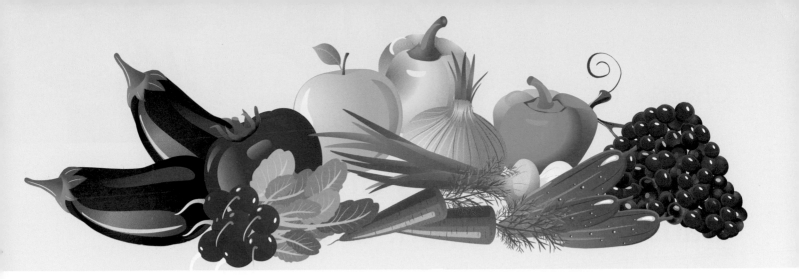

PART III

Nutritional Aspects of Oral Health

18   Nutritional Aspects of Dental Caries: Causes, Prevention,
     and Treatment, 364
19   Nutritional Aspects of Gingivitis and Periodontal Disease, 381
20   Nutritional Aspects of Alterations in the Oral Cavity, 393
21   Nutritional Assessment and Education for Dental Patients, 406

Chapter 18

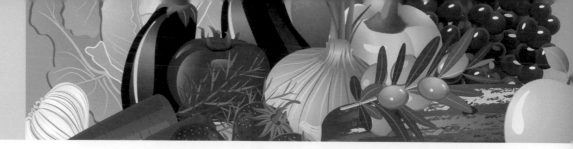

Nutritional Aspects of Dental Caries: Causes, Prevention, and Treatment

Student Learning Outcomes

Upon completion of this chapter, the student will be able to achieve the following student learning outcomes:

- Explain the role each of the following play in the caries process: tooth, saliva, food, and plaque biofilm.
- Identify foods that stimulate salivary flow.
- Suggest food and beverage choices and their timing to reduce the cariogenicity of a patient's diet.

- Describe characteristics of foods having noncariogenic or cariostatic properties.
- Provide nutrition education to a patient at risk for dental caries.

Key Terms

Caries Management by Risk Assessment
Casein

Macrodontia

◉ Test Your NQ

1. **T/F** Cariogenic carbohydrates are the only reason for development of carious lesions.
2. **T/F** Nutrients have a role in the composition and structure of teeth during development.
3. **T/F** Bicarbonates, phosphates, and proteins in saliva dilute and neutralize plaque acids in the mouth.
4. **T/F** Sucrose, fructose, glucose, and maltose have equal potential to cause dental caries.
5. **T/F** Most sugar alcohols, including sorbitol, mannitol, and xylitol, are cariogenic.
6. **T/F** For a tooth to demineralize, the plaque pH needs to be 6 or higher as a result of consuming cariogenic foods.

7. **T/F** The total quantity of sugar is of greatest importance when assessing the patient's diet.
8. **T/F** A fermentable carbohydrate consumed with a meal is less cariogenic than the same food consumed as a snack.
9. **T/F** The revised Recommended Dietary Allowances provide helpful nutrition information for patients trying to reduce dental caries.
10. **T/F** Providing patients with information about the caries process leads to desirable dietary and oral behavior changes.

Nutritional status and oral health have a strong interrelationship. Countless research studies have shown the importance of diet in the development, maintenance, and repair of hard and soft oral tissues. Dental caries is an oral infectious disease that is multifactorial, transmissible, and of bacterial origin (Fig. 18-1).

Diet and nutrients play a role in dental caries. Some foods exert a cariogenic effect, whereas others are cariostatic or anticariogenic and offer protection to reduce caries. Nutrients also have topical and systemic effects, which can be primary or secondary factors in the development of dental caries. However, many factors must be considered if the situation is to be defined as cariogenic. A list of cariogenic foods would be misleading because no food is cariogenic in all situations.

The primary oral health goals of *Healthy People 2020* are to reduce the number of caries in children and adolescents by 10%, and to reduce untreated decay in this population group and adults by 10%.[1] Thirty-three percent of preschool-age children and more than 50% of children and adolescents have experienced decay. Regarding untreated decay, 24% of preschool-age children, 29% of children, 17% of adolescents, and 28% of adults up to age 44 years have at least one untreated area.[1]

Even with advancements in the quality of digital radiography, emerging technology for early detection of caries, improved restorative materials, multiple fluoride options, application of sealants, frequent dental care appointments, dental health education, and increased access to care, dental caries remain the most common chronic childhood disease. Although a remarkable reduction in caries has been observed in school-age children since the 1970s, certain racial, ethnic, and lower-income population groups continue to be problematic. *Healthy People 2020* estimates that only 44.5% of the U.S. population older than age 2 years have had a dental appointment within the past year.[1] Barriers to dental care include cost; lack of dental insurance, public programs, or providers for underserved groups; fear of dentistry; difficulties in accessing services; or poor awareness of the importance of oral health maintenance.

MAJOR FACTORS IN THE DENTAL CARIES PROCESS

No single parameter is responsible for formation of a carious lesion (Fig. 18-2). A combination of factors is involved, including a susceptible host or tooth surface, a sufficient quantity of cariogenic microorganisms in the mouth, the presence of fermentable carbohydrates, and a particular composition or flow of saliva. All of these must be present simultaneously for an adequate time to allow decay to occur.

Tooth Structure

Increasing resistance of the tooth against demineralization begins in the preeruptive phase. It is essential to maintain an adequate intake of nutrients during growth and development of enamel and dentin. The most influential nutrients include calcium; phosphorus; vitamins A, C, and D; fluoride; and protein. Indirectly, some fermentable carbohydrates play a role in the formation of caries before tooth eruption. Consider a child who snacks on cookies, candy, or ice cream throughout the day and is not hungry for meat, vegetables, fruit, and milk offered at mealtime. A child's diet high in low-nutrient (or calorie-dense) carbohydrates may be deficient in required nutrients for optimal growth and development of the dentition. Other factors, such as genetic or metabolic disturbances, can be responsible for poor tooth formation. Dental anomalies include macrodontia (abnormally large teeth) and enamel hypoplasia.

After the tooth erupts, the depth of the natural anatomical pits and fissures and the position of the teeth are relevant factors in the development of dental caries. Deep pits and fissures increase susceptibility for dental caries because of the potential for plaque biofilm and food entrapment. Overlapping and crowding of teeth also offer areas for these materials to collect and ferment, compounded by difficulty of keeping these areas clean.

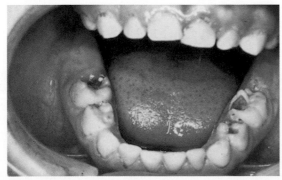

FIGURE 18-1 Dental caries. (Courtesy of Alton McWhorter, DDS, MS, Associate Professor of Pediatric Dentistry, The Texas A&M University System, Baylor College of Dentistry, Dallas, TX.)

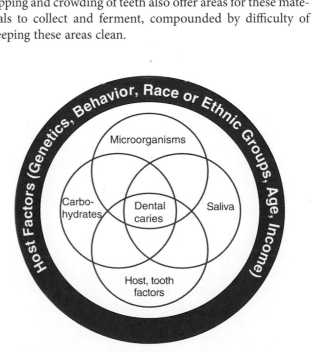

FIGURE 18-2 Major factors that interact in the dental caries process.

Host Factors

Food selection, dietary patterns, oral hygiene habits, genetics, race or ethnicity, age, and income are factors that determine susceptibility to caries.

Saliva

Availability of essential nutrients during the development of salivary glands, which begins during the fourth week in utero, has a significant impact on the amount of saliva and its composition. Of particular importance are vitamin A, iron, and protein, which have a role in normal growth, development, and secretion of saliva.

The protection provided by an adequate salivary flow and buffering capacity of saliva ultimately reduce the destructive capabilities of fermentable carbohydrates on teeth. This fact is recognized in patients with xerostomia, who are at high risk for development of caries because of decreased salivary production.

Saliva provides protection against caries in several ways. First, saliva acts as a buffer by neutralizing much of the acid produced by plaque biofilm as a result of carbohydrate metabolism. Second, normal saliva contains bicarbonate, phosphate, and protein, which dilute and neutralize acids to maintain a neutral oral pH, which is around 7. After an acidic drink is consumed, the pH of the oral cavity is rapidly normalized by the components of saliva. However, if the frequency or duration of the acidic drink is extended, it becomes more difficult for saliva to buffer the continuous supply of acid, and it loses its caries protection.

Particularly important to the prevention of dental caries is the flow of saliva. An adequate salivary flow enables rapid transport of foods from the mouth, decreasing the length of time harmful bacteria and food particles are able to attach to teeth and cause caries to develop. Consumption of citrus fruits (e.g., orange juice and lemonade) promotes saliva formation by means of their citric acid content, so intake needs to be monitored because of the potential to cause enamel erosion.

Because saliva is saturated with calcium, phosphate, and fluoride ions, the potential for remineralization (restoration of damaged enamel) and resistance to enamel dissolution exists. Finally, antimicrobial elements in saliva, such as immunoglobulin A, either interfere with adherence of bacteria or compete with bacteria to attach to the tooth surface. An alkaline saliva offers protection, whereas an acidic saliva increases susceptibility to caries.

Plaque Biofilm and Its Bacterial Components

Plaque biofilm is a complex environment of bacteria, polysaccharides, proteins, and lipids. Plaque biofilm forms a local barrier on enamel and may interfere with demineralization. However, acids produced in plaque biofilm have harmful properties that offset the benefit of its barrier effect.

Composition of plaque biofilm is altered as it matures and is strongly influenced by the diet. As a by-product of the metabolism of sucrose and glucose, bacteria produce acids that lower the pH, resulting in a more favorable environment for development of certain bacteria, such as *Streptococcus mutans*. *S. mutans,* a gram-positive, anaerobic, spherical bacterium, is widely implicated in initiation of dental caries. Other microorganisms, such as bacteria from other mutans streptococci and the *Lactobacillus* species, are capable of fermenting carbohydrates. They also thrive in an acidic environment.

When a carbohydrate has been ingested, its metabolism by salivary amylase begins within 2 to 3 minutes and can persist for hours. The metabolic products are acetic, butyric, formic, lactic, and propionic acids. Concentration of the acids escalates as carbohydrate intake continues, whereas the pH of the plaque decreases. Demineralization of enamel occurs when the "critical pH" of 5.5 is reached. The pH can increase to 6.7 for incipient demineralization of cementum and dentin to occur; this is a real concern for areas of gingival recession. In addition, demineralization is faster on root surfaces than on enamel because dentin contains less mineral content. In interproximal areas or in deep pits and fissures, the pH can decrease to 4 and remain at that pH for an hour. The pH of acids produced by bacteria in plaque biofilm is eventually neutralized after elimination of cariogenic foods as saliva exerts its protective action.

 Dental Considerations

- Evaluate the patient for deep pits and fissures, amount of plaque biofilm in the oral cavity, and composition and flow of saliva. Encourage use of sealants in deep pits and fissures of young patients to prevent plaque biofilm accumulation.
- Encourage meticulous oral hygiene habits, including regular recare visits.
- For patients with a high caries rate, recommend use of chlorhexidine or other antimicrobial agents. Educate the patient that this practice can suppress harmful plaque and organisms. Counsel the patient regarding the potential of chlorhexidine staining teeth.
- Caution parents to avoid sharing utensils with children, a practice allowing transfer of the cariogenic microorganism *S. mutans.*
- Recommend a combination of fluoride sources for patients at high risk for caries. Fluoride in plaque biofilm and saliva inhibit demineralization and enhance remineralization of tooth surfaces.

 Nutritional Directions

- Eating a variety of foods in moderation ensures adequate nutrient intake, and forming healthy eating habits is a factor in growth, development, and maintenance of teeth; prevention of dental caries; and general good health.
- Firm, fibrous foods, such as raw fruits and vegetables; chewing gum; sour foods; and citrus fruits stimulate salivary flow. An increase in the flow rate has a positive impact on resistance of teeth to caries.

Cariogenic Foods

As previously discussed, fermentable carbohydrates are a factor in the development of caries. The average daily consumption from added sugars among 2- to 18-year olds is 365 kcals (over 90 g, or approximately 23 tsp).[2,3] The major sources of added sugars, in descending order, are sugar-sweetened beverages (e.g., sodas or fruit drinks), grain desserts (e.g., cookies or cakes), dairy desserts (e.g., ice cream), candy, and cold cereals.[2-4] Nondiet sports and energy drinks are other fast growing sugar-sweetened beverage choices. Almost 1 in 4 U.S. adults consumes sports and energy drinks at least one time per week.[5] A 20-oz bottle of a regular sports drink contains 32 g of added sugars, a 12-oz can of energy drink contains 37 g, and 12 oz sugar-sweetened soda may contain as much as 40 g sugar.[6]

The small size of sugar molecules allows salivary amylase to split the molecules into components that can be easily metabolized by plaque bacteria. Sucrose is not the only culprit; other monosaccharides and disaccharides, such as fructose, glucose, and maltose, all produce similar amounts of substrate for metabolism by plaque bacteria to produce acid. Sucrose is used to produce glucans, facilitating the adherence of bacteria, such as *S. mutans,* to the dental pellicle. Glucose and other carbohydrates are also used to produce extracellular polysaccharides. Therefore diets containing sucrose, glucose, and other disaccharides can increase plaque biofilm mass and facilitate its retention and colonization. "Natural sugars," such as honey (fructose and glucose), molasses (sucrose and invert sugar), and brown sugar (sugar and molasses), have cariogenic potential similar to sucrose.

Polysaccharides—starchy foods such as rice, potatoes, and corn—are less cariogenic than monosaccharides and disaccharides. Physical and chemical properties of starches are very different from the properties of simple carbohydrates, and render complex carbohydrates less damaging to enamel. In contrast to sucrose, the large number of glucose units needed to form a starch make it almost insoluble. Because starch must be hydrolyzed (split into smaller glucose units) before acid can be produced, the time a starch is in the mouth is usually not long enough for it to be completely metabolized if oral self-care is promptly completed. Normal saliva flow readily neutralizes any acids produced by polysaccharides.

These unique properties prevent starch from providing a readily available energy source for cariogenic microflora, and it is less likely to produce caries than mono- or disaccharides. When starches and simple carbohydrates are combined (as in pastries or sugar-coated cereals), their potential to produce caries is equal to or greater than that of sucrose. Also, processed starches, as found in instant oatmeal, are often more fermentable than their nonprocessed counterparts because of partial hydrolysis or diminution of particle size. The cariogenic activity is also related to the form of starch.

Fresh fruit is another food group of low cariogenicity because of its low percentage of carbohydrate and

> **BOX 18-1   Foods That Can Cause the pH of Human Interproximal Plaque to Fall Below 5.5**
>
> - Alcohol
> - Bananas
> - Beans, baked
> - Bread
> - Candy
> - Cereals, non–presweetened, ready-to-eat
> - Cereals, presweetened, ready-to-eat
> - Chips
> - Cookies
> - Crackers
> - Doughnuts, plain
> - Energy drinks
> - Flavored coffees and teas
> - Fruit, dried
> - Fruit drinks
> - Fruit smoothies
> - Gelatin, flavored
> - Honey
> - Ice cream
> - Jams and jellies
> - Marshmallows
> - Oatmeal, instant cooked
> - Pasta
> - Peanut butter
> - Pretzels
> - Rice, cooked
> - Snack cakes
> - Soft drinks
> - Sports drinks

high percentage of water. Firm fruits such as apples play a protective role by stimulating saliva flow. The high concentration of fructose found in juices is potentially a source of substrate for plaque bacteria that may influence caries risk; this is shown in early childhood caries (formerly known as baby bottle tooth decay), which occurs in children given unlimited amounts of fruit juice and other fermentable carbohydrate beverages. The sticky nature of dried fruit (e.g., raisins) also increases risk of decay. Each of these foods is important in its nutritional value, however, and should not be completely eliminated.

Box 18-1 lists examples of fermentable carbohydrates potentially increasing risk to dental health. The role of the dental hygienist is to know which foods and situations have the potential to be cariogenic, create awareness of the potential harm, and offer suggestions for appropriate consumption of sweetened foods or alternative choices for sugar-containing foods.

Anticariogenic Properties of Food

Sugar Alcohols

Some food components can protect teeth by decreasing demineralization, enhancing remineralization, or increasing salivary flow, even in the presence of a fermentable carbohydrate. Sugar alcohols, such as mannitol and sorbitol, are often used as substitute sweeteners. They are viable alternatives to sugar because of their sweet taste but have the added benefit of being noncariogenic (see Table 4-1 in Chapter 4). Sugar alcohols ferment more slowly in the mouth than monosaccharides and disaccharides; buffering effects of saliva competently neutralize destructive acids produced by plaque bacteria.

Another sugar alcohol, xylitol, is found naturally in plants and is equal to or sweeter than sucrose. Xylitol is classified as anticariogenic because oral flora do not contain enzymes to ferment it, and metabolizing microorganisms, such as *S. mutans,* are inhibited. Chewing gums, mints, and candies containing xylitol inhibit enamel demineralization. This inhibitory effect is enhanced by increased salivary flow, increased oral clearance, and greater buffering capabilities. Compounded by increased mastication, the outcome can be remineralization of incipient decay.

Nonnutritive Sweeteners

Aspartame, saccharin, sucralose, neotame, and acesulfame are a few examples of nonnutritive sweeteners. These sweeteners are not metabolized by microorganisms and do not promote dental caries. Foods made from these sweeteners are generally higher in cost, however, and may not be feasible for low-income patients. Other components of foods using these substitutes, such as raisins, may offset the benefits of using nonnutritive sweeteners to prevent dental caries.

Protein and Fat

Protein and fat are two nutrient classes that may be considered cariostatic because they do not lower plaque pH. Generally, protein may contribute to buffering effects of saliva. Consuming foods with fat and protein following a fermentable carbohydrate may increase plaque pH. Meat, seafood, poultry, eggs, nuts, seeds, margarine, and oils are examples of potentially cariostatic foods.

Phosphorus and Calcium

Phosphorus and calcium also provide qualities protecting against caries. Dispersion of these minerals throughout plaque biofilm may provide a buffering effect, increasing plaque pH. Ultimately, this action curtails demineralization of enamel.

Protein, especially the principal protein in milk, casein, and the minerals phosphorus and calcium. are all ingredients of other anticariogenic—or even cariostatic—foods, such as cheese and milk. Despite the fact lactose is cariogenic (although the least cariogenic of all saccharides), these other elements in milk and dairy products decrease risk of dental caries (Fig. 18-3). Cheese, produced from milk, contains several anticariogenic properties and has the potential to reduce demineralization (or enhance remineralization) of tooth enamel.

An increase of salivary flow occurs when chewing hard cheeses. This increased salivary flow provides a neutral environment and increases clearance of carbohydrates from the oral cavity. Following the *MyPlate* recommendation for the milk and milk products group (using low-fat dairy products) is prudent advice for a dental patient. Eating these foods as snacks or at the end of a meal can provide anticariogenic effects.

Other Foods with Protective Factors

A constituent in chocolate, known as the cocoa factor, has shown anticariogenic properties. The classic Vipeholm study compared the caries rate of individuals consuming chocolate with the rate for individuals consuming other types of "nonchocolate" candies under similar circumstances. The results indicated a slightly lower caries incidence in individuals consuming chocolate.[7]

Glycyrrhiza, the active ingredient in licorice, can also be considered anticariogenic. However, glycyrrhiza is contraindicated with some antihypertensive medications, has a staining capability, and can cause sodium retention and increased blood pressure. Grapefruit and other fruits containing citric acid can stimulate saliva production. However, they are generally not considered noncariogenic because of their ability to lower salivary pH and increase caries risk. Emerging research indicates consumption of cranberries, tea, coffee, wine and probiotics have properties that may interrupt caries formation.[8,9] Probiotics are live bacteria that are beneficial to the host.

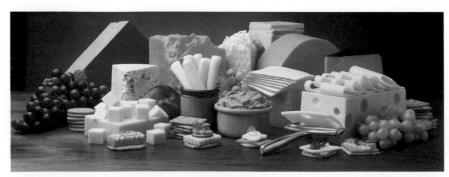

FIGURE 18-3 Milk and dairy products contain anticariogenic properties. (Courtesy of National Dairy Council.)

Dental Considerations

- Educate patients about the caries process and how to prevent demineralization of enamel, including the role diet plays in initiation and progression of decay. Use terms that are appropriate and understandable for the patient.
- Use of topical and systemic fluoride, and products containing adequate levels of xylitol, and application of sealants increase tooth resistance.
- Consider using an antimicrobial agent to control existing plaque biofilm, reduce the number of *S. mutans*, and prevent the formation of new plaque biofilm.

Nutritional Directions

- Using the *Dietary Guidelines* and *MyPlate*, evaluate the patient's diet for adequate nutritional intake and frequency of fermentable carbohydrate consumption.
- Substitute nonnutritive sweeteners for sucrose, if practical. Use aspartame to sweeten coffee and tea instead of table sugar, especially if the beverage is consumed between meals.
- "Natural sugars," such as honey and molasses, are as cariogenic as refined carbohydrates.
- Encourage the consumption of healthy beverages, such as water, skim milk, and vegetable and 100% fruit juices.
- Food sources of probiotics include yogurt, kefir, buttermilk, tempeh, miso, and sauerkraut.
- Educate the patient regarding sports and energy drinks. Although these beverages are promoted to support intense physical activity since they contain electrolytes, vitamins and minerals, remind patients that excessive consumption can lead to dental decay.
- Educate the patient regarding energy drinks. Although these beverages may contain vitamins and minerals, the main ingredients are added sugars and a stimulant (e.g., caffeine). The amount of caffeine varies widely among drinks, but can be as high as 500 mg caffeine/can which is comparable to approximately 14 cans of caffeinated soda. The consumption of energy drinks has been associated with insomnia, nervousness, and headache, and can lead to tachycardia, seizures and cardiac arrest.[5]
- Caution the patient against excessive intake of beverages or other products containing caffeine because of the potential interaction with certain drugs (e.g., bronchodilators, antibacterials, and antipsychotics).[5]
- Caution against frequent use of medications containing fermentable carbohydrates, including antacids and cough drops.
- Increased use of products containing sugar alcohols (e.g., chewing gum, hard candy, dentifrices, and some medications) can cause gastrointestinal distress.
- Although sorbitol and mannitol ferment slowly in the mouth, which allows saliva to neutralize the acids produced, frequent use has the potential to cause caries. This occurs especially in a patient with xerostomia using these products for relief of symptoms.
- Xylitol-containing chewing gums inhibit growth of microorganisms, reducing caries rate. Use of these gums after eating when patients cannot brush is recommended.
- High-sugar foods are generally high in fat as well. *MyPlate* recommends intake of high-sugar and high-fat foods should be limited.
- The *Dietary Guidelines* and *MyPlate* recommend 10% of the total calories to be added sugar. The Institute of Medicine recommends that added sugars should not exceed 25% of the total kilocalories.[10]

- Popular sugar-sweetened beverages include sodas, fruit drinks, sport drinks, energy drinks, chocolate milk, and many vitamin waters.
- Compare some low-fat or nonfat foods that compensate for flavor by increasing sugar or sodium content (e.g., frozen dairy products).
- Exercise caution in recommending high-fat foods for their potential anticariogenic properties to patients with chronic diseases such as heart disease or diabetes mellitus because of their deleterious effects on these conditions.
- Because physical properties of milk are comparable to saliva, increasing low-fat milk intake as a saliva substitute may also offer protection against caries for a patient experiencing xerostomia.
- Encourage proper oral hygiene techniques to avoid complications associated with exposure to the lactose in milk, as seen in early childhood caries.

OTHER FACTORS INFLUENCING CARIOGENICITY

The amount and type of carbohydrates are not the only determinants of food intake that influence caries prevalence and severity. Other considerations include retentiveness of the carbohydrate, how often or how long teeth are exposed, sequence in which a carbohydrate is consumed, and whether food is eaten with a meal or as a snack. Some foods thought to have low cariogenic potential (e.g., cornflakes, crackers, or potato chips) may be more acidogenic than simple-carbohydrate foods because of their retentiveness in embrasures, pits, and fissures. Preventive practices, such as regular recare appointments, appropriate oral hygiene practices, sealants, xylitol, and fluoride use, should also be considered when discussing cariogenicity.

Physical Form

How quickly a cariogenic food is cleared from the mouth is a factor related to caries development. Ingestion of hard candy results in prolonged exposure. A sticky and retentive carbohydrate (e.g., chewy fruit snacks) remains in contact with the enamel surface for a longer period than sweetened fluids. Slow oral clearance of fermentable carbohydrate means longer exposure of the tooth to acid attack.

Fermentable carbohydrates that are chewy, such as caramels, adhere to teeth. However, the additional mastication required to process these foods stimulates saliva flow, making them less retentive and less damaging than dry, sticky foods, such as pretzels. Caramels are higher in sucrose than pretzels, supporting the concept of quantity of fermentable carbohydrates having a limited impact.

Frequency of Intake

Closely related to the physical form of a food in caries potential is frequency of fermentable carbohydrate intake. Longer periods of oral exposure to a fermentable carbohydrate lead to a greater risk of demineralization and less opportunity for teeth to remineralize. Two individuals can eat equal amounts of fermentable carbohydrates, but the one who eats more

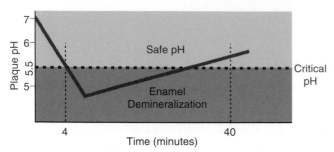

FIGURE 18-4 Stephan curve: time involvement of carbohydrate consumption and enamel demineralization.

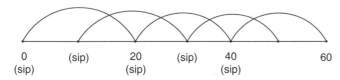

Minutes of acid exposure per sip of soda

FIGURE 18-5 The increased consumption of soft drinks and sports drinks results in an enhanced caries risk. Although oral clearance is rapid, consuming such drinks over an extended time creates a cariogenic environment. If only soda is consumed, each sip results in at least 20 minutes of acid exposure. In this example, the patient took a sip at approximately 10-minute intervals and finished the drink in 5 sips for a total of 60 minutes of acid exposure.

frequently throughout the day has the greatest potential for decay. With each exposure, a decrease in pH begins within 2 to 3 minutes; at a pH of 5.5 or less (the critical pH), enamel decalcification occurs. Within 40 minutes, the pH has increased to its initial value. The classic Stephan curve shows the pH changes of dental plaque after rinsing with a sugar solution (Fig. 18-4). Using a similar scenario, if a person eats a candy bar within a 5-minute period, the teeth would be exposed to a critical pH that lasts for approximately 40 minutes before the pH returns to the original level. If another person eats the same candy bar in five bites, but only takes a bite every hour until it is gone, the total acid exposure would be approximately 200 minutes (5 bites × 40 minutes = 200 minutes of acid exposure).

Frequent consumption of soft drinks, sports drinks, energy drinks, and flavored coffees and teas compounded with a decline in dairy products can also influence caries risk and erosion despite the rapid oral clearance of these beverages (Fig. 18-5). The pH of diet and regular soft drinks, bottled iced teas, and sports drinks ranges from 2.5 to 3.5. Although these drinks are popular snacks, low-fat dairy products, 100% fruit juice, and water are preferable beverage alternatives. Fruit juice should be limited to 4 to 6 oz per day for children 1 to 6 years old and 8 to 12 oz per day for children 7 to 18 years old.[11]

Timing and Sequence in a Meal

Another consideration is whether the cariogenic food is eaten with meals or snacks. Participants in the Vipeholm

---

BOX 18-2   Foods That May Produce Little or No Plaque Acid

- Cheeses*
  - American
  - Blue cheese
  - Brie
  - Cheddar
  - Cheese spread
  - Cream cheese
  - Gouda
  - Monterey jack
  - Mozzarella
  - Swiss
- Yogurt†
- Nuts
- Chewing gum with xylitol
- Cocoa products
- Protein foods‡
  - Meat
  - Seafood
  - Poultry
  - Eggs
- Fats‡
  - Margarine
  - Butter
  - Oils

*These natural cheeses are high in fat. Reduced-fat or low-fat cheeses can be recommended.
†Encourage use of low-fat or skim versions, sugar-free or plain.
‡Follow *MyPlate* and *Dietary Guidelines* for serving sizes and low-fat choices and preparation methods.

study who ate foods high in sugar between meals in addition to mealtime had a significantly higher decay rate than participants who consumed these foods at mealtime only.[7] Despite these results, recommendations to eliminate snacks are not always realistic. Children cannot eat enough food in three meals to get all the nutrients they need, and snacks are warranted. Foods chosen for snacks should produce little or no acid (Box 18-2), and oral self-care should follow a snack.

The location of an acidogenic food within a meal presents another consideration for caries potential. Drinking coffee with sugar after a meal has been determined to lower plaque pH, whereas consuming cheese after a fermentable carbohydrate within a meal prevents the decrease of plaque pH that would occur if this fermentable carbohydrate were eaten alone. Cariogenic foods create less risk of enamel demineralization if followed by a noncariogenic or cariostatic food.

Dental Considerations

- Review diet history for patterns of fermentable carbohydrate consumption, frequency, form, and time consumed.
- Further questioning can reveal dietary habits the patient failed to recognize as being relevant to oral health.

Nutritional Directions

- Consume fermentable carbohydrates at mealtimes (when possible) to allow other foods to neutralize acids in saliva.
- Foods that require chewing (e.g., chewing gum, raw fruits and vegetables) help increase salivary flow. This aids in providing additional buffering effects and accelerated removal of retentive foods.
- Noncariogenic snacks include raw fruits and vegetables, low-fat cheese, skim milk, low-fat yogurt, peanuts, popcorn, whole-grain bagels, seeds, pizza, and tacos.
- Cariogenic snacks before bedtime should be omitted or followed by careful oral hygiene. Salivary flow is reduced when sleeping; clearance of plaque acids is limited. Uninterrupted acid production for 2 hours can be harmful.
- Consume fermentable carbohydrates within a meal, or eat a noncariogenic food last.
- Carbohydrate foods that are retentive (e.g., graham crackers or potato chips) are retained in the mouth longer, creating a greater potential for decay.
- Products made with a nonnutritive sweetener, such as aspartame or sucralose, should be used in moderation (two to three products per day). Some patients may not tolerate large amounts of aspartame or other nonnutritive sweetener, or choose not to use them. Recommend alternative noncariogenic food items and oral self-care.
- Encourage the patient to limit purchasing soft drinks and sports and energy drinks in large, resealable containers in an effort to decrease the frequency and duration of consumption.
- Athletes require fluid for hydration. In most events lasting less than 4 hours, water is the preferred source of hydration rather than high-carbohydrate sports drinks.

BOX 18-3   Situations Presenting High Caries Risk

Early Childhood Caries
- Parents before pregnancy
- Parents during pregnancy
- Parents of young children

Root Caries and Xerostomia
- Older adults
- Periodontal patients
- Chronic disease states, e.g., diabetes mellitus, chronic renal disease
- Polypharmacy
- Radiation therapy
- Gingival recession

Habits
- Frequent use of hard candy or chewing gum, cough drops, chew tobacco, medication containing a fermentable carbohydrate source
- Frequent vomiting
- Poor oral hygiene
- Patients with orthodontic appliances
- Adolescents
- Patients with dexterity challenges

Dental Issues
- Intake of low-fluoridation or nonfluoridated water
- Unsealed deep pits and fissures
- Family history of high caries risk
- Levels of cariogenic bacteria

DENTAL PLAN

Providing nutrition information is an essential component of the preventive program. Although all patients benefit from nutrition education, certain populations (Box 18-3) require special attention by the dental hygienist. As mentioned, the quantity of fermentable carbohydrates consumed is of concern, especially nutritionally. However, the form of the carbohydrate, how often it is consumed, and whether it is eaten with meals or snacks, are more important for oral health than the amount consumed.

Assessment

When a dental nutrition care plan is necessary, many factors must be considered. Anthropometric measures (i.e., height and weight), clinical signs, dental and dietary assessment, health and dental history, and laboratory data (if applicable) are addressed in Chapter 21. In addition, an assessment takes into account a patient's learning style, literacy level, cultural heritage, and socioeconomic status.

Caries Management by Risk Assessment is a popular protocol used by dental professionals to identify risk of caries and to determine preventive and therapeutic goals for both children and adult patients. Figures 18-6 and 18-7

show risk forms, approved by the American Dental Association and the American Academy of Pediatric Dentistry, differentiated by age. The patient or caregiver can answer the questions prior to the dental appointment or upon arrival at the dental office. The first step is to identify disease indicators (e.g., low income), caries risk factors (e.g., frequent snacks), and caries protective factors (e.g., use of products with xylitol) along with the clinical evaluation (e.g., number of existing restorations). Note that the age 6-to-adult form (Fig. 18-6) includes identification of medications associated with xerostomia while the 0-to-6 years form (Fig. 18-7) highlights acid exposure associated with childhood caries, such as the availability of bottles or sippy cups between meals or in the bed. The second step is to create and implement a treatment plan of action based on the risk outcome. The risk form can be used as a pedagogical tool by the dental professional to educate the patient. Risk factors are color coded for ease in explanation. For example, green designates *low risk*. A risk score can be obtained and compared to future risk forms. Detailed instructions on use of the form and educating patients are available on the American Dental Association website. Accompanying patient education material and sources are also provided.

Caries Risk Assessment Form (Age >6)

ADA American Dental Association®
America's leading advocate for oral health

Patient Name:

Birth Date: | **Date:**

Age: | **Initials:**

		Low Risk	Moderate Risk	High Risk
	Contributing Conditions	Check or Circle the conditions that apply		
I.	**Fluoride Exposure** (through drinking water, supplements, professional applications, toothpaste)	☐Yes	☐No	
II.	**Sugary Foods or Drinks** (including juice, carbonated or non-carbonated soft drinks, energy drinks, medicinal syrups)	Primarily at mealtimes ☐		Frequent or prolonged between meal exposures/day ☐
III.	**Caries Experience of Mother, Caregiver and/or other Siblings** (for patients ages 6-14)	No carious lesions in last 24 months ☐	Carious lesions in last 7-23 months ☐	Carious lesions in last 6 months ☐
IV.	**Dental Home**: established patient of record, receiving regular dental care in a dental office	☐Yes	☐No	
	General Health Conditions	Check or Circle the conditions that apply		
I.	**Special Health Care Needs** (developmental, physical, medical or mental disabilities that prevent or limit performance of adequate oral health care by themselves or caregivers)	☐No	Yes (over age 14) ☐	Yes (ages 6-14) ☐
II.	**Chemo/Radiation Therapy**	☐No		☐Yes
III.	**Eating Disorders**	☐No	☐Yes	
IV.	**Medications that Reduce Salivary Flow**	☐No	☐Yes	
V.	**Drug/Alcohol Abuse**	☐No	☐Yes	
	Clinical Conditions	Check or Circle the conditions that apply		
I.	**Cavitated or Non-Cavitated** (incipient) **Carious Lesions or Restorations** (visually or radiographically evident)	No new carious lesions or restorations in last 36 months ☐	1 or 2 new carious lesions or restorations in last 36 months ☐	3 or more carious lesions or restorations in last 36 months ☐
II.	**Teeth Missing Due to Caries in past 36 months**	☐No		☐Yes
III.	**Visible Plaque**	☐No	☐Yes	
IV.	**Unusual Tooth Morphology** that compromises oral hygiene	☐No	☐Yes	
V.	**Interproximal Restorations - 1 or more**	☐No	☐Yes	
VI.	**Exposed Root Surfaces** Present	☐No	☐Yes	
VII.	**Restorations with Overhangs** and/or **Open Margins**; **Open Contacts** with Food Impaction	☐No	☐Yes	
VIII.	**Dental/Orthodontic Appliances** (fixed or removable)	☐No	☐Yes	
IX.	**Severe Dry Mouth (Xerostomia)**	☐No		☐Yes

Overall assessment of dental caries risk: ☐ Low   ☐ Moderate   ☐ High

Patient Instructions:

FIGURE 18-6 Caries Risk Assessment form for ages 6 to adult. (American Dental Association. Accessed September 11, 2013. Available at: http://www.ada.org/sections/professionalResources/pdfs/topic_caries_over6.pdf)

ADA American Dental Association®
America's leading advocate for oral health

Caries Risk Assessment Form (Age >6)

Circle or check the boxes of the conditions that apply. Low Risk = only conditions in "Low Risk" column present; Moderate Risk = only conditions in "Low" and/or "Moderate Risk" columns present; High Risk = one or more conditions in the "High Risk" column present.

The clinical judgment of the dentist may justify a change of the patient's risk level (increased or decreased) based on review of this form and other pertinent information. For example, missing teeth may not be regarded as high risk for a follow up patient; or other risk factors not listed may be present.

The assessment cannot address every aspect of a patient's health, and should not be used as a replacement for the dentist's inquiry and judgment. Additional or more focused assessment may be appropriate for patients with specific health concerns. As with other forms, this assessment may be only a starting point for evaluating the patient's health status.

This is a tool provided for the use of ADA members. It is based on the opinion of experts who utilized the most up-to-date scientific information available. The ADA plans to periodically update this tool based on: 1) member feedback regarding its usefulness, and; 2) advances in science. ADA member-users are encouraged to share their opinions regarding this tool with the Council on Dental Practice.

FIGURE 18-6, cont'd

Gathering information about the quality of the patient's meal pattern and eating habits is an important step in assessing the cariogenic potential of a diet. A food diary (Fig. 18-8), which provides food data for one day, can be obtained through an interview by the dental hygienist, or the patient can be asked to return the completed form at a recare appointment. This practical assessment tool is helpful in determining adequacy of the overall diet and habits related to carbohydrate intake. Several food records are available on the Internet. Choose one that meets the needs of the dental environment. Figure 18-9 shows a second example of a food diary.

Using *MyPlate* as a guide, the dental hygienist can review adequacy of food intake with participation of the patient. Actively involving the patient in as many steps as possible enhances motivation and adherence. Ask the patient to highlight all fermentable carbohydrates on the food diary (Figs. 18-8 and 18-9). Review the food diary, and discuss any oversights with the patient as needed. Classify each fermentable carbohydrate as cariogenic or noncariogenic to assess caries potential (Fig. 18-10). This classification requires identifying the carbohydrate according to its form, frequency of consumption, and when it was eaten. More than two hours of acid exposure in one day is generally considered high.

Goals

When all the facts are gathered, help the patient develop realistic goals. These goals need to be flexible to meet the patient's needs, preferences, and lifestyle. Achievement of long-term goals is possible only if the patient is able and motivated to make behavioral changes, such as altering choices of cariogenic snacks or limiting frequency of cariogenic foods.

Education

Providing current information about detrimental dietary habits is instrumental in determining appropriate goals. Education alone does not guarantee behavioral change. For example, a patient may recite the process of decay and list components responsible for caries development, but if several areas of decay are evident at each 6-month recare visit, change has not occurred. Individualize dietary advice based on the patient's lifestyle, rather than requesting a change in lifestyle to accommodate recommendations. The patient's assessment and goals are the basis for any recommendations. The dental professional should attempt to dispel myths, redirect inappropriate habits, and provide new thoughts.

ADA American Dental Association®
America's leading advocate for oral health

Caries Risk Assessment Form (Age 0-6)

Patient Name:

Birth Date: Date:

Age: Initials:

		Low Risk	Moderate Risk	High Risk
	Contributing Conditions	Check or Circle the conditions that apply		
I.	**Fluoride Exposure** (through drinking water, supplements, professional applications, toothpaste)	☐ Yes	☐ No	
II.	**Sugary Foods or Drinks** (including juice, carbonated or non-carbonated soft drinks, energy drinks, medicinal syrups)	Primarily at mealtimes ☐	Frequent or prolonged between meal exposures/day ☐	Bottle or sippy cup with anything other than water at bed time ☐
III.	**Eligible for Government Programs** (WIC, Head Start, Medicaid or SCHIP)	☐ No		☐ Yes
IV.	**Caries Experience of Mother, Caregiver and/or other Siblings**	No carious lesions in last 24 months ☐	Carious lesions in last 7-23 months ☐	Carious lesions in last 6 months ☐
V.	**Dental Home**: established patient of record in a dental office	☐ Yes	☐ No	
	General Health Conditions	Check or Circle the conditions that apply		
I.	**Special Health Care Needs** (developmental, physical, medical or mental disabilities that prevent or limit performance of adequate oral health care by themselves or caregivers)	☐ No		☐ Yes
	Clinical Conditions	Check or Circle the conditions that apply		
I.	**Visual or Radiographically Evident Restorations/Cavitated Carious Lesions**	No new carious lesions or restorations in last 24 months ☐		Carious lesions or restorations in last 24 months ☐
II.	**Non-cavitated** (incipient) **Carious Lesions**	No new lesions in last 24 months ☐		New lesions in last 24 months ☐
III.	**Teeth Missing Due to Caries**	☐ No		☐ Yes
IV.	**Visible Plaque**	☐ No	☐ Yes	
V.	**Dental/Orthodontic Appliances Present** (fixed or removable)	☐ No	☐ Yes	
VI.	**Salivary Flow**	Visually adequate ☐		Visually inadequate ☐

Overall assessment of dental caries risk: ☐ Low   ☐ Moderate   ☐ High

Instructions for Caregiver:

FIGURE 18-7 Caries Risk Assessment form for up to age 6 years. (American Dental Association. Accessed September 11, 2013. Available at: http://www.ada.org/sections/professionalResources/pdfs/topics_caries_under6.pdf)

Circle or check the boxes of the conditions that apply. Low Risk = only conditions in "Low Risk" column present; Moderate Risk = only conditions in "Low" and/or "Moderate Risk" columns present; High Risk = one or more conditions in the "High Risk" column present.

The clinical judgment of the dentist may justify a change of the patient's risk level (increased or decreased) based on review of this form and other pertinent information. For example, missing teeth may not be regarded as high risk for a follow up patient; or other risk factors not listed may be present.

The assessment cannot address every aspect of a patient's health, and should not be used as a replacement for the dentist's inquiry and judgment. Additional or more focused assessment may be appropriate for patients with specific health concerns. As with other forms, this assessment may be only a starting point for evaluating the patient's health status.

This is a tool provided for the use of ADA members. It is based on the opinion of experts who utilized the most up-to-date scientific information available. The ADA plans to periodically update this tool based on: 1) member feedback regarding its usefulness, and; 2) advances in science. ADA member-users are encouraged to share their opinions regarding this tool with the Council on Dental Practice.

FIGURE 18-7, cont'd

Food Diary

Day _____

Time	Place	Food Eaten	Amount Eaten	How Prepared
Example: 6:00 A.M.	Kitchen	Orange juice Whole wheat bread Diet margarine Egg	1/2 c 2 slices 1 tsp 1	Unsweetened Toasted Tub Fried in oil

Instructions:
1. List EVERYTHING you eat or drink on 3 consecutive, typical days.
2. Use 2 weekdays and 1 weekend day.
3. Include extras such as chewing gum, sugar and cream in coffee, or mustard on a sandwich.

FIGURE 18-8 Food diary. Typically used for 1 to 7 days. (A customizable version is available on Evolve.)

Daily Food and Activity Diary

	Monday	Tuesday	Wednesday	Thursday	Friday	Saturday	Sunday
Breakfast							
Lunch							
Dinner							
Activity							

GOALS: DIET   **PHYSICAL ACTIVITY**

BEHAVIOR

FIGURE 18-9 Another example of a food diary. (U.S. Department of Health and Human Services. National Heart, Lung and Blood Institute. Accessed September 11, 2013. Available at: http://www.nhlbi.nih.gov/health/public/heart/obesity/lose_wt/diary.pdf)

Carbohydrate Intake Analysis Worksheet

Fermentable CHO	Cariogenic?	Reason	Period of Exposure to Enamel
Banana and coffee with sugar	Yes	2 carbohydrates eaten at the same time; banana is retentive.	40 minutes
Pizza and regular soda (consumed together)	No	If soda is consumed with meal, carbohydrates in pizza (crust, sauce) and soda will be neutralized by fat and protein of other components of pizza.	0 minutes
Pizza and regular soda (consumed separately)	Yes	If consumption of soda is continued after the meal, there are no components to neutralize the carbohydrates in the soda.	20 minutes

TOTAL EXPOSURE TIME: _____

FIGURE 18-10 Example of a carbohydrate intake analysis. (A customizable version is available on Evolve.)

HEALTH APPLICATION 18   Genetically Modified Foods

Genetically modified organisms (GMOs) consist of taking genetic material (DNA) from one plant, animal, or microorganism and inserting it into the permanent genetic code of another. This technology is also referred to as "genetic engineering" and "biotechnology."

The first genetically modified (GM) food, introduced in the mid-1990s, was herbicide-resistant soybeans. Currently, more than 85% of corn, soybeans, cotton, and sugar beets in the United States are genetically engineered. Additionally, other GM plants include quinoa, canola (rapeseed), rice, potatoes, and bananas. While the United States is the leading producer of GM foods, developing countries are planting GM crops at a more rapid rate than rich countries. Currently GM foods are mostly plants, but foods derived from GM microorganisms or GM animals may be introduced in the near future. Very few fresh fruits and vegetables are GM, but highly processed foods, such as vegetable oils or breakfast cereals, most likely contain some percentage of GM ingredients.

GM plants are modified in the laboratory and marketed because of a perceived advantage either to the farmer or consumer, such as lower price, improved durability, or nutritional value. The purposes of genetic engineering are to (a) speed growth, (b) resist disease, (c) repel insects, (d) withstand harsh growing conditions, and (e) improve nutritional quality. The world faces serious problems in feeding 9 billion people by 2050. Agriculture production must be increased and ecosystem services maintained at a time when conditions for growing crops are predicted to worsen in many parts of the world.[12]

Malnutrition in developing countries is a consequence of a dearth of certain vitamins in staple foods, losses during crop processing, and overreliance on a single primary food source. Golden Rice is a GM rice that provides vitamin A. The beta-carotene in this rice is effectively converted to vitamin A and can be used to improve the vitamin A status of young children in developing countries.[13]

Insect resistance is accomplished by incorporating the gene for a toxin from the bacterium *Bacillus thuringiensis*. This toxin, used as a conventional insecticide in agriculture, is safe for human consumption. Viral resistance makes plants less susceptible to diseases caused by viruses, resulting in higher crop production. The potential for GM seeds to result in bigger yields should lead to lower prices.

A systematic review of 24 studies of GM foods found no statistically significant differences or any health hazards in animal feeding trials.[14] Overall, peer-reviewed studies on GM food safety have not found significant health risks, with few exceptions. A couple of studies indicated health risks, but these were disregarded by the scientific community because of incorrect experimental designs and statistical analysis.[15,16]

On the other hand, altering the genetic makeup of plants and animals has been very controversial with concerns from many experts about the long-term effects on humans and the environment. Some of the concerns voiced include the potential for GM foods to cause (a) organ damage, (b) disrupt endocrine functions, (c) decrease fertility, (d) increase allergies, (e) increase pesticide resistance, (f) accelerate aging, and (g) promote immune system disorders. Indeed, no studies have tracked the long-term effect GMOs may have on humans.

The main issues widely debated are the potential for GM foods to provoke allergic reaction, gene transfer, and cross contamination. In response to the allegation that GM crops may increase allergenicity, foods that are considered highly allergenic are highly discouraged in producing GM products. When foods are digested and absorbed, a possibility exists that the genes can transfer through the digestive system, increasing antibiotic resistance and pesticide residues in the body. The World Health Organization indicates the probability of transfer occurring is low, but using technology without antibiotic-resistant genes has been encouraged by an expert World Health Organization panel.[17] Some are fearful that modified plants or animals may have genetic changes that are unexpected and harmful. Some are concerned that the protein that was intended to be created during the manufacturing process may be different than what is actually created. Any minor error in a DNA sequence could cause various unintended effects and health issues.

A few of the concerns are legitimate. Whereas GM technology was supposed to decrease the need for pesticides to fight weeds and insects, herbicides in the production of three GM crops (cotton, soybeans, and corn) has actually increased approximately 25%.[18] Resistant weeds have become a major problem for farmers using GM seeds. Genes from GM plants have cross-pollinated into conventional crops or related wild species as well as mixing with crops derived from conventional seeds with those grown using GM crops. This occurred when traces of maize approved for animals appeared in maize products produced for human consumption in the United States.[19]

The United States and Canada modified existing regulatory statutes to control GM foods. In the United States, three different government agencies have jurisdiction of GM foods. The U.S. Environmental Protection Agency (EPA) evaluates GM plants for environmental safety. The U.S. Department of Agriculture evaluates whether the plant is safe to grow; they are concerned with potential hazards of the plant itself. They ensure that the function of the introduced gene is known, and the gene does not cause plant disease. The FDA evaluates whether the plant is safe to eat. The FDA has no control over the production of corn, but they regulate a box of cornflakes because it is a food product. To the FDA, GM foods are substantially equivalent to unmodified, "natural" foods, and are not subject to FDA regulations. Companies who create new GM foods are not required to consult the FDA, nor are they required to follow any recommendations made by the FDA.

In contrast, many European countries have strict restrictions on growing GM crops, but they allow importation of GM foods. Despite strong consumer concerns, the European Food Safety Authority recently declared that GMOs pose no health risks.[20]

GM foods currently available have passed risk assessments and are not likely to present risks for human health. Conversely, there is little scientific data tracking the long-term effects GMOs may have on humans, and the information available does not ensure complete safety. It is possible that GM foods may cause unexpected health consequences that will not be evident for years. Furthermore, it is impossible to design a long-term safety test in humans. Each new GM food should be assessed on an individual basis before being allowed on the market. General statements regarding the safety of all GM foods are inappropriate.

Most Americans would prefer that GM foods be labeled. Very low concentrations of GMOs in foods often cannot be detected. Proponents of labeling genetically engineered foods

Continued

HEALTH APPLICATION 18   Genetically Modified Foods—cont'd

feel consumers have a right to know where products come from when making food purchases. If all GM foods and food products are to be labeled, Congress must enact sweeping changes in the existing food labeling policy, and establish acceptable limits of GM contamination in non-GM products. Labeling is mandatory in the European Union. Organic foods do not contain GM products.

There are many challenges for GM products, in the areas of safety testing, regulation, international policy, and food labeling. This technology has enormous potential benefits, but caution is needed to avoid causing unintended harm to human health and the environment.

Case Application for the Dental Hygienist

At his 6-month recare visit, John S. presented with six new areas of decay: one occlusal area (class I carious lesion), two proximal surfaces of posterior teeth (class II), and three proximal surfaces of anterior teeth (class III). There is bleeding on probing, suggesting active periodontal disease. John admits his busy schedule prevents him from flossing his teeth. He stopped smoking and replaced it with chewing gum and hard candy since his last appointment. When asked about work, John states he takes antacids to settle his stomach because of added pressures of his job.

Nutritional Assessment
- Food, nutrient, and caloric intake
- Frequency of eating between meals
- Eating habits
- Motivation level
- Knowledge level

Nutritional Diagnosis
Altered nutrition: frequent intake of chewing gum, hard candy, and antacids at various intervals throughout the day compounded by an increased plaque index, a measure of the quantity and location of plaque biofilm.

Nutritional Goals
The patient will improve his overall nutrient intake and make substitutions or modify the habits increasing his caries risk.

Nutritional Implementation
Intervention: Provide a food diary (see Figs. 18-8 and 18-9) with an explanation for its use and instructions emphasizing the importance of listing everything put into his mouth.
Rationale: The food record provides additional information about John's intake and reveals habits that he may have neglected to mention, thinking they were not relevant to his dental needs.
Intervention: Review the food record with John to identify health aspects and aspects needing revision. Allow John to make the necessary changes.
Rationale: The probability of a patient adhering to a recommended regimen is enhanced when the patient is actively involved in the decision-making process. The dental hygienist can suggest possible solutions and direct misguided changes. The patient ultimately makes required changes.
Intervention: Explain the caries process, factors involved, and that several of the carious lesions are in places usually unaffected.
Rationale: Understanding the total picture of his particular dental status can be motivating for John and may help him make needed changes.

Intervention: Stress that not only the quantity of fermentable carbohydrates in his diet, but also spacing, duration, frequency, and form of intake lead to caries. Use the example, Carbohydrate Intake Analysis (see Fig. 18-10) as an educational tool to enhance the explanation.
Rationale: Each time the patient consumes a fermentable carbohydrate, even if it is a small mint, he is decreasing the plaque pH to an acidic level for 40 minutes. By consuming sugar-containing mints six times throughout the day, the acid produced by plaque bacteria may be present for 4 hours.
Intervention: Educate John about the cariogenic potential of sugar-containing antacids, and discuss options to avoid or reduce use of antacids. Another option may be to use sugar-free antacids, although his condition should be evaluated by his healthcare provider if it persists.
Rationale: Sugar-containing antacids contain simple carbohydrates and have cariogenic potential. Antacids are high in sodium and can interfere with absorption of many nutrients. Suggestions to decrease use of antacids include consuming small, frequent meals; eating slowly; avoiding excessive amounts of caffeine products and alcohol; and reducing stress. Referral to the healthcare provider is necessary for persistent heartburn to ensure diagnosis and management of gastroesophageal reflux, which may increase the risk for caries and dental erosion and esophageal cancer.
Intervention: Praise John for his ability to quit smoking. (See Chapter 19, *Health Application 19*).
Rationale: Smoking is a very difficult habit to break; many who stop smoking will start again, especially in stressful situations.
Intervention: Recommend fluoride treatments in the office and at home; sealants, if applicable; an antimicrobial rinse; and optimum oral self-care practices.
Rationale: Omitting the carbohydrate source is not the only factor involved in the caries process. In John's situation, protecting susceptible tooth surfaces and removing plaque biofilm also serve to eliminate the potential for caries.

Evaluation
The patient returns for his 6-month recare appointment caries-free with a reduction in gingival bleeding. He is still not smoking and uses a chewing gum and mints with xylitol. He has begun an exercise program, which is helping to relieve his stress, and he has decreased his use of antacids.

STUDENT READINESS

1. Explain the role of firm, fibrous foods in protecting the tooth against caries.

2. List several noncariogenic substitutions for fermentable carbohydrate snacks.

3. What are the different roles carbohydrates, protein, and fat play in the decay process?

4. Identify at least four nutritional foods contraindicated for a caries-active patient.

5. Complete a 1- to 3-day food diary (see Fig. 18-8). Assess for nutrient adequacy, comparing it with *MyPlate*. Highlight the fermentable carbohydrates.

6. Based on the food diary from question 5, complete the example Carbohydrate Intake Analysis worksheet (see Fig. 18-10). Determine your cariogenic behaviors and the number of minutes of acid production. Based on this intake record, create a realistic and appropriate meal pattern. Discuss the rationale for modifications and substitutions.

7. Compare the pH, grams of sugar and mg of caffeine for an 8-oz serving of 100% apple juice, skim milk, an energy drink, a sports drink, soda, a fruit drink, and water. Provide a conclusion based on your findings.

CASE STUDY

Carol is a 42-year-old married high school graduate with three teenage children. She is a homemaker and does all the cooking and grocery shopping. Each member of Carol's family continues to have new areas of decay at each recare visit. The dental hygienist decides to have Carol write down her food consumption from the previous day while waiting for her appointment. Her food record showed the following:

Breakfast: skipped

Morning snack: glazed doughnut, coffee with cream and sugar

Lunch: grilled cheese sandwich, taco chips, gelatin salad with fruit and whipped cream, coffee with cream and sugar

Afternoon snack: candy bar and two or three homemade cookies throughout the afternoon

Dinner: meat loaf, fried potatoes, buttered carrots, roll with margarine

Evening snack: chocolate chip ice cream

1. What other information needs to be obtained before starting to educate the patient?
2. What dental information does Carol need to have?
3. What dietary recommendations should a dental hygienist suggest? What are some specific substitutions and modifications that can be made?
4. Approximately how many minutes of acid production occurred on the enamel surfaces this day?

CASE STUDY

As a new mother, Barbara wanted to take precautionary measures to prevent her daughter from having rampant dental decay like the neighborhood children. She breastfed the infant until 9 months of age and refused to allow any sugar-containing foods, including ice cream. The daughter was frequently observed carrying a box of crackers and her sippy cup around the house. By age 3, she has six caries.

1. When should nutrition education have first been initiated for Barbara? Explain.
2. Describe the procedure a dental professional would take to educate Barbara.
3. What suggestions would you recommend?

References

1. U.S. Department of Health and Human Services: *Healthy People 2020: Last updated October 30, 2012*. Accessed September 11, 2013. Available at: http://www.healthypeople.gov/2020/default.aspx.

2. Han E, Powell LM: Consumption patterns of sugar-sweetened beverages in the United States. *J Acad Nutr Diet* 113(1):43–53, 2013.

3. Reedy J, Krebs-Smith SM: Dietary sources of energy, solid fats, and added sugars among children and adolescents in the United States. *J Am Diet Assoc* 110(10):1477–1484, 2010.

4. Kosova EC, Auinger P, Bremer AA: The relationships between sugar-sweetened beverage intake and cariometabolic markers in young children. *J Acad Nutr Diet* 113(2):219–227, 2013.

5. Park S, Onufrak S, Blanck HM, et al: Characteristics associated with consumption of sports and energy drinks among US adults: National Health Interview Survey, 2010. *J Acad Nutr Diet* 113(1):112–119, 2013.

6. U.S. Department of Agriculture. Agricultural Research Service: *USDA national nutrient database for standard reference, release 26*. 2013, Nutrient Data Laboratory. Accessed September 10, 2013. Available at: http://ndb.nal.usda.gov/.

7. Gustaffson BE, Quensel CE, Lanke LS, et al: The Vipeholm dental caries study: the effect of different levels of carbohydrate intake on caries activity in 436 individuals observed for 5 years. *Acta Odontol Scand* 11:232–364, 1954.

8. Van Loveren C, Broukal Z, Oganessian E: Functional foods/ingredients and dental caries. *Eur J Nutr* 52(Suppl 2):S15–S25, 2012.

9. Chuang LC, Huang CS, Ou-Yang LW, et al: Probiotic *Lactobacillus paracasei* effect on cariogenic bacterial flora. *Clin Oral Investig* 15(4):471–476, 2011.

10. Institute of Medicine: *Dietary reference intakes for energy, carbohydrates, fiber, fat, fatty acids, cholesterol, protein, and amino acids (macronutrients)*. Washington, DC, 2005, National Academies Press.

11. American Academy of Pediatrics, Committee on Nutrition: The use and misuse of fruit juice in pediatrics. *Pediatrics* 107(5):1210–1213, 2001.

12. Raybould A, Poppy GM: Commercializing genetically modified crops under EU regulations: objectives and barriers. *GM Crops Food* 3(1):9–20, 2012.

13. Tang G, Qin J, Dolnikowski GG, et al: Golden Rice is an effective source of vitamin A. *Am J Clin Nutr* 89(6):1776–1783, 2009.

14. Snell C, Bernheim A, Bergé JB, et al: Assessment of the health impact of GM plant diets in long-term and multigenerational

animal feeding trials: a literature review. *Food Chem Toxicol* 50(3-4):1134–1148, 2012.

15. Martinelli L, Karbarz M, Siipi H: Science, safety, and trust: the case of transgenic food. *Croat Med J* 54(1):91–96, 2013.

16. Arjó G, Portero M, Piñol C, et al: Plurality of opinion, scientific discourse and pseudoscience: an in depth analysis of the Séralini et al. study claiming the Roundup™ Ready corn or the herbicide Roundup™ Ready cause cancer in rats. *Transgenic Res* 22(2):255–267, 2013.

17. World Health Organization: *Food safety—20 questions on genetically modified foods.* Accessed September 6, 2013. Available at: http://www.who.int/foodsafety/publications/biotech/20questions/en/.

18. Benbrook CM: Impacts of genetically engineered crops on pesticide use in the U.S.–the first sixteen years. *Environ Sci Eur* 24:24, 2012.

19. World Health Organization: *Food safety—20 questions on genetically modified foods.* Accessed September 6, 2013. Available at: http://www.who.int/foodsafety/publications/biotech/20questions/en/.

20. Kupferschmidt K: Amid Europe's food fights, EFSA keeps its eyes on the evidence. *Science* 338(6111):1146–1147, 2012.

ⓔ EVOLVE RESOURCES

Please visit http://evolve.elsevier.com/Stegeman/nutritional for additional practice and study support tools.

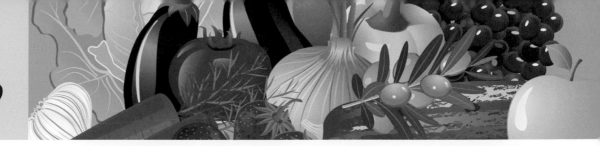
Nutritional Aspects of Gingivitis and Periodontal Disease

Student Learning Outcomes

Upon completion of this chapter, the student will be able to achieve the following student learning outcomes:

- Describe the role nutrition plays in periodontal health and disease to a patient.
- List the effects of food consistency and composition in periodontal disease.
- Describe nutritional factors associated with gingivitis and periodontitis.

- Discuss components of nutritional education for a periodontal patient.
- List major differences between full liquid, mechanically altered, bland, and regular diets.

Key Terms

Clinical attachment loss
Fibrotic
Full liquid diet

Mechanically altered diet
Purulent exudates
Suppuration

 Test Your NQ

1. **T/F** Vitamin-mineral supplementation beyond recommended levels is ineffective in controlling or preventing periodontal disease.
2. **T/F** Firm, fibrous foods physically remove plaque biofilm from the gingiva and tooth surface.
3. **T/F** A deficiency of vitamin C causes gingivitis.
4. **T/F** A bland, soft diet is commonly prescribed for a patient with necrotizing ulcerative gingivitis (NUG)/necrotizing ulcerative periodontitis (NUP).
5. **T/F** An appropriate instruction to a patient after periodontal surgery is, "Eat whatever foods you can manage."
6. **T/F** An individual with uncontrolled diabetes should be referred to a registered dietitian nutritionist for nutrition counseling if the diet needs to be modified because of oral discomfort, such as with NUG/NUP or after a periodontal procedure.

7. **T/F** Whole milk and milkshakes mixed with an instant breakfast mix are acceptable on a full liquid diet.
8. **T/F** A mechanically altered diet is similar to a regular diet except in consistency and texture.
9. **T/F** It is acceptable for a dental hygienist to recommend an Instant Breakfast drink or liquid supplement to a periodontal patient who is temporarily following a full liquid diet.
10. **T/F** The dental hygienist should complete the nutritional assessment and provide nutritional education immediately after periodontal surgery.

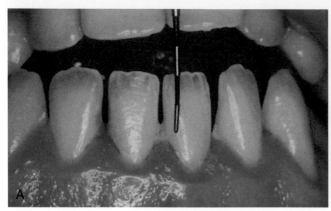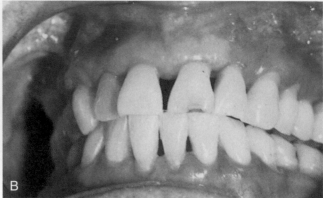

FIGURE 19-1 A, Gingivitis. **B,** Periodontal disease. (**A,** From Perry DA, Beemsterboer P, Essex G: *Periodontology for the dental hygienist,* ed 4, St Louis 2014, Saunders Elsevier. **B,** Courtesy Barbara D. Altshuler, BSDH, MS, Clinical Assistant Professor, Caruth School of Dental Hygiene, The Texas A&M University System, Baylor College of Dentistry, Dallas, TX.)

Gingivitis is characterized by inflammation, swelling, changes in contour or consistency, presence of plaque biofilm or calculus or both, no evidence of attachment loss, and bleeding on probing (Fig. 19-1, *A*). Connective tissue and bone support are intact. Gingivitis is often reversible with appropriate oral hygiene techniques. If left untreated, gingivitis can progress to periodontal disease.

Periodontal disease is a chronic, inflammatory, and infectious disease (see Fig. 19-1, *B*). It is the result of a loss of connective tissue and alveolar bone. Common findings are gingival bleeding, pain, infection, **suppuration** (formation or discharge of pus), tooth mobility, and tooth loss. Two targets for *Healthy People 2020* are (1) to reduce the prevalence of moderate and severe periodontitis from nearly 13% to 11% in people ages 45-74 years and (2) to reduce the prevalence of tooth loss from periodontal involvement.[1]

The inflammatory process of gingivitis and periodontal disease is affected by the host's immune response—the body's ability to protect itself from destructive periodontal pathogens and infection. Nutritional deficiencies, which may occur from adolescence through adulthood, can modify the body's response to periodontal disease. Periodontal disease is the leading reason for tooth loss for individuals older than age 45 years. Bacteria associated with periodontal disease increase the risk of cardiovascular disease, stroke, premature births, respiratory infections, and uncontrolled diabetes (Fig. 19-2).

The involvement of nutrition in periodontal disease is not as clear as it is for dental caries. Predisposing, etiological, and contributing factors of periodontal disease are diverse; however, the primary initiating agent is plaque biofilm accumulation around teeth and gingiva. Nutrient deficiencies, excesses, or imbalances do not initiate periodontal disease, and megadoses of vitamin-mineral supplements do not cure or prevent periodontal disease. Indirectly, nutritional status may alter development, resistance, or repair of the periodontium (Fig. 19-3), which ultimately affects severity and extent of the disease. In addition, a patient's health, medications, and food choices influence the properties of plaque biofilm

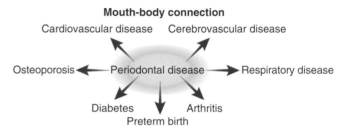

FIGURE 19-2 The possible connections between periodontal disease and other systemic diseases or conditions.

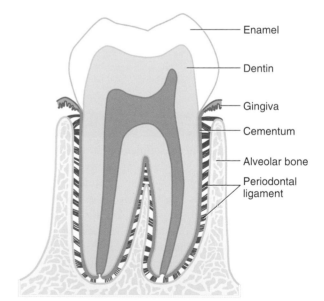

FIGURE 19-3 The periodontium consists of the gingiva, alveolar bone, cementum, and periodontal ligament. (From Bath-Balogh M, Fehrenbach MJ: *Illustrated dental embryology, histology, and anatomy,* ed 3, St Louis, 2011, Saunders Elsevier.)

and saliva. The buffering and antimicrobial effects of saliva are significant factors in periodontal disease. A change in composition or amount of saliva can influence development and maturation of plaque biofilm (see discussion of xerostomia in Chapter 20).

PHYSICAL EFFECTS OF FOOD ON PERIODONTAL HEALTH

Food Composition

The classes of macronutrients and micronutrients that have physiological roles in growth, maintenance, and repair include carbohydrates, proteins, fats, vitamins, minerals, and water. At least 50 nutrients are provided by food, most of which are required for a healthy periodontium. An imbalance of one or more nutrients can be a factor in the disruption of tissue integrity and immune response. Consuming adequate amounts of each is the ultimate goal.

Normal growth and development of periodontal and oral mucosal tissues depend on sufficient intake of vitamin A (salivary glands, epithelial tissue), vitamin C (collagen, connective tissue), and vitamin B complex (epithelial and connective tissue). Calcification of the alveolus and cementum requires amino acids, calcium, phosphorus, vitamin D, and magnesium. Maintenance of oral tissues and integrity of the host's immune and repair responses requires sufficient amounts of vitamins A, C, D, and E; proteins; carbohydrates; calcium; iron; zinc; folic acid; and omega-3 fatty acids. Higher kilocalorie ranges also are indicated for increased metabolic needs for individuals with periodontal disease. (Refer to Chapters 4 through 12 for more descriptive information on the effects of specific nutrients on the periodontium.) Figure 19-4 depicts gingivitis-related malnutrition; note the inflammation, bulbous tissue, edema, and suppuration.

Supragingival plaque biofilm adhesion and formation is influenced by frequent dietary consumption of monosaccharides (e.g., glucose) and disaccharides, particularly sucrose. Subgingival plaque biofilm seems to be protected from local effects of sugars.

Nutritional intervention needs to be a component of the treatment plan for periodontal disease because poor nutrition can affect the entire body and has an adverse effect on the periodontium. In combination with local irritating factors, such as plaque biofilm or tobacco use, systemic factors can increase risk or severity of periodontal disease of a host, but is not solely responsible for periodontal disease. A nutrition assessment by the dental hygienist can reveal dietary deficiencies that should be corrected for optimal healing. Referral to a registered dietitian nutritionist (RDN) may be indicated, particularly for compromised patients requiring medical nutrition therapy, such as patients with diabetes.

Food Consistency

Another factor affecting periodontal health is the texture of food. Chewing firm, coarse, and fibrous foods, such as raw fruits and vegetables, stimulates salivary flow. The increase in saliva enhances oral clearance of food, reducing food retention: i.e., the less food debris that remains in the mouth, the less debris accumulates on the teeth. Plaque biofilm is not physically removed by eating firm foods, however. Soft, sticky foods increase accumulation of food, which enhances dental biofilm growth.

NUTRITIONAL CONSIDERATIONS FOR PERIODONTAL PATIENTS

Increased nutrients and energy are required by periodontal patients experiencing stress, tissue catabolism, or infection. A thorough assessment of the periodontal patient, as described in Chapter 21, provides valuable data needed to formulate a nutrition plan.

A medical and social history can indicate whether a patient is at risk of nutrient deficiencies because of alcoholism, anorexia, or other health problems. These patients would benefit from medical nutrition therapy by a RDN to normalize nutrient levels before treatment. Dietary education of all periodontal patients by the dental hygienist facilitates tissue repair and wound healing, improves resistance to infection, and reduces the number and severity of complications. Optimally, good nutritional status results in a shorter recovery and a more rapid return to health (Box 19-1).

GINGIVITIS

Gingivitis is a progressive inflammatory process beginning in the interdental papillae and advancing to the attached gingiva. The color of the gingiva varies from slight redness

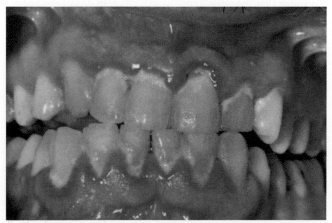

FIGURE 19-4 Gingivitis-related malnutrition. (From Perry DA, Beemsterboer P, Essex G: *Periodontology for the dental hygienist,* ed 4, St Louis 2014, Saunders Elsevier.)

BOX 19-1	Nutritional Involvement in Periodontal Disease

A patient's dietary intake plays a role in periodontal health, directly and indirectly affecting:
- Growth and development, maintenance, and repair of the periodontium
- Amount and type of supragingival plaque biofilm
- Inflammation and immune response for optimal healing
- Amount and type of saliva
- Host resistance to decrease the susceptibility to infection

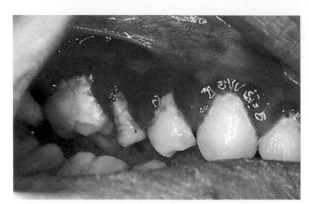

FIGURE 19-5 Gingivitis, with heavy calculus present. (From Darby ML, Walsh MM: *Dental hygiene: theory and practice*, ed 4, St Louis, 2015, Saunders Elsevier.)

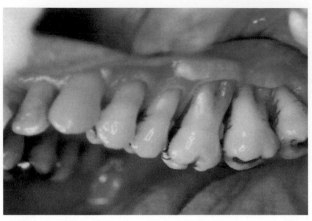

FIGURE 19-6 Clinical attachment loss. (From Perry DA, Beemsterboer P, Essex G: *Periodontology for the dental hygienist*, ed 4, St Louis 2014, Saunders Elsevier.)

to a darker reddish blue. The gingiva bleeds easily and is either edematous and spongy or **fibrotic** (formation of fibrous tissue of the gingiva owing to chronic inflammation). The stippling of the gingiva disappears, and probing depths may increase without loss of attachment. Gingivitis is associated with a large accumulation of plaque biofilm and calculus on teeth (Fig. 19-5), which is exacerbated by frequent exposure to fermentable carbohydrates and retentive foods.

Gingival disease may be an indication of metabolic disease, such as diabetes mellitus. In combination with local factors, systemic factors, including an immunocompromised system (e.g., AIDS); use of certain medications (e.g., antihistamines, antidepressants); hormonal changes (e.g., pregnancy, puberty); and a vitamin C deficiency can be elements in the development of gingivitis. Scurvy, a disease associated with vitamin C deficiency, is rarely seen in the United States because of the availability of fruits, vegetables, and foods fortified with vitamin C. Hemorrhage, bluish red gingiva, a widened periodontal ligament, and tooth mobility are characteristic oral symptoms of scurvy. Correcting the vitamin C deficiency through appropriate food choices, and sometimes supplementation, improves gingival health.

A lack of nutrients does not cause gingival inflammation, but may be a predisposing factor by disrupting the process of tissue repair. Adequate nutrients can hasten healing and repair processes. Controlling or modifying the etiological factors can reverse clinical characteristics. Nutritional interventions for varying severities of gingivitis are the same as those for promoting overall health by encouraging adequate intake of all food groups and analyzing fermentable carbohydrate intake to determine potentially damaging habits that intensify the gingivitis.

Dental Considerations

Assessment
- *Physical*: gingival tissue is red to reddish blue, or pink if fibrotic; interdental papillae are often bulbous; spontaneous bleeding on probing; the gingival margin is coronal to the cementoenamel junction; periodontal condition may be asymptomatic.

- *Dietary*: adequate nutrient and kilocalorie intake; frequency and amount of alcohol consumption.

Intervention
- Educate the patient that tissue damage associated with gingivitis is reversible.
- Encourage tailored oral self-care regimens.
- Provide oral prophylaxis, including biofilm and endotoxin debridement.

Evaluation
- Satisfactory response to therapy, resulting in healthy tissue; patient is able to demonstrate adequate oral hygiene techniques; adequate dietary intake.

Nutritional Directions

- Encourage nutrient-dense foods that are not retentive. Soft foods are followed by appropriate oral hygiene.
- Encourage vitamin C–rich foods and a well-balanced diet using *MyPlate* as a guide.

CHRONIC PERIODONTITIS

Periodontitis involves **clinical attachment loss** (Fig. 19-6), separation of collagen fibers from the cementum and apical movement of the junctional epithelium onto the root surface. This destructive process results in bone loss. Inflammation is also present, affecting gingiva and other components of the periodontium. Severity of the gingival inflammation, recession, bone loss (Fig. 19-7), tooth mobility, and periodontal pocket formation varies according to duration of disease and the individual's resistance level or immune response. It can be localized or generalized in the mouth possibly with **purulent exudates**, or drainage of fluids from the gingival sulcus.

Initiation and progression of periodontitis do not occur unless plaque biofilm and calculus are present. As with gingivitis, certain types of food (e.g., soft, retentive, or fermentable carbohydrate) can enhance food retention and severity of gingival inflammation. In addition to retentive

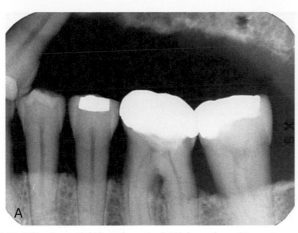
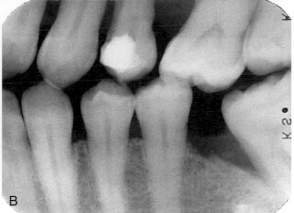

FIGURE 19-7 Horizontal (**A**) and vertical (**B**) bone loss. (From Iannucci JM, Howerton LJ: *Dental radiography: principles and techniques,* ed 4, St Louis, 2012, Saunders Elsevier.)

carbohydrates, excess glucose and sucrose have been shown to increase rate of bacterial growth in the early stages of biofilm development. Biofilm development eventually reaches a steady state at this point, and the influence of diet is thought to be less important in the process of maturation of plaque biofilm.

Systemically, nutritional status determines immunocompetence of the periodontium. A deficiency of calcium, phosphorus, and vitamin D can contribute to severity of bone loss (although the deficiency is not the primary cause). Recovery from periodontitis also is enhanced by the positive effect of adequate nutrient reserves and intake on the immune system. Adequate vitamin C reserves can help ensure wound healing.[2] Nutrient intake exceeding the Recommended Dietary Allowances (RDA) may not improve or accelerate the healing process and can be detrimental because of interference with other nutrients or drugs. With assistance from the dental professional, the patient can make dietary adjustments necessary to meet the stresses and increased nutrient requirements of the disease and to ensure optimal wound healing.

Nutritional recommendations for a patient with gingivitis can be adapted to meet the needs of a patient with periodontitis. Emphasis is placed on maintaining a nutritionally adequate diet; the *Dietary Guidelines* and *MyPlate* are valuable educational tools. The patient maintains a nutritionally adequate diet, while avoiding retentive foods; the dental hygienist analyzes food intake for the amount and frequency of fermentable carbohydrate intake (see Fig. 18-10 in Chapter 18). By working toward improving or eliminating etiological factors related to periodontitis, the healing process can minimize irreversible damage.

Periodontal Surgery
Preoperative
If periodontal surgery is indicated, the body's immunological competency is important for optimal healing and preventing or minimizing infections. The dental hygienist should conduct a preliminary assessment of the patient for adequate nutrient reserves before the dental procedure. If the recommendations of the *Dietary Guidelines* and *MyPlate* are

met, the patient's dietary intake is considered adequate. Generally, minor periodontal surgical procedures on a healthy patient with an adequate intake do not require special dietary modification. Surgery on a chronic alcoholic or a patient with an eating disorder could require preoperative replenishment of nutrient reserves. An elective surgery may need to be postponed for 1 or 2 weeks to allow improvement in nutritional status. A medically compromised patient is best served by an RDN who can appropriately assess and determine energy and other nutrient requirements.

Recommendation of a liquid nutritional supplement (e.g., instant breakfast) or multivitamin with minerals may be warranted. Coordinating efforts with an RDN provides the patient with continuity of care. To enhance compliance, the dental professional can provide a clear understanding of the relationship of nutrition to periodontal status.

Before surgery, the patient should be given a tailored meal plan listing nutrient-dense foods and beverages to consume during the recovery period. Milk and 100% fruit juices contain many more nutrients than soft drinks, even if caloric value is similar. The dental hygienist should consider the extent of the surgery, its potential discomfort, and the patient's ability to eat after the periodontal procedure, and encourage the patient to make food choices that avoid tissue trauma. The patient's food preferences and dislikes are other factors to be taken into consideration.

Postoperative
Because of blood loss, increased catabolism, tissue regeneration, and host defense activities after periodontal surgery, adequate nutrient intake is required. Meeting the requirements for kilocalories, proteins, vitamins, minerals, and decaffeinated fluids (8 to 10 glasses a day) enhances recovery.

Dietary intake can be influenced by complications of anorexia, nausea, dysphagia, and oral discomfort. The texture of foods depends on extent of the surgery and symptoms of the patient. A full liquid diet may be required the first 1 to 3 days (Box 19-2). A **full liquid diet** provides food in a liquid form for patients who are unable to chew. It should consist

---

BOX 19-2	Full Liquid Diet: Oral Surgery

Purpose

To provide a high-protein, high-kilocalorie liquid diet to promote healing in cleft lip and cleft palate repair, oral surgery (when chewing is difficult), or mouth irritations when solid foods are not tolerated.

Adequacy

This diet meets the Dietary Reference Intakes for energy, carbohydrates, protein, fat, calcium, and vitamin C for children and adults. It may be inadequate in all other nutrients. Nutritional adequacy can be improved by the addition of a commercial nutritional supplement. For prolonged use, a multivitamin-mineral supplement should be considered.

Description

All foods are liquid or semisolid at room temperature. All foods are of a consistency that can be drunk from a cup without a spoon or straw (to avoid penetrating the repaired palatal tissue).

Guidelines

This is a transitional diet: followed by the mechanically altered diet to a regular diet. Oral nutritional supplements are recommended after 48 hours. Refer to an RDN or a healthcare provider if the patient requires longer time on this diet. A multivitamin-mineral supplement may be needed. Six small meals are recommended.

Sample Menu for Full Liquid Diet for Oral Surgery Patients

BREAKFAST	SNACK	LUNCH	SNACK	DINNER SNACK	SNACK
½ cup apple juice	8 oz malted milk	½ cup cranberry juice	½ cup ice cream with chocolate syrup	½ cup grape juice ½ cup gelatin	
8 oz smoothie made with yogurt and fruit		8 oz strained cream of pea soup with pureed ham		8 oz tomato soup made with milk and additional milk powder	
1 cup Cream of Wheat with butter		12 oz milkshake mixed with instant breakfast powder		8 oz vanilla yogurt	
1 cup whole milk		8 oz whole milk ½ cup custard		1 cup eggnog ½ cup of pudding	

Approximate Nutrient Composition for Sample Full Liquid Menu for Oral Surgery

Kilocalories 2649

Carbohydrate 345 g

Protein 102 g

Fat 100 g

Cholesterol 484 mg

Dietary fiber 13 g

Sodium 3622 mg

Potassium 5191 mg

Calcium 3019 mg

Iron 18 mg

Vitamin A 2086 μg RAE (retinol activity equivalents)

Vitamin C 113 mg

With permission of Texas Academy of Nutrition and Dietetics: *Texas Academy of Nutrition and Dietetics MNT Manual*, Dallas, TX, 2013.

---

of high-protein, high-kilocalorie fluids and semi-solid foods to promote optimal healing. Fluids can be drunk from a cup without the use of a spoon or straw. A full liquid diet is used only temporarily because nutrient and caloric value is usually inadequate. Any special diet modifications (e.g., low sodium, low fat) and patient preferences should be considered.

The full liquid diet can progress to a mechanically altered diet when tolerated. A **mechanically altered diet** (Box 19-3) is a regular diet altered in consistency and texture for ease in mastication when chewing may be compromised. This diet includes soft, ripened, chopped, ground, mashed, and pureed foods. Foods are generally moist. Most raw fruits (except bananas) and vegetables are avoided, as are any foods containing seeds or nuts. The mechanically altered diet is recommended for 3 to 7 days until the patient can tolerate regular foods. Consuming small, frequent meals (e.g., six small

feedings one-half the size of a regular meal) may provide adequate intake and is easier for the patient. Bland foods (Box 19-4) may be necessary to avoid irritating sensitive tissue. A liquid nutritional supplement, a multivitamin with minerals, or both may be recommended to ensure adequate nutrients and accelerate recovery.

Periodontal dressing may be used to cover and protect the surgical site; shield the tissue from irritation; help control postoperative bleeding, edema, and infection; and prevent accumulation of food debris and bacteria. Instruct the patient to avoid hard, sticky, and brittle foods, and to follow the guidelines for a mechanically altered diet for 1 to 2 days. Also, encourage cool liquids and foods for the first 24 hours to allow the dressing to harden and prevent swelling. Discourage smoking and the use of straws because sucking pressure could dislodge a blood clot.

**BOX
19-3**   **Mechanically Altered Diet**

Purpose

To provide a well-balanced diet, soft in texture and consistency, for patients with chewing difficulties due to poor or missing dentition, oral surgery or radiation of the head and neck area which may make the mouth sore.

Adequacy

If a variety of foods are selected, this diet meets the Dietary Reference Intakes for nutrients for most adults.

Description

1. The diet consists of a regular diet with alterations in consistency and texture.
2. Foods are generally tender, finely chopped, ground, or pureed, although very soft whole foods may be eaten as tolerated.
3. Patient tolerance to food texture and consistency may vary; modifications should be made accordingly.

Mechanically Altered Diet Food List

FOOD	ALLOWED	AVOID
Soup	Broth or creamed soups made with allowed foods, or strained	Soup with large pieces of food or whole meats or crunchy vegetables
Meat and meat substitutes	Any chopped or ground meat or poultry, very tender baked, broiled, creamed or stewed whole meat, fish, or poultry; bacon, cheese and cottage cheese; eggs; smooth peanut butter; soft dried beans and peas; boiled, creamed, poached, scrambled, soufflé eggs; soft casseroles	Whole cuts of meat; fried meat, fish, poultry and eggs; hot dogs and other meat in casings; crunchy peanut butter; pizza with thick, tough crust
Potato and substitutes	Any white or sweet potatoes, mashed, baked, creamed, scalloped, or boiled; macaroni, noodles, rice, pasta	Fried potatoes, potato chips, potato skins; whole grain or brown rice
Vegetables	Vegetable juice; any well-cooked, soft vegetable without seeds or skins; peeled raw tomatoes	Corn and other raw vegetables, unless tolerated
Bread	Any enriched or whole grain breads, soft rolls, doughnuts, pancakes, crackers and biscuits	Hard crusty bread; bread containing nuts, or dried fruit; bagels; taco shells; popcorn
Cereals	Cooked cereals, cereals that require minimal chewing	Cereals containing nuts, coconut, dried fruit; shredded wheat cereal; granola; cereals that remain crunchy in milk
Fats	Any	None
Fruits	Any fruit juice; all canned or cooked fruit, soft fresh fruit	All other raw fruits and fruits with skins, dried fruits
Milk	Any	None
Desserts	Any except those to "Avoid"	Desserts containing coconut, nuts, dried fruits; fried, tough, or chewy items
Beverages	Any	None
Miscellaneous	Honey, iodized salt, sugar, sugar substitutes, syrup, jelly, ketchup, mustard, pepper, herbs, ground spices, cream sauces and gravies, chocolate, vinegar, lemon juice, cranberry sauce	Whole spices, pickles, popcorn, nuts, coconut

Sample Menu for Mechanically Altered Diet

BREAKFAST	LUNCH	DINNER	SNACK
½ cup orange juice	3 oz ground beef	3 oz broiled salmon	1 tbsp smooth peanut butter
1 cup oatmeal with brown sugar	½ cup mashed potatoes with gravy	1 medium baked potato (no peel)	3 squares graham crackers
1 slice whole wheat toast	½ cup well-cooked green beans	½ cup well-cooked broccoli	½ cup apple juice
1 tsp margarine	2 slices peeled tomato	1 slice whole-wheat bread	
1 cup skim milk	1 ripe banana	1 tsp margarine	
	1 whole wheat bun	1 small brownie without nuts	
	1 tsp mayonnaise	1 cup chocolate skim milk	
	½ cup ice cream	½ cup vegetable juice	
	1 cup skim milk		

Continued

BOX 19-3 **Mechanically Altered Diet—cont'd**

Approximate Nutrient Composition for Mechanically Altered Diet

Kilocalories 1898

Carbohydrate 287 g

Protein 154 g

Fat 60 g

Cholesterol 307 mg

Dietary fiber 26 g

Sodium 3114 mg

Potassium 5700 mg

Calcium 1587 mg

Iron 16 mg

Vitamin A 1199 μg RAE (retinol activity equivalents)

Vitamin C 186 mg

Adapted from Texas Academy of Nutrition and Dietetics: *Texas Academy of Nutrition and Dietetics MNT Manual*, Dallas, TX, 2013.

BOX 19-4 **Bland Diet**

Purpose

To provide a temporary well-balanced diet for dental patients with ulcerations.

Foods and Fluids to Avoid

- Caffeine-containing beverages (coffee, tea, cola, cocoa)
- Alcohol
- Peppermint
- Chocolate
- Black and red pepper
- Chili pepper
- Chili powder
- Acidic foods
- Citrus fruits

  Intolerance to these and other foods varies. Foods that cause discomfort should be avoided.

Dental Considerations

Assessment

- *Physical:* pale pink to purplish red gingival tissue (firm to spongy); interdental papillae may not fill the interdental spaces; bleeding on probing and suppuration may occur; probing depths of 4 mm or more; tooth mobility, furcation involvement, and pain may be present.
- *Dietary:* adequacy of dietary and fluid intake; avoidance of alcohol; use of vitamin-mineral supplements.

Interventions

- Oral prophylaxis to debride and deplaque teeth to eliminate or suppress infectious microorganisms.
- Recommend an antimicrobial (systemic or site-specific).
- Encourage appropriate techniques for optimal oral self-care.
- Provide smoking cessation counseling, if needed (see *Health Application* at the end of this chapter).
- Control of systemic disease, such as diabetes.
- Identify and recommend modification of open margins, overhangs, inadequate restorations.
- Recommend or provide fluoride therapy for desensitization, if needed.

Evaluation

- Absence of inflammation and other signs of periodontal issues, such as pain and ulcerations; patient adhering to an adequate diet, avoiding alcohol and smoking; patient maintaining regular recare appointments with a healthy periodontal clinical assessment.

Nutritional Directions

- Postsurgical patients may require a full liquid or mechanically altered diet until the patient can chew comfortably.
- To meet energy and nutrient needs, postsurgical patients typically require small, frequent meals and nutrient-dense foods and beverages.
- A patient requiring a therapeutic meal plan, such as for diabetes, may need a referral to an RDN.
- Discuss with the patient how alcohol abuse may contribute to periodontal issues because of enhanced bleeding tendencies and a propensity toward malnutrition.
- There is emerging evidence that probiotics may inhibit the growth of plaque biofilm and bacteria associated with periodontal disease (see Table 20-1 in Chapter 20). Probiotics vary in the means of administration, including foods, tablets, chewing gums, and lozenges. Probiotics differ in strains and strengths; therefore, selecting the correct strain for a specific oral issue is essential and complex. Other considerations for selecting a probiotic include mode and time of administration; health of the patient; and retention and exposure times in the oral cavity. Further rigorous research is needed in this area.[3-6]

NECROTIZING PERIODONTAL DISEASES

Necrotizing Ulcerative Gingivitis and Necrotizing Ulcerative Periodontitis

Necrotizing ulcerative gingivitis (NUG) and necrotizing ulcerative periodontitis (NUP) are classified as acute periodontal diseases and are prevalent in young adults. NUG is characterized by red and shiny marginal labial and lingual gingivae that bleed when probed, and by cratered interdental papillae, grayish sloughing of marginal gingiva, foul breath, metallic taste, occasional fever, and pain (Fig. 19-8). Common complaints include a burning mouth and anorexia. The etiology of NUG involves bacteria (e.g., *Borrelia vincentii*); systemic factors (e.g., increased susceptibility to infection, as in patients with diabetes or HIV/AIDS); local factors (e.g., smoking, poor oral hygiene); and psychological factors (e.g., stress, fatigue) predisposing a patient to the disease.

Nutrient deficiencies, such as protein or vitamin C or B complex deficiency, are contributing factors to NUG because of lowered host resistance. These deficiencies commonly occur in young adults with poor eating habits, consuming

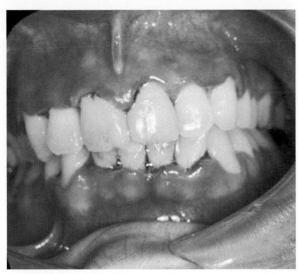

FIGURE 19-8 Necrotizing gingivitis. (From Ibsen OAC, Phelan JA: *Oral pathology for the dental hygienist,* ed 6, St Louis, 2014, Saunders Elsevier.)

primarily low nutrient-dense foods, who rely primarily on convenience or fast food meals. Also, patients with NUG may lose the desire to eat because of pain, or they may choose soft foods that are easier to eat. Excessive alcohol intake and food impacted in the interproximal areas of open contacts are other possible factors related to the condition.

Tissue infection and destruction increase physiological requirements for all nutrients. When fever is present, a 12% increase in total nutrient and energy intake is recommended for each degree above normal body temperature. Also, additional nutrients and energy are necessary for optimal tissue repair and healing. If left untreated, NUG can progress to NUP, in which attachment loss is present.

Obtaining the patient's health, dental, and social histories is the first step in nutritional management, followed by an extraoral and intraoral examination. In addition, a 24-hour food recall (see Chapter 18, Figs. 18-8 and 18-9) provides important insights into dietary practices and potential nutrient deficiencies. A 3- to 7-day food record may help provide a more accurate picture of food intake. Information gathered provides valuable clues regarding nutritional factors needing to be altered or eliminated. Dietary information allows the dental hygienist to make recommendations suited to the patient's eating patterns with consideration of the patient's food preferences and habits, and financial resources. Maintaining food intake as closely as possible to the regular eating pattern generally results in greater compliance.

The severity of NUG determines initial dietary recommendations. The goal is to provide adequate nutrients and kilocalories, avoid alcohol, and consume noncaffeinated fluids to maintain hydration. Based on the food record, a liquid nutritional supplement, such as Carnation Instant Breakfast, Ensure (Abbot Nutrition), and Boost (Nestlē), or a multivitamin with minerals supplement may be suggested to ensure nutrient and caloric adequacy during acute periods of the disease. As soon as a nutritionally adequate diet is

regularly consumed, any supplements recommended can be eliminated.

Lip and tongue ulcers, extremely painful inflamed gingival tissue, and possibly initial removal of calculus may warrant a full liquid diet for 1 to 3 days (see Box 19-2). As tolerated, the patient progresses to a mechanically altered diet (see Box 19-3). A patient's tolerance to consistency varies; the dental hygienist needs to tailor the dietary information to the patient. A patient with ulcerations may need to eliminate nuts and seeds because they can lodge in the ulcer and cause further discomfort. Encourage fluids with meals to make chewing foods easier.

Provide examples of acceptable bland and soothing foods (e.g., gelatin, puddings), while recommending avoidance of spicy and acidic foods (e.g., citrus fruits and tomatoes), which can irritate the oral mucosa (see Box 19-4). Frequent, small meals are beneficial for a patient who is having difficulty eating; choosing a variety of foods from each of the food groups is important. Additional protein intake (in the form of beans, low-fat cottage cheese, or skim milk) is effective in meeting the increased needs related to fever and infection. Adequate decaffeinated fluid intake is essential. When a regular diet can be reinstated, concentrate efforts on continuing to follow the *Dietary Guidelines* and *MyPlate*. Recurrence of NUG is possible, and preventive guidelines should be emphasized. Each episode of NUG increases the risk of progression to NUP.

Dental Considerations

Assessment
- *Physical:* inflamed, hemorrhagic, and red labial and lingual gingivae; cratered interdental papillae; grayish sloughing of the marginal gingivae; metallic taste; foul odor; pain; fever; malaise.
- *Dietary:* adequate nutrient, kilocalorie, and fluid intake; amount and frequency of alcohol consumption.

Interventions
- Explain extrinsic and intrinsic etiological factors associated with the type and severity of periodontal disease the patient is experiencing.
- Educate the patient on appropriate self-care procedures, and recommend use of non–alcohol-containing antimicrobial mouth rinses.
- Explain how fermentable carbohydrates enhance plaque biofilm formation by providing substrates for bacterial growth and biofilm maturation. Also, explain how soft, retentive foods cling to the tooth, allowing adherence of plaque biofilm.
- When nutrient requirements are increased because of a periodontal condition, and therapeutic treatment is needed, a multivitamin supplement may be recommended. Care should be taken to ensure the nutrients in the supplement do not exceed 100% of the RDA unless recommended by an RDN.
- Many foods on a full liquid diet are milk-based. Consider the needs of a patient who is lactose intolerant. A referral to an RDN may be needed.
- A proper balance of calcium and phosphorus is associated with bone mineralization (see Chapter 9). A calcium-to-phosphorus ratio of 1:1 is recommended; however, higher

Continued

Dental Considerations—cont'd

amounts of phosphorus are common. One hypothesis suggests that inadequate dietary intake of calcium combined with excessive amounts of phosphorus creates a nutritional secondary hyperparathyroidism. Bone stores (e.g., alveolar bone) may release calcium to maintain this ratio. Nutritional secondary hyperparathyroidism may be associated with abnormal absorption of the alveolar bone.

• Ask the patient about any allergies to antibiotics.

• The methyl red sugar test can be incorporated into nutrition education as a practical motivational and educational tool. Its purpose is to determine a low pH (acid environment) in the oral cavity. Plaque is removed from the oral cavity and placed on a porcelain tile. Add a few drops of methyl red indicator to cover the plaque, and sprinkle sugar on top. A change of color from red to yellow within 10 to 30 minutes indicates a decrease in the pH level. The patient should be taught not only about caries production, but also how carbohydrates increase plaque biofilm adhesion and maturation.

Evaluation

• The patient improves nutritional adequacy of foods chosen; limits or avoids smoking and alcohol consumption; oral hygiene improves with each visit; and clinical signs and symptoms of NUP/NUG improve.

 Nutritional Directions

• Initially, a liquid diet may be needed; advancement to a mechanically altered diet is followed by a regular diet, depending on the patient's tolerance and comfort.

• Antibiotics (e.g., tetracycline or penicillin) may be prescribed for oral infection to suppress oral microorganisms, such as periodontal pathogens.

• Liquid nutrition supplements may be needed. Most of these products contain cariogenic sweeteners; these should be followed by appropriate oral hygiene care.

• Cooler temperature foods are more soothing when ulcerations are present in the oral cavity.

HEALTH APPLICATION 19   Tobacco Cessation

Throughout this text, there are multiple references to the impact of smoking on health, including a negative influence on nutrient absorption. This health application focuses on one of the essential roles of dental professionals: implementing tobacco cessation protocols for dental patients.

Approximately 46.6 million U.S. adults smoke cigarettes, with cigarettes being responsible for 443,000 deaths each year. Furthermore, exposure to second-hand smoke affects 88 million nonsmoking Americans, 54% of whom are younger than age 11 years.[7] Cigarette smoke contains more than 4800 chemicals, 69 of which are known to cause cancer. Second-hand smoke is the number one cause of cancer in household pets. It is linked to premature births, low-birth-weight babies, and cleft lip or palates in infants of women who smoke during pregnancy. Tobacco use is associated with cancer, CHD, stroke, respiratory diseases and diabetes. In the oral cavity, tobacco use increases the risk of periodontal disease, oral cancers, leukoplakia, hairy tongue, delayed healing and extrinsic staining.

The addictive ingredient of cigarettes is nicotine. Nicotine is a stimulant that increases the heart rate and blood pressure. All forms of tobacco have health consequences (Box 19-5).

The American Dental Hygienists' Association (ADHA) has developed a tobacco-cessation action plan with accompanying education tools. This 3-minute plan is divided into three steps: *Ask, Advise* and *Refer. Ask* involves identifying and documenting tobacco use at every visit. Tobacco use should be a part of every health history. The dental hygienist should determine if the patient is a current, former, or never-used tobacco, as well as the form, frequency and duration of tobacco use.[8] Box 19-6 provides questions the dental hygienist can ask.

Advise advocates all tobacco users to quit. The dental hygienist is to send a clear message about health risks at every appointment. It can be as simple as providing basic information about tobacco use. The message should be tailored to the patient.[2] A helpful statement may be, "I can't see what tobacco is doing to your heart, lungs, brain, and other organs, but I would like to show you some changes in your mouth." This opens opportunities to educate the patient on the importance of oral self-examinations in order to recognize abnormal situations.

In the final step, the dental hygienist will *Refer* the patient to support services. Popular resources include quitlines, online programs, pamphlets or local smoking cessation programs.[8] During the tobacco-cessation process, the dental hygienist should encourage and praise the patient.

Tobacco quitlines are available in most states with a toll free number. It is a free cessation service that includes coaching, self-help kits, cessation information, and referrals to local programs. The coaching is on an individual basis and anonymous. The ADHA quitline is a single access to the National Network of Tobacco Cessation quitlines: 1-800-QUIT-NOW.

Online smoking cessation assistance is also anonymous, but group support is also available. A popular program is available at http://www.smokefree.gov/. Except in the presence of contraindications, pharmacotherapy can be an effective support for patients going through smoking cessation (Box 19-7). A combination of tobacco cessation methods increases the likelihood for success.

Dental professionals are distinctly situated to provide tobacco education and promote abstinence or cessation. It is the responsibility and obligation of all dental professionals to intervene and educate patients. The ADHA supports and encourages the dental hygienist to assess patients at each recare visit.

BOX 19-5 Tobacco Products

- Regular cigarettes
- Low-tar (light) cigarettes
- Smokeless tobacco
  - Spitless tobacco products
  - Moist snuff
  - Sticks
  - Orbs
  - Strips
- Cigars
- Pipes
- Electronic cigarettes
- Imported tobacco products
  - Hookah
  - Flavored tobacco

BOX 19-7 Pharmacotherapy for Tobacco Cessation

- Nicotine Replacement
  - Gum
  - Lozenges
  - Patch
  - Nasal spray
  - Inhaler
- Nonnicotine Replacement
  - Bupropion
  - Clonidine
  - Nortriptyline
  - Varenicline
- Combination therapy

BOX 19-6 Questions for Tobacco Cessation

- Do you use any tobacco products?
- Have you ever used tobacco in the past?
- How much do you smoke?
- What forms of tobacco do you use?
- How many cigarettes do you smoke each day?
- Why do you continue to smoke?
- How soon after you wake do you smoke your first cigarette?
- Do others in your household smoke?
- Do you smoke inside your home or car?
- Do you want to quit?
- Tell me about your last quit attempt(s).
  - Did you use a smoking cessation medication?
  - Did you receive any professional support?

Case Application for the Dental Hygienist

Jenny is a 20-year-old college student. It has been 9 months since her last recare visit because of her busy school and work schedule. She continues to smoke despite the dental hygienist's encouragement to quit. An oral examination exhibits inflamed gingiva bleeding on touch and a grayish pseudomembrane covering the marginal gingiva. The dental hygienist also notices an unusual odor from the patient's mouth. A 24-hour dietary recall is as follows:

    7:30 AM: large coffee with cream and sugar; pastry
    10:00 AM: 12 oz cola; potato chips
    2:30 PM: 3 slices pizza; 12 oz cola
    7:30 PM: 12 oz can of ravioli; 8 oz milk
    11:30 PM: hot chocolate; 8 sandwich cookies

Nutritional Assessment
- Food, nutrient, caloric intake
- Eating habits
- Social history
- Motivation level
- Knowledge level

Nutritional Diagnosis
Identify the patient's irregular eating patterns; choices of high-kilocalorie, low nutrient-dense foods; stress from school and work; and smoking.

Nutritional Goals
Jenny will attempt to discontinue smoking or avoid smoking during periods of acute inflammation. With the help of the dental hygienist, she will review her busy schedule and prioritize events to incorporate a variety of foods, including some choices that are quickly prepared, or more nutritious selections from vending machines.

Nutritional Implementation
Intervention: Question Jenny further on the level of oral discomfort she is experiencing. Determine whether a relationship exists between oral health and food choices. Depending on her response, a full liquid diet may initially be suggested, followed by a mechanically altered diet within 1 to 3 days, as tolerated.

Rationale: Oral conditions can interfere with chewing or swallowing. Jenny might be eating too little or omitting foods too painful to eat. Consequently, she may be experiencing a deteriorating nutritional status, which is negatively affecting her oral status. Altering the consistency of her diet can increase nutrient intake by minimizing the task of chewing and swallowing. Every patient's oral situation is unique, and tolerance levels vary greatly. The dental hygienist should listen closely to Jenny's response to individualize recommendations to meet her needs.

Intervention: Encourage Jenny to eat a variety of foods, making choices as similar to her normal eating patterns as possible.

Rationale: Systemic factors, such as nutrient deficiencies, influence inflammatory response of the gingiva. The dental hygienist should explain the role of nutrients in maintaining a healthy periodontium, suggesting food choices that vary only slightly from Jenny's regular food intake to enhance compliance.

Continued

Case Application for the Dental Hygienist—cont'd

Essential education tools include *MyPlate* and *Dietary Guidelines.* Temporary use of a multivitamin supplement may be recommended.

Intervention: Identify the frequency and form of fermentable carbohydrates in Jenny's diet, along with soft and sticky foods.

Rationale: Foods and drinks, such as coffee with sugar, pastries, potato chips, and cookies, influence formation of plaque. With Jenny's cooperation, practical and realistic modifications can be established in her diet that are compatible with the demands of her busy lifestyle. The dental hygienist should discuss use of dairy products (e.g., cheese on pizza and hot chocolate) in her diet.

Intervention: Continue efforts to eliminate smoking. Evaluate Jenny's readiness to quit tobacco use. Refer her to the National Network of Smoking Cessation quitlines at 1-800-QUITNOW, or www.smokefree.gov, or the state quitline.

Rationale: Smoking may promote plaque biofilm accumulation and inhibit the healing process. Heat, staining, and smoke from cigarettes can lead to unfavorable gingival changes. According to

the ADHA, evidence suggests that quitlines are convenient, effective, and preferred by smokers.

Intervention: During an oral examination, note any areas of ulceration.

Rationale: Depending on the patient's tolerance, a bland diet may be recommended because discomfort may be experienced from highly seasoned or acidic foods. Nuts, popcorn hulls, and seeds are avoided because they can become lodged in an ulcerated area and become painful. Finally, cooler temperature foods are more soothing.

Evaluation

The patient comes to each of her recare appointments, with improvement in oral health noted each time. At a 1-month reevaluation appointment, Jenny is (a) consuming a regular diet including a variety of foods; (b) eating fermentable carbohydrates only with meals; (c) choosing firm, fibrous foods more frequently; and (d) attending a smoking-cessation program. She is also able to verbalize reasons for these lifestyle changes.

STUDENT READINESS

1. List at least four factors detrimentally affecting nutritional status in a periodontally involved patient. Why is it important to concentrate on nutrient intake?

2. Discuss the difference between a mechanically altered and a full liquid diet. What dental situations benefit from use of each of these diets?

3. Describe a periodontal situation in which small, frequent meals should be recommended. Explain the rationale to a patient.

4. What dietary strategies can be offered to a patient experiencing oral discomfort?

CASE STUDY

A 43-year-old man comes to his recare appointment complaining of "sore and bleeding gums, especially after brushing." He is a busy executive and entertains his clients frequently. Consequently, he dines out often and averages two to three alcoholic drinks each day. His medical history is uneventful—no medications or health alerts. An oral examination reveals bleeding on probing with pocket depths generalized at 4 to 6 mm with moderate gingival inflammation.

The dental hygienist asks him to recall everything he has eaten on the previous day. His food consumption is high in fat, kilocalories, and sodium because of heavy reliance on dining out. His diet also lacks variety and is low in nutrient value.

1. List several secondary factors precipitating the periodontal problem. What changes in his lifestyle could be suggested?

2. From the limited information presented, what additional data can the dental hygienist gather to help him modify his diet?

3. What vitamins and minerals might be deficient that could cause progression of his periodontal condition?

4. What diet should be suggested? What is the rationale? Provide a realistic menu for one day on the recommended diet.

References

1. U.S. Department of Health and Human Services: *Healthy People 2020: Last updated August 28, 2013.* Accessed September 17, 2013. Available at: healthypeople.gov/2020/topicsobjectives 2020/TechSpecs.aspx?hp2020id=OH-5.

2. Van der Velden U, Kuzmanova D, Chapple ILC: Micronutritional approaches to periodontal therapy. *J Clin Periodontol* 38(Suppl 11):142–158, 2010.

3. Koduganti RR, Sandeep N, Guduguntla S, et al: Probiotics and prebiotics in periodontal therapy. *Indian J Dent Research* 22(2):324–330, 2011.

4. Gupta G: Probiotics and periodontal health. *J Med Life* 4(4):387–394, 2011.

5. Chatterjee A, Bhattacharya H, Kandwal A: Probiotics in periodontal health and disease. *J Indian Soc Periodontol* 15(1):23–28, 2011.

6. Dhingra K: Methodological issues in randomized trials assessing probiotics for periodontal treatment. *J Periodontal Res* 47:15–26, 2012.

7. Centers for Disease Control and Prevention: *Tobacco use: Targeting the nation's leading killer.* Last updated November 16, 2012. Accessed September 15, 2013. Available at: http://www.cdc.gov/chronicdisease/resources/publications/aag/osh.htm.

8. American Dental Hygienists' Association: *Tobacco cessation protocols for the dental practice.* Accessed September 15, 2013. Available at http://www.askadviserefer.org/.

ⓔ EVOLVE RESOURCES

Please visit http://evolve.elsevier.com/Stegeman/nutritional for additional practice and study support tools.

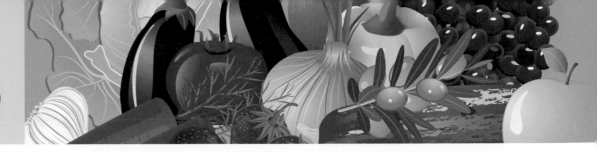

Chapter 20

Nutritional Aspects of Alterations in the Oral Cavity

Student Learning Outcomes

Upon completion of this chapter, the student will be able to achieve the following student learning outcomes:

- Describe the common signs and symptoms of xerostomia and glossitis.
- Synthesize appropriate dietary and oral hygiene recommendations for a patient with orthodontics, xerostomia, root caries, dentin hypersensitivity, glossitis, temporomandibular disorder, or removable prosthetic appliances.
- Identify dietary guidelines appropriate for a patient undergoing oral surgery and a patient with a new denture, before and after insertion.

Key Terms

Abrasion
Crepitus
Dentin hypersensitivity
Erosion

Functional food
Lichen planus
Temporomandibular disorder
Tinnitus

 Test Your NQ

1. **T/F** While charting for dental caries, the dental hygienist notes several root surface caries and documents xerostomia as the cause. This is a correct assessment.
2. **T/F** Xerostomia is a consequence of the aging process.
3. **T/F** Xerostomia can be a contributing factor to malnutrition in an older patient.
4. **T/F** Root caries are frequently seen in adolescents.
5. **T/F** The primary component of alveolar bone is compact cortical bone.
6. **T/F** Glossitis can be a symptom of a nutrient deficiency.
7. **T/F** Masticatory efficiency, or chewing, is a factor in providing a well-structured, alveolar process.
8. **T/F** A relationship exists between nutritional status of a patient and tooth mobility, missing teeth, and denture performance.
9. **T/F** Hard, fibrous, nutrient-dense foods are recommended for the first few days after insertion of new dentures to promote healing and prevent loss of alveolar bone.
10. **T/F** To maintain a normal serum calcium level, calcium is obtained from the alveolar process when the patient is in negative calcium balance.

Instructing patients to follow the *Dietary Guidelines* and *MyPlate* is practical nutrition advice for optimum general and oral health. Various oral conditions can interfere with food intake and influence a patient's nutritional status. These situations require modifications of eating patterns based on individual needs. The oral health team is in an ideal position to provide dietary advice to a patient or to be a valuable member of a multidisciplinary team in complicated cases, such as patients with renal disease.

ORTHODONTICS

Orthodontic treatment presents unique nutritional implications. Risk of decalcification and gingival inflammation are a concern that may compromise orthodontic outcomes and long-term oral health. The treatment time varies widely and is dependent on the complexity of the situation and patient compliance. The level of comfort and duration of discomfort also varies with common complaints of pain localized to the teeth, soft tissues, and tongue, particularly in the first days after placement or adjustment. Pain can last from 1 day to 2 weeks.[1] These symptoms have an impact on food choices, quantity of foods, and food preparation. Eating foods that require biting and chewing may be difficult.

Chaotic meal patterns and snack habits typical of many adolescents create an additional challenge during orthodontic treatment. Health and science courses at school provide adolescents with sufficient knowledge to make better choices, but this information is often ignored. Choosing snacks or meals from vending machines, convenience stores, or fast food restaurants is commonplace.

Dental Considerations

Assessment
- *Physical:* gingival inflammation, dental caries, decalcification of teeth, soft tissue lesions from sharp appliances, root resorption, and accumulation of food debris around brackets.
- *Dietary:* frequency and times fermentable carbohydrates are consumed, form of food chosen.

Interventions
- Individualize nutrition education to motivate adolescents to improve their eating and oral hygiene habits. For any plan to succeed, the adolescent must be willing to change. Remind adolescents this procedure is to help improve their appearance.
- After initial placement, adjustments or repairs in orthodontic care may require a liquid or mechanical soft diet for 1 to 2 days.
- Emphasize the importance of oral self-care, daily fluoride use, and possibly an alcohol-free antimicrobial rinse.
- Because fermentable carbohydrates are a factor in demineralization and plaque biofilm formation, counsel the orthodontic patient to use caution, including recommendations to modify the frequency of consuming fermentable carbohydrates.

- Remind the patient that appliances can be damaged with sticky, hard, or firm foods, or chewing ice.
- Soft-tissue trauma caused by sharp appliances can lead to discomfort and avoidance of certain foods. Warm saltwater rinses (8 oz water with 1 tsp salt) and utility wax (to cover the offending surface of the appliance) provide comfort for the patient until the situation can be resolved.

Evaluation
- The patient has demonstrated acceptable plaque biofilm control abilities; the soft tissues are free of trauma; the patient is choosing a variety of foods based on *MyPlate*.

Nutritional Directions

- Although a mechanically-altered diet allows for ease of chewing and is less painful, it consists of soft, sticky, and retentive foods that can adhere around the brackets, contributing to plaque biofilm formation. Consequently, this diet can result in gingival inflammation and increased caries risk. Encourage and educate the patient regarding an optimal oral self-care regimen.
- Commonly chosen soft foods include mashed potatoes, rice, pasta, bananas, soups, cheese, and boiled vegetables.[1]
- Liquids such as milkshakes or smoothies may also be well tolerated.
- Foods such as carrots and apples should not be avoided, but cut into small pieces.
- Corn on the cob, meat dishes, nuts, chewing gum, chewy candy, and crackers are foods commonly identified as difficult to consume with orthodontic bands.[1]
- Soft drinks, energy drinks, specialized coffee drinks, and sports drinks with fermentable carbohydrate along with citric acid should be avoided to minimize enamel decalcification.
- Adequate nutritional intake is indispensable for maintenance and repair of hard and soft tissue, and to withstand the stresses of tooth movement.
- Foods with a low nutrient value and fermentable carbohydrates minimize success of orthodontic treatment and increase the risk of oral complications.

XEROSTOMIA

Good oral health depends on adequate salivary flow. Common factors contributing to xerostomia are listed in Box 20-1. Because xerostomia is characterized by diminished or absent salivary flow or a change in the viscosity of saliva, xerostomia has a negative impact on oral tissues and dietary intake (Fig. 20-1). Chapter 3 provides some basic information about the functions of saliva and xerostomia.

The dental professional should determine from the medical history the patient's risk for xerostomia. Salivary flow does not significantly decrease as a result of aging. Adults most frequently experience xerostomia in relation to taking multiple medications (see Box 20-1). Xerostomia can also be a result of one or more chronic diseases, such as

> **BOX 20-1 Factors Contributing to Xerostomia**
>
> **Medications**
> - Analgesics
> - Antianxiety agents
> - Anticholinergics
> - Anticonvulsants
> - Antidepressants
> - Antihistamines
> - Antihypertensives
> - Antiinflammatories
> - Antiobesity agents
> - Antiparkinson agents
> - Antipsychotics
> - Bronchodilators
> - Decongestants
> - Diuretics
> - Gastrointestinal agents
> - Narcotics
>
> **Other Considerations**
> - Antineoplastic therapy (chemotherapy and radiation)
> - Systemic diseases (diabetes, Sjögren syndrome)
> - Stress and depression
> - Significant nutrient deficiency (e.g., vitamins A and C, protein)
> - Liquid diets, due to lack of mastication
> - Dehydration
> - Females—smaller salivary glands and produce less saliva[2]

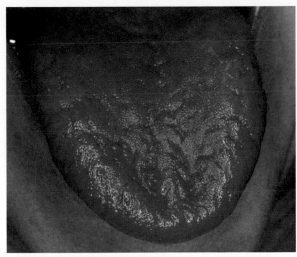

FIGURE 20-2 Sjögren syndrome. Xerostomia. Note the absence of filiform papilla. (From Ibsen OAC, Phelan JA: *Oral pathology for the dental hygienist*, ed 6, St Louis, 2014, Saunders Elsevier.)

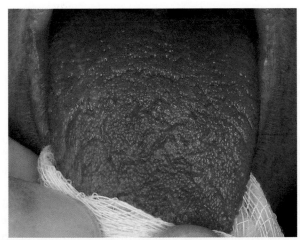

FIGURE 20-1 Xerostomia. (From Ibsen OAC, Phelan JA: *Oral pathology for the dental hygienist*, ed 6, St Louis, 2014, Saunders Elsevier.)

> **BOX 20-2 Consequences of Xerostomia Influencing Nutrient Intake**
>
> - Increased rate of root caries and oral infections
> - Inability to keep mouth moist
> - Sticky or tacky saliva
> - Absence of salivary pooling
> - Difficulty in chewing and swallowing
> - Burning or sensitive oral mucosa
> - Dry, crusty, smooth, or shiny mucosa
> - Low tolerance to spicy and acidic foods
> - Ulcerations
> - Food sticks to hard palate or tongue
> - Painful tongue—atrophied, fissured, inflamed, edematous, burning sensation
> - Angular cheilosis—cracking or burning at the corners of the mouth
> - Altered or lack of taste—lack of interest in eating, possible unintentional weight loss
> - Difficulty wearing dentures
> - Dentin hypersensitivity—hot, cold, sweet, touch
> - Dry nose—impairment of sense of smell
> - Dry throat—difficulty with swallowing

Sjögren syndrome (Fig. 20-2). An estimated 5% to 39% of the general population and 17% to 40% of older adults experience some level of xerostomia. This jumps to as high as 72% in older adults residing in nursing home care.[2] Xerostomia results in various oral complications compromising a patient's nutrient intake (Box 20-2). Overall, the goals for a patient with xerostomia are to protect the oral cavity from the destructive effects of xerostomia, treat existing conditions, and provide relief from the dryness to improve the quality of the diet and quality of life. The dental professional should be able to recognize and provide suggestions for patients experiencing xerostomia.

Dental Considerations

Assessment

- *Physical:* dry mouth; dysgeusia; burning sensation of the tongue or oral mucous membranes; dry and crusty mucosa; difficulty in swallowing and speaking (see Box 20-2); medications (see Box 20-1); antineoplastic therapy (chemotherapy and radiation); systemic diseases (diabetes, Sjögren syndrome, AIDS); stress and depression; dehydration; and weight loss.
- *Dietary:* inadequate intake of vitamins A and C, fluid, fiber, potassium, vitamin B$_6$, iron, calcium, zinc, and protein; taste changes; lack of interest in eating; and poor appetite.

Interventions

- If the patient complains of oral dryness, the dental hygienist can place a mouth mirror or tongue blade on the oral mucosa and watch for stickiness on removal. Milking the major salivary glands (submandibular, sublingual, and parotid) to observe the amount of saliva produced is another assessment option.
- After a thorough oral examination of the patient with oral dryness, a sialometric test can be performed. Saliva flow tests take approximately 10 to 15 minutes and provide fast results of not only the flow, but also consistency, pH, and quantity of saliva. A low salivary rate with this type of test may raise suspicion and indicate systemic disease. A more invasive procedure, scintigraph, can be performed in the hospital to observe salivary function if necessary. Examples include tumors, cysts, salivary stones, duct blockage, and trauma.
- Because burning mouth syndrome cannot be identified clinically, listen to the patient's symptoms. Patients may compare the burning sensation to consumption of hot peppers, typically complaining of having an intense burning sensation on the anterior two-thirds of the tongue or oral mucous membranes; this is commonly associated with taste changes and xerostomia.
- Discomfort with a removable appliance may occur because of the tongue sticking to the prosthesis, an inability to retain the appliance properly, and gingival lesions created by an improperly fitting denture.

- A complete assessment, as described in Chapter 21, allows the dental professional to formulate appropriate intervention strategies for xerostomia.
- Each patient's situation is unique, and oral therapy must be individualized.
- Educate the patient about techniques and procedures to relieve symptoms of xerostomia effective in minimizing oral discomfort and related conditions, especially increased dental caries.
- After assessing food intake, note any changes in appetite affecting overall dietary adequacy resulting in weight changes.
- More than 400 over-the-counter and prescription medications indicate xerostomia is a possible side effect. Because drugs are a common cause of xerostomia, review the patient's medications to identify any drugs associated with xerostomia (see Box 20-1). The patient may want to discuss an alternative medication or a reduction in dosage with the healthcare provider. If the medication cannot be changed, or the dosage cannot be reduced, provide alternative options for maintaining oral health.
- Enhance appetite by presenting foods in interesting, appealing, and appetizing ways. Suggestions to improve the appearance and appeal of food can involve colorful combinations of foods. Imagine the lack of appeal of a plate with cauliflower, mashed potatoes, and baked white fish compared with a colorful plate of baked salmon, steamed broccoli, and a baked yam.
- Frequent recare appointments to monitor the oral cavity.
- Discuss the importance of excellent daily oral hygiene.
- Fluoride therapy to reduce the risk of caries.
- Pilocarpine or cevimeline may be prescribed by the healthcare provider for relief of xerostomia.

Evaluation

- The patient uses oral hygiene and dietary interventions to relieve xerostomia.

Nutritional Directions

- Use products formulated to relieve xerostomia (e.g., sprays or oral rinses).
- Use unflavored or mildly flavored oral hygiene products that have a neutral pH.
- Use lip balm to help keep lips moist.
- Consume fluids with meals and between meals; frequent sips of fluids between bites facilitate chewing and swallowing.
- Use a humidifier to maintain the humidity in the air.
- Choose nutrient-dense, soft, moist foods (e.g., macaroni and cheese, cottage cheese, or applesauce).
- Use gravies and sauces to moisten dry foods (e.g., roast beef).
- Choose foods principally made with a non-nutritive sweetener or sugar alcohols (e.g., gum, hard candy, lozenges, or popsicles), especially between meals.
- Avoid or limit dry (e.g., saltines), crumbly (e.g., whole-wheat muffins), sticky (e.g., peanut butter), and spicy (e.g., salsa or chili peppers) foods; alcohol; commercial mouthwashes containing alcohol; tobacco; and caffeine.
- Suck on ice chips between meals.
- Carry a water bottle during the day.
- Tart, sour, and citrus foods and drinks may help stimulate saliva flow (e.g., sugar-free lemonade, sour candy, and dill pickles).

ROOT CARIES AND DENTIN HYPERSENSITIVITY

Because the population of older adults who have retained their teeth is increasing, root caries are increasingly common. New carious lesions in adults are typically located on the root, below the cementoenamel junction, in areas of gingival recession. The area around the cementoenamel junction is particularly susceptible because it often has an anatomically thin layer of enamel. The cementum, which is thinner and contains fewer minerals than enamel, is also more susceptible. Adequate removal plaque biofilm from exposed root surfaces is very difficult because of root morphology allowing the bacteria and cariogenic material to accumulate, thus increasing caries risk. Xerostomia frequently compounds the risk for root caries because of limited buffering and dilution capacity of decreased amounts of saliva along with poor oral clearance. Also, prevalence of root caries is increased when carbohydrates are consumed frequently.

In addition to root caries, other problems often associated with gingival recession are abrasion and erosion of enamel and cementum. **Erosion** is the permanent depletion of tooth

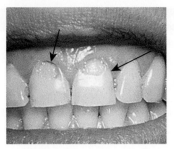

FIGURE 20-3 Erosion caused by frequently sucking on lemons. (From Darby ML, Walsh, MM: *Dental hygiene theory and practice,* ed 4, St Louis, 2014, Saunders Elsevier.)

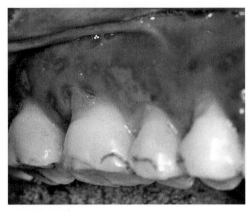

FIGURE 20-4 Toothbrush abrasion. (From Newman MG, Takei HH, Klokkevold PR, Carranza FA: *Carranza's clinical periodontology,* ed 11, St Louis, 2012, Saunders Elsevier.)

surfaces due to the action of an external or internal chemical substance (Fig. 20-3). Erosion is the major cause of hypersensitivity and often occurs as a consequence of exposure to acids such as those found in food and beverages (extrinsic), and acid from gastroesophageal reflux or excessive vomiting (intrinsic). **Abrasion** is the permanent depletion of tooth surfaces as a result of pathologic tooth wear, such as toothbrush abrasion (Fig. 20-4). Erosion and abrasion produce dentin exposure, which can lead to dentin hypersensitivity. **Dentin hypersensitivity** is an extremely painful feeling resulting from a stimulus to the exposed dentin.

Dental Considerations

Assessment
- *Physical*: gingival recession, oral infections, a narrow region of attached gingiva, toothbrush abrasion, use of fluoridated water, oral hygiene status, and xerostomia.
- *Dietary*: diet history, frequency of eating, use of sugar-sweetened medications (cough syrup or lozenges), or intake of hard candy.

Interventions
- Patients who complain of a sudden, sharp pain in areas where dentin is exposed and recession exists may be experiencing dentin hypersensitivity.

- Onset of dentin hypersensitivity is often related to temperature, primarily cold, or touch.
- Recommend 3-month recare visits, meticulous oral hygiene, topical fluoride treatments at home, and fluoridated water. Self-applied fluoride gels reduce enamel solubility and oral bacteria.
- For patients with areas of hypersensitivity, recommend the following: (a) brushing before consuming acidic foods to neutralize the pH of saliva; (b) using a straw for acidic drinks; (c) decreasing frequency of intake or following with a chewing gum containing xylitol or a noncariogenic food (e.g., cheese or milk); or (d) avoiding foods causing discomfort (e.g., hot coffee or iced beverages).
- Brushing immediately after consuming acidic foods can hasten the erosion process. Wait at least 40 minutes to brush.
- Recommend use of soft-bristled tooth brushes.
- Saliva is one of the best protective measures for the demineralizing effects of erosion by neutralizing the acid. Tips to increase saliva flow should be recommended.[3]

Evaluation
- The patient is free of pain, can eat comfortably, has avoided controllable risk factors, and has incorporated appropriate oral hygiene procedures into a home care regimen.

 Nutritional Directions

- Consumption of carbonated beverages (regular and diet), sports drinks, energy drinks, pickled products, wine, citrus products (e.g., grapefruit juice), and ciders are acidic and should be minimized because they can contribute to erosion.
- Because dairy products, especially cheddar cheese, are cariostatic, their consumption with or without cariogenic foods can decrease the risk of caries. A reduced-fat cheese (5 g of fat per oz or less) or smaller portion size is appropriate for many patients.

DENTITION STATUS

Over the decades, a steady reduction in tooth loss has occurred. However, 18% of individuals older than age 65 years still incur loss of all natural teeth.[4] Although many mistakenly believe tooth loss is a normal element of aging, education level and race/ethnicity of the patient are the strongest determinants of tooth loss.[5,6] Smoking status has also been identified as a variable.[6] Although complete dentition is not required for adequate nutrient intake, loss of teeth or supporting periodontium and/or an improperly fitting prosthesis are frequently associated with poor food selection and limited chewing ability. Compromised nutritional intake may be a result of tooth loss, tooth mobility, edentulous status, and discomfort from removable appliances. Malnutrition or inability to comply with nutrition recommendations may result from declining dentition status.

A patient with complete dentures, less than 20 functioning teeth, or few pairs of opposing teeth has lower nutrient intakes than a patient with adequate dentition.[6,7] The patient's masticatory efficiency and biting force increasingly decline with each tooth lost. The number of teeth and presence of advanced mobility determine food choices. Well-fitting dentures and/or implants may improve quality of the diet, but with loss of chewing ability, the patient may choose predominantly soft foods with less variety.[6] Because of the number of variables that can have an impact on nutrient intake, it is imperative for the dental professional to provide personalized nutrition education for patients who are edentulous, wear a dental prosthesis, or have missing or compromised teeth.

Dental Considerations

Assessment

- *Physical*: masticatory efficiency, biting force, number of teeth and location, and fit of dentures.
- *Dietary*: adequacy of kilocalories and nutrients, especially protein, fiber, vitamins A, B$_{12}$, and C, folic acid, iron, magnesium, zinc, and fluids; interest in foods.

Interventions

- Most tooth loss is a result of caries or periodontal disease. Tooth loss can be prevented with education, early diagnosis, and regular care. As a dental health educator, it is important to educate the patient and community continuously regarding prevention and recognition of signs and symptoms of oral disease.
- Nutrient deficiencies frequently interfere with maintenance and repair of oral soft and hard tissues.
- During the appointment preceding placement of a new denture, educate the patient about the initial days of adaptation so that appropriate foods can be available for the adjustment period.
- Swallowing foods may initially present a challenge to a new denture wearer because a full upper denture interferes with the ability to determine the location of food in the mouth. Days 1 and 2 of placement may necessitate a full liquid diet (see Chapter 18, Box 18-2) to allow the patient to master swallowing with the new prosthesis before having to deal with chewing or biting firmer textured foods.
- A liquid nutrition supplement may be needed to meet caloric and nutrient needs to promote healing from extractions or sore spots or both.
- Encourage intake of dairy products fortified with vitamin D to slow the rate of bone loss.
- During the next 2 to 3 days, the patient should advance as tolerated to a mechanically-altered diet (see Chapter 19, Box 19-3), which slowly introduces foods that require limited mastication.
- Discuss the possible decline in taste and a limited ability to identify texture and temperature of foods for complete denture patients.
- As sore spots heal, the patient should add firmer-textured foods. This process is essential for masticatory efficiency and stability of the denture and to enhance the patient's nutritional status.
- Examine the denture for fit. An appointment to reline or make new dentures may be needed. Explain the significance of a properly fitting denture to the patient, including its relationship to a poor-quality diet.
- Patients with a compromised dentition status frequently have inadequate intake of whole grains, fruits, vegetables, and meats.
- Chewy, hard, or fibrous foods are often avoided because of low masticatory performance.
- Ensure adequate nutrient intake by encouraging a variety of food based on *MyPlate* guidelines.

Evaluation

- The patient is choosing a variety of foods from each of the *MyPlate* groups, and understands the importance of a complete and functioning dentition to overall general health.

Nutritional Directions

- Fortified foods may improve nutrient intake.
- Cut food into small pieces.
- Peel and chop fruits and vegetables; cooked fruits and vegetables may be better tolerated.
- Chew food well and longer.
- Evenly distribute food on both sides of the mouth.
- Chew in a straight up-and-down motion rather than a rotary motion and avoid biting with anterior teeth.
- Avoid foods such as chewing gum, sticky foods (e.g., caramels), berries with seeds, and nuts.

ORAL AND MAXILLOFACIAL SURGERY

Oral and maxillofacial surgeries include extractions, orthognathic surgery, dental implants, and maxillomandibular fixation. The dental hygienist is a vital part of the dental team providing comprehensive treatment to a patient for optimal outcomes.

The role of the dental hygienist includes obtaining an assessment of the nutritional needs for patients before a surgical procedure to cope better with the postsurgical demands and to minimize complications. The patient must have an adequate nutrient and fluid intake to meet the stress of surgery (e.g., blood loss and catabolism), provide for optimal healing, and increase resistance to infection, which shortens the recovery period. Patients who are malnourished as a result of various chronic diseases and conditions, such as anorexia nervosa, chemotherapy, or alcoholism, are at increased risk because they are likely to be immunosuppressed. A compromised immune response may compound the severity of complications. These patients should be referred to a registered dietitian nutritionist (RDN) for medical nutrition therapy before the procedure. Based on a nutrition assessment and consideration of the procedure, recommendations can be developed to help the patient plan and purchase appropriate food for the recovery period. Postoperative recommendations should also be addressed by the dental professional.

Dental Considerations

Assessment

- *Physical:* oral dysfunction that affects speech, mastication, or swallowing; medical history.
- *Dietary:* dietary intake, including decaffeinated fluids.

Interventions

- When general anesthesia is used for the surgical procedure, the stomach should be empty of food at the time of the operation to avoid aspirating vomitus.
- If the patient loses weight unintentionally, healing seems delayed, history of bisphosphonate use exists, or overall health declines, the patient should be referred to a healthcare provider or RDN.

Dental Considerations—cont'd

- Provide written instructions to reinforce nutrition education. Tailor the information to meet the patient's needs, attitudes, and behaviors.
- For successful nutrition intervention, it is important to obtain information before discussing dietary interventions, including food preferences, eating patterns, living conditions, economic status, lifestyle, and physical capabilities.
- Recommendations for oral surgery such as extractions include reminding the patient to avoid alcohol and smoking, avoid sipping through a straw, drink adequate decaffeinated fluids, and refrain from brushing during the first 24 hours to avoid a dry socket.
- Emphasize meeting the recommendations of *MyPlate*. The key factor for optimal healing during the recovery process is adequate intake of kilocalories, carbohydrates, protein, fat, vitamins, minerals, and fluids.
- Depending on severity of the operative procedure, the patient may tolerate solid foods after surgery. If not, the dental hygienist can suggest a full liquid diet (see Chapter 19, Box 19-2) for 1 to 2 days with progression to a mechanically-altered diet (see Chapter 19, Box 19-3) and then to a regular diet when tolerated.
- Suggest nutrient-dense and fortified foods that the patient enjoys.
- Because nutrient requirements increase after surgery, patients may find it difficult to consume adequate amounts of food. A liquid nutritional supplement or multivitamin with minerals may be necessary.

Evaluation

- The patient is able to verbalize the problem and discuss ways to continue maintaining a healthy oral cavity and an adequate nutrient intake.

Nutritional Directions

- Cold foods may be soothing to the oral cavity post-surgically.
- Frequent small meals with nutrient-dense foods help meet nutrient needs.

LOSS OF ALVEOLAR BONE

Several factors, including poor calcium intake over a lifetime, create a physiological negative calcium balance. To maintain a normal serum calcium level, the body obtains calcium from other internal sources. The calcium from spongy trabecular bone, the primary component of the alveolar process, can readily be absorbed. The status of the alveolus, which may undergo resorption before other bones, may be an early indicator of osteoporosis. When osteoporotic change in the alveolus is detected, the dental professional should refer the patient to a healthcare provider for further evaluation. Progressive loss of the alveolar ridge leads to tooth loss.

After tooth extractions, accelerated atrophy of alveolar bone occurs (within months). A reduction in masticatory efficiency, as occurs in individuals with dentures, also increases resorption, loss of bone mass, or alveolar

osteoporosis. As the alveolar ridge reduces in height and volume, it becomes increasingly difficult to fit dentures properly, and relined or new dentures are necessary. Management of osteoporosis is discussed in *Health Application 9* in Chapter 9.

GLOSSITIS

Inflammation of the tongue, or glossitis, is very painful. Glossitis may be caused by bacteria, fungus, virus, or disease, and unknown causes. Nutrient deficiency (e.g., B vitamins) or an allergic reaction to food or drugs can result in glossitis. Additionally, psychological stress can be related to psychogenic glossitis. There are many forms of glossitis. One of the most common forms of glossitis is "geographic tongue" or benign migratory glossitis. Although usually asymptomatic, having a patient avoid dietary triggers such as hot, spicy, or acidic foods is recommended. Dental professionals should also closely examine the oral cavity for any signs of lichen planus, considering a potential link.[8] **Lichen planus** is a disease with an itchy rash most often in the mouth. If lichen planus is observed, natural therapies such as green tea and aloe vera may help relieve pain, as well as customary topical steroid treatments.[9,10] A mouthwash, consisting of Maalox, Benadryl, and dexamethasone (Decadron)—or similar variations—is another commonly prescribed treatment for pain and irritation for patients with glossitis, lichen planus, and geographic tongue (Fig. 20-5). Ultimately more options for pain control provide a better quality of life for the patient. Once pain is controlled, patients can continue with normal eating, consuming the Recommended Dietary Allowances.

Glossitis typically appears as slight to total atrophy of the filiform and fungiform papillae. Depending on the degree of atrophy, the tongue inevitably appears shiny, smooth, and red (see Chapter 11, Fig. 11-6). The atrophy can be localized

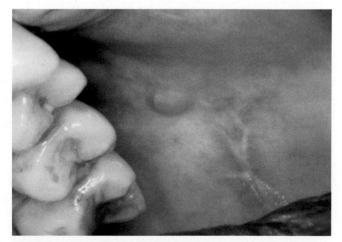

FIGURE 20-5 Mild lichen planus on the buccal mucosa. The patient was prescribed a mouthwash and pain subsided within 24 hours. (Courtesy of Amy L. Sullivan, University of Mississippi Medical Center, Jackson, MS.)

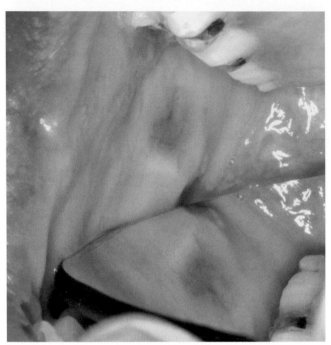

FIGURE 20-6 The irritation on the buccal mucosa appeared after eating acidic and spicy foods. (Courtesy of Amy L. Sullivan, University of Mississippi Medical Center, Jackson, MS.)

Dental Considerations

Assessment
- *Physical:* burning sensation, pain, or tenderness of the tongue; atrophy of papillae on the dorsum of the tongue; tongue size (microglossia or macroglossia); appearance of the tongue (e.g., shiny, smooth, red); diminished, altered, or lost taste sensation; change in the alveolus.
- *Dietary:* nutritional status.

Intervention
- Macroglossia is commonly observed in edentulous mouths.
- Individualize dietary instructions with the goal of improving nutritional quality of the diet.
- Suggest enhancing the taste and appearance of foods on the plate.

Evaluation
- The patient is developing or maintaining healthful eating and exercise patterns and behaviors and has met with the healthcare provider for further evaluation.

Nutritional Directions

- Choose soft, nutrient-dense foods (e.g., tuna salad, cream soups, cottage cheese).
- Liquid nutrition supplements, such as instant breakfast, may help provide adequate nutrients.

or generalized. The tongue size can shrink because of dehydration or become enlarged (macroglossia) as a result of edema. A thorough assessment determines the extent and cause of glossitis.

With benign migratory glossitis, an assessment of the tongue might reveal erythematous or atrophic patches surrounded by a yellow-white border, often changing pattern or appearance. These erythematous patches may extend onto the buccal mucosa (Fig. 20-6). When patients do engage in the previously mentioned triggers (spicy foods), antihistamine or corticosteroid rinses may be suggested.[11] In those cases where lichen planus is also observed, an assessment might reveal whitish plaques on the dorsal of the tongue and even the buccal mucosa.

TEMPOROMANDIBULAR DISORDER

When a patient complains of orofacial pain, frequent headaches, impaired mandibular movement, or tinnitus (ringing in the ears), and the extraoral examination reveals clicking, crepitus (crackling or crunching sound), and popping of the temporomandibular joint, the resultant diagnosis can be temporomandibular disorder. Clenching, grinding, stress, malocclusion, injury, and bone abnormalities are common conditions that result in temporomandibular disorder. Limited jaw opening and associated discomfort can inhibit intake. Recommendations may include avoiding gum chewing and foods that require significant chewing, such as caramels, taffy, and bagels. A mechanically-altered diet (see Chapter 19, Box 19-3) may also be warranted.

HEALTH APPLICATION **20**   Functional Foods

The term functional food is a relatively new concept. "Functional" implies that the food has value in providing some type of health benefits beyond basic nutrition and may function to optimize health by reducing or minimizing the risk of certain diseases and other health conditions. The term "functional foods" has no legal meaning in the United States. In fact, the Academy of Nutrition and Dietetics, the International Food Information Council, Institute of Food Technologists, the European Commission, Health Canada, European Commission, and the Japanese Ministry of Health, Labour, and Welfare all define functional foods slightly differently.

Foods have always been known to provide therapeutic benefits, so all foods, because they provide nutritive value, are functional to some extent. After determining the role for essential elements (e.g., protein, carbohydrates, vitamins) of foods in deficiency diseases, scientists began to recognize physiologically active components in plant and animal products that can reduce risk for various chronic diseases or otherwise provide desirable physiological effects. Functional foods are found in virtually all food categories and can include conventional foods; and fortified, enriched, or enhanced foods with potentially beneficial effects on health when consumed as a part of a varied diet. Implying that some foods are "good" and others are "bad" leads to misinformed food choices. Dietary supplements are not foods. Some food components, not the traditional nutrients of carbohydrate, protein, fat, vitamins, and minerals, may provide positive health benefits. Foods containing these components are defined by the Academy of Nutrition and Dietetics as functional foods.[12]

The scientifically sound approach to labeling and marketing a functional food is through the use of FDA-approved health claims as outlined by the Nutrition Labeling and Education Act (1990) discussed in Chapter 1. Under the Nutrition Labeling and Education Act, a health claim can be authorized by the FDA with the consensus of qualified experts acknowledging scientific studies support the validity of the relationship described in that claim. Scientific agreement requires consistent findings from well-designed clinical, epidemiological studies, and expert opinions from independent scientists. Strong evidence supports some of the claims, but only weak evidence for others. When research confirms links between food components and health, the FDA will permit additional health claims.

Health-related statements or claims allowed on labels include[13]:
- nutrient content claims that indicate a specific nutrient at a certain level;
- structure and function claims that describe the effect of dietary components on the normal structure or function of the body;
- dietary guidance claims in reference to health benefits of broad categories of foods or diets, not a disease or health-related condition;
- qualified health claims that convey a relationship between components in the diet and reduced risk of disease.

Examples of functional foods include natural components of fruits and vegetables, milk, fortified or enhanced foods, and even some foods previously thought of as unhealthy, such as chocolate and red wine. More than a dozen classes of biologically-active plant chemicals are known as phytochemicals and antioxidants (Table 20-1). These natural components found in vegetables such as cabbage, carrots, broccoli, and tomatoes may reduce the risk of cancer. Foods that have been fortified to enhance the level of a specific food component include products such as calcium-fortified orange juice, fiber-supplemented snack bars, or folate-enriched cereals. Oat products reduce serum cholesterol, reducing risk of coronary heart disease. Food products are constantly being developed with beneficial components, such as cholesterol-lowering margarine and products with soy protein.

Frequently, the press reports about a perfectly legitimate scientific study, or a firm will begin marketing a functional food on the basis of "emerging evidence." (For more information, see Chapter 16.) Conversely, consumers worry that new technological developments may influence the safety of the food. For instance, many prefer natural additives as opposed to synthetics. Lack of nutritional knowledge may limit the acceptance of functional foods. However, people should not automatically assume that consuming functional foods will necessarily improve their health. Adding a food containing a particular nutrient does not mean the nutrient will always have the desired effect.

Research regarding how foods or food components and dietary supplements may promote health and reduce chronic disease is providing a steady stream of new information. Dietary recommendations from established scientific authorities are slow to react because of the need for a strong, consensus-based body of evidence before changing dietary advice for the public. Increasing intake of selected foods may not be wise without considering potential negative consequences, and whether or not these specific elements are needed. Factors such as overall nutritional value and kilocalorie intake of an individual's diet, and whether sound scientific evidence backs the claims on package labels should be considered before routinely encouraging or choosing these foods. When evaluating functional foods, safe levels of intake must be considered. In many cases, optimal levels of nutrients and other physiologically-active components in the foods have yet to be determined.

A person who does not have cardiovascular disease or an elevated cholesterol level would not benefit from using sterol-enhanced products. The vitamins in vitamin-enhanced drinks are probably well absorbed, but the vitamins may not be the ones deficient in the diet, and most of these products have more sugar than a regular soda. Many products that are available indicate improvement of athletic performance, conditioning, recovery from fatigue after exercise, and avoidance of injury. Some of these claims may be valid. However, these foods should be used only when scientific evidence clearly supports the claim and when the physiological changes caused by the functional ingredient are understood. The best way a consumer can evaluate the effectiveness of a food product is by trying it for several weeks to observe for benefits.

Functional foods are an important part of wellness because they offer great potential for consumers to optimize their health through diet, but they are not "magic bullets" or a universal panacea for poor health habits. Functional foods are not a substitute for a well-balanced diet and regular physical activity within the framework of a healthy lifestyle. Consumers will probably continue to choose functional foods they enjoy eating, with which they are familiar, and which are readily accessible. When referring to functional foods, the important thing is that what *is* eaten may be more important to health than what *is not* eaten. The best advice is to discuss appropriate intake of functional foods and strategies for achieving dietary intake goals in the context of a healthful diet based on *MyPlate* to optimize health and potentially decrease the risk of chronic diseases.

Table 20-1	Examples of functional components*	
Class/Component	**Source***	**Potential Benefit**
Carotenoids		
Beta-carotene	Carrots, pumpkin, sweet potato, cantaloupe, spinach, tomatoes	Neutralizes free radicals that may damage cells; bolsters cellular antioxidant defenses; can be made into vitamin A in the body
Lutein, zeaxanthin	Kale, collard, spinach, corn, eggs, citrus fruits, asparagus, carrots, broccoli	Supports maintenance of eye health
Lycopene	Tomatoes and processed tomato products (more effective after heating), watermelon, red/pink grapefruit	Supports maintenance of prostate health
Dietary (Functional and Total) Fiber		
Insoluble fiber	Wheat bran, corn bran, fruit skins	Supports maintenance of digestive health; may reduce risk of some types of cancer
Beta glucan†	Oat bran, oatmeal, oat flour, barley, rye	May reduce risk of coronary heart disease (CHD)
Soluble fiber†	Psyllium seed husk, peas, beans, apples, citrus fruit	May reduce risk of CHD and some types of cancer
Whole grains†	Cereal grains, whole-wheat bread, oatmeal, brown rice	May reduce risk of CHD and some types of cancer; may contribute to maintenance of healthy blood glucose levels
Fatty Acids		
Monounsaturated fatty acids (MUFAs)†	Tree nuts, olive oil, canola oil	May reduce risk of CHD
Polyunsaturated fatty acids (PUFAs)-Omega-3 fatty acids—delta-aminolevulinic acid (ALA)	Walnuts, flaxseeds, flaxseed oil	Supports maintenance of heart and eye health; supports maintenance of mental function
PUFAs—Omega-3 fatty acids—docosahexaenoic acid (DHA)/eicosapentaenoic acid (EPA)	Salmon, tuna, marine, other fish oils	May reduce risk of CHD; contributes to maintenance of eye health and mental function
Conjugated linoleic acid (CLA)	Beef and lamb; some cheese	Supports maintenance of desirable body composition and immune health
Flavonoids		
Anthocyanins—cyanidin, delphinidin, malvidin	Berries, cherries, red grapes	Bolster cellular antioxidant defenses; supports maintenance of healthy brain function
Flavonols—catechins, epicatechins, epigallocatechin	Tea, cocoa, chocolate, apples, grapes	Supports maintenance of heart health
Procyanidins and proanthocyanidins	Cranberries, cocoa, apples, strawberries, grapes, red wine, peanuts, cinnamon, tea, chocolate	Supports maintenance of urinary tract health and heart health
Flavanones—hesperetin, naringin	Citrus fruits	Neutralizes free radicals which may damage cells; bolster cellular antioxidant defenses
Flavonols—quercetin, kaempferol, isorhamnetin, myricetin	Onions, apples, tea, broccoli	Neutralizes free radicals that may damage cells; bolster cellular antioxidant defenses
Isothiocyanates		
Sulforaphane	Cauliflower, broccoli, broccoli sprouts, cabbage, kale, horseradish	May enhance detoxification of undesirable compounds; bolsters cellular antioxidant defenses
Minerals		
Calcium†	Sardines, spinach, yogurt, low-fat dairy products, fortified foods and beverages	May reduce the risk of osteoporosis
Magnesium	Spinach, pumpkin seeds, whole grain breads and cereals, halibut, almonds, brazil nuts, beans	Supports maintenance of normal muscle and nerve function, immune health and bone health
Potassium†	Potatoes, low-fat dairy products, whole grain breads and cereals, citrus juices, beans, banana, leafy greens	May reduce risk of high blood pressure and stroke, in combination with a low sodium diet
Selenium	Fish, red meat, whole grains, garlic, liver, eggs	Neutralizes free radicals which may damage cells; supports maintenance of immune and prostate health

Table 20-1	Examples of functional components—cont'd	
Class/Component	**Source***	**Potential Benefit**
Phenolic Acids		
Caffeic acid, ferulic acid	Apples, pears, citrus fruits, some vegetables, whole grains, coffee	Bolsters cellular antioxidant defenses; supports maintenance of eye and heart health
Plant Stanols/Sterols		
Free stanols/sterols†	Corn, soy, wheat, fortified foods and beverages	May reduce risk of CHD
Stanol/sterol esters†	Stanol ester dietary supplements, fortified foods and beverages, including table spreads	May reduce risk of CHD
Polyols		
Sugar alcohols†—xylitol, sorbitol, mannitol, lactitol	Some chewing gums and other food applications	May reduce risk of dental caries
Prebiotics		
Inulin, fructooligosaccharides (FOS), polydextrose	Whole grains, onions, some fruits, garlic, honey, leeks, fortified foods and beverages	Supports maintenance of digestive health; supports calcium absorption
Probiotics		
Yeast, *Lactobacilli*, *Bifidobacteria*, other specific strains of beneficial bacteria	Certain yogurts and other cultured dairy and nondairy products	Supports maintenance of digestive and immune health; benefits are strain specific
Phytoestrogens		
Isoflavones—daidzein, genistein	Soybeans and soy-based foods	Supports maintenance of bone and immune health, and healthy brain function; for women, supports menopausal health
Lignans	Flax seeds, rye, some vegetables, seeds and nuts, lentils, triticale, broccoli, cauliflower, carrot	Support maintenance of heart and immune health
Soy Protein		
Soy protein	Soybeans and soy-based foods like milk, yogurt, cheese and tofu	May reduce risk of CHD
Sulfides/Thiols		
Diallyl sulfide, allyl methyl trisulfide	Garlic, onions, leeks, scallions	May enhance detoxification of undesirable compounds; supports maintenance of heart, immune and digestive health
Dithiolthiones	Cruciferous vegetables	May enhance detoxification of undesirable compounds; supports maintenance of healthy immune function
Vitamins		
A‡	Organ meats, milk, eggs, carrots, sweet potato, spinach	Supports maintenance of eye, immune and bone health; contributes to cell integrity
Thiamin (vitamin B₁)	Lentils, peas, brown or enriched white rice, pistachios, certain fortified breakfast cereals	Supports maintenance of mental function; helps regulate metabolism
Riboflavin (vitamin B₂)	Lean meats, eggs, green leafy vegetables, dairy products and certain fortified breakfast cereals	Supports cell growth; helps regulate metabolism
Niacin (vitamin B₃)	Dairy products, poultry, fish, nuts, eggs, certain fortified breakfast cereals	Supports cell growth; helps regulate metabolism
Pantothenic acid (vitamin B₅)	Sweet potato, organ meats, lobster, soybeans, lentils, certain fortified breakfast cereals	Helps regulate metabolism and hormone synthesis

*Examples are not an all-inclusive list.
†FDA-approved health claim for component.
‡Preformed vitamin A is found in foods that come from animals. Provitamin A carotenoids are found in many darkly colored fruits and vegetables and are a major source of vitamin A for vegetarians. Data from International Food Information Council Foundation: Functional Foods, July 2011. Accessed September 15, 2013. Available at: http://www.foodinsight.org/Content/3842/Final%20Functional%20Foods%20Backgrounder.pdf.

Case Application for the Dental Hygienist

Mrs. Owen is a 73-year-old patient with complete dentition in the maxillary arch and a removable mandibular partial denture. The mandibular canines and incisors are present, all of which have periodontal involvement with 3 to 5 mm of gingival recession. Root caries are present on the mandibular right and left canine. Examination reveals dry, cracked lips; a lack of salivary pool; and an ill-fitting mandibular prosthesis. The medical history reveals high blood pressure and a 10-year history of antihypertensive drug use. Mrs. Owen complains of difficulty in swallowing dry food, xerostomia, and taste alterations.

While obtaining a 24-hour food recall, the dental hygienist realizes that Mrs. Owen has lost interest in food. She states: "I just don't feel like eating. Food doesn't taste good, and I don't like cooking for myself." If she eats breakfast, she typically has orange juice and a doughnut; for lunch, she has canned soup; and before bedtime, part of a frozen dinner. A jar of hard candy sits in her living room from which she periodically takes a piece throughout the day, and she is constantly drinking soda for relief of xerostomia.

Nutritional Assessment
- Food intake for possible nutrient deficiencies
- Oral factors affecting motivation to eat
- Social and medical factors affecting nutrient intake
- Knowledge and motivation level
- Financial status

Nutritional Diagnosis
Several factors are involved with Mrs. Owen's poor nutrient intake: xerostomia; root caries; an ill-fitting prosthesis; frequent intake of hard candy; lack of variety in food; choice of soft, low nutrient-dense foods; and social isolation.

Nutritional Goals
Mrs. Owen has agreed to improve her overall nutritional status gradually by replacing soft, low nutrient-dense foods with high-fiber foods and using sugar-free candies and soda to prevent root caries.

Nutritional Implementation
Intervention: Increase intake of calcium-rich foods, such as low-fat milk, yogurt, and cheese.

Rationale: Adequate calcium and vitamin D intakes help to protect the alveolar bone from resorption.

Intervention: Provide education on xerostomia and its effects on the oral cavity and dietary process.

Rationale: An understanding of the cause and effect of xerostomia can help Mrs. Owen make necessary changes.

Intervention: Limit the intake of commercial frozen prepared meals and other processed foods high in sodium. Suggest that she could prepare several meals and freeze them in individual portion sizes when she feels like cooking.

Rationale: An occasional frozen meal is quick and effortless and a better choice than not eating. However, they are expensive and generally need to be supplemented with other foods for adequate nutrients. Because many are high in sodium, an important factor because of Mrs. Owen's hypertension, remind her to read labels and to purchase ones that contain less than 500 mg of sodium per serving.

Intervention: Suggest (a) frequent sips of a nutritious beverage (e.g., milk or juices) or a noncariogenic fluid (e.g., water or diet soda) throughout the day; (b) use of products designed for patients with xerostomia, such as Biotène® or Oral Balance®; (c) foods containing nonnutritive sweeteners or sugar alcohols (e.g., products containing xylitol); and (d) foods that stimulate saliva flow, such as citrus, tart, or sour foods (e.g., sugar-free lemon drops). Remind the patient of gastrointestinal distress associated with excessive consumption of products containing sugar alcohols.

Rationale: High-nutrient or noncariogenic fluids keep the mouth moist to relieve xerostomia. Products containing xylitol consumed after a meal can deter demineralization and promote remineralization. Citrus, tart, or sour foods and chewing gum stimulate saliva flow.

Intervention: Emphasize the importance of practicing proper oral hygiene techniques, and explain the caries and periodontal disease process.

Rationale: Because dentition status is related to nutritional status, Mrs. Owen would benefit by retaining each natural tooth as long as possible. Xerostomia is also a contributing factor to root caries; however, plaque biofilm must be present for xerostomia to play a role in caries development. Proper daily oral hygiene care would improve her oral status and prevent further complications.

Intervention: Apply topical fluoride in the office, and instruct the patient on self-applied home fluoride treatments.

Rationale: Topical fluoride application reduces caries risk by disrupting destructive bacteria from metabolizing fermentable carbohydrates. Application of fluoride is based on caries risk, not age.

Intervention: Instruct the patient to use a daily antimicrobial rinse for 2 weeks after each treatment.

Rationale: Antimicrobial agents are used as an adjunct to other strategies for caries reduction. Antimicrobial agents effectively control plaque biofilm formation and maturation.

Intervention: Avoid dry, spicy, and some acidic foods; alcohol; caffeine; and tobacco.

Rationale: These choices can worsen xerostomia or irritate the mucosa.

Intervention: Encourage involvement with a local senior group and provide information for food assistance programs for older adults, such as Meals on Wheels.

Rationale: An older adult who lives alone may experience a decreased appetite and lack motivation to prepare appropriate meals. Socializing with others during meals enhances the enjoyment of eating.

Evaluation
Mrs. Owen's mandibular partial denture has been adjusted. The nutrition goals established with the dental hygienist are gradually being met. She has substituted a few pieces of sugar-free candy for the hard sugar-containing candy, prepares more meals, and has joined the community senior citizen center. She recently began using home fluoride treatments, completed the antimicrobial rinse, and remains caries-free. She appears to be a much happier individual.

STUDENT READINESS

1. To understand what a patient with xerostomia experiences, eat several saltine crackers with no fluid, and note the dryness of the oral cavity. Imagine this situation indefinitely and its impact on a patient's food intake. Now try a product designed to relieve xerostomia to understand its effect before recommending it to a patient.

2. Discuss at least two changes in the oral cavity that can change a patient's taste sensation. What recommendations can a dental hygienist provide?

3. Prepare an educational program for interdisciplinary healthcare professionals on recognizing changes in the oral cavity affecting nutrient intake and, ultimately, general health. List at least three healthcare professionals who would benefit from this knowledge.

References

1. Al Jawad FA, Cunningham SJ, Croft N, et al: A qualitative study of the early effects of fixed orthodontic treatment on dietary intake and behavior in adolescent patients. *Eur J Orthod* 34:432–436, 2011.

2. Liu B, Dion MR, Jurasic M, et al: Xerostomia and salivary hypofunction in vulnerable elders: prevalence and etiology. *Oral Surg Oral Med Oral Pathol Oral Radiol Endod* 114(1):52–60, 2012.

3. Ignjatović Z, Stojšin I, Brkanić T, et al: The effect of excessive Coca-Cola consumption on the development of dental erosions. *Serbian Dent J* 59(3):148–150, 2012.

4. Centers for Disease Control and Prevention, Oral Health Resources: *Complete tooth loss.* Accessed September 15, 2013. Available at: http://apps.nccd.cdc.gov/nohss/ListV.asp?qkey=8&DataSet=2.

5. Kim JK, Baker LA, Seirawan H, et al: Prevalence of oral health problems in US adults, NHANES 1999-2004: exploring differences by age, education, and race/ethnicity. *Spec Care Dentist* 32(6):234–241, 2012.

6. Ervin RB, Dye BA: Number of natural and prosthetic teeth impact nutrient intakes of older adults in the United States. *Gerodontology* 29:e693–e702, 2012.

7. Cousson PY, Bessadet M, Nicolas E, et al: Nutritional status, dietary intake and oral quality of life in elderly complete denture wearers. *Gerodontol* 29:e685–e692, 2012.

8. Boozer CH, Langland OE, Guillory MB: Benign migratory glossitis associated with lichen planus. *J Oral Med* 29(2):58–59, 1974.

9. Salazar-Sanchez N, Lopez-Jornet P, Camacho-Alonso F, et al: Efficacy of topical aloe vera in patients with oral lichen planus: a randomized double-blind study. *J Oral Pathol Med* 39(10):735–740, 2010.

10. Zhang J, Zhou, G: Green tea consumption: an alternative approach to managing oral lichen planus. *Inflamm Res* 61(6):535–539, 2012.

11. Huber MA: White oral lesions, actinic cheilitis, and leukoplakia: confusions in terminology and definition: Facts and controversies. *Clin Dermatol* 28(3):262–268, 2010.

12. Crowe KM, Francis C: Position of the Academy of Nutrition and Dietetics: functional foods. *J Acad Nutr Diet* 113(8):1096–1103, 2013.

13. International Food Information Council Foundation: *Functional foods.* 2011 July. Accessed September 15, 2013. Available at: http://www.foodinsight.org/Content/3842/Final%20Functional%20Foods%20Backgrounder.pdf.

ⓔ EVOLVE RESOURCES

Please visit http://evolve.elsevier.com/Stegeman/nutritional for additional practice and study support tools.

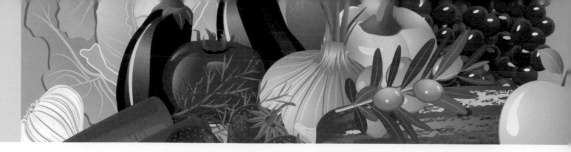

Chapter 21

Nutritional Assessment and Education for Dental Patients

Student Learning Outcomes

Upon completion of this chapter, the student will be able to achieve the following student learning outcomes:

- Discuss the importance of a thorough health, social, and dental history in relation to assessment of nutrition status.
- Describe the components needed to assess the nutrition status of a patient.
- Explain the types of diet histories, and determine situations in which each is used effectively.
- Formulate a dietary treatment plan for a dental problem influenced by nutrition.
- Identify steps and considerations in implementing a dietary treatment plan.
- Assimilate the steps of a nutrition education session.
- Practice several communication skills the dental professional should employ when educating a patient.
- Integrate EXPLORE-GUIDE-CHOOSE techniques of motivational interviewing into a clinical setting.

Key Terms

Anthropometry
Diet history
Explored
Food frequency questionnaire

Goal
Guide
Motivational interviewing
24-Hour recall

⊙ Test Your NQ

1. **T/F** When health and dental histories have been reviewed, the dental professional has adequate information to begin nutrition education with the patient.
2. **T/F** A clinical oral examination is a very sensitive tool for identifying nutritional deficiencies.
3. **T/F** Using food models helps the patient to learn how to determine portion sizes quickly and accurately.
4. **T/F** When providing nutrition education, the dental professional should change the patient's usual intake as little as possible and reinforce positive practices.
5. **T/F** Results of dietary discussion sessions do not need to be documented or communicated with other dental staff members.
6. **T/F** Providing a standardized low-carbohydrate menu is sufficient for most patients with a high caries rate.

7. **T/F** The dental professional should highlight all foods on the food diary that may contribute to increasing the risk for caries.
8. **T/F** After the nutrition education session, the patient should have enough information and motivation to make the necessary changes.
9. **T/F** "What type of snacks do you eat?" is an example of an open-ended question.
10. **T/F** Listening involves interpreting the words said, the manner in which they are said, and nonverbal actions directly observed.
11. **T/F** In motivational interviewing, patients are confronted about their inappropriate behavior and presented with a course of treatment by the dental expert.
12. **T/F** It is better to elicit a patient's motivation and thoughts than to present the dental professional's opinions.

Health is a multidimensional and interprofessional concept, encompassing the interaction of many elements. Dissemination of information to a patient does not guarantee that the patient will establish healthier patterns. For example, millions of people start or continue smoking despite innumerable documented health risks. To facilitate positive changes toward a desired health behavior, the healthcare educator must tailor the message to meet the patient's needs, practices, habits, attitudes, beliefs, and values.

The relationship between nutrition and the oral cavity has already been established in this book. As you have learned, signs of a nutrient deficiency, excess, or imbalance are detectable in the mouth. Conversely, integrity of the oral cavity is a factor in nutrient intake. Nutrition education should be patient-centered, should emphasize prevention, and should provide evidence-based information. Through the dental hygiene process of care (assessment, diagnosis, planning, implementation, and evaluation), the dental hygienist is ideally situated to address nutrition status as it relates to oral health.[1] The position of the Academy of Nutrition and Dietetics states, "The Academy supports the integration of oral health with nutrition services, education, and research. Collaboration between dietetics and oral healthcare professionals is recommended for oral health promotion and disease prevention and intervention."[2] Nutrition is essential for general health and dental health. The American Dental Hygienists' Association *Standards for Clinical Dental Hygiene Practice*[1] state one of the dental hygienist's responsibilities is assessment of nutrition history and dietary practices with integration of nutrition counseling into comprehensive dental hygiene care. Poor eating habits are widespread among Americans; nutrition education as it relates to oral care is justifiable for most patients. When the instruction requires more than general nutrition information or complex medical nutrition therapy, the patient is to be referred to the healthcare provider or registered dietitian nutritionist (RDN).

A nutrition assessment involves compiling and comparing data about the patient from various resources to provide meaningful evaluation and effective education. Providing nutritional information without a complete assessment is inappropriate. All steps in the assessment require critical thinking by the dental professional. The evaluation tools to be discussed in this chapter include health, social, and dental histories; clinical evaluations; dietary intake evaluation; and biochemical analysis.

EVALUATION OF THE PATIENT

For effective education, a comprehensive picture of the patient is essential. If information gathered is incomplete, the treatment plan is distorted and may be ineffective or even detrimental to the patient's overall health. Consider this scenario: a patient with rampant caries is told to substitute sugar-free candy for mints. The patient agrees to try this until she discovers that sugar-free mints cost more money and are unrealistic with her limited income. The patient is unaware of other acceptable alternatives and continues with the mints. Thus, information essential for making appropriate recommendations for the patient was overlooked. Another example: a dental hygienist recommends a fluoride supplement to a young patient who drinks only bottled water, without assessing all fluoride sources being consumed. This could potentially lead to fluorosis.

Health History

The health history is designed to identify health-related considerations and side effects from medications putting a patient at nutritional risk. The presence of some medical conditions could affect nutrition status by interfering with a patient's ability to chew, digest, absorb, metabolize, or excrete nutrients. Medications (over-the-counter and prescription), herbs, and supplements have numerous side effects and interactions altering eating behaviors or affecting nutrition status or both. A patient taking an antihypertensive medication may experience drug-induced xerostomia and its consequent dental complications. Changes in taste and appetite, increased risk of dental problems, gastrointestinal distress, nausea or vomiting, and xerostomia are just a few drug-induced side effects. Many medications also have drug-nutrient interactions (e.g., prednisone), which may influence nutrient needs.

By reviewing the health history and clarifying statements with the patient, the clinician can discover additional health-related information. Patients may not report valuable information because they (a) perceive it as irrelevant for dental professionals, (b) have forgotten it, (c) are confused by the question, or (d) are apprehensive about their visit to the dental office. Patients frequently neglect to disclose the use of oral contraceptives, antiobesity drugs, or dietary supplements, which can have several dental and nutrition implications. A few minutes of further questioning by the dental professional can save hours of time and effort spent trying to treat the complications. A thorough health history provides the dental professional with a strong foundation for developing a plan for dietary education. In addition, a blood glucose level on a patient with diabetes and a blood pressure measurement for all patients can be obtained to augment the assessment.

Screening tools, such as a nutrition assessment questionnaire (see Evolve), are helpful. When a nutritional screening is obtained during the initial steps of the assessment, the dental professional can detect warning signs to investigate further.

Psychosocial History

A social history identifies factors influencing food intake. Personal, environmental, or economic influences can imply nutritional problems (Box 21-1). The dental professional obtains much of this information through conversation and further questioning. In addition, by asking a patient to describe a "typical day," the dental professional can determine routine activities reflective of the patient's lifestyle. Understanding reasons for food choices and considering emotional patterns provide directions for suggesting dietary modifications. Considerations in choosing foods or eating patterns can be found in Chapter 16.

Dental History

A knowledge of how patients perceive or value their oral health assists the dental professional in developing strategies for education. Such information is part of a dental history. Explanations of past and current dental practices, past dental treatment, and behaviors that impact oral care (e.g., clenching teeth, biting fingernails, sinus trouble) should also be collected. Tobacco and alcohol use, fluoride history, and snacking patterns are also important components.

The most effective technique for gathering a medical, social, and dental history is for the dental professional to interview the patient.

ASSESSMENT OF NUTRITIONAL STATUS

A thorough assessment provides the dental professional with enough information to determine the nutrition status of the patient. An assessment of a healthy patient may identify nutritional aspects that can be improved or "fine-tuned" for optimal health. When patients are experiencing medical or dental complications, the assessment provides information alerting the dental professional to nutritional factors that can impede responses to dental treatment or recovery (e.g., a patient with anorexia nervosa, whose fragile nutrition status would delay recovery after periodontal surgery). During the assessment, the dental professional can also identify the level of patient readiness for change to provide appropriate guidelines directed toward modifying behavior. Overall, assessment provides the basis for the dental professional's well-informed recommendations or referrals.

Clinical Observation

Clinical observation begins as soon as the patient walks through the door. General appraisal should include posture, gait, mobility, skin tone and color, general weight status, significant loss or gain of weight since previous visit, emotional state, personal hygiene, and physical limitations. Unintentional weight loss can be indicative of numerous disease states or even oral problems.

Extraoral and Intraoral Assessments

Visual inspection during an extraoral and intraoral examination identifies abnormal clinical signs. Table 21-1 lists physical signs and symptoms that may indicate an alteration in nutrition. These findings are not sensitive tools for determining nutrient deficiencies or excesses because they can mirror non-nutritional complications or the possibility of several nutritional difficulties. For example, cheilosis can be the result of a vitamin B complex, iron, or protein deficiency; uncontrolled diabetes, excess or lack of saliva; constantly licking lips; allergies; yeast or fungal infections; or environmental exposure. Observations are used as an adjunct to supplement other assessment techniques.

Examples of extraoral signs and symptoms for the dental professional to document are multiple skin bruises or pallor, excessively dry or easily plucked hair, dry eyes, and cracked or spoon-shaped fingernails. Intraoral inspection of the integrity of soft tissues, status of the periodontium, and presence of plaque biofilm and calculus are examples of valuable indicators of the need for nutrition intervention. Data obtained during an extraoral and intraoral examination can supply valuable evidence of a nutrition problem that can be confirmed with other assessment procedures.

Other health professionals, such as RDNs, provide a physical assessment that includes the performance of a basic oral screening. A dental professional is capable of sharing expertise related to oral health concepts. Educating other health professionals to recognize normal and non-normal oral conditions that interfere with dietary intake and encouraging performance of oral screenings can lead to identifying potential problems with oral issues and an increase in referrals to dental professionals.[2] Ultimately, the patient benefits from the strategies formulated by an interdisciplinary team.

Anthropometric Evaluation

Anthropometry involves measurements of physical characteristics such as height, weight, and change in weight. Indirectly, an anthropometric evaluation provides an image of body composition and helps to monitor progress of pregnant women; and growth of infants, children, and adolescents. This assessment alone is not sensitive enough to determine nutrition status; however, anthropometric measures may be useful in diagnosis.

Although measuring height and weight is unrealistic and inappropriate in most dental environments, it is appropriate to request a patient's height and weight because this information is needed to determine appropriate dosage for

Table 21-1	Nutrition-related complications of the oral cavity
Nutrient	**Deficiency Symptoms**
Thiamin (B_1)	Increased sensitivity and burning sensation of oral mucosa; burning tongue; loss of taste and appetite
Riboflavin (B_2)	Angular cheilosis; blue to purple mucosa; glossitis, magenta tongue, enlarged fungiform papillae, atrophy and inflammation of filiform papillae, burning tongue
Niacin (B_3)	Glossitis, ulcerations of tongue, atrophy of papillae; cheilosis; thin epithelium; burning of oral mucosa, stomatitis, erythematous marginal and attached gingiva; loss of appetite
Pyridoxine (B_6)	Cheilosis; glossitis, atrophy and burning of tongue; stomatitis
Cobalamin (B_{12})	Stomatitis; hemorrhaging; pale to yellow mucosa; glossitis, atrophy and burning of tongue; altered taste; loss of appetite
Folic acid	Glossitis with enlargement of fungiform papillae, ulcerations along edge of tongue; gingivitis; erosion and ulcerations on buccal mucosa, pale mucosa
Biotin	Glossitis; gray mucosa; atrophy of lingual papillae
Vitamin C	Odontoblast atrophy; porotic dentin formation; alterations in pulp; gingival inflammation with easy bleeding, deep red to purple gingiva; ulceration and necrosis; slow wound healing; muscle and joint pain; defects in collagen formation
Vitamin A	Ameloblast atrophy; faulty bone and tooth formation; accelerated periodontal destruction; hypoplasia; xerostomia; cleft lip; keratinization of epithelium; drying and hardening of salivary glands *Toxicity symptoms:* Hypertrophy of bone; cracking and bleeding lips; thinning of epithelium; erythematous gingiva; cheilosis
Vitamin D, calcium, and phosphorus	Failure of bones to heal; mild calcification to enamel hypoplasia; loss of alveolar bone; delayed dentition; increased caries rate; loss of lamina dura around roots of tooth; reduced plasma calcium levels
Vitamin K	Gingival hemorrhaging
Iron	Painful oral cavity; stomatitis; thinned buccal mucosa with ulcerations; pale to gray mucosa, lips, and tongue; angular cheilosis; burning tongue; reddening at lip and margins of tongue; salivary gland dysfunction
Zinc	Thickening of epithelium; thickening of tongue with underlying muscle atrophy; impaired taste
Protein	Smooth, edematous tongue; angular cheilosis; fissures on lower lip; smaller teeth; delayed eruption; salivary gland dysfunction

medications and local anesthesia used during dental care. The height and weight information can easily be put into a body mass index (BMI) calculator (available the Evolve website). The BMI, as described in the *Dietary Guidelines* (see Chapter 1 or http://www.usda.gov/cnpp), provides the general weight category and associated health risk, and is a guide toward measuring nutrition status. However, BMI does not consider variables such as body composition and should not be the only anthropometric measure assessed. BMI is not used for pregnant or lactating women, older adults, or athletes. Visual inspection also assists in detecting unusual leanness, indicating undernutrition, or notable obesity.

Concern arises when weight loss is unintentional. A reduction of 10% of usual weight over 6 months is significant, and a loss of 20% of body weight or greater may indicate depletion of body mass, which may affect the immune response and the patient's ability to heal after invasive dental treatment.

Laboratory Information

When available, laboratory tests provide another piece of the puzzle in determining nutrition status. Generally, blood and urine samples supply the most sensitive data. As with other assessment techniques, a laboratory test alone should not be used to diagnose malnutrition because non-nutritional

factors also can influence these data. A healthcare provider or RDN generally interprets nutrition-related laboratory tests. Dental professionals generally do not have access to this information, and it is not commonly used in a dental nutrition assessment.

In a dental environment, laboratory evaluations can include measuring salivary flow, plaque indices, caries risk assessment, determining the number of destructive bacterial cells, testing the pH of saliva, or monitoring blood glucose. Each of these tests provides valuable information to be included in the assessment.

Dental Considerations

Assessment

- *Physical:* deviations from normal anatomy, particularly of the head and neck areas; diseases or conditions; emotional state; activity level; abnormal anthropometric measurements; blood pressure; if accessible or practical, laboratory tests, such as blood glucose values for individuals with diabetes.
- *Dietary:* medications responsible for difficulties in eating; conditions that interfere with obtaining adequate nutrients (e.g., financial status, ability to shop for or prepare food); oral health issues interfering with food intake.

Continued

Dental Considerations—cont'd

Interventions

- To be an effective nutrition educator, the dental professional must understand eating habits of local cultural, ethnic, or religious groups (see Chapter 16).
- Questioning the patient about mode of transportation and mobility in the community may reveal difficulties in food procurement related to immobility or isolation.
- Have the patient describe past dental experiences to gauge knowledge level, and perception and attitude toward dentistry.
- Information about previous fluoride exposure provides valuable indicators for the assessment. Additional questions include the following: "Were you raised in an area with fluoridated water?" "Did you take fluoride supplements growing up?" "How often did the dentist provide fluoride treatments?" "Were fluoride treatments given at school?" "Have you used fluoridated rinses or gels at home?"
- Observations of the patient's attentiveness, anxiety level, motivation, previous dental treatment, and present oral conditions provide direction when initiating a nutrition treatment plan.
- A simple method to determine a patient's readiness for behavior change is to ask, "On a scale from 1 to 10, how ready are you to substitute 12 oz of milk for 12 oz of soda?" (1 being not ready to change and 10 being ready to change).[4]
- Questions and comments made by the patient reflect existing knowledge and understanding of information presented, and their needs and desires. A dental professional should practice active listening skills to gain valuable information needed in the assessment.
- While interviewing, maintain verbal and nonverbal neutrality in response to the patient's statements.

Evaluation

- When histories and other information about the patient have been obtained, and the clinical examination has been performed, the dental professional should have some understanding of the patient's preferences and needs.

Nutritional Directions

- Take the time to gather as much nutrition information about the patient as possible to provide individualized suggestions for greater patient compliance. Generic and vague health messages and meal plans are ineffective.

Determining Diet History

To assess the patient's nutrition status further, the evaluation process should include a screening of the diet history, or a review of usual patterns of food intake and various factors that determine food selection. The overall goal is to determine usual dietary habits to individualize recommendations and suggest minor changes, while improving the dietary quality. Reviewing intake of the parent, guardian, or caregiver is necessary to understand food choices of a child or adolescent. Questioning may be necessary to clarify information provided. Explain the need for a nutrition assessment before asking the patient to complete the diet history form. Additional questioning may be necessary to clarify the information provided. Inquire about food preparation, whether

foods chosen are nonfat or dietetic, and use of beverages or condiments. Also, use of food models, pictures of foods in measured portions, and measuring devices are helpful to easily and precisely identify the patient's usual serving sizes.

The diet history can be evaluated based on *MyPlate* and the *Dietary Guidelines* for adequacy and variety of nutrients. There is no charge to use this U.S. Department of Agriculture government-operated website. Other nutrition software programs, such as is available on the Evolve website, are available. An analysis of daily carbohydrate exposures identifies cariogenic potential of the diet. Practical tools used to collect data on dietary intake include the 24-hour recall, food frequency questionnaire, and 3- to 7-day food diary.

Twenty-Four-Hour Recall

The 24-hour recall (see Fig. 18-8; Figs. 21-1 and 21-2) allows the dental professional to collect data on food consumed during a single day. It is easy, quick, and presents a representative sample of the patient's dietary intake. The information is most accurate when interviewing the patient or the parent or guardian of a child and requesting intake from the previous day; this requires little time and is easy to obtain. The patient is generally able to recreate the dietary intake from the preceding day with minimal effort. Obtaining as much detail as possible elicits an accurate view of usual food and beverage intake. The use of food models or visuals of common serving sizes (Box 21-2) helps the patient provide a more accurate estimation of portion size. Snacking patterns and spacing of meals may also be revealed in a 24-hour recall. Another advantage is it allows a general analysis of basic nutrient adequacy, variety, and cariogenicity.

An account of the previous day may not be optimal, however, if it was not a typical day. For example, the patient may have been extremely busy the day before and ate only

---

BOX 21-2 How to Keep Your Food Record

- Record foods and beverages as soon after eating as possible.
- Record on days when *not* sick or fasting.
- Record all meals and snacks for each day, including one weekend day.
- Estimate portion sizes (e.g., 3 oz fish, 1 cup of cereal, ½ cup of milk, 1 tsp of vegetable oil) as closely as possible.
- Document the food preparation method (e.g., baked, broiled, fried, or grilled).
- Include amounts of added sugar, creamer, sauces, gravies, and condiments (e.g., mayonnaise or mustard).
- For combination dishes such as casseroles, soups, chili, or pasta, record all the ingredients and the amounts accurately, and the portion eaten.
- Record brand names (e.g., Cheerios or Promise Margarine).
- Enter the time of consumption.
- Include miscellaneous items, such as mints, gum, and cough drops.

My Daily Food Plan

Based on the information you provided, this is your daily recommended amount for each food group.

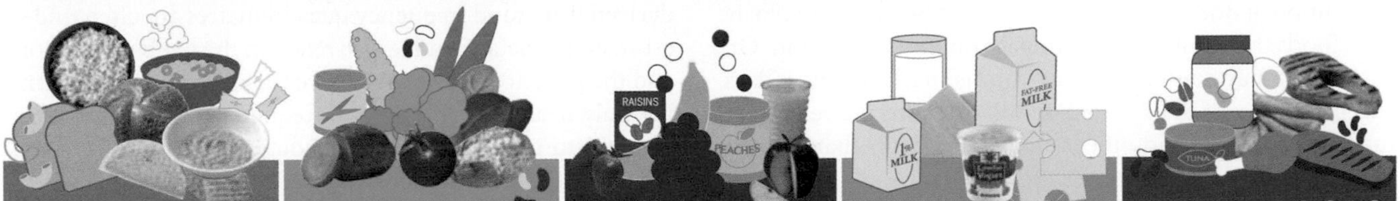

GRAINS	VEGETABLES	FRUITS	DAIRY	PROTEIN FOODS
6 ounces	2 1/2 cups	2 cups	3 cups	5 1/2 ounces

Make half your grains whole	**Vary your veggies**	**Focus on fruits**	**Get your calcium-rich foods**	**Go lean with protein**
Aim for at least **3 ounces** of whole grains a day	Aim for these amounts **each week:** **Dark green veggies** = 1 1/2 cups **Red & orange veggies** = 5 1/2 cups **Beans & peas** = 1 1/2 cups **Starchy veggies** = 5 cups **Other veggies** = 4 cups	Eat a variety of fruit Choose whole or cut-up fruits more often than fruit juice	Drink fat-free or low-fat (1%) milk, for the same amount of calcium and other nutrients as whole milk, but less fat and Calories Select fat-free or low-fat yogurt and cheese, or try calcium-fortified soy products	Twice a week, make seafood the protein on your plate Vary your protein routine— choose beans, peas, nuts, and seeds more often Keep meat and poultry portions small and lean

Find your balance between food and physical activity

Be physically active for at least **150 minutes** each week.

Know your limits on fats, sugars, and sodium

Your allowance for oils is **6 teaspoons** a day.
Limit Calories from solid fats and added sugars to **260 Calories** a day.
Reduce sodium intake to less than **2300 mg** a day.

Your results are based on a 2000 Calorie pattern.

Name: _____

This Calorie level is only an estimate of your needs. Monitor your body weight to see if you need to adjust your Calorie intake.

FIGURE 21-1 *MyPlate* food record worksheet for a 2000-calorie intake goal. (From U.S. Department of Agriculture (USDA) Center for Nutrition Policy and Promotion. Available at: http://www.choosemyplate.gov.)

CDC

My Food Diary   Day _____

Meal/Snack (Indicate time of day)	What You Ate and Drank	Where and With Whom	Notes (Feelings, hunger, etc.)
Breakfast			
Snack			
Lunch			
Snack			
Dinner			

FIGURE 21-2 Food record worksheet. (From the Centers for Disease Control. Available at: http://www.cdc.gov/healthyweight/pdf/food_diary_cdc.pdf.)

one meal, instead of the usual three meals and two snacks. In addition, it does not capture long-term behaviors and may miss foods that could have an impact on the assessment.[3] Or, the patient may consume raw carrots as snacks on most days except the day of the 24-hour recall. The interviewer would miss the carotenes and other valuable nutrients that are part of this patient's dietary intake. Requesting recall of a typical day also may result in unreliable estimates because the patient is more likely to supply information about a "fictitious" day with optimal nutrient intake. It is an option, however, for obtaining a typical day's intake when the past 24 hours were atypical. Another problem may be that a patient has difficulty recollecting the previous day's food intake. Take a minute to write down what you ate yesterday to understand how arduous this task can be, and how easy it is to omit snacks and other foods of lesser importance.

Food Frequency Questionnaire

Another dietary evaluation tool is the food frequency questionnaire. The purpose of this questionnaire is to determine how often a patient consumes foods from groupings containing similar nutrient content. A list of commonly-eaten foods is provided with instructions for the patient to circle the number of times per day, week, or month the food is chosen (Table 21-2). It requires limited explanation and little time; the questionnaire can be completed in the waiting room. The data gained allow for an analysis of food group consumption and carbohydrate intake. It is specifically relevant in determining caries risk.

Because of the lack of a comprehensive food list, the food frequency questionnaire is not specific and does not garner enough data to evaluate nutrient content. Nutrient intakes derived from food frequency questionnaires are often underestimated.[3] Dietary intake also relies on the patient's memory, and the patient can easily improve the choices by documenting only healthy foods. A food frequency questionnaire can be used to supplement the 24-hour recall to increase reliability of the information collected. For instance, a patient may have had a glass of milk yesterday; however, the food frequency questionnaire indicates this is unusual. The dental professional may not have concentrated on dairy products with only the 24-hour recall, but in combination with the food frequency questionnaire, it becomes a component of the nutrition education session.

Food Diary

The patient (or parent or guardian) may also be asked to record food and drink consumption for 3 to 7 days, including a weekend day, to evaluate intake. Figure 21-3 is an example of 1 day of a food diary (see Fig. 18-8 for another example). Verbal and written instructions for using the food diary can be provided at the prophylaxis appointment (see Box 21-2). For accuracy, important points to stress include recording the intake when it is consumed, as well as weighing and measuring foods and beverages. The patient can return the diary at the recare or follow-up appointment. Overall, this is the most effective method of obtaining dietary information because the data are more likely to be representative of actual intake, and the analysis of nutrient and fermentable carbohydrate intake is more accurate. In addition, the patient becomes actively involved when recording the information and may see obscure eating patterns emerge.

Table 21-2	Food frequency questionnaire						
Directions: The following questions will help show your (or your child's) normal eating behavior. This information will allow the dental health team to thoroughly evaluate your (or your child's) dental status. Please mark how often you (or your child) ate or drank each of these items in the past week.							
Food Item	Never	1 to 3 Times per Month	1 to 3 Times per Week	5 or More Times per Week	1 to 2 Times per Day	3 to 4 Times per Day	5 or More Times per Day
Fruit and juices							
Vegetables, other than starchy choices							
Potatoes and other starchy choices							
Milk and yogurt							
Meat, fish, poultry, eggs							
Cheese							
Cereals (cold and hot)							
Cookies, cake, pies, pastries							
Candy							
Regular soda							
Diet soda							
Gum							
Sugar-free gum							
Alcohol							

From Thompson FE, Byers TB: Dietary Assessment Resource Manual. J Nutr 1994; 124(II Suppl):2297S.

DIETARY ANALYSIS					NAME _____			
					AGE _____			
					ACTIVITY LEVEL *SEDENTARY MODERATE ACTIVE*			
					CALORIE LEVEL _____			

Food Groups	Day 1	Day 2	Day 3	Daily Average	Recommended Daily Amounts (Based on appropriate calorie level)	Comparison		
						Adequate	Low	High
Milk					_____ cups			
Protein Foods					_____ oz. equivalents			
Vegetables					_____ cups			
Fruits					_____ cups			
Grains					_____ oz. equivalents			

FIGURE 21-3 Assessment of dietary intake form. This tool can also be used as an educational tool for patient understanding. (A customizable version is available on Evolve.)

Patient compliance is a deterring factor. Requesting records for too many days may decrease cooperation. The validity of the food diary is threatened when the patient underestimates food intake and neglects to record all foods or accurate portion sizes. The patient also may adjust the food diary to reflect healthier eating patterns. By emphasizing this is not a test, but an instrument to evaluate actual food patterns and to identify areas for potential modifications to improve overall health and oral health, the dental professional can concentrate on applying the data or may be able to dispel myths and misinformation that surface from the food diary. Finally, the food diary represents food consumed only for the time period documented, which does not always reflect usual intake.

The dental hygienist and other members of the dental team can cooperatively establish the most practical and realistic approach for determining food intake in their setting. Along with other components of assessment, the dental professional can generally evaluate the nutrition status of the patient and be knowledgeable about the effect of food habits on oral status.

Dental Considerations

Assessment
- *Physical:* age or status of patient may require a caregiver to provide information.
- *Dietary:* current dietary practices and requirements, adequacy of diet, fermentable carbohydrate intake.

Interventions
- When interviewing a patient for a 24-hour recall, you may want to begin with, "What was the first thing you ate or drank after you got up?" or "What was the first thing you ate or drank yesterday morning?" Do not assume breakfast was eaten. Other questions commonly used are the following: "Do you use gum, mints, antacids, or cough drops?" "Do you eat snacks?" "Tell me what you do to clean your mouth." "What do you usually drink?"
- Allow as much participation by patients as possible, encouraging them to make their own decisions and to prescribe their own dietary modifications. Active involvement in problem solving is more effective in changing patients' habits and making them more accountable for their actions.

Evaluation
- The patient participates in the nutrition assessment process, asking appropriate questions and making statements that reflect understanding.

Nutritional Directions

- Nutrition analysis of food intake, even if it is computer generated, cannot be used exclusively for diagnosing a deficiency and cannot replace nutrition education. Many software programs do not have complete or current data, and they do not consider other factors such as overcooking or caries risk. Nutrient intakes may not be accurately estimated. Nutritional analysis provides only an approximation of nutrient content and should be used only as an assessment tool and a guide in educating patients.

IDENTIFICATION OF NUTRITIONAL STATUS

When all of the information is collected, the dental professional can begin to identify nutrition status and cariogenicity of the dietary intake and help the patient establish goals. (Chapter 18 describes the cariogenic potential of the diet.)

A thorough understanding of the nutrients in each group of *MyPlate* helps to identify nutrients that may be deficient or excessive. For example, a commonly-omitted food group is the dairy group, which, if evaluated, would alert the dental professional to possible inadequate intake of calcium, vitamin D, protein, and riboflavin. If such inadequacies are found, the dental hygienist could concentrate on helping the patient identify suitable food choices that are appetizing, accessible and affordable. Preferably, choices providing these nutrients would be from foods, rather than supplements.

Several methods are available to evaluate a dietary intake. Figure 21-3 provides an example to use as an assessment and/or education tool. The foods from the 24-hour recall or 3-day food record (Table 21-3) are transferred to the appropriate food categories with assistance from the patient. It is helpful to have the parent or guardian present when educating a child or adolescent, encouraging the child or adolescent to participate as much as possible. The patient easily determines adequacy of intake, and ideas for modifications or substitutions can follow. The number of servings consumed from each group is totaled. Average intakes are determined by dividing the totals by the number of days in the diary, and the averages are compared with *MyPlate*. As described in Chapter 18, the patient should be encouraged to circle or highlight each carbohydrate exposure and identify form, frequency, and time eaten (i.e., with a meal or as a snack), to evaluate the cariogenic potential of the diet.

Combination foods can be problematic for the patient because of numerous ingredients and difficulties of assigning different components into appropriate food groups. Each ingredient is considered separately and placed in the appropriate food group with servings. A 1-cup serving of spaghetti and meatballs generally is categorized as two grain servings (spaghetti), one protein serving (meatballs), one oil serving (if oil is present in spaghetti sauce or meatballs are fried), and one vegetable serving (tomato sauce).

Computer dietary analysis software packages, online programs, websites, and phone applications are available to assess dietary intake. Patients should be advised to investigate these tools before relying on them completely. Because anyone can publish on the Internet, professionals and patients should examine accuracy, authority, credibility, currency, objectivity, and coverage when using these tools (see "Relevant Websites" on Evolve). Several packages are specifically designed for the dental office. Nutrients usually available include kilocalories, vitamins, minerals, protein, fiber, fat, and cholesterol. Programs vary in complexity, visuals, efficiency, number of food items, and accuracy. A printout of the comparison with the Recommended Dietary Allowances, dietary goals, and exchanges provides a useful and "eye-opening" adjunct to the nutrition education session.

Use of a computer software program is limited by the cost of the hardware and software and the time factor. Not all software is reliable and accurate. Before relying on the data, randomly compare the nutrient content of several foods to U.S. Department of Agriculture nutrient data (http://www.nal.usda.gov/fnic/foodcomp) or the manufacturer's information. Most importantly, use computer feedback to supplement nutrition education sessions but not to replace them.

Table 21-3	Checklist for food records*
Type of Food	**Did You Specify**
All	Amount eaten? By cup, tablespoon, or teaspoon? By size, giving dimensions (length, width, thickness, or diameter)? By number, for standard-size items? By weight?
Cereals	Size of servings? Brand name? Additions, such as milk, sugar, or fruit? Instant or ready-to-eat type?
Baked goods	Homemade or commercial? From scratch or mix? Topping or frosting? Portion size? Number eaten? Low fat? Low carbohydrate?
Fruits and juices	Cooked, raw, or dried? Peeled? Fresh, frozen, or canned? Sweetened? Size of serving? 100% Fruit juice?
Vegetables	Cooked or raw? Fresh, frozen, or canned? Sauces, other additions? Serving size?
Milk products	Percent fat? Made with sweetener? Regular, low fat, or nonfat? Powder or liquid?
Meat, fish, poultry	Type of cut? Oil or water packed? Fat, skin removed? Preparation method? Additions? Cooked weight or dimensions of amount eaten?
Eggs	Added fat? Egg substitutes? Quantity? Preparation method?
Mixed dishes	Homemade or commercial? From scratch or mix? Brand? Major ingredients and proportions? Cooking method?
Soups	Homemade or commercial? Brand? Broth or milk base? Type of milk? Principal ingredients?
Fats and oils	Stick, tub, diet, whipped, liquid, or nonfat margarine? Brand? Major oil? Type of shortening? Homemade or commercial salad dressing? Low kilocalorie or nonfat? Creamy?
Beverages	Brand? Sweetened? Diet? Decaffeinated? Alcohol content? Additions? Amount?
Snacks	Brand? Size, weight, or number eaten?
Restaurant meals	Type? Fast food, ethnic, seafood, steak? How often?
Vitamin-mineral supplements	Type? Reasons? Amount?

From Aronson V: Checklist for food records. In *Guidebook for Nutrition Counselors*, Englewood Cliffs, NJ, 1990, Prentice Hall.
*Use this list to help clarify and increase accuracy of a food diary.

These approaches to determining dietary intake are adequate and practical for most dental patients. The primary goal of a dietary assessment in dentistry is to identify patients with oral concerns related to eating and to improve these habits to prevent dental disease. If a more thorough assessment is required, the patient should be referred to an RDN.

FORMATION OF NUTRITION TREATMENT PLAN

After evaluation of data, the results can be shared with the patient and parent or guardian, if appropriate. The dental professional and patient can begin to establish an individualized dietary plan and course of action. The patient should be involved in as many processes as possible to improve compliance. When assisting the patient in preparing an altered meal pattern, several strategies need to be considered. As discussed earlier, accommodating factors affecting food intake, whenever possible, are advantageous. The goal is patient adherence so that oral health is improved. Other important considerations are food preferences, habits and behaviors, allergies, and prescribed diets. Compliance is more likely if changes are minimal or deviate as little as possible from the patient's normal pattern of eating. The patient should verify other results indicated by the assessment. For instance, if a patient's intake seems deficient in fruits, further questioning may reveal no fruit was available during the days of recording because of the patient's inability to go to the grocery store. The dental professional would interpret this deficiency as atypical, or the situation may occur frequently because of lack of transportation.

Integration and Implementation

The purpose of nutrition education is to provide accurate, evidence-based information, and motivate and encourage positive changes in behavior and continue healthful practices. Obtaining knowledge and changing a personal habit requires a patient to internalize and accept that modifying a specific behavior is beneficial for overall health. A large gap exists between gaining information and applying the information because of difficulties in changing eating patterns. The patient and dental hygienist work together to bridge the gap. Knowledge alone does not determine desired behavior. Providing a sheet with a textbook diet or a list of nutrition "dos and don'ts" is unlikely to effect change. These written guidelines are not meaningful because they do not account for each patient's individuality and unique nutrition needs, and for the difficulty in changing established eating patterns. Consider a patient who accurately describes *MyPlate*, but continues to omit vegetables. This patient is knowledgeable but does not change behavior; learning is ineffective.

Effective nutrition education involves the patient and dental professional working together to define the diet/dental problem and formulate solutions. An education session in which the dental professional points out each negative behavior is not conducive to learning. The dental professional's responsibility is to supply accurate information and guide the patient in making healthful decisions toward improving the diet/dental situation. The dental professional can offer some suggestions and encouragement; however, it is the patient's responsibility to make changes in food patterns.

Motivational Interviewing

As far back as the early 1980s and early 1990s in medical settings, motivational interviewing was initiated as an education tool for changing behaviors.[5,6] Motivational interviewing is a respectful, collaborative conversation about change. A three-component model is proposed to help dental professionals educate patients using motivational interviewing.[7,8] First, the patient's behavior must be explored (Fig. 21-4). Professionals do this by building rapport, asking open-ended questions, listening, affirming patient's thoughts and feelings (without judgment), and summarizing what the patient is saying. It is ideal to find out what is important to patients, their concerns and values, and their health and nutrition history.

The second step after this enlightening conversation is to guide. Professionals should inquire about the patient's own motivation and commitment rather than imposing ideas and suggestions. Dental professionals could easily ask, "On a scale from 1 to 10, how interested are you in changing your eating behavior?" The power for change resides solely in the hands of the patient not the dental professional. When patients recognize a difference between where they are and where they want to be, they become more motivated (Fig. 21-5). If the patient expresses some interest in a commitment to change, then the final step in the model is to choose. Dental professionals assist the patient by identifying specific, patient-oriented goals to build an action plan. Multiple options should be offered to avoid patient rejection (Fig. 21-6). Rolling with any resistance may help the patient not feel judged or pressured. Professionals can reflect back on things the patient has previously mentioned and use that information to move forward, focusing on reasons of the

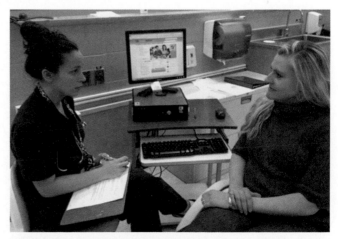

FIGURE 21-4 Motivational interviewing: exploring, establishing good rapport, and listening. (Courtesy of Amy L. Sullivan, University of Mississippi Medical Center, Jackson, MS.)

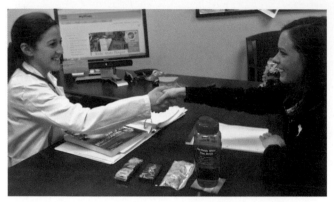

FIGURE 21-5 Motivational interviewing: guiding—getting a commitment. (Courtesy of Amy L. Sullivan, University of Mississippi Medical Center, Jackson, MS.)

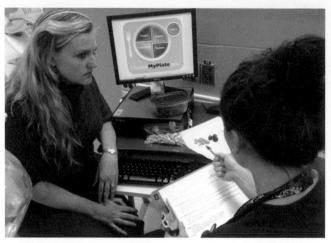

FIGURE 21-6 Motivational interviewing: choosing—offering multiple options. (Courtesy of Amy L. Sullivan, University of Mississippi Medical Center, Jackson, MS.)

BOX 21-3

Motivational Interviewing: Three-Component Model

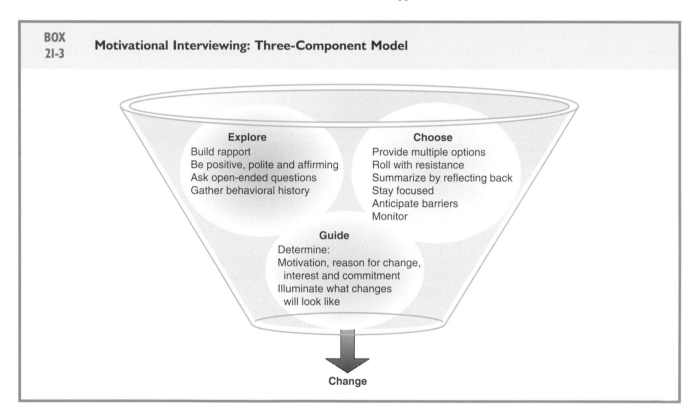

Explore
Build rapport
Be positive, polite and affirming
Ask open-ended questions
Gather behavioral history

Choose
Provide multiple options
Roll with resistance
Summarize by reflecting back
Stay focused
Anticipate barriers
Monitor

Guide
Determine:
Motivation, reason for change,
 interest and commitment
Illuminate what changes
 will look like

Change

---

importance of changing. Professionals can also help foresee potential barriers the patient may encounter and monitor the patient's follow through (Box 21-3).

Setting Goals

Resistance to change, despite knowledge, is a natural response of an individual. Consider the dental health professional who does not floss regularly yet encourages patients to floss. Box 21-4 presents an exercise to further understanding. Establishing a goal is an important aspect of changing behaviors because it sets a concrete standard for change. A meaningful and realistic goal should be something achievable by the patient. The goal chosen should be difficult enough to be

BOX 21-4 **Exercise to Understand Resistance to Change**

Fold your arms in front of you. Do not glance down to identify which arm rests on top. Quickly unfold your arms and refold them the opposite way. For example, if the right arm was initially on top, it should be under the left arm after the switch.

Note the awkwardness. Does this reflect a change in an established behavior? If even this slight physical change leads to some resistance, think of the implications for more substantial behavioral changes asked of a patient.

Adapted from Newstrom JW, Scannell EE: *Games Trainers Play*, New York, 1980, McGraw-Hill.

challenging, but not so difficult as to seem impossible. Occasionally, behaviors may need to be prioritized; a behavior with the most significant impact on oral health is addressed first. Perhaps frequent use of cough drops has led to an increased caries rate. The dental professional should emphasize the reason this behavior is detrimental and guide the patient in establishing goals to decrease use of or eliminate cough drops. This guidance may include referring the patient to a healthcare provider to determine what is causing the sore throat or cough, or explaining why the mouth is so dry.

A goal needs to be measurable or observable. "Eat one vegetable each day" is a very specific goal that can readily be measured. However, "improve oral health" is vague and difficult to observe; this goal should be more specific. Creating goals for multiple behavior changes at one time could be overwhelming. Gradual changes in behavior are more successful and can be accomplished by breaking goals into small steps. The dental professional can work with the patient to select and develop a realistic goal. When established, the goal should be modified as needs change. For example, "Eat one vegetable every other day" may be more appropriate for someone eating no vegetables at all than "Eat three to five servings of vegetables each day as recommended." The latter example may prove to be too difficult, and the patient may give up. Successful achievement of smaller steps motivates the patient toward larger changes. When smaller steps are accomplished, the patient can modify the goal to eating one vegetable every day and eventually work toward eating three to five vegetables per day.

Menu Creation

When the patient has a grasp of the dietary need and has direction as to how to accomplish it, he or she should create a realistic menu for a day. The dental professional assists the patient in documenting a menu that follows the principles discussed, including nutritionally adequate and non-cariogenic situations (Fig. 21-7). It should vary as little as

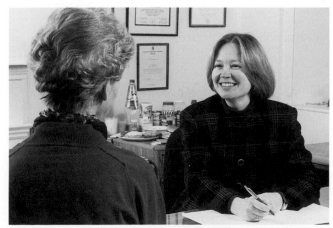

FIGURE 21-7 Menu planning. (A customizable version is available on Evolve.)

possible from the original intake and include foods the patient likes. Often the patient may suggest an ideal intake, modeling *MyPlate*. The dental professional can intervene and suggest individualized or personalized options to improve long-term compliance. For instance, most individuals know it is unwise to eat frequently at fast food restaurants, but it is unrealistic to instruct patients never to eat there. The dental professional can help the patient determine the best food selections available if fast food establishments are necessary several times each week.

The feedback given by the patient to formulate a menu is one indicator for determining whether learning has occurred. An ideal menu reflects knowledge-based skills, but the patient may need to be redirected toward more realistic modifications.

Follow-up

A follow-up appointment to monitor progress and to evaluate the care provided can be scheduled separately or in conjunction with another dental appointment. Primary approaches for the dental professional include supporting continued change, establishing challenging goals or revising existing goals, and clarifying information. Reviewing a new food record with the patient promotes feedback of progress, particularly when compared with the original. Rather than expressing disappointment over failure to achieve a goal, the dental professional praises any positive behaviors, no matter how small. Praise and encouragement are more motivating. Perhaps the initial interventions established did not meet the patient's needs. Follow-up appointments can be used to listen, reassess the plan, identify new needs, and formulate new goals.

Review

The dental professional concludes the session by summarizing the pertinent points and giving the patient a sense of accomplishment and direction after leaving the appointment. A firm commitment toward change may not always occur, but an agreement to think about it can be a successful conclusion. Providing a work phone number, email address or other social media forum, and encouraging the patient to contact you with questions also helps him/her recognize your concern.

Evaluation

Evaluation is an ongoing process that occurs in all stages of assessment and education. The dental hygienist needs to revise the nutrition assessment and educate continuously, and make appropriate changes as needed (Fig. 21-8).

Documentation

The nutrition assessment process must be documented in the treatment record. Because this is a permanent legal document, if it is not recorded, presumably the intervention did not occur. Also, the treatment record serves as a tool to communicate with other members of the dental team and healthcare professionals. At a restorative appointment,

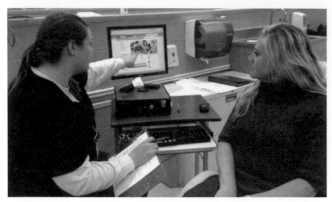

FIGURE 21-8 Educating. (Courtesy of Amy L. Sullivan, University of Mississippi Medical Center, Jackson, MS.)

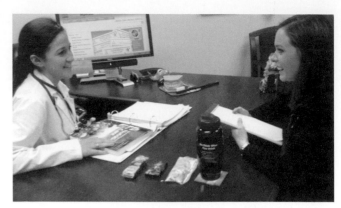

FIGURE 21-9 Listening. (Courtesy of Amy L. Sullivan, University of Mississippi Medical Center, Jackson, MS.)

another dental team member can reinforce the nutrition message already initiated from the information provided on the treatment record. Documentation should include the dental issues, assessment, plan, and outcomes.

FACILITATIVE COMMUNICATION SKILLS

Intertwined with implementing an effective nutrition care plan is the interpersonal communication skills of the dental professional. An atmosphere of sincerity, trust, and empathy should be established to help the patient relax and feel more comfortable in revealing accurate information and be more cooperative in working toward a goal. Good rapport is the foundation; without it, very little is accomplished. Using nonjudgmental and noncritical responses encourages a patient to provide accurate accounts of food intake without the threat of being reprimanded. If a patient's food record reveals donuts and soda for breakfast, it would be judgmental to say, "I can't believe you eat that for breakfast!" Instead, a noncommittal verbal and nonverbal acknowledgment of the food, such as, "Is this usual?" would elicit a more accurate reply. Phrases discounting a patient's feelings do not promote the warm and caring atmosphere essential for good rapport. Phrases such as, "You're making a mountain out of a molehill," "Don't be ridiculous," or "It is good, but…," are guaranteed to inhibit the patient's participation.

Listening

Listening to the patient is an important and distinguishing feature of effective communication that the dental professional must practice. Listening involves more than hearing. It includes interpreting what is said, how it is said, and nonverbal actions observed. Active listening is difficult and requires full attention of the dental hygienist. Active listening can actually save time, however, because it gains a better understanding of a situation (Fig. 21-9).

Impediments to active listening include interrupting, preparing a response while the other person is speaking,

distracting mannerisms, daydreaming, multitasking with devices such as phones or computers, and finishing the speaker's sentences. Awareness of personal barriers to listening allows the dental professional to focus on establishing appropriate alternatives for more effective communication.

To improve listening skills, the dental professional can practice being attentive by shutting out external distractions or not interrupting (e.g., decreasing the number of questions asked, not taking the subject in another direction). A patient feels more comfortable and important when the patient is being heard.

Nonverbal Communication

Facial expressions, eye contact, body movements, personal distance, head nodding, and vocal cues are nonverbal behaviors serving to enhance verbal behavior. Positive nonverbal communications increase the effectiveness of the message and create a comfortable atmosphere for the patient. Eye contact is a significant interaction between the dental professional and patient. Good eye contact communicates interest, understanding, and warmth, whereas a lack of eye contact or staring can be interpreted as indifference or preoccupation. Eye contact and other nonverbal signals can communicate what cannot be verbalized.

Verbal Communication

Asking open-ended questions encourages the patient to expand on the answers, which can include much more information about food choices than anticipated. "What is your evening routine?" would evoke a more detailed response than a question with a yes or no reply, such as, "Do you snack in the evening?"

Dental hygienists can also demonstrate effective communication by reflecting back on what a patient has previously mentioned. This demonstrates that the professional has heard what the patient stated and offers a sense of understanding to the patient. An example might be, "If I heard you correctly, you said that snacking in the evenings is your biggest downfall."

Dental Considerations

Assessment
- *Physical:* attitude and interest of patient toward behavior change; nonverbal signs from patient.
- *Dietary:* completed and analyzed dietary intake.

Interventions
- Avoid scheduling nutrition education sessions after a long or difficult dental appointment.
- The operatory causes anxiety for many patients; when possible, choose a quiet and private location for nutrition education so that the patient feels more relaxed and less apprehensive.
- The room designated for nutrition education should be equipped with a computer with Internet access and educational material such as pertinent literature, posters, flannel boards, food packages, food models, and measuring utensils to enhance the learning experience. In underprivileged scenarios, this may be the dental operatory.
- Explain to the patient you will be taking notes of what is being discussed so that you will not forget important information.

- Resist the temptation to create an ideal diet prescription and solve all nutrition problems. Help patients to adapt and develop a less than perfect menu plan that is more likely to be followed routinely.
- When appropriate, request that a family member or friend participate with the patient in the education session, especially an individual who is responsible for the cooking and food shopping. Assistance is also warranted when a physical or mental impairment interferes with the patient's understanding.

Evaluation
- The patient is an active participant, making a change toward food choices and behaviors agreed to in the nutrition education session; at the follow-up visit or next recare appointment, there is successful achievement of the first set of goals and advancement to implement other, more difficult suggestions; many questions are asked and comments are made that verify interest and understanding.

Nutritional Directions

- Establishing good eating habits is a wise investment toward lifelong positive health and dental status. Prevention, alleviation, or postponing the onset of a disease is possible with good nutrition.

HEALTH APPLICATION **21** Health Literacy

Snrettap reihtlaeh hsilbatse lliw tneitap eht that eetnaraug ton seod tneitap a ot noitamrofni fo noitanimessid. Stnemele ynam fo noitcaretni eht gnissapmocne, tpecnoc lanoisnemiditlum a si htlaeh.

While reading this passage, how did you feel? Are you confused; frustrated; uncertain; too embarrassed to ask what it means; sense of shame; or did you stop trying to understand the two sentences? These are examples of feelings that people with low-proficiency health literacy skills may experience during our discussions with them. *Fermentable carbohydrates, gingiva, suppuration, xerostomia, periodontal disease,* and *calculus* may be unfamiliar, complex, and technical terms that we frequently use with our patients. The above passage simulates what a patient may view on a printed page or the gibberish they may hear in conversation. (*Note:* It is the first two sentences of this chapter written backwards.) Miscommunication is recognized for failure to follow health instructions.

Healthy People 2020 defines health literacy as the "degree to which individuals have the capacity to obtain, process and understand basic health information and services needed to make appropriate health decisions." An objective of *Healthy People 2020* is: (a) to improve health literacy of the population by increasing the number of people receiving easy-to-understand instructions about what to do to take care of their health, (b) being asked to repeat healthcare instructions, and (c) being offered help in filling out the health history or other dental forms.[9] It is the responsibility of all dental health professionals to recognize misunderstanding of patients and to work toward presenting information to match their needs and abilities.

Thirteen percent of English-speaking adults in the United States have proficient health literacy skills, while 44% have basic or below-basic literacy skills (Box 21-5).[10] Low health literacy has been linked to poor health outcomes, such as less frequent use of preventive services. However, the dental hygienist should appreciate that any patient can have difficulty understanding the health information provided. A well-educated individual in a non-healthcare discipline, for example, may not fully understand complex dental information. Situations in which comprehension of health information may be a challenge include those individuals with limited English proficiency; obvious cultural differences; a lack of knowledge and experience; communication or developmental disorders. Populations at risk of low health literacy include older adults, racial and ethnic groups, people with less than a high school education, people with low income levels, and non-native English speakers. The dental hygienist should tailor the dental health information to meet the learning needs of the patient (Box 21-6).

Look at the description below provided by the dental hygienist. The information is at a college level. Box 21-7 provides a list of terms that can be used in place of complex terms. What are examples of simple words that you have used in place of complex words?

Hyperglycemia can cause many complications including nephropathy, retinopathy, neuropathy, and periodontal disease.

How can you get the message across to a patient with basic or below basic levels of health literacy?

High blood sugar can be dangerous to your health. It can cause problems with your kidneys, your eyes, your ability to walk, and your gums.

BOX 21-5   Levels of Heath Literacy

Below Basic
- Able to sign name
- Do simple addition
- Find a country in an article
- Read or complete a brief and uncomplicated document

Basic
- Able to do one-step arithmetic problems
- Locate information in a newspaper article
- Make low level inferences from a text
- Integrate easily identifiable pieces of information

Intermediate
- Can apply information from a moderately-dense text and make simple inferences
- Determine appropriate arithmetic operations
- Identify quantities needed to perform the arithmetic operation

Proficient
- Demonstrate proficiencies associated with long and complex documents and text

National Assessment of Adult Literacy: Health literacy of America's adults: results of the National Assessment of Adult Literacy (NAAL) 2003 Accessed September 6, 2013. Available at http://nces.ed.gov/naal/multimedia.asp.

BOX 21-6   Strategies the Dental Professional Can Utilize to Minimize or Avoid Misunderstanding

- Simple, short, common and plain terms
- Short sentences
- Jargon-free language
- Break complex information into understandable chunks
- Supplement the discussion with relevant and simple pictures and other visual cues
- Use concrete examples rather than abstract principles
- Avoid numbers and statistics
- Present essential information first
- Clear messages
- Limit the number of messages at one time
- Repeat key messages
- Have the patient repeat instructions
- Modify the explanation until it is clear to the patient
- Ask open-ended questions
- Provide the information in multiple ways
- Provide forms in multiple languages
- Provide written instructions
- Offer assistance to the patient in completing the paperwork
- Arrange for a medically trained interpreter

BOX 21-7   Substituting Simple Words for Complex Words

COMPLEX	SIMPLE	COMPLEX	SIMPLE
Administer	Give	Periodontal disease	Gum disease
Anesthetic	Numbing medicine	Plaque	Germs
Bacteria	Germs	Physician	Doctor
Calculus	Tartar, germs that are hard	Procedure	Test
Diagnosis	Problem, condition	Prone	Lying down
Discontinue	Stop	Purulent, suppuration	Pus
Facial, buccal	Cheek side	Remain	Stay
Fermentable carbohydrates	Foods that can cause cavities	Requirement	Need
Gingiva	Gums	Substantial	Large, much
Identify	Find, name, show	Supine	Lay back
Lesion	Cut, injury	Suture	Stitch
Lingual	Tongue side	Validate	Confirm
Minimum	Least, smallest	Xerostomia	Dry mouth

Adapted from: Improving Communication from the Federal Government to the Public. Accessed September 16, 2013. Available at: http://www.plainlanguage.gov/howto/wordsuggestions/simplewords.cfm.

Case Application for the Dental Hygienist

As 70-year-old Mr. B walks into the operatory, it is noted he continues to lose weight and has less energy than at his previous 4-month recare visit. His health history reveals no significant findings except one daily medication to control hypertension. The social history reveals his wife has been deceased for 2 years, and his limited income makes it difficult to purchase the foods he needs. He complains of a loose-fitting maxillary denture and xerostomia.

Nutritional Assessment
- Medical, dental, and social history
- Nutrition assessment questionnaire (see Evolve)
- Extraoral and intraoral examination
- Periodontal evaluation
- Anthropometric evaluation for weight changes
- Three-day food record

Case Application for the Dental Hygienist—cont'd

Nutritional Diagnosis

Social and oral factors are affecting the desire and ability to obtain adequate nutrition.

Nutritional Goals

The patient will seek support from suggested referrals and begin to improve his caloric intake and variety of food.

Nutritional Implementation

Intervention: Ask open-ended questions pertaining to his late wife.

Rationale: Weight change can stem from lack of transportation and education. Mr. B's late wife may have done all the shopping (primary driver) and cooking previously. Educating Mr. B on finding transportation or educating him on what foods should be included in a meal may be appropriate.

Intervention: Examine the oral cavity for any deviation from normal and the fit of the maxillary denture.

Rationale: Ill-fitting dentures can be a result of weight loss, which can be responsible for creating sore spots. The presence of oral infections can decrease the ability and desire to eat, ultimately affecting nutrition status. Identifying such areas can allow for treatment and education on prevention.

Intervention: Provide instruction for completing a 3-day food record.

Rationale: This component completes the assessment process. Determining typical eating habits and patterns and the variety of foods gives direction to the nutrition education. Look for the predominant use of soft foods, highly salted foods, convenience foods, and fermentable carbohydrates; variety; low kilocalories; and number of meals daily.

Intervention: Educate Mr. B regarding basic information about nutrient needs and the relationship between diet and health status.

Rationale: Depression over a spouse's death and dining alone are two factors decreasing an older individual's desire to eat.

Referral to a community-based senior citizen program may provide support and companionship needed to improve his desire to eat.

Intervention: Explain to Mr. B that frequent consumption of acid-containing beverages (e.g., sodas, citrus juices) can put him at high risk for caries. Due to his xerostomia, the lack of protection by saliva may even allow sugar alcohols to create a cariogenic environment, especially if his remaining teeth have gingival recession.

Rationale: Patients with xerostomia have limited cleansing and buffering capabilities because of reduced quantities of saliva. Even foods generally noncariogenic when saliva flow is adequate can be detrimental when saliva flow is diminished. Suggest rinsing with water to dilute the effects of citrus juices or to remove carbohydrates (e.g., rinsing away remnants of crackers or pretzels).

Intervention: Provide positive feedback on any changes, even small ones, Mr. B makes.

Rationale: An older adult may be more resistant to modifications in well-established habits. Small goals are more realistic. Allow him to make the goals based on the information presented to him. Recognize any change is a sign of effort. A follow-up on his progress is important to establish new goals or modify goals as necessary.

Evaluation

At a return visit, Mr. B's new 24-hour recall reveals adequate caloric intake and improvement in variety of food choices. He has slowly begun to gain back some of his weight. He has sought the support of various local senior citizen groups. His denture has been repaired, and he presents a healthy oral cavity.

STUDENT READINESS

1. Examine your own health, social, and dental histories, and identify health-related factors a dental professional would find useful in developing a dietary plan.

2. Interview a partner to obtain health, social, and dental histories. What questions were effective in clarifying or obtaining additional pertinent information?

3. Establish a nutrition goal you can realistically apply this week, and have a partner evaluate. Review progress with the partner at the conclusion of the week. Would you do anything differently to increase the likelihood of accomplishing the goal?

4. Select and explain at least two reasons why a dental professional should conduct a nutrition assessment for patients.

5. Describe the components needed for an assessment of a patient's nutrition status, and explain the rationale of each.

6. The following 24-hour recall was obtained by a dental hygienist. What questions need to be asked to get a more accurate estimate of the patient's intake?

    Breakfast: Bagel and cream cheese, coffee

    Lunch: Hamburger, french fries, soda

    Snack: Candy bar

    Dinner: Roast beef, potatoes, salad, corn

7. Explain why the following question asked during a nutrition education session is undesirable: "Do you realize omitting fruits and vegetables from your day could lead to a deficiency in vitamins A and C?" Reword the question to enhance effectiveness.

CASE STUDY

The dental hygienist has reviewed Jim S's medical, dental, and social histories at the prophylaxis appointment, indicating no significant changes. Jim presents with observable weight gain since the last 6-month recare appointment and three new areas of dental caries. He has no idea why the areas of decay occurred. A 3-day food diary is explained, and a nutrition education session is established following his restorative treatment. At the restorative appointment, the patient forgot to bring his completed food diary. The dental hygienist attributed this to a lack of interest. A 24-hour recall is obtained, and the session is conducted in the operatory.

Continued

CASE STUDY—cont'd

1. Prioritize the diet and dental information that Jim S needs.
2. Explain why and how a nutrition education session could be beneficial to Jim.
3. What questions should be asked before and during the session to gain additional information?
4. State several reasons why the education session may not be effective to motivate behavior change. How could these situations be modified to enhance motivation?

References

1. American Dental Hygienists' Association: *Standards for Clinical Dental Hygiene Practice*, Chicago, 2008, ADHA. Accessed September 15, 2013. Available at: http://www.adha.org/resources-docs/7261_Standards_Clinical_Practice.pdf.
2. Touger-Decker R, Mobley C: Position of the Academy of Nutrition and Dietetics: Oral health and nutrition. *J Acad Nutr Diet* 113(5):693–701, 2013.
3. Kaye EK: Nutrition, dietary guidelines and optimal periodontal health. *Periodontol 2000* 58:93–111, 2012.
4. Chapman-Novakofski K: Education and counseling: behavioral change. In Mahan LK, Escott-Stump S, Raymond JL, editors: *Krause's food and the nutrition care process*, ed 13, St Louis, 2012, Saunders Elsevier.
5. Miller WR: Motivational interviewing with problem drinkers. *Behav Psychother* 11:147–172, 1983. doi: 10.1017/S0141347300006583.
6. Rollnick S, Heather N, Bell A: Negotiating behaviour change in medical settings: the development of brief motivational interviewing. *J Ment Health* 1(1):25–37, 1992. doi: 10.3109/09638239209034509.
7. Resnicow K, McMaster F: Motivational interviewing: moving from why to how with autonomy support. *Int J Behav Nutr Phys Act* 9:19, 2012.
8. Resnicow K, McMaster F, Rollnick S: Action reflections: a client-centered technique to bridge the WHY-HOW transition in Motivational Interviewing. *Behav Cogn Psychother* 40(4):474–480, 2012.
9. U.S. Department of Health and Human Services: *Healthy People 2020*. Health communication and health information technology. Accessed September 17, 2013. Available at: http://www.healthypeople.gov/2020/topicsobjectives2020/objectiveslist.aspx?topicId=18.
10. National Assessment of Adult Literacy: Accessed September 17, 2013. Available at: http://nces.ed.gov/naal/kf_demographics.asp#3.

ⓔ EVOLVE RESOURCES

Please visit http://evolve.elsevier.com/Stegeman/nutritional for additional practice and study support tools.

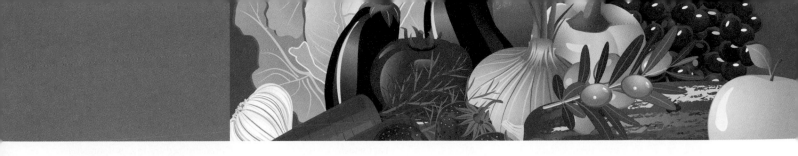

Glossary

abrasion permanent depletion of tooth surfaces as a result of pathologic tooth wear, such as toothbrush abrasion.

acceptable macronutrient distribution ranges (AMDRs) a part of the latest dietary reference intakes (DRIs); established for the macronutrients (fat, carbohydrate, protein, and two polyunsaturated fats) to ensure sufficient intakes of essential nutrients while reducing risk of chronic diseases.

accessory organs organs, such as salivary glands, liver, gallbladder, and pancreas, that provide secretions essential for the digestive process.

achlorhydria absence of hydrochloric acid in the stomach, a condition that occurs primarily in older patients.

active site the region of an enzyme that selectively binds a substrate and contains the amino acids that directly participate in the chemical transformation that converts a substrate into a product.

ad libitum as desired, at will.

added sugars sugars added to foods during processing or at the table.

adenosine triphosphate (ATP) main form of energy used by the cells.

adequate intake (AI) average amount of a nutrient that seems to maintain a defined nutritional state; derived from mean nutrient intakes by groups of healthy people.

adipose tissue body fat.

aerobic lives and grows in the presence of oxygen.

age-related macular degeneration (AMD) deterioration in the central area of the retina (back of the eye) in which lesions lead to loss of central vision.

aldosterone hormone secreted by the adrenal cortex to signal the kidney to retain sodium and water, and excrete potassium and hydrogen ions; ultimately causes edema and high blood pressure.

alimentary canal all the body parts through which food passes, extending from the mouth to the anus.

alopecia hair loss.

α-linolenic acid organic compound found in many vegetable oils.

alternative medicine use of medical and health care systems that are not considered part of conventional Western medicine.

alveolar process crest of the maxilla and mandible.

ameloblasts tall columnar epithelial cells in the inner layer of the enamel.

amenorrhea absence of menses.

amino acids basic building blocks or monomer units for proteins.

amorphous having no definite form.

amphiphilic compound with molecules with a water-soluble group attached to a water-insoluble grouping.

amylase an enzyme that begins the process of digesting dietary carbohydrates.

anabolism use of absorbed nutrients to build or synthesize more complex compounds.

anencephaly absence of a major portion of the brain and skull.

aneurysm bulge or ballooning in the wall of an artery. When an aneurysm becomes too large, it may burst and cause dangerous bleeding or death.

anhydrous contains no water.

anion ion carrying a negative charge as a result of an accumulation of electrons.

anorexia lack or loss of appetite.

anosmia loss of smell.

anthropometric measurements of physical characteristics such as height, weight, and change in weight.

anticariogenic reducing the risk of caries by preventing plaque from recognizing a cariogenic food.

anticholinergic medication used to block parasympathetic nerve impulses.

anticoagulant drug or substance that delays or prevents the clotting of blood (e.g., heparin).

antidiuretic hormone (ADH) hormone released by the pituitary gland to act on the kidneys to control urine output.

antigenic having the properties of an antigen (substance that comes in contact with target cells, inducing an immune response or sensitivity).

antioxidant synthetic or natural substance that prevents or delays the damaging effects of a reactive substance seeking an electron.

apatite calcium phosphate complex that forms crystalline salts within the matrix of bone and teeth.

appetite external factors that influence people to seek and eat food even when not hungry.

ariboflavinosis symptoms associated with riboflavin deficiency (angular cheilitis, glossitis, dermatitis, and anemia).

ataxia gait disorder characterized by uncoordinated muscle movements.

atherosclerosis degenerative disease caused by progressive accumulation of fatty materials on smooth inner walls of arteries of the heart, narrowing the arteries and disrupting blood flow.

atrophic gastritis chronic stomach inflammation with atrophy of the mucous membrane and glands, resulting in diminished hydrochloric acid production.

atrophic gingivitis condition characterized by redness, pain, and wasting of the gingival tissue owing to local and systemic causes.

atrophic glossitis atrophy of the filiform and fungiform papillae beginning at the tip and lateral borders of the tongue and gradually spreading to the entire dorsum of the tongue.

autoimmune disorder condition in which the body produces antibodies against one's own tissues (e.g., celiac disease).

avidin biotin-binding glycoprotein substance present in raw egg white.

baby bottle tooth decay (BBTD) see *early childhood caries*.

bariatric surgery surgical procedure that promotes weight loss by restricting food intake or interrupting the digestive process to prevent absorption of some kilocalories and nutrients.

basal energy expenditure person's total caloric requirement.

basal metabolic rate energy required for involuntary physiological functions to maintain life, including respiration, circulation, and maintenance of muscle tone and body temperature.

beriberi dietary deficiency of thiamin characterized by neuropathy, diarrhea, weight loss, fatigue, and poor memory.

bile emulsifier that helps in the digestion of fats.

binges periods of overeating.

bioavailability amount of nutrient available to the body based on its absorption.

biological value measure of protein quality, with a higher score for proteins of higher quality.

biomolecule any molecule that is produced by a living cell or organism, as well as other organic compounds found in living organisms.

bisphosphonates medications primarily prescribed for osteoporosis, multiple myeloma, and used intravenously during cancer chemotherapy; decrease bone turnover and inhibit the bone's reparative ability.

body mass index (BMI) mathematical calculation using a person's height and weight to determine weight status and to predict health risks that increase at higher levels of overweight and obesity (see p. v).

bolus mass of food that is swallowed and passed into the stomach.

bradycardia low or slow heart rate.

bradykinesia slowness of movement.

brown tumors giant cell tumor replacement of bone evidenced radiologically.

bruxism clenching and grinding of teeth that erodes and diminishes the height of dental crowns.

calcitonin polypeptide hormone regulating the balance of calcium and phosphate in the blood by direct action on bone and kidney. It is secreted by the parathyroid, thyroid, and thymus tissue.

calorie see *kilocalorie*.

calorie-dense foods term used for food usually high in fats (or fat and sugar) and low in vitamins and minerals and other nutrients. A characteristic of calorie-dense foods is less volume of food is needed to furnish energy requirements.

calorimeter device used to measure kilocalories.

cancellous bone internal bone that appears spongy with little hollows that contain bone marrow.

Candida invasive fungal microorganism.

carbohydrate a biomolecule containing carbon, hydrogen, and oxygen with twice as much hydrogen as oxygen; 1 g yields 4 kcal; produced by plants through photosynthesis.

Caries Management by Risk Assessment (CaMBRA) used by dental professionals to identify risk of caries and to determine preventive and therapeutic goals for both children and adult patients.

cariogenic fermentable carbohydrate that causes a reduction of salivary pH to less than 5.5.

cariostatic caries-inhibiting; not metabolized by microorganisms in plaque biofilm.

casein principal protein in cow's milk and chief constituent of cheese.

catabolism breakdown of complex substances into simpler substances.

cation ion carrying a positive charge as a result of a deficiency of electrons.

celiac disease malabsorption syndrome in which individuals are hypersensitive to gluten, a protein inherent to wheat, rye, barley, and triticale.

chelation therapy use of specific chemicals to bind and eliminate heavy metals from the body.

cheilosis unilateral or bilateral presence of cracks and dry scaling around the vermilion border of lips and corners of the mouth; the skin is scaly with red fissures.

chemical bonds hold together atoms in a compound.

chemotherapy treatment of disease by chemical agents.

cholesterol waxy lipid found in all body cells; found only in animal products.

cholinergic parasympathetic (autonomic) nerves stimulated by acetylcholine.

chyme bolus entering the stomach, a semifluid material produced by gastric juices on ingested food.

circumvallate lingual papillae 8 to 10 large and distinctive structures forming a V shape on the posterior end of the anterior two-thirds of the dorsum of the tongue.

cleft lip/palate split where parts of the upper lip or palate fail to grow together.

clinical attachment loss (CAL) loss of periodontal attachment.

coenzyme molecule needed to activate an enzyme.

cofactor element similar to an enzyme in that it is necessary to activate reactions, but the molecule required is a mineral or electrolyte.

coliforms a bacterial indicator of sanitation, universally present in the feces of animals.

collagen basic protein substance of connective tissue helping support body structures such as skin, bones, teeth, and tendons.

colonics a method to cleanse the lower intestines is based on the assumption that years of bad diet causes the colon to become caked with layers of accumulated toxins.

complementary foods foods that do not contain adequate amounts of all the essential amino acids, but when eaten together make up for insufficient amounts of specific essential amino acids, so that adequate amounts of all the essential amino acids are available.

complementary medicine use of untraditional medical and health care systems and products along with conventional medical treatments.

complex carbohydrates see *polysaccharides*.

compound lipids triglycerides with at least one of the fatty acids replaced with carbohydrate, phosphate, or nitrogenous compounds.

compressional forces actions in which the pressure attempts to diminish a structure's volume, which usually increases density.

condensation reaction biochemical reaction in which two molecules combine, eliminating water or some other simple molecule.

conditionally essential amino acids amino acids that are essential in the diet during certain stages of development or in certain nutritional or disease states.

conditionally indispensable amino acids amino acids normally not required by the body, but in certain physiologic conditions, become indispensable.

conjugated linoleic acid (CLA) family of at least 13 isomers (or forms) of linoleic acid, found especially in meats and dairy products.

constipation having a bowel movement fewer than three times per week with hard, dry, small, and difficult to pass stools.

covalent bond bond formed when electrons are equally shared between two nonmetals.

crepitus crackling or grating sound made by a joint, such as the temporomandibular joint.

cretinism stunting of growth often characterized by mental deficits and deaf mutism; a result of inadequate iodine intake during pregnancy.

Daily Reference Values (DRVs) desirable levels of nutrients considered important for health: total fat, saturated fatty acids, protein, cholesterol, carbohydrate, fiber, and sodium.

Daily Value (DV) term used on food labels indicating the percentage of the DV provided by a serving to show the amount of nutrients provided as a percentage of established standards; based on a 2000-kcal diet.

demineralization removal or loss of calcium, phosphate, and other minerals from tooth enamel, causing tooth enamel to dissolve.

dental erosion chemical removal of minerals from the tooth structure that occurs when an acidic environment causes the enamel to dissolve gradually; occurs with frequent exposure to foods with a pH below 4.2.

dentin hypersensitivity extremely painful feeling of exposed dentin resulting from a stimulus, such as temperature or tactile.

detoxification ("detox") the biochemical process that transforms non-water-soluble toxins and metabolites into water-soluble compounds that can be excreted in urine, sweat, bile, or stool.

dextrins intermediate products of the digestive enzymes on starch molecules; they are long glucose chains split into shorter ones.

dialysate material that passes through the membrane during dialysis.

diaphoresis excessive sweating.

diet history detailed dietary record; may include 24-hour recall; food frequency questionnaire; and other information such as weight history, previous diet changes, use of supplements, and food intolerances.

dietary acculturation dietary changes that occur as a result of adapting to food resources of a new location.

dietary fiber several different types of nondigestible carbohydrates and lignin intrinsic and intact in plants.

Dietary Reference Intakes (DRIs) set of nutrient-based reference values that identify amounts of required nutrients for various stages of life.

dietetic technician, registered (DTR) nutritional professional having completed a 2-year degree in a Dietetic Technician Program or a 4-year degree from an approved (Accreditation Council for Education in Nutrition and Dietetics) program.

dipeptide two amino acids together.

diplopia perception of two images of a single object; also known as *double vision*.

disaccharides double sugars (two simple sugars joined together) containing 12 carbon atoms.

docosahexaenoic acid (DHA) omega-3 fatty acid with 22 carbons and 6 double bonds synthesized by the body from linolenic acid; present in fish oils.

dysesthesia condition in which a burning sensation is produced by ordinary stimuli.

dysgeusia persistent, abnormal distortion of taste, including sweet, sour, bitter, salty, or metallic.

dysphagia difficulty in swallowing.

early childhood caries (ECC) early rampant tooth decay associated with inappropriate feeding practices.

edentulous without teeth or lacking some or all teeth.

eicosapentaenoic acid (EPA) omega-3 fatty acid with 20 carbon atoms and 5 double bonds synthesized by the body from linolenic acid; present in fish oils.

emulsification the breakdown of fats into smaller particles by lowering the surface tension.

enamel hypoplasia developmental disturbance of the teeth characterized by defective formation of the enamel matrix.

energy ability or power to do work.

enrichment process of restoring nutrients removed from food during processing.

enteral feedings feeding that delivers liquid food through a tube; may be used for infants and children with a functioning gastrointestinal tract unable to ingest nutrients orally to meet their metabolic needs.

enteric general term for the intestines.

enzymes complex proteins enabling metabolic reactions to proceed at a faster rate without being exhausted themselves.

epilepsy transient disturbance of brain function that results in episodic impairment or loss of consciousness.

epinephrine the "fight or flight" hormone secreted in time of immediate energy need; activates glycogen degradation for energy.

epiphyses growing points at ends of long bones.

epithelialization natural healing process in which the area is covered with or converted to epithelium.

erosion permanent depletion of tooth surfaces due to the action of an external or internal chemical substance.

erythema marginated redness of mucous membranes caused by inflammation.

erythropoiesis formation of red blood cells.

esophagitis inflammation of the lower esophagus.

essential amino acids (EAAs) amino acids that must be supplied by the diet. Also known as indispensable amino acids.

essential fatty acids (EFAs) fatty acids (linoleic acid and linolenic acid) that must be supplied by the diet.

essential hypertension elevated blood pressure of unknown cause.

Estimated Average Requirement (EAR) amount of a nutrient estimated to meet the needs of half of the healthy individuals in a specific age and gender group.

Estimated Energy Requirement (EER) dietary energy intake that is predicted to maintain energy balance in healthy normal-weight individuals of a defined age, gender, weight, height, and physical activity level consistent with good health.

Evidence Analysis Library (EAL) a process in which an expert work group identifies practice-related questions, performs a systematic literature review, and develops and rates a conclusive statement for each question; such a library was developed by the Academy of Nutrition and Dietetics (AND).

evidence-based medical practices that have been thoroughly evaluated using scientific methods.

explore the first step of motivational interviewing, the patient's behavior is to be explored.

extracellular fluid (ECF) fluid outside the cells.

fatty acids structural component of fats.

fermentable carbohydrate carbohydrates that can be metabolized by bacteria in plaque biofilm to decrease the pH to a level causing demineralization; this includes all sugars and cooked or processed starches.

fibroblasts collagen-forming cells.

fibrotic formation of fibrous tissue of the gingiva and other mucous membranes because of chronic inflammation; tissue may clinically appear to be healthy, concealing the disease.

filiform papillae smooth threadlike structures, which are covered by a nonkeratinized epithelium, on the anterior two-thirds of the dorsum of the tongue.

flavin adenine nucleotide (FAD/FADH$_2$) a redox coenzyme derived from riboflavin.

flexitarian person who primarily follows a plant-based diet, but occasionally eats small amounts of meat, poultry or fish; also known as a *semivegetarian*.

fluid volume deficit (FVD) relatively equal losses of sodium and water in relation to their gains.

fluid volume excess (FVE) relatively equal gains of water and sodium in relation to their losses.

fluorapatite fluoride-containing crystalline substance produced during bone and tooth development; resistant to acid.

fluorosis hypomineralization of enamel.

foliate papillae vertical ridges or grooves scattered along the lateral borders of the tongue.

follicular hyperkeratosis condition characterized by the appearance of cone-shaped, horny, hyperkeratinized, scaly eruptions resulting from blocked pores as a result of vitamin A deficiency.

food deserts located in lower-income, inner-city and rural areas, with few supermarkets but numerous small stores that stock limited nutritious food items, particularly produce, at affordable prices.

food fad catch-all term covering all aspects of nutritional nonsense, characterized by exaggerated beliefs about the value of nutrition in health and disease.

food frequency questionnaire checklist of many foods used to determine how often specific foods are consumed.

food insecurity lack of access to enough food to fully meet basic needs at all times.

food jags refusing to eat anything except one food for several days.

food pattern customary way of eating, reflecting a person's ethnic or cultural, social, religious, geographical, economic, and psychological components and family lifestyle.

food quackery promotion of nutrition-related products or services having questionable safety or effectiveness, or both, for the claims made.

fortification process of adding nutrients not present in the natural product or to increase the amount above that in the original product.

full liquid diet nutrients provided in a liquid form when solid food is not tolerated. Provides a transition between a clear liquid and soft diet.

functional fiber isolated, nondigestible carbohydrates with beneficial physiological effects in humans.

functional foods foods that contain potentially healthful products, including any modified food or food ingredients providing a health benefit beyond its traditional nutrients.

functional group a group of atoms that gives a family of molecules its characteristic chemical and physical properties.

fungating producing fungus-like growth.

fungiform papillae red, knoblike structures on the tongue scattered throughout the filiform papillae.

gastroesophageal reflux disease (GERD) return of gastric contents into the esophagus, causing a severe burning sensation under the sternum.

gastrostomy establishment of a new opening into the stomach to insert a tube for nutrition, foods, or medications directly into the stomach, bypassing the mouth and esophagus.

genome all of the DNA contained in an organism or cell, which includes the chromosomes in the nucleus and DNA in the mitochondria.

genomics scientific discipline of mapping, sequencing, and analyzing the genome.

ghrelin peptide hormone secreted in the gastrointestinal tract by exocrine cells.

ginseng fleshy root of a plant; stimulant used in energy drinks that may improve concentration and thinking, physical stamina, and athletic endurance, but may cause abdominal pain and headaches.

gingivitis inflammation of the gingival tissue.

glossitis inflammation of the tongue.

glossodynia pain in the tongue.

glossopyrosis pain, burning, itching, and stinging of the tongue with no apparent lesions.

glucagon a signal of the "starved" state; secreted when blood glucose levels are low.

glucogenic amino acids can be converted into glucose as a fuel for the body.

gluconeogenesis synthesis of glucose from noncarbohydrate sources.

gluten protein found mainly in wheat and to a lesser degree in rye, oat, and barley.

gluten sensitivity a condition in which individuals are unable to tolerate gluten; not an allergic or auto-immune response.

glycemic effect amount a carbohydrate increases the blood glucose level.

glycogen carbohydrate storage form of energy in humans.

glycogenesis process by which sugars, including fructose, galactose, sorbitol, and xylitol, are stored as glycogen.

glycolysis anaerobic conversion of glucose to produce energy in the form of adenosine triphosphate (ATP).

glycosidic bond a bond that combines two monosaccharides into a disaccharide.

goal achievable aim or target that would be meaningful in changing behaviors by setting a concrete standard for change.

goiter chronic enlargement of the thyroid gland occurring most frequently in areas with low iodine in the soil.

goitrogens naturally occurring substances in foods that interfere with the synthesis of thyroid hormone production; may cause goiter if consumed in large amounts.

gravida pregnant woman; gravida followed by a Roman numeral or preceded by a Latin prefix (e.g., "primi-," "secundi-") designates the number of pregnancies for the woman (e.g., gravida I or primigravida is a woman in her first pregnancy).

guarana a seed containing four times as much caffeine as coffee beans.

guide the second step of motivational interviewing in which the patient's motivation and commitment is identified.

gustatory sense of taste.

health claim claim that describes a health relationship between a food, food component, or dietary supplement ingredient and reduced risk of a disease or a health-related condition.

hematopoiesis formation of red blood cells.

heme iron iron provided from animal sources.

hemochromatosis an uncommon disorder in which iron is absorbed at a high rate despite elevated iron stores in the liver.

hemosiderin storage form of iron in the liver when the amount of iron in the body exceeds storage capacity.

herbs leafy green parts of a plant.

herpetic related to the herpes virus; ulceration on the tongue or esophagus or both.

hiatal hernia partial protrusion (herniation) of the stomach through the esophageal opening into the chest cavity.

high-energy phosphate compounds instant source of energy for cells; also called *ATP*.

high-quality proteins foods that contain adequate amounts of the nine essential amino acids to maintain nitrogen balance and permit growth.

hirsutism excessive hair growth.

homeopathy treatment of diseases and conditions with minute doses of drugs that cause symptoms of a disease in healthy people to cure similar symptoms in sick people.

homeostatic mechanisms body's ability to correct nutritional imbalances, for instance, decreased nutrient intake accompanied by an increase in absorption or efficiency or use.

hormone compound produced and secreted by cells of the body, transported in the blood to another site where it has a specific regulatory function.

hormone replacement therapy (HRT) therapy using medication that contains one or more female hormones, usually estrogen and progestin.

hunger physiological drive to eat or an uneasy or painful sensation caused by lack of food.

hydrocarbon the hydrophobic chain "tail" of a fatty acid that contains only carbon and hydrogen atoms.

hydrogenation process in which polyunsaturated vegetable oil is converted to a solid by a commercial process whereby hydrogen is added to the oil; increases the proportion of saturated fatty acids, alters the shape of the fatty acid, and creates *trans* fatty acids.

hydrolysis splitting of a large molecule into smaller water-soluble ones that can be used by cells; the reaction requires water.

hydrolysis reactions cleavage of a compound with the addition of water.

hydrolyzed protein proteins broken down into amino acids.

hydrophilic "water-loving" biomolecules.

hydrophobic "water fearing" compounds that do not readily combine with water.

hydroxyapatite inorganic component of bones and teeth.

hypercalcemia excessive levels of calcium in the blood.

hypercalciuria high levels of calcium in the urine.

hypercarotenemia excessive levels of carotene in the blood, characterized by yellowing of the palms of the hands and soles of the feet.

hypergeusia heightened taste acuity.

hyperglycemia elevated blood sugar.

hyperkalemia elevated potassium concentrations in the blood.

hyperlipidemia elevated concentrations of any or all of the serum lipids, especially triglycerides or cholesterol or both.

hypernatremia elevated serum sodium level.

hypertension persistent high arterial blood pressure; considered a risk factor for heart and kidney disease, and stroke.

hypervitaminosis A condition resulting from the ingestion of excessive amounts of vitamin A.

hypocalcemia deficient levels of calcium in the blood.

hypodipsia diminished thirst.

hypogeusia loss of taste.

hypoglycemia low blood sugar (less than 70 mg/dL).

hypokalemia low potassium concentrations in the blood.

hyponatremia lowered sodium in the blood.

hypotonic solution having less osmotic pressure than another solution.

iatrogenic adverse condition resulting from treatment (e.g., medications, irradiation, or surgery) by a healthcare provider.

immune response body's ability to protect itself from destructive bacteria and infection present in the body.

immunocompromised immune response weakened by a disease or pharmacological agent.

immunoglobulins antibodies, the body's main protection from disease.

incontinence inability to control urinary excretion.

indirect calorimetry method to estimate metabolic energy by measuring oxygen consumption, carbon dioxide production, respiratory quotient, and resting energy expenditure as a means to assess and manage a patient's nutrition.

innate inborn.

insulin hormone that lowers blood sugar levels.

interesterified fats a new type of customized fat suitable for commercial preparation produced to replace *trans* fats; affect blood lipids, but not as much as *trans* fats.

interstitial spaces between cells within a tissue or organ.

interstitial fluid fluid located between cells and in body cavities, including joints, pleura, and gastrointestinal tract.

intracellular fluid (ICF) liquid within cells.

intrinsic factor glycoprotein synthesized by parietal cells in the stomach; required for vitamin B_{12} absorption.

ionic bond bond formed between a positively charged metal ion and a negatively charged nonmetal ion.

irradiated foods process of treating food with controlled amounts of ionized radiation to kill the spoilage-causing and disease-causing bacteria and molds in food.

ischemia inadequate blood flow and lack of oxygen because of constriction or obstruction of arteries.

Kaposi's sarcoma malignant tumor of blood vessel origin that occurs on skin and oral mucosa.

Kayser-Fleischer ring greenish yellow pigmented ring encircling the cornea; consists of copper deposits in the Descemet membrane.

keratinized epithelium a protein, main component of epidermis and horny tissues on the skin.

Keshan disease cardiomyopathy (disease of the heart muscle) resulting from deficiency of selenium found in women and children, primarily in Keshan, China.

ketoacidosis accumulation of ketone bodies in the blood.

ketogenic amino acid giving rise to ketones.

ketone bodies soluble forms of lipids that can be used as fuel for the body.

ketones normal products of lipid metabolism in the liver; can be used by muscles for energy if adequate amounts of glucose are available.

ketonuria ketones excreted in the urine as a result of high levels in the blood.

ketosis accumulation of ketone bodies in the blood.

kilocalorie (calorie, Calorie) amount of heat needed to increase the temperature of 1 kg of water 1° C; measurement of the potential energy value of foods and energy within the body, equivalent to 1000 calories; more frequently referred to as calorie.

kwashiorkor nutritional deficiency disease due to inadequate protein but adequate kilocalories.

lactovegetarian person who consumes only products from plants and dairy products.

large intestine cecum, colon, and rectum.

leukemia generalized malignant disease characterized by distorted proliferation and development of white blood cells.

leukoplakia white, yellow, or gray thickened patches on mucous membranes of the oral mucosa that cannot be wiped away; appearance may be wrinkled, fissured, nodular, or smooth.

lichen planus a disease with an itchy rash most often in the mouth.

linoleic acid essential fatty acid with 18 carbon atoms and 2 double bonds; also called *omega-6 fatty acid*.

lipase an enzyme that begins the process of digesting dietary lipids.

lipids compounds that contain carbon, hydrogen, and oxygen with less oxygen in proportion to hydrogen and carbon than carbohydrates; provide 9 kcal/g; a biomolecule that is produced by a living cell or organism.

lipoatrophy loss of fat from specific areas of the body, especially the face, arms, legs, and buttocks.

lipodystrophy rearrangement of fat cells in the face.

lipogenesis process of converting glucose to fats.

lipohypertrophy accumulation of fat on the back or the neck between the shoulders.

lipolysis fat breakdown.

lipoprotein compound lipids composed of triglycerides, phospholipids, and cholesterol combined with protein; produced by the body.

Listeriosis serious infection caused by food contaminated with the bacterium *Listeria monocytogenes*, principally affects infants and adults with weakened immune systems.

long-chain fatty acids fatty acid that contains 12 or more carbon atoms.

longitudinal fissure slits or wrinkles that extend lengthwise on the tongue.

low birth weight (LBW) weighing less than $5\frac{1}{2}$ lb (2500 g) at birth.

lower esophageal sphincter (LES) group of very strong circular muscle fibers located just above the stomach.

low nutrient density foods having a high fat, alcohol, or sugar content with nominal amounts of vitamins and minerals.

low-quality proteins plant proteins that lack one or more essential amino acids or may lack a proper balance of amino acids; also called *incomplete proteins*.

lymphatic system comprised of lymph (plasma-like tissue fluid), the lymph nodes, and lymph vessels that are not connected to the blood system; carries fat-soluble nutrients through the thoracic duct and into venous blood at the left subclavian vein.

lysosomes intracellular bodies containing hydrolytic enzymes that promote breakdown of materials taken into the cells.

macrodontia larger than normal teeth.

macronutrients nutrients needed in large amounts by the body to provide energy—carbohydrates, protein, and fats.

macules flat lesions of abnormal color.

manganese madness severe psychotic and neuromuscular symptoms that resemble the symptoms of parkinsonism.

marasmus nutritional deficiency caused by inadequate protein and kilocaloric intake.

mastication process in which teeth crush and grind food into smaller pieces to initiate digestion.

masticatory efficiency how well the patient prepares the food for swallowing.

mechanically altered diet regular diet altered in consistency during periods when chewing is difficult; may provide a transition between a full liquid diet and a regular diet.

medium-chain fatty acids fatty acid with 6 to 10 carbon atoms.

megaloblastic anemia condition in which red blood cells are extra large in size but fewer in number.

melting point temperature at which a product becomes a liquid.

menopausal gingivostomatitis changes in the oral mucosa that result in a dry, shiny gingiva that bleeds easily; color ranges from an abnormally pale pink to a deep red may be alleviated with estrogen hormone replacement.

menopause cessation of the menses; occurs when production of the hormones estrogen and progesterone ceases.

meta-analysis systematic analysis that is applied to separate experiments on a related topic involving pooling the data to provide larger study samples that generate information about statistically significant results from the cumulative research on a topic.

metabolism continuous processes whereby living organisms and cells convert nutrients into energy, body structure, and waste.

microflora microorganisms living in the large intestine.

macroglossia large, protruding tongue.

materia alba soft white deposit around the necks of teeth.

micrognathia abnormally small jaw.

micronutrients nutrients needed by the body in small amounts (e.g., vitamins and minerals).

microvilli minute cylindrical processes located on the surface of the intestinal cells, greatly increasing their absorptive surface area.

mineralization deposition of inorganic minerals on an organic matrix.

mitochondria the power source of the cell.

modified barium swallow assessment to measure the physiological and anatomical abnormalities associated with swallowing.

molecule the smallest particle of a substance that retains all the properties of the substance.

monomer the smallest repeating unit present in a polymer.

monosaccharides simple sugars containing two to six carbon atoms.

monounsaturated fatty acid (MUFA) fatty acid containing one double bond; found in olive, peanut, and canola oil.

motivational interviewing an education tool for changing behaviors involving a respectful, collaborative conversation.

mucositis ulcerations and sores of the mucous membrane in the mouth or throat, usually caused by chemotherapy or radiation.

myelin lipid substance that insulates nerve fibers and affects transmission of nerve impulses.

myxedema severe hypothyroidism.

nanotechnology the ability to measure and detect molecular structures nanometers or smaller, allowing determination and manipulation of minute amounts of substances in the food supply.

naturopathy support of the body's inherent ability to maintain and restore health, using non-invasive treatments with minimal use of surgery and drugs.

necrosis degeneration and death of cells.

necrotizing enterocolitis (NEC) condition in neonates with development of cellular dead patches in the intestines interfering with digestion and absorption.

necrotizing ulcerative gingivitis (NUG) oral condition caused by nutritional deficiencies, stress, infection, and depressed immune responses; characterized by erythema and necrosis of the interdental papillae.

neoplasia an abnormal mass of tissue, more frequently referred to as a tumor.

neural tube defects (NTD) birth defects of the skull, brain, and spinal cord.

neurotransmitters substance released at the end of a nerve cell when a nerve impulse arrives there, which diffuses across to the next cell to excite or inhibit it.

neutropenia diminished number of neutrophils in the blood; also called *leukopenia* or *agranulocytosis*.

nicotinamide adenine dinucleotide (NAD+/NADH) a redox coenzyme derived from niacin

night blindness inability to adapt to bright lights when the eyes are adapted to darkness.

nitrogen balance balance of reactions in which protein substances are broken down and rebuilt.

nocturia excessive urination at night.

noma severe gangrenous process usually manifesting as a small ulcer on the gingiva that becomes necrotic and spreads to the lips, cheek, and tissues covering the jaw; caused by inadequate amounts of protein.

nondigestible enzymes in the gastrointestinal tract cannot digest and absorb the substance; plant cells that remain largely intact through the digestive process.

nonessential amino acids (NEAAs) amino acids essential to the body, but not required in the diet. Also know as dispensable amino acids.

nonheme iron iron provided primarily from plant sources and supplements; less efficiently absorbed than heme iron.

non-nutritive sucking sucking on objects that do not provide nutrition (i.e., pacifier, fingers).

normoglycemia normal blood glucose range.

nucleic acid a biomolecule that is produced by a living cell or organism forms the genetic material in the cell; synthesizes cellular protein.

nucleotide the building blocks for nucleic acids.

nutrient content claim characterizes the level of a nutrient in a food; terms used are "free," "low," "high," and "reduced."

nutrient-dense containing a high percentage of nutrients in relation to the number of kilocalories provided.

nutrient density amount of nutrients in a food relative to its kilocalories.

nutrients biochemical substances that can be supplied in adequate amounts only from an outside source, normally from food.

nutrigenomics/nutritional genomics scientific study of how foods or their components interact with genes, and how individual genetic differences affect response to nutrients (and other naturally occurring compounds).

nutrition study of foods and nutrients and their effect on health, growth, and development.

nutrition facts panel label on food products providing nutrient content of food and the number of servings in the package.

nutritional deficiency inadequate amounts of a nutrient available to sustain biochemical functions.

nutritional insult deficiency or excessive amounts of specific nutrients.

nutritionist person who may have a 4-year degree in foods and nutrition and usually works in a public health setting; may be legally defined in some states denoting licensure or certification.

nystagmus involuntary rapid movement of the eyeball.

obesity excess weight for height, with a BMI above 30.0.

observational studies epidemiological research studies with no type of intervention or experiment.

odontoblasts tissue cells that deposit dentin and form the outer surface of dental pulp adjacent to the dentin.

odynophagia pain associated with swallowing.

oils fats liquid at room temperature.

olfactory nerves receptors for smell.

omega-3 fatty acid unsaturated fatty acid with its first double bond at the third carbon atom from the methyl end; includes eicosapentaenoic acid and docosahexaenoic acid.

omega-6 fatty acid unsaturated fatty acid with its first double bond at the sixth carbon atom from the methyl end; includes linoleic acid and linolenic acid.

organic foods that meet U.S. Department of Agriculture (USDA) standards and do not contain parts of other slaughtered animals, were not given growth hormones or antibiotics, and allowed outdoors; not genetically engineered or irradiated; grown on land that has not been fertilized with sewage sludge or chemical fertilizers or treated with pesticides.

osmoreceptors neurons in the hypothalamus stimulated by increased osmolality, enhancing the release of ADH.

osmosis movement of water from an area of lower solute concentration to a higher solute concentration. When solute concentrations in the body are different, water moves across the membrane.

osteoblasts assists in production of collagen; helps in building and reformation of new bone.

osteocalcin vitamin K–dependent, bone-specific protein that is released into blood from the resorbed bone matrix and from the originating osteoblasts.

osteoclasts resorbed bone in microscopic cavities.

osteodystrophy abnormal bone development, similar to osteomalacia.

osteoid young bone that has not undergone calcification.

osteomalacia softening of bones.

osteonecrosis a condition in which bone dies or undergoes necrosis.

osteoporosis age-related disorder characterized by decreased bone mass, causing bones to be more susceptible to fracture.

osteosclerosis increased bone formation resulting in reduced marrow spaces and increased radiopacity.

overweight excess accumulation of body fat, or a BMI between 25.0 and 29.9.

ovolactovegetarian vegetarian diet supplemented with milk, eggs, and cheese.

ovovegetarian type of vegetarian whose diet consists of foods from plants with the addition of eggs (no meat, poultry, fish, or dairy products).

oxidation process of hydrolyzing triglycerides into two-carbon entities to enter the TCA (Krebs) cycle for energy production.

oxidation-reduction reaction a chemical reaction that can convert functional groups into other functional groups.

oxidative phosphorylation a metabolic process that synthesizes phosphoric bonds from the energy released by the oxidation of various substrates.

pancreatic enzymes enzymes that hydrolyze carbohydrates, protein, and fats.

papillae epithelium surrounding taste buds; papillae appear on the tongue as little red dots, or raised bumps, and are most prevalent on the dorsal epithelium.

parasympathetic nerves division of autonomic nervous system.

Parkinson disease progressive neurological condition characterized by involuntary muscle tremors, muscular weakness, rigidity, stooped posture, and peculiar gait.

parotitis inflammation of the parotid gland.

pathogenic harmful.

pedometer instrument used by a walker; measures approximate distance walked by recording steps.

pellagra deficiency resulting from inadequate intake of niacin, which results in the four D's (diarrhea, dermatitis, dementia, and death).

peptide bond a strong covalent bond that forms polypeptides.

periapical area around the root apex.

perimenopause time leading up to menopause, in which the ovaries begin to shut down, making less of certain hormones, such as estrogen and progesterone.

periodontal disease infections and lesions affecting tissues that form the attachment apparatus of a tooth or teeth.

periodontitis inflammatory process involving interproximal and marginal areas of two or more adjacent teeth.

periodontium hard and soft tissues that surround and support teeth: gingiva, alveolar mucosa, cementum, periodontal ligament, and alveolar bone.

peripheral edema in the extremities, such as the legs and feet.

peristalsis involuntary rhythmic waves of contraction traveling the length of the alimentary tract.

pernicious anemia megaloblastic anemia with a decrease in red blood cells; occurs when the body cannot properly absorb vitamin B_{12} in the gastrointestinal tract.

petechia (*pl.* petechiae) small, pinpoint, round red spot caused by submucous hemorrhage.

phantom taste dysgeusia without identifiable taste stimuli.

phenylketonuria genetic disorder characterized by inability to metabolize the amino acid phenylalanine.

phospholipid fat-related substances that contain phosphorus, fatty acids, and a nitrogen-containing base; constituent of every cell.

photosynthesis compounding or building up of chemical substances under the influence of light; green plants use chlorophyll and energy from sunlight to produce carbohydrates from water and carbon dioxide and to liberate oxygen.

phytochemical biologically active substances found in plants.

pica abnormal consumption of specific food and nonfood substances, such as dirt, clay, starch, or ice; occurs more frequently during pregnancy.

plant sterols essential components of plant membranes resembling the chemical structure of cholesterol and perform similar cellular functions in plants; naturally present in small quantities in fruits, vegetables, nuts, seeds, legumes, and oils.

plaque biofilm well-organized community of bacteria embedded in a slime layer and adheres tenaciously to tooth surfaces, restorations, and prosthetic appliances.

plethora red appearance resulting from an excess of blood.

pocketed foods foods retained in the mouth, especially in the vestibule.

polycythemia sustained increase in number of red blood cells; may result in iron-deficiency anemia.

polymer a large molecule containing numerous repeating units.

polyols sugar alcohols formed from or converted to sugar; sorbitol, xylitol, and mannitol are present in the body or added to foods.

polypeptide several amino acids joined together.

polysaccharides (complex carbohydrates) sugars containing more than 12 carbon atoms.

polyunsaturated fatty acid (PUFA) fatty acid containing two or more double bonds.

portal circulation passage of nutrients from the gastrointestinal tract and spleen through the portal vein to the liver.

postabsorptive state time when digestive and absorptive processes are minimal, not affecting the basal metabolic rate.

ppb parts per billion.

prebiotics nondigestible food ingredients having beneficial effects on the host by stimulating growth or activity of probiotics in the colon.

precursor substance from which another biologically active substance is formed.

preeclampsia development of hypertension as a result of pregnancy or the influence of recent pregnancy; usually occurs after the 20th week of pregnancy.

premature born before the state of maturity, occurring with a gestational age (length of pregnancy) of less than 37 weeks.

primigravida woman in her first pregnancy.

probiotics products containing live bacteria that aid in restoring and maintaining an intestinal balance of healthful bacteria.

prognathism overgrowth of the mandible.

prostaglandins hormone-like compounds derived from unsaturated fatty acids.

protease an enzyme that begins the process of digesting dietary proteins.

protein a biomolecule that is produced by a living cell or organism; chains of amino acids joined by peptide linkage; essential for physiological structure and function; contains nitrogen.

protein digestibility corrected amino acid score (PDCAAs) official assay for evaluating protein quality in humans.

protein-energy malnutrition (PEM) nutritional deficiency condition caused by consistently consuming inadequate amounts of energy and protein.

protein-sparing energy source that allows protein to be used for building and repairing (i.e., fats and carbohydrates).

proteolytic enzymes enzymes that hydrolyze proteins.

prothrombin first stage in forming an insoluble clot; a deficiency results in impaired blood coagulation.

purging use of laxatives, enemas, emetics, diuretics, or exercise to negate effects of overindulgence.

purpura condition characterized by hemorrhaging into tissues, under the skin, and through the mucous membranes; the three types are petechiae, ecchymoses, and hematomas.

purulent exudates consisting of or containing pus; generally the result of inflammation.

pyogenic producing pus.

qualified health claims statements on food labels that are supported by some evidence, but do not meet the scientific standard; must be accompanied by a disclaimer specified by the FDA.

quercetin bioflavonoid reported to energize muscles (unsubstantiated claim).

radical group of atoms forming a fundamental constituent of a molecule.

R-binder protein produced by salivary glands necessary for absorption of vitamin B_{12}.

Recommended Dietary Allowances (RDAs) specific amounts of essential nutrients that adequately meet the known nutrient needs of 97% to 98% of healthy Americans.

redox coenzymes coenzymes that capture and transfer electrons.

reduction a gain of electrons, a decrease in charge, a loss of oxygen atoms, or a gain of hydrogen atoms.

Reference Daily Intakes (RDIs) term used on food labels, based on the former RDAs. There are five sets of RDIs, which are designed for special foods for infants, children younger than 4 years, pregnant women, lactating women, and children older than 4 years and adults.

registered dietitian-nutritionist (RDN) person who has completed a bachelor's degree in foods and nutrition with training in normal and clinical nutrition, food science, and food service management, and advanced training in medical nutrition therapy.

remineralization restoration or return of calcium, phosphates, and other minerals into areas that have been damaged, as by incipient caries, abrasion, or erosion.

remodeling resorption and reformation of bone.

renal failure inability of the kidneys to maintain normal function of excreting toxic waste materials.

renal osteodystrophy changes in bones associated with renal failure.

renin enzyme synthesized in the kidney; released in response to low blood pressure.

residue total amount of fecal solids, including undigested or unabsorbed food, and metabolic (bile pigments) and bacterial products.

resistant starch starch that resists digestive enzyme action and reaches the colon; a starch that is encased in a nondigestible plant seed coat or modified by cooking or processing can be resistant.

respiration a process in which animals hydrolyze glucose into carbon dioxide and water, and plants use these products for photosynthesis.

retinoic acid form of vitamin A that can be produced by the body and can be made in the laboratory; used in combination with other drugs to treat leukemia and acne.

rhodopsin light-sensitive pigment that allows the eye to adjust to changes in light.

rickets condition resulting from vitamin D deficiency, especially in infancy and childhood; causes disturbance of normal bone formation.

sarcopenia progressive loss of muscle mass, strength, and function, due to the aging process.

satiety feeling of fullness.

saturated fatty acid fatty acid that does not contain any double bonds.

scorbutic similar to scurvy.

sealants clear or shaded plastic material applied to the occlusal surfaces of permanent teeth.

secretory immunoglobulin antibody present in oral, nasal, intestinal, and other mucosal secretions; provides the first line of defense in the oral cavity.

sensory neuropathy impairment of the ability to feel.

severe early childhood caries (SECC) see early childhood caries (ECC).

severe sensory neuropathy impairment of the ability to sense touch, vibration, temperature, and pinprick.

short-chain fatty acid fatty acid that contains fewer than six carbon atoms.

side chain (R group) the part of the amino acid that varies to form 22 different amino acids that varies from one amino acid to another.

spices botanical seasonings from seeds, berries, fruit, bark, or roots.

signs objective evidence of disease perceptible to the clinician.

small intestine duodenum, jejunum, and ileum.

solutes dissolved substances in fluid.

solvent fluid in which substances are dissolved.

sphincter muscles any of the ringlike muscles encircling an opening that is able to contract to close the opening, such as the sphincter pylori between the stomach and small intestine.

squamous metaplasia change in oral cavity cell structures with keratin production in the duct cells of salivary glands, caused by vitamin A deficiency.

stable nutrients nutrients of which more than 85% is retained during processing and storage.

stannous containing tin.

stomatitis inflammation of the oral mucosa.

Streptococcus mutans bacteria found in dental plaque biofilm.

structural lipids fats that are a component of cell membranes, tooth enamel, and dentin (e.g., phospholipids).

structural polysaccharides see *dietary fiber.*

substrate the substance acted upon and changed by an enzyme.

suckling process the infant uses to extract breastmilk by moving the jaws back and forth and squeezing with the gingiva; this encourages mandibular development by strengthening the jaw muscle.

sugar alcohols formed from or converted to sugar; also called *polyols.*

suppuration discharge or formation of pus.

sympathetic nerves exhibiting a mutual relationship between two organ systems or parts of the body.

symptoms subjective evidence of abnormality as perceived by the client.

symbiotic intimate relationship of two dissimilar organisms in a mutually beneficial relationship; prebiotics stimulate growth or activity of beneficial bacteria from probiotics in the gut.

synergistic effect combined sweeteners yield a sweeter taste than each sweetener alone.

syrup of ipecac cardiotoxic drug induces vomiting after accidental ingestion of a chemical or poison.

systematic reviews reliable information based on all relevant published and unpublished evidence, selecting studies for inclusion, assessing the quality of each study, then compiling the findings, and interpreting them to present a balanced and impartial summary while defining limitations of the evidence.

systemic condition disease or disorder that affects the whole body.

tachycardia rapid heartbeat.

taste buds receptors for sense of taste.

taurine an amino acid with antioxidant properties.

temporomandibular disorder (TMD) group of symptoms that cause pain and dysfunction in the head, face, and temporomandibular region.

tensional forces actions in which pressure stretches or strains the structure.

tetany neuromuscular disorder of uncontrollable muscular cramps and tremors.

theanine an amino acid used to treat anxiety and high blood pressure.

thermic effect increase in metabolism that occurs during digestion, absorption, and metabolism of energy-yielding nutrients.

thermogenesis process of heat production in warm-blooded organisms; occurs when the metabolic rate increases above normal, influenced by many factors, including digestion of food and activity.

thiaminase active enzyme found naturally in foods (e.g., raw fish) inactivating thiamin.

thromboembolism plug or clot in a blood vessel formed by coagulation of blood.

thrombus blood clot.

tinnitus noise in the ears, which sometimes may be heard by others.

tocopherols name given to vitamin E and compounds chemically related to it.

tocotrienols component of vitamin E.

Tolerable Upper Intake level (UL) maximum daily level of nutrient intake that probably would not cause adverse health effects or toxic effects for most individuals.

total fiber sum of dietary fiber and added fiber.

total parenteral nutrition (TPN) nutrition provided to a patient with impaired digestive tract; special liquid food mixture administered into the blood through a vein.

toxoplasmosis infection caused by a parasite; gravida may be symptom-free because the immune system prevents the parasite from causing illness, but the infection is passed on to the fetus.

trabecular bone spongy internal bone.

trans **fatty acid** unsaturated fatty acid that is usually monounsaturated; may be formed during hydrogenation, in which the hydrogen ions rotate so that the hydrogens stick out on opposite sides of the bond.

transferrin serum protein transports iron in the blood.

tricarboxylic acid cycle (TCA cycle) the central metabolic pathway that produces energy, also known as the citric acid cycle or Krebs cycle.

triglycerides major form of lipid in the body and food composed of three fatty acids bonded to glycerol, an alcohol.

24-hour recall a method of assessing everything a person has consumed (foods, supplements, and beverages) in a 24-hour period; may or may not reflect a typical day.

unqualified health claims statements allowed on food labels by FDA; must be supported by qualified experts agreeing scientific evidence is available determining a relationship between a nutrient and a specific disease.

unsaturated fatty acid (UFA) of or related to an organic compound, especially fatty acids, containing one or more double or triple bonds between carbons.

Upper Level (UL) see *tolerable upper intake level.*

uremic condition in which too much urea and other nitrous waste products are present in the blood.

valves/sphincter muscles circular muscles regulating the flow of bolus between different segments of the gastrointestinal tract.

variants different forms of genes.

varicose veins unnaturally and permanently distended veins.

vegan person who eats only plant foods.

vegetarian people who puposefully do not eat meat (beef, pork, poultry, seafood, and the flesh of any animal, and sometimes animal by-products).

very low food security at times food intake of household members is reduced and normal eating patterns disrupted because of insufficient funds or other resources to obtain food.

viscous fiber water-soluble fibers, including pectins, gums, psyllium, mucilages, and algal polysaccharides, which are physiologically important for their gel-forming ability.

vitamins general term for numerous related organic, noncaloric substances present in foods in small amounts.

wheat allergy adverse immunological reaction to wheat proteins.

whole grains grains and grain products made from the entire grain seed, usually called the kernel (consisting of bran, germ, and endosperm); a cracked, crushed, or flaked kernel must retain nearly the same relative proportions of bran, germ, and endosperm as the original grain to be called whole grain.

xeroderma dry, rough, scaly skin.

xerophthalmia abnormally dry and thickened surface of the conjunctiva and cornea of the eye.

xerostomia dryness of the mouth resulting from inadequate salivary secretion.

xylitol sugar alcohol used as a sugar substitute; considered a nutritive sweetener; provides four calories per gram.

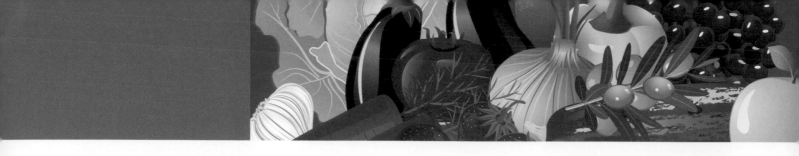

Answers to Nutritional Quotient Questions

CHAPTER 1: OVERVIEW OF HEALTHY EATING HABITS

1. False. No single food contains all the essential nutrients in amounts needed for optimal health.
2. False. Only consumption of added sugars should be reduced. Naturally occurring sugars, especially from milk and fruits, are desirable.
3. True.
4. False. DRIs are a set of nutrient-based reference values that include the Estimated Average Requirements, Recommended Dietary Allowances, Adequate Intakes, and Tolerable Upper Intake Levels intended to be used for planning and assessing diets of healthy Americans and Canadians.
5. True.
6. False. Three to five servings are recommended for vegetables, and two to four servings are recommended for fruit.
7. True.
8. False. Sugar is implicated as a cause of dental caries, but not in other major diseases, such as hypertension, cardiovascular disease, or diabetes mellitus.
9. True.
10. False. The nutrients that provide energy are fats, carbohydrates, and proteins.

CHAPTER 2: CONCEPTS IN BIOCHEMISTRY

1. False. A hydrolysis reaction requires H_2O as a reactant to degrade molecules. A condensation reaction produces H_2O as a product.
2. False. Amino acids are the building blocks of proteins. Nucleotides are the building blocks of nucleic acids.
3. True.
4. False. Sucrose is a disaccharide containing glucose and fructose.
5. True.
6. True.
7. True.
8. False. Catabolism involves the oxidation of carbohydrates into CO_2 and H_2O. Oxidation is the loss of electrons. The electrons released in catabolism are captured by NADH and $FADH_2$ and used to synthesize ATP in oxidative phosphorylation.
9. False. Insulin is a signal of the "fed" state and is secreted when blood glucose levels are high. It activates metabolic pathways that will lower blood glucose levels, like glycolysis and glycogen biosynthesis, not glycogen degradation.
10. True.

CHAPTER 3: THE ALIMENTARY CANAL: DIGESTION AND ABSORPTION

1. True.
2. False. This is the hydrolysis of lipids or fat; carbohydrate yields monosaccharides.
3. False. Absorption occurs primarily in the small intestine.
4. False. Long-chain triglycerides enter the lymphatic system; short-chain and medium-chain triglycerides enter the portal circulation.
5. True.
6. False. Most enzymes end in -ase (e.g., lactase); lactose is a sugar found in milk.
7. True.
8. False. Villi are located in the small intestine.
9. True.
10. True.

CHAPTER 4: CARBOHYDRATE: THE EFFICIENT FUEL

1. False. The FDA has labeled raw sugar as unfit for direct use as a food or a food ingredient because of the impurities it contains.
2. True.
3. False. Oral bacteria are unable to metabolize xylitol, which is a calorie-containing sugar alcohol.
4. False. The desire for sweetness is not considered an acquired taste because newborn infants exhibit a preference for it.
5. True.
6. True.
7. False. Excessive caloric intake leads to obesity, whether from carbohydrates, proteins, fats, or alcohol.
8. False. Sucrose is table sugar.

9. False. Many other factors, including consumption of other fermentable carbohydrates, contribute to development of caries.
10. True.

CHAPTER 5: PROTEIN: THE CELLULAR FOUNDATION

1. True.
2. False. The breed of hen determines the color of eggshell, and color is not related to its nutritional value.
3. False. Gelatin does not contain all the indispensable amino acids.
4. False. The protein requirement is at least equal to that of a young adult and may be increased.
5. False. Adequate amounts of protein are needed for development of healthy teeth, but increasing protein beyond the RDA would not have any effect on tooth enamel.
6. True.
7. True.
8. False. It is a protein-deficiency and kilocalorie-deficiency disorder.
9. False. In addition to foods from plants, dairy products are consumed. Eggs are excluded.
10. True.

CHAPTER 6: LIPIDS: THE CONDENSED ENERGY

1. False. The overall average of fat intake is important; foods, such as margarine and oils, are 100% fat, but can be used safely in the diet.
2. False. As an antioxidant, vitamin E protects the oil to which it is added to some degree; however, in doing so, vitamin E may be inactivated, so it cannot be used by the body.
3. True.
4. False. The AMDR for fat is estimated to be 20% to 35% of energy intake for adults.
5. False. Bananas contain a trace of fat; avocados are 88% fat. However, they are both plant products, so they do not contain any cholesterol.
6. False. All fats produce 9 kcal/g.
7. True.
8. False. Even though they are nutritious foods, for most Americans, their use should be limited because of their high fat content.
9. True.
10. True.

CHAPTER 7: USE OF THE ENERGY NUTRIENTS: METABOLISM AND BALANCE

1. True.
2. True.

3. False. BMR stands for basal metabolic rate, which is the amount of energy needed to maintain involuntary physiologic functions.
4. True.
5. True.
6. False. Hunger is the physiological drive to eat, whereas appetite implies a desire for specific types of food.
7. False. Fats are stored by the body for energy, but they must first be converted into a form the body can use. Glycogen stores, which depend on carbohydrate intake, are readily available for energy.
8. True.
9. True.
10. False. Only fats, carbohydrates, proteins, and alcohol provide energy (kcals).

CHAPTER 8: VITAMINS REQUIRED FOR CALCIFIED STRUCTURES

1. True.
2. True.
3. True.
4. True.
5. False. Retinol is obtained from animal foods; beta carotene is found in fruits and vegetables.
6. True.
7. True.
8. False. A deficiency of vitamin D causes rickets.
9. False. Vitamin K is essential for blood clotting; vitamin D functions to regulate blood calcium and phosphorus levels.
10. True.

CHAPTER 9: MINERALS ESSENTIAL FOR CALCIFIED STRUCTURES

1. True.
2. False. Many nutrients work together in building strong healthy bones, including protein, calcium, phosphorus, magnesium, fluoride, and vitamins C and D.
3. True.
4. True.
5. False. Based on the DRIs, teenagers need 1300 mg of calcium. To obtain adequate amounts of calcium, 4½ cups equivalent of foods and beverages containing calcium. If milk is the only calcium source, a teen would need to consume 4½ cups.
6. False. Fluoridation of community water supplies is the most effective method of preventing dental caries.
7. False. Although many women take calcium supplements to prevent osteoporosis, they are not essential for all women. Excessive calcium intake may increase the risk of CHD and symptoms including dizziness, kidney stone formation, and irregular heartbeat.
8. True.
9. False. Caffeine decreases calcium absorption.
10. False. Bottled waters vary in fluoride content.

CHAPTER 10: NUTRIENTS PRESENT IN CALCIFIED STRUCTURES

1. False. The IOM has established ULs for copper, manganese, and molybdenum, but not for chromium.
2. True.
3. True.
4. False. Alzheimer disease and aluminum toxicity are two different conditions.
5. True.
6. False. Unrefined foods generally provide more trace minerals.
7. False. Aluminum is cariostatic, especially in combination with fluoride.
8. True.
9. False. Sugar is not a good source of any nutrients except kilocalories. Good sources of chromium include meats, whole-grain cereals, mushrooms, green beans, and broccoli.
10. False. Selenium supplements are not recommended because selenium can be toxic.

CHAPTER 11: VITAMINS REQUIRED FOR ORAL SOFT TISSUES AND SALIVARY GLANDS

1. True.
2. False. Vitamin D is called the sunshine vitamin because sun facilitates the body's production of vitamin D; vitamin B_6 is also called pyridoxine, pyridoxal, and pyridoxamine.
3. False. Beriberi is caused by a thiamin deficiency; niacin deficiency causes pellagra.
4. True.
5. False. Flushing and intestinal disturbances are symptoms of niacin toxicity. No toxicity symptoms have been observed for thiamin.
6. True.
7. True.
8. False. Liver, leafy vegetables, legumes, grapefruit, and oranges are rich sources of folate.
9. True.
10. True.

CHAPTER 12: WATER AND MINERALS REQUIRED FOR ORAL SOFT TISSUES AND SALIVARY GLANDS

1. True.
2. True.
3. True.
4. True.
5. False. The IOM has established an AI for total fluid (beverages, water, and food) requirements to be 15 to 16 cups per day for men and 11 to 12 cups per day for women.
6. False. The minimum requirement for sodium is 500 mg per day for adults, but no RDA has been established for sodium.
7. True.
8. False. Potassium is principally within the cells (intracellular).
9. True.
10. False. Oral pallor is a sign of iron-deficiency anemia.

CHAPTER 13: NUTRITIONAL REQUIREMENTS AFFECTING ORAL HEALTH IN WOMEN

1. False. These cravings do not reflect natural instincts for required nutrients.
2. True.
3. False. If the diet is deficient in calcium, the fetal calcium requirements would be met first, but some of the calcium may come from her bones, not from her teeth.
4. False. Although she is "eating for two," normal energy requirements are not doubled. Depending on the prepregnancy weight, approximately 300 k calories more than her usual caloric requirement are needed during the second and third trimesters.
5. True.
6. False. Iron and folate are usually the nutrients needing supplementation.
7. True.
8. False. Breast milk is normally thin and is nutritionally adequate.
9. False. The more often an infant nurses, the more milk is produced. Milk production is most active during infant sucking.
10. True.

CHAPTER 14: NUTRITIONAL REQUIREMENTS DURING GROWTH AND DEVELOPMENT AND EATING HABITS AFFECTING ORAL HEALTH

1. True.
2. False. Fluoride supplements are not recommended for infants before age 6 months even though breast milk and artificial breast milk are low in fluoride.
3. False. Solid foods are introduced between 4 and 6 months of age, not at 6 weeks.
4. False. Orange juice is one of the last juices to be introduced because of the high frequency of allergies.
5. True.
6. True.
7. False. Breastfed infants need a supplement of 200 IU vitamin D beginning during the first 2 months to prevent rickets.
8. False. Suckling, as occurs when extracting milk from the breast, encourages maximum development of the genetically defined jaw and chin; breastfed infants are less likely to develop malocclusion.

9. True.
10. False. Toddlers and children need snacks because of their high energy needs; however, wholesome snacks (e.g., cheese cubes, fresh fruit, raw vegetable sticks, milk, or yogurt) that do not promote tooth decay are recommended.

CHAPTER 15: NUTRITIONAL REQUIREMENTS FOR OLDER ADULTS AND EATING HABITS AFFECTING ORAL HEALTH

1. False. Because of changes in nutrient requirements secondary to physiological changes, the IOM has developed DRIs for individuals 51 to 70 years old and older than 70 years.
2. True.
3. True.
4. False. The texture for edentulous patients is determined by their own preferences.
5. False. Dehydration is a frequent occurrence in elderly individuals for many reasons—impaired homeostatic mechanisms, decreased thirst sensation, inability of the kidney to concentrate urine, changes in functional status, side effects of medications, and mobility disorders.
6. True.
7. False. Intake requirement is lower because of menopause.
8. True.
9. False. Although it is highly likely that an elderly individual may benefit from taking a dietary supplement, toxicity or nutrient imbalances may occur. An older individual should consult a healthcare provider before deciding to take a vitamin supplement.
10. False. Physical activity can help ameliorate some chronic health problems, improve physiological well-being, and relieve symptoms of depression and anxiety.

CHAPTER 16: OTHER CONSIDERATIONS AFFECTING NUTRIENT INTAKE

1. True.
2. False. Patterns and attitudes internalized during childhood promote a sense of stability and security for older patients.
3. False. No culture has ever been known to make food choices solely on the basis of nutritional values of food. The factors that seem to predominate in food choices are cultural and economic.
4. False. Only about 10% of the American food dollar is spent on food.
5. False. Fad diets may be physically harmless, but they are usually not based on sound nutritional principles.
6. False. Scientific research to date has not shown any nutritional benefits from the use of organically grown foods.

7. False. Although some food processing is detrimental to the nutritive value of foods, the goal of food processing is to maintain optimum qualities of color, flavor, texture, and nutritive value.
8. True.
9. True.
10. True.

CHAPTER 17: EFFECTS OF SYSTEMIC DISEASE ON NUTRITIONAL STATUS AND ORAL HEALTH

1. True.
2. True.
3. False. Supplements for anemia should not be prescribed without the results of blood testing to determine the type of anemia. High intakes of iron could possibly complicate the situation.
4. False. Because of the various considerations involved in constructing a meal plan and lifestyle changes for a patient with diabetes, the patient must be referred to a certified diabetes educator.
5. True.
6. True.
7. False. Kaposi's sarcoma is a tumor that occurs frequently in immunocompromised patients.
8. True.
9. False. Although a patient with an eating disorder should be referred to a physician or an eating disorder program, it is the dental hygienist's responsibility to approach the patient with the objective findings.
10. False. Bulimics are generally of normal weight or sometimes above recommended body weight.

CHAPTER 18: NUTRITIONAL ASPECTS OF DENTAL CARIES: CAUSES, PREVENTION, AND TREATMENT

1. False. A combination of diet, host, environment, and saliva are necessary for initiation of dental decay.
2. True.
3. True.
4. True.
5. False. Sugar alcohols are fermented slowly by oral bacteria, and they are noncariogenic. Xylitol is cariostatic because of its ability to inhibit production of *Streptococcus mutans*.
6. False. An acid environment is required to demineralize a tooth; a cariogenic food causes the plaque pH to decrease to less than 5.5.
7. False. It is the least important factor to consider. Identifying frequency of intake, physical form, and spacing of food within a day or meal would provide a more accurate assessment.
8. True.
9. False. Although the RDAs provide a lot of factual information, they are too overwhelming for most

patients. *MyPlate* and *Dietary Guidelines for Americans* provide practical and general nutrition information relevant to preventing dental decay and improving overall health.

10. False. Information alone does not guarantee a behavioral change.

CHAPTER 19: NUTRITIONAL ASPECTS OF GINGIVITIS AND PERIODONTAL DISEASE

1. True.
2. False. Indirectly, firm, fibrous foods reduce the amount of bacterial plaque biofilm by stimulating salivary flow, which promotes oral clearance of food and lessens food retention.
3. False. A nutrient deficiency can be a contributing factor to gingivitis, but local irritants (plaque biofilm and calculus) must be present. The inflammation can be exaggerated by a nutrient deficiency, and by reduced resistance and recovery time.
4. True.
5. False. A patient may interpret this advice as condoning ice cream, gelatin, and chicken noodle soup, which would not provide enough nutrients or kilocalories for quick recovery. The dental hygienist should provide a specific list of nutrient-dense foods for the patient to purchase before the periodontal surgery.
6. True.
7. True.
8. True.
9. True.
10. False. If surgery is indicated for a periodontal patient, optimally, the nutritional assessment and counseling should be completed before the procedure to increase nutrient reserves that would expedite the recovery period.

CHAPTER 20: NUTRITIONAL ASPECTS OF ALTERATIONS IN THE ORAL CAVITY

1. False. Although root surface caries can be a complication of xerostomia, other causes are possible, such as frequent intake of hard candy. Also, a complete and thorough assessment of the patient is essential. No single factor is adequate to diagnose the presence, extent, or cause of root caries. An inaccurate evaluation can lead to inappropriate recommendations.
2. False. Although xerostomia is a common complaint in an older adult, the changes in saliva in a healthy older individual are minimal. Xerostomia has been strongly associated with multiple factors, such as use of medications, one or more systemic diseases, and radiation, all of which are common to this population.
3. True.
4. False. Root caries appear on the root surface, in areas of gingival recession. This condition is seen more often

in older adults who have experienced periodontal disease or toothbrush trauma.
5. True.
6. False. It is important to have nutrient-dense foods available, but in different consistencies. A full liquid diet, progressing to a mechanically altered diet and then to a regular diet would allow the patient to adjust to swallowing, chewing, and biting with the new appliance.
7. True.
8. False. Spongy cancellous bone is the major component of alveolar bone.
9. True.
10. True.

CHAPTER 21: NUTRITIONAL ASSESSMENT AND EDUCATION FOR DENTAL PATIENTS

1. False. Although the health and dental histories provide valuable information, they are not enough to determine the patient's nutritional status. Other evaluation tools include clinical assessment and dietary intake.
2. False. Clinical oral examinations detect physical signs and symptoms of many nutrient deficiencies. However, deficiencies generally do not appear until an advanced state exists. An oral examination should be used as an adjunct in identifying potential nutritional deficiencies.
3. True.
4. True.
5. False. Dietary counseling must be documented and other staff members informed about the nutritional counseling for consistency and reinforcement of the information at future appointments.
6. False. Changing a dietary habit is difficult and requires a meal plan and lifestyle behavior changes tailored to meet the patient's needs. A thorough assessment identifies many factors that should be considered. Active involvement of the patient in establishing a meal pattern enhances compliance.
7. False. The dental hygienist is responsible for providing information and guiding the patient to make healthier decisions. Active participation, problem solving, and decision making allow for greater compliance. The patient should highlight the fermentable carbohydrates.
8. False. Changing food habits is very difficult. The first attempt established by the dental hygienist and patient may not have been successful, and other alternatives may need to be established. Follow-up is an essential component of the nutritional counseling process.
9. True.
10. True.
11. False. The patient's behavior is "explored" by building rapport and not being confronted; the patent is then "guided" by the dental professional; and the patient "chooses" the course of treatment.
12. True.

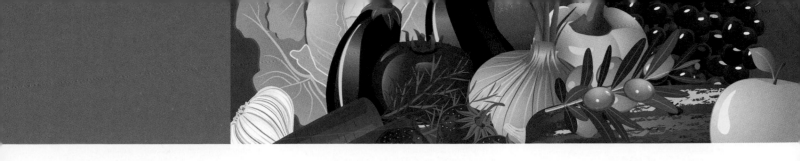

Index

A

Abdominal obesity, 28b-30b
Acceptable macronutrient distribution ranges
    (AMDRs), 6
    for carbohydrates, 74
    dietary, for children older than two years, 274, 275b
    for fat, 108
Accessory organs, of alimentary canal, 51
Acesulfame, 368
Achlorhydria, 204
Acids, as food additives, 324t-325t
Acquired immunodeficiency syndrome (AIDS)
    dental hygiene considerations in, 356b-357b
    nutritional directions in, 357b
    oral manifestations in, 341t, 355-356
Active sites, 39-40, 40f
Ad libitum, 95
Ad libitum, 95
Additives, food, 322-323
Adenosine 5'-monophosphate (AMP), structure of,
    42f
Adenosine triphosphate (ATP), 45, 127
Adequate intake (AI), 6
    of biotin, 205, 205t
    of calcium, 163t
    of chloride, 225t, 228
    of chromium, 181, 181t
    of fats, 109t
    of manganese, 182, 182t
    of pantothenic acid, 197, 198t
    of potassium, 228-229, 228t
    of sodium, 223, 225t
    of water, 214, 215t
Adequate nutrients within kilocalorie needs,
    recommendation for, 10
Adipose tissue, 106
Adolescents, 282-284
    fluoride supplementation for, 267t
    growth and nutrient requirements of, 282-283
    influential factors in eating habits of, 283-284
    nutritional counseling, 284
        dental hygiene consideration in, 284b
        nutritional directions in, 285b
    nutritional insult to bone growth in, 283
    obesity in, health application, 285b-287b
Adult, general, community nutrition resources for,
    330t
Age
    and basal metabolic rate, 127, 127f
    and susceptibility to caries, 366
Age-related macular degeneration, 302
AI. see Adequate intake (AI)
Alcohol
    as folic acid antagonist, 246-247
    metabolism of, 125
Alcoholic beverage(s)
    energy value of, 125b
    intake of, *Dietary Guidelines for Americans*
        recommendations for, 13
Aldosterone
    and sodium levels, 223, 224f
    and water regulation, 215
Alimentary canal, 50-65
    esophagus, 56
    gastric digestion in, 56-57

Alimentary canal *(Continued)*
    large intestine, 60-61
    oral cavity, 52-56
    small intestine, 57-59
Alopecia, 143
Alpha (α)-linoleic acid, 104
Alternative medicine, 206b-209b
Aluminum, 184
Alveolar bone loss, 399
Alveolar process, 55
Alzheimer's disease, 185b-186b
    warning signs of, 186b
AMDRs. see Acceptable macronutrient distribution
    ranges
Ameloblasts, 141
American Academy of Pediatrics (AAP), dietary
    guidelines for children older than 2 years,
    274-277
American Cancer Society, 142
American Cleft Palate Association, 274
American Dental Association, 77
American Dental Hygienists' Association (ADHA),
    390
American Diabetes Association, 95
    exchange system of nutrition of, 132b-135b
    nutritional recommendations of, 136t-137t
American Heart Association
    on controlling hyperlipidemia, studies and
        recommendations, 116b-117b
    diet and lifestyle recommendations of, for
        cardiovascular risk reduction, 117b
    tips to implement lifestyle recommendations of,
        118b
American Medical Association, 275-276
Amino acid metabolic pool, 124
Amino acid supplements, 89b
Amino acid(s), 38-39, 87-88
    carbohydrate conversion to, 71
    conditionally indispensable, 88
    dental hygiene considerations of, 89b, 91b-92b
    dipeptide linkage of, 88
    in human diet, 88t
    metabolism of, 124
    nutritional directions for, 89b, 93b
    structure of, 39f, 87f
Amorphous calcium, 161
Amylases, 39
Amylopectin, 38
    branched structures of, 39f
α-amylose, 38
    linear structure of, 39f
Anabolic processes, 122
Anabolism, 122, 124
    characteristics of, 45
    energy flow in, 46f
Anemia(s)
    iron deficiency, 232, 252, 342-343, 343b, 343f
    megaloblastic, 202, 343, 343b-344b
    oral manifestations in, 341t, 342-343,
        342f-343f
    pernicious, 204, 204f, 343, 344f
    in young children, 277
Anencephaly, 252
Aneurysm, bleeding
    dental hygiene considerations in, 347b
    nutritional directions for, 347b
    oral manifestations in, 346-347
Anions, 223
Anorexia, 54
    and appetite, 340-342

Anorexia nervosa
    diagnostic criteria for, 357, 358f
    oral manifestations in, 357-359
Anosmia, 54, 294
Anthropometric evaluation, 408-409
Anthropometry, 408
Anticaking agents, as additives, 324t-325t
Anticariogenic foods, 367-368
    non-nutritive sweeteners in, 368. see also Sugar
        substitutes.
    phosphorus and calcium in, 368
    proteins and fats as, 368
    sugar alcohols in, 367-368. see also Sugar
        alcohols.
Anticariogenic substance, 79
Anticholinergic medications, 342
Anticoagulant, 151
Antidiuretic hormone (ADH), in water regulation,
    215, 216f
Antigenic substances, in oral cavity, 191
Antioxidant intake, and macular degeneration,
    302
Antioxidants, 44, 142, 156b
    as food additives, 324t-325t
Apatite, 161
Appetite, 129-130
Arachidonic acid, 106, 267
Area Information Center(s), 329
Ariboflavinosis, 195
Ascorbic acid. see Vitamin C
Aspartame, 368
Assessment, patient, 407-408
    see also Nutritional assessment and counseling
Ataxia, 193
Atherosclerosis, 104, 106f
    dental hygiene considerations in, 347b
    nutritional directions for, 347b
    oral manifestations in, 346-347
ATP (adenosine triphosphate), 45, 127
Atrophic gastritis, 295
Atrophic gingivitis, 259
Atrophic glossitis, 342-343
Attention deficit-hyperactivity disorder, nutrition
    for children with, 280
Avidin, and biotin deficiency, 205

B

Baby bottle tooth decay (BBTD), 271-272
Bariatric surgery, 28b-30b
Basal energy expenditure (BEE), 128
Basal metabolic rate (BMR), 127-128
    dental hygiene considerations of, 129b
    factors affecting, 127-128
    measurement of, 127, 127f
    normal, at different ages for each sex, 127f
    nutritional directions for, 129b
    in older adults, 296, 297f
Bases, as food additives, 324t-325t
Basic convenience foods, 319
B-complex vitamins
    see also specific vitamin
    in oral soft tissue health, 189-212
        cobalamin (vitamin B_{12}), 203-204
        folate/folic acid, 200-202
        niacin (vitamin B_3) in, 195-197
        pyridoxine (vitamin B_6), 198
        riboflavin (vitamin B_2), 194-195
        thiamin (vitamin B_1) in, 192-193
        water solubility of, 141
    in pregnancy, 251-252

Page numbers followed by f indicate figures; t, tables;
b, boxes.

BEE (basal energy expenditure), 128
Behavior modification
   in obese and overweight children, 285b-287b
   as part of healthy weight control, 28b-30b
Beriberi, 193
Beta-carotene
   see also Vitamin A
   over-consumption of, 143, 144f
Beverages
   consumption of, 217, 218f
   destructive effects of, 78t
   recommended, and frequency, 12t
Bile, secretion of, 57
Binge-eating disorder, diagnostic criteria for, 359b
Binges, 357
Bioavailability, of nutrients, 91, 164-165
Biochemistry, 35
   concepts in, 34-49, 35b
   fundamentals of, 35-36
Biological information transfer, central dogma of, 40,
   41f
Biomolecules, 36t
Biotechnology, 377
Biotin, 205
   deficiency symptoms of, 409t
   dental hygiene considerations of, 205b
   hypo states of, 205
   nutritional directions for, 205b
   nutritional requirements for, 205, 205t
   physiological roles of, 205
   sources of, 205
Bisphosphonates, and development of osteonecrosis,
   348, 349f
Bland diet, 386, 388b
Bleaching agents, as additives, 324t-325t
Blood glucose level, metabolic maintenance of, 123
Blood lipid levels, 113-114
   dental hygiene considerations of, 114b
   desirable/optimal, 117t
   nutritional directions for, 114b
Blood pressure, classification of, 238t
BMI. see Body mass index
BMR. see Basal metabolic rate (BMR)
Body composition, and basal metabolic rate, 128
Body fluid distribution, 214
Body mass index (BMI), 9-10, 28b-30b
   changes in, in older adults, 296
   and childhood obesity, 285b-287b
   in patient assessment, 408-409
Bolus, 56
Bone mineralization, and growth, 161
   see also Calcified structures
Bone remodeling, 161
Bone resorption, in older adults, 295
   see also Osteoporosis
Boron, 183
Bottled water
   added ingredients in, 217
   consumption of, 172, 217
Bradycardia, 192b
Bradykinesia, 352
Brain health, maintaining, 186b
Breast milk, in nutritional requirements of infants,
   266-267, 266t
Breastfeeding
   advantages of, 256b. see also Lactation.
   and allergy prevention of, 267f, 269
   nutritional recommendations for, 256
Brown tumors, 351
Bruxism, 281
Buccal mucosa, irritation on, 400f
Bulimia nervosa
   diagnostic criteria for, 358f
   oral manifestations in, 357-359, 359f

C
Caffeine, 218
   myths and facts of, 219b-220b
Calciferol poisoning, 148
Calcified structures, 160-177
   see also Dental caries; Dentition
   changes in, oral manifestations of, 348
   mineral physiology of, 160-177, 368. see also
      Calcium; Fluoride; Magnesium;
      Phosphorus.

Calcified structures (Continued)
   case application in, 176b
   case study for, 177b
   health application of, 175b
   trace mineral physiology of, 178-188. see also
      Chromium; Copper; Manganese; Selenium;
      Ultratrace elements.
   vitamin physiology of, 139-159, 140b. see also
      Vitamin A; Vitamin C; Vitamin D; Vitamin E;
      Vitamin K.
   case application in, 157b
   deficiencies in, 140-141
   dental hygiene considerations in, 141b
   health application in, 156b
   nutritional directions for, 141b
   requirements in, 140, 140b
Calcitonin, 145
Calcium, 162-166
   absorption and excretion of, 163-164, 164f. see also
      Calcium balance.
   in calcified structures, 368. see also Calcified
      structures.
   deficiency symptoms of, 409t
   dental hygiene considerations of, 166b
   food labeling for, 165t
   hyper-state and hypo-states of, 165-166
   nutritional directions for, 167b
   nutritional requirements for, in pregnancy, 250-251
   physiological roles of, 162
   recommended dietary allowance (RDA) for, 162-163
   in saliva, 162
   sources of, 164-165, 165t
Calcium balance, 163
   hormones in maintenance of, 163
   in older adults, 294
   and vitamin D, 145
Calcium equivalents, 164b
Calcium intake
   adequate, 163t
   excessive, 166
   inadequate, 166
   during pregnancy, 250-251
Calcium-to-phosphorus ratio, 163
Caloric intake
   see also Kilocalorie(s) (kcal)
   adequate nutrients within, 10
   excess, metabolic pathways of, 125, 126f
Calorie, 4
Calorie-dense foods, 105
Calorimetry, indirect, 127, 127f
Canada's Food Guide, 20, 22f-23f
Cancellous bone, 55
Cancer prevention
   vitamin A in physiology of, 142
   vitamin D in, 150
Cancer risk, and fat intake, 114
Cancer treatments
   dental hygiene considerations in, 355b
   nutritional directions for, 355b
   oral manifestations in, 355
Candidiasis, oral, 349, 349f
Carbohydrate intake, Dietary Guidelines for Americans
   recommendations, 12-13
Carbohydrates, 66-85, 67f
   see also Dietary fiber; Starch(es); Sugar(s)
   case application for, 83b-84b
   case study, 84b
   classification of, 67-71
   complex, 67
   consumption of, excessive, 77
   conversion of, 71
   deficiency, 77
   and dental caries, 77-79
   dental hygiene considerations, 69b
   in fat metabolism, 71
   fermentable, 67
      in demineralization of enamel, 366, 367b
      food sources of, 367b
      and severe early childhood caries, 272b
   metabolism of, 47, 123-124
      in diabetes mellitus, 132b-135b
   in nutrition and health
      hyper-states and hypo-states, 77-80
      nutritional directions, 69b
      requirements for, 74

Carbohydrates (Continued)
   physiological roles, 71-72
   sources, 74-75
   structure and function of, 36-38
Carbon cycle, 36f
Cardiovascular disease
   community nutrition resources for patients with,
      330t
   dental hygiene considerations in, 347b
   and hyperlipidemia, 116b-117b
   nutritional directions for, 347b
   oral manifestations in, 341t, 346-347
Cardiovascular risks, vitamin D in, 150
Caries. see Dental caries
Caries management by risk assessment, 371
Caries risk assessment form, 372f-375f
Cariogenic foods, 367
   see also Fermentable carbohydrates
Cariogenic sweetener(s), 68t, 77-78
Cariostatic activity, of stannous fluoride, 171f, 184
Cariostatic foods, 370, 370b
Carotene. see Vitamin A
Casein, anticariogenic properties of, 368
Catabolism, 122, 124
   characteristics of, 45
   energy flow in, 46f
   of foods, 125
   summary of, 46f
Cations, 223
Cellulose, 70, 71t
Cementum, 161
Cephalin, 104
Cereals, recommended, and frequency, 12t
Cerebrovascular accident
   dental hygiene considerations in, 347b
   nutritional directions for, 347b
   oral manifestations in, 346-347
Cheese. see Milk and dairy products
Cheilitis, angular, in riboflavin deficiency, 195,
   195f
Cheilosis, 192b
Chelation therapy, 326
Chemotherapy
   dental hygiene considerations in, 355b
   nutritional directions for, 355b
   oral manifestations in, 355
Children, 331
   adolescents, 282-284
      dental hygiene considerations of, 284b
      growth and nutrient requirements of, 282-283
      influential factors in eating habits of, 283-284
      nutritional counseling, 284
      nutritional directions for, 285b
   attention deficit-hyperactivity disorder in, 280
   case application in nutrition for, 287b-288b
   case study for, 288b-289b
   community nutrition resources for, 330t
   dietary recommendations for, 274-277
   health application in nutrition for, 285b-287b
   MyPlate guide for, 274
   obesity in, health application, 285b-287b
   oral health and dental development in, 271
   school-age, 281-282
      dental carries in, 281-282
      dental hygiene considerations of, 282b
      nutritional directions for, 282b
   special needs, 281
      dental hygiene considerations of, 281b
      nutritional directions for, 281b
   toddler and preschool, 277-279
      dental hygiene considerations of, 279b
      food-related behaviors of, 278-279
      growth of, 277
      nutrient requirements of, 277, 278t
      nutritional directions for, 280b
Chloride, 228
   hyper states and hypo states of, 228
   physiological roles of, 228
   regulation of, 228
   requirements for, 225t, 228
   sources of, 228
Chlorophyll molecule, magnesium within, 169f
Cholesterol, 44, 105
   in selected foods, 110t
   structure of, 45f

Cholesterol intake, average, 116b-117b
Cholinergic nerves, 192b
Chromium, 181-182
    dental hygiene considerations of, 182b
    hyper-states and hypo-states of, 182
    nutritional directions for, 182b
    nutritional requirements for, 181, 181t
    physiological roles of, 181
    sources of, 181
Chronic disease
    and obesity, 28b-30b
    oral manifestations in, 340-342
Chronic periodontitis, 384-388, 385f
Chylomicrons, 104-105, 105f
    metabolism of, 124
Circumvallate lingual papillae, 191f, 192
cis fatty acids, physiologic actions of, 106t
Citric acid cycle, 45-47, 103
CL (ConsumerLab.com), 206b-209b
Cleft palate
    and cleft lip, 273, 273f
        dental hygiene considerations in, 273b
        nutritional directions for, 274b
    feeding suggestions for infant with, 274b
    with prosthesis, 274f
Clinical attachment loss (CAL), 384, 384f
Clinical observation, 408-409
    anthropometric, 408-409
    extraoral and intraoral assessments in, 408, 409t
Cobalamin (vitamin B₁₂), 203-204
    absorption and excretion of, 203
        in older adults, 300
    deficiency symptoms of, 409t
    dental hygiene considerations of, 204b-205b
    hyper states and hypo states of, 204
    nutritional directions for, 205b
    nutritional requirements for, 203
    physiological roles of, 203
    recommended dietary allowance (RDA) for, 203, 203t
    sources of, 203, 204t
Cocoa factor, anticariogenic properties of, 368
Coenzyme(s), 39, 41t, 103
    biotin, 205
    niacin, 195-197
    pyridoxine, 198
    thiamin, 192-193
    vitamin C, 154
Cofactor(s), 103
    selenium, 180
Coffees and teas, 218
Cold pasteurization, 319-320
Coliforms, 217
Collagen, 89, 161
    vitamin C and production of, 154
Colonics, 326
Colorings, as food additives, 324t-325t
Communication, in patient learning, 418-421
    listening and, 418
    nonverbal, 418
    questioning and, 418-421
Community nutrition resources, 330t
Complementary foods, 95b-96b
Complementary medicine, 206b-209b
Complex carbohydrates, 67, 69-71
Complex convenience foods, 319
Compound lipids, 102, 104-105
Compressional forces, 161
Condensation, 36
Conjugated linoleic acid (CLA), 110
Constipation, in older adults, 295
ConsumerLab.com (CL), 206b-209b
Convenience foods, 319
Cooking food. *see* Food preparation
Copper, 179-180
    absorption and excretion of, 179
    dental hygiene considerations of, 180b
    hyper-states and hypo-states of, 180
    nutritional directions for, 180b
    nutritional requirements for, 179
    physiologic roles of, 179
    recommended dietary allowance (RDA) for, 179, 179t
    sources of, 179
Corn sugar, 68

Counseling. *see* Nutritional assessment and counseling
Cow's milk, 267
    see also Milk and dairy products
Crepitus, 400
Cretinism, 235
Crohn's disease, oral manifestations in, 346
Cultural influences, on diet, 309, 312t-314t
Curing agents, as additives, 324t-325t
Cushing's syndrome, oral manifestations in, 350

D

Daily reference values (DRVs), 24-25, 24t
Daily value (DV), 24-25
Dairy products, risk for osteoporosis, 48b-49b
DASH (Dietary Approaches to Stop Hypertension), 236b-237b
DASH eating plan, 238b, 238t
Delaney clause, 322
Demineralization, 55
Dental caries, 77-79, 364-380, 365f
    case study for, 379b
    contributory factors in, 365-368, 365f
        cariogenic foods, 367, 367b
        food intake frequency, 369-370
        host factors, 366
        other, 368-370
        physical form of cariogenic food, 369
        plaque biofilm, 366
        saliva, 366
        timing and sequence in meal, 370
        tooth structure, 365
    fluoride deficiency and, 173
    in infants and young children, 271. *see also* Severe early childhood caries.
    in school-age children, 281-282
Dental caries prevention, 364-380
    anticariogenic foods, 367-368
    considerations in, 366b, 369b-370b
    dental plan, 371-373, 371b
        assessments in, 371-373
        case application in, 378b
        goals of, 373
        patient education in, 373
    nutritional directions for, 366b, 369b, 371b
Dental decay, vitamin D status and, 150
Dental erosion, 78, 221
Dental fluorosis, 173, 173f
Dental history, 408
Dental hygiene profession, promotion of health and wellness in, 3
Dental hygienist, role of, 332
Dentin, 161
    trace elements in, 179t
Dentin hypersensitivity, 396-397
    and dental abrasion, 396-397, 397f
    and dental erosion, 396-397, 397f
    dental hygiene considerations in, 397b
    nutritional directions for, 397b
Dentition
    see also Calcified structures; Dental caries
    development of, 161
        childhood oral health in, 271, 365
        chronology of, 248t
        nutritional deficiencies and, 248t
        nutritional status in utero and, 247
    loss of, 397-398, 398b
    and orthodontic treatment, 394
Dentures, patients with, 397-398
    dental hygiene considerations for, 398b
    and masticatory efficiency, 295
    nutritional directions for, 398b
Desserts, recommended, and frequency, 12t
Detoxification, 326
Developmental disabilities, oral manifestations and oral-motor impairment in, 341t, 353
Dextrins, 70
Diabetes mellitus, 132b-135b
    case application in, 137b
    comparison of carbohydrate use in patients without and with, 133f
    comparison of type I and type II, 135t
    dental hygiene considerations in, 349b-350b
    nutritional directions for, 350b
    oral manifestations in, 341t, 348-349, 349f

Diabetic patients, community nutrition resources for, 330t
Diaphoresis, 221
Diet history
    dental hygiene considerations of, 413b
    determining, 410-413
        food diary in, 412-413, 413f
        food frequency questionnaire in, 412, 412t
        twenty-four hour recall in, 410-412, 410b, 411f
    nutritional directions for, 413b
Dietary acculturation, 310-311
Dietary Approaches to Stop Hypertension (DASH), 20
    see also Popular diets
Dietary counseling. *see* Diet history; Nutritional assessment and counseling
Dietary fiber, 67f, 69-71
    for children older than two years, 277
    dental hygiene considerations of, 72b, 75b
    and gastrointestinal motility, 72
    guidelines for, 73t
    nondigestible carbohydrates, 70
    nutritional directions, 73b, 76b
    other nutrients, 72
    in sample menu, 76t
Dietary (food) patterns, 309-310
    cultural influences in, 309
    dental hygiene considerations of, 311b
    effecting changes in, 310-311
    food budget influence on, 311-316
    during lactation, 257, 258f
    nutritional directions for, 311b
    of older adults, 301
    religious food restriction in, 311
    respecting cultural differences in, 310
    status and symbolic influences in, 309-310
    and susceptibility to caries, 366
    unusual, in pregnancy, 244-245
Dietary Guidelines for Americans, 6-16, 7f, 9f, 75, 75b, 90
    recommendations of, 8b
        for adequate nutrients within kilocalorie needs, 10
        for alcoholic beverages, 13
        for carbohydrate intake, 12-13
        for fat intake, 11
        for food groups, 11-15, 12t
        for food safety, 15-16
        for physical activity, 10-11
        for sodium intake, 11
        for weight management, 9-11
Dietary intake. *see* Diet history
Dietary reference intakes (DRIs), 5-6
    for children through adolescence, 278t
    dental hygienist's use of, 6b
    for infants, 266-267, 266t
    nutritional directions for, 6b
    for older adults, 298, 299t
    in pregnancy, 249-250, 249t
    for saturated fatty acids and *trans* fats, 108
    summary of, 6
Dietary Supplement Health and Education Act, 206b-209b
Dietetic technician, registered (DTR), 3
Digestion, 57-59
    and absorption, 50-65
        case application in, 63b
        case study, 64b
        chemical action, 51
        mechanical action, 51
    and nutrition
        dental hygiene considerations of, 52b
        health application in, 62b-63b
        process of, 52f
            large intestine, 60-61
            in oral cavity, 52-56
            in small intestine, 57-59
Diplopia, 143
Disaccharides, 69
Docosahexaenoic acid (DHA), 110-111, 250, 267
    in infant formulas, 267-268
DRIs. *see* Dietary reference intakes; Dietary reference intakes (DRIs)
Drug interactions, with dietary supplements, 206b-209b
Drug use, during pregnancy, 246-247

DRVs (daily reference values), 24-25, 24t
Dry beans and peas
    contributions of, in daily nutrition, 19t
    in *MyPyramid Food Guidance System*, 19
Dry tongue, 221
DV (daily value), 24-25
Dysesthesia, 259
Dysgeusia, 54
Dysphagia, 295, 352

E

EAR (estimated average requirement), 5
Early childhood caries (ECC), 271-272, 271f
    contributing factors to, 272
Eating disorders
    dental hygiene considerations in, 359b
    nutritional directions for, 359b
    oral manifestations in, 357
Eating patterns, 15-16, 16b
    see also Dietary (food) patterns
Edentulism, in older adults, 294
Edentulous patients, 397-398
    dental hygiene considerations for, 398b
    and masticatory efficiency, 295
    nutritional directions for, 398b
EER (estimated energy requirement), 6, 128
Eggs
    contributions of, in daily nutrition, 19t
    in Food Pyramid Guidance System, 97f
    in *MyPyramid Food Guidance System*, 19
Eicosapentaenoic acid (EPA), 104, 110-111
Electrolytes, 223
    see also Mineral electrolytes
Electronic Benefit Card (EBT), 329
Emulsification, 57
Emulsifiers, as food additives, 324t-325t
Enamel, 161
    demineralization of, by carbohydrate fermentation, 365-366, 370f
    trace elements in, 179t. *see also* specific element.
Enamel hypoplasia, 145, 150, 365
Endocrine glands, and basal metabolic rate, 128
Energy, 71
    and protein, in older adults, 298
Energy balance, 129-131
    dental hygiene considerations of, 132b
    expenditure factors in, 131
    factors affecting, 130f
    inadequate food intake and, 131
    intake factors in, 129
    nutritional directions for, 132b
    physiological factors in maintaining, 130-131
    psychological factors in maintaining, 131
Energy-dense foods, 311
Energy drinks, 218-220
Energy expenditure, 131
    during various activities, 129t
Energy intake, inadequate, 131
Energy production, 127
    from alcohol, 125
    basal metabolic rate in, 127-128
    from carbohydrates, 123-124
    dental hygiene considerations of, 126b
    and energy balance, 129-131. *see also* Energy balance.
    and estimated energy requirements, 128
    from lipids, 124-125
    metabolism and, 127. *see also* Metabolism.
    nutritional directions for, 126b
    from proteins, 124
    and total energy requirements, 128
    and unusual work and play, 128
Energy sources, food, fats (lipids) in, 105
Enriched products, and whole grains, nutrient values of, 14t
Enrichment, definition of, 12-13
Enteral feeding, 185b-186b
Enzymes, 103
    copper component of, 179
Epilepsy, oral manifestations of phenytoin use in, 353-354, 353f
Epinephrine, 47, 47t
Epiphyses, 148
Epithelialization, 206b
Erythema, 93-94

Erythropoiesis, 252
Escherichia coli, 317
Esophagitis
    dental hygiene considerations in, 345b
    nutritional directions for, 345b
    oral manifestations in, 345
Esophagus, 56
    dental hygiene considerations of, 56b
    nutritional directions for, 56b
Essential amino acids (EAAs), 47-48, 48t
Essential fatty acid (EFA), 105
Essential hypertension, 236b-237b
Essential nutrients, 4
Estimated average requirement (EAR), 5
Estimated energy requirement (EER), 6, 128
Evaluation, patient, 407-408
Expanded Food and Nutrition Education Program, 331-332
Extracellular fluid (ECF), 214
Extraoral and intraoral assessments, 408, 409t

F

Fad diets, 325
Fast foods, 322
Fasting and starvation, and basal metabolic rate, 128
Fat intake
    Dietary Guidelines for Americans recommendations, 11
    during pregnancy, 250
Fat replacers, 115, 115t
    dental hygiene considerations of, 116b
    nutritional directions for, 116b
Fat soluble vitamins, 40, 105, 141
Fat storage, 71, 106-107
Fats, 67f, 102, 102f
    see also Lipids
    absorption of, in small intestine, 59
    anticariogenic properties of, 368
    case application of, 118b-119b
    characteristics of, based on composition, 104
    choosing dietary, 111b
    as energy source, 105, 107, 125
    health application of, 116b-117b
    for insulation, 107
    metabolism of, 71
    over-consumption of, and health-related problems, 113-114
    and palatability of foods, 105
    physiological roles of, 105-107, 106t
    for protection of organs, 107
    recommendations for adults, 109t
    recommended daily, for specific caloric levels, 108b
    recommended sources of, and frequency, 12t
    satiety value of, 105
    sources of, 106t, 108-113, 110t
    storage of, 106-107
        carbohydrates and, 71
    total, in U.S. food supply, per capita per day, 108f
    under-consumption of, and health-related problems, 114
Fatty acids, 41, 102
    see also Lipids
    characteristics of, 104
    melting point of, 43
    monounsaturated, 103
    omega numbering system of, 43f
    polyunsaturated, 104, 250
    saturated, 103
    in selected foods, 108-113, 110t
    summary of common, 43t
    trans, 103-104
    unsaturated, 103
FDA. *see* U.S. Food and Drug Administration (FDA)
Feeding problems, in neuromuscular disabilities, 353, 353t
Fermentable carbohydrates, 67
    in demineralization of enamel, 365
    dental hygiene considerations of, 370b
    food sources of, 367, 367b
    nutritional directions for, 371b
    and severe early childhood caries, 272b
Fermentable carbohydrates intake, analysis worksheet, 376f
Fetal alcohol spectrum disorder, 260b-261b

Fetal alcohol syndrome, signs of, 261b, 261f
Fetal birth defects
    alcohol exposure during pregnancy, 260b-261b
    excessive supplementation during pregnancy and, 253-254, 253t
    vitamin A toxicity and, 143
Fetal development
    factors affecting, 244-247
        age, 245
        drugs and medications during, 246-247
        food safety, 247
        healthcare, 245
        oral health, 246
        preconceptional nutritional status, 244
        unusual dietary patterns, 244-245
        weight gain, 245-246
    and nutrients available during pregnancy, 249-254
    nutritional requirements during, 249-254
        B vitamins, 251-252
        calcium and vitamin D, 250-251
        energy and kilocalories, 250, 251f
        fat, 250
        iodine, 252-253
        iron, 252
        protein, 250, 251f
        zinc, 252
Fiber
    dietary, 70-71
    functional, 70-71
    soluble, 72
    total, 71
    viscous, 72
Fiber-rich food, 72
Fibroblasts, vitamin C and formation of, 154
Fibrotic tissue formation, 383-384
Filiform papillae, of tongue, 191, 191f
Firming agents, as additives, 324t-325t
Fissured tongue, 221, 222f
Flavin adenine dinucleotide (FAD/FADH2), 45-47
Flavorings, as food additives, 324t-325t
Flexitarians, 95b-96b
Fluid intake, for older adults, 298
Fluid volume deficit (FVD), 221
Fluid volume disturbances, 222f
Fluid volume excess (FVE), 221
    conditions causing, 221
Fluids
    absorption of, 215
    hyper states and hypo states of, 221
    oral soft tissue requirements for, 213-241, 215t
        dental hygiene considerations of, 221b-222b
        nutritional directions for, 223b
    physiological roles of, 214
    regulation of, 214-215
    requirements for, 214-215, 216f
    sources of, 215-221, 217t, 218f
Fluorapatite, 170
Fluoride, 170-174
    absorption and excretion of, 171-172
    age-specific guidelines for, 175b
    in calcified structures, 170-174
        concentration gradients of, 170f
        dental hygiene considerations of, 174b
        nutritional directions for, 174b
        protective effect of, 173
    hyper-states and hypo-states of, 173
    nutritional requirements for, 171, 172t
    physiologic roles of, 170-171
    safety of in water supply, 174
    sources of, 172
        food, 172, 173t
        water, 172
    supplementation of
        and birth defects, 253t
        for infants, 267t, 270
    topical application of, 172, 282
Fluorosis
    and bone health, 173
    in infants, 268
Folate/folic acid, 200-202
    absorption and excretion of, 201
    deficiency symptoms of, 409t
    dental hygiene considerations of, 202b
    hyper states and hypo states of, 202
    nutritional directions for, 203b

Folate/folic acid *(Continued)*
  nutritional requirements for, 200
  physiological roles of, 200
  recommended dietary allowance (RDA) for, 200, 201t
  recommended dietary allowance (RDA) for, in pregnancy, 252
  sources of, 201, 201t
  supplementation of, during pregnancy, 253
Folate status, drugs that may negatively affect, 202b
Foliate papillae, of tongue, 191f, 192
Folic acid, alcohol as antagonist, 246-247
Follicular hyperkeratosis, 144-145, 144f
Follow-up, on nutrition treatment goals, 417
Food additives, 322-323
  benefits of, 323
  and hyperactivity, 280
Food and Drug Administration (FDA)
  allowance for *trans* fat labeling, 112
  bottled water regulation by, 217
  and detention of suspect foods, 318
  and implementation of good manufacturing practices for supplements, 206b-209b
  infant formula standards of, 267
  and mandated addition of folic acid to cereal and grain products, 201
Food budget(s), 311-316
  economical purchases in, 315b
  low-income, economical purchasing in, 316t
Food choice (selection)
  and dentition, 295
  factors affecting, 4
  and oral problems, 293
  and susceptibility to caries, 366
Food deserts, 315
Food diary, 373, 375f-376f
  in determining diet history, 412-413, 413f
Food fad, 323-329
  case application in, 335b
  case study for, 336b
  definition of, 325
Food frequency questionnaire, in diet history, 412, 412t
Food groups
  descriptions of, in *MyPyramid Food Guidance System. see MyPyramid Food Guidance System.*
  Dietary Guidelines for Americans recommendations for, 11-15, 12t
  in-depth information on, in *MyPyramid*, 16-19
  nutrients contributions of, 17t
  representation in *MyPyramid Food Guidance System*, 17f
Food guidance system(s)
  American Cancer Society, 20
  American Diabetes Association, 20
  American Heart Association, 20
  Canadian, 20
  Dietary Approaches to Stop Hypertension (DASH), 20
  Healthy Eating Pyramid, 20, 21f
  Mexican, 311f
  National Cholesterol Education Program Expert Panel on Detection, Evaluation and Treatment of High Blood Cholesterol in Adults, 20
  other, 20-21
  USDHHS Pyramid, 6-7. *see also MyPyramid Food Guidance System.*
Food insecurity, 333
  trends in, 334f
Food insecurity in the United States, 333b-335b
Food intake
  factors influencing, social, 410b
  inadequate, 131, 132f
  inadequate, effects of, in United States, 333b-335b
  in older adults, 295. *see also* Older adults.
  physical activity and, 131
  stimuli affecting, 131, 131t
  twenty-four hour recall of, 410-412, 410b, 411f
Food jags, 279
Food label(s), 7
  see also Nutrition Facts label
  health claims on, 25
  qualified health claims on, 25
  terms and definitions on, 26b

Food patterns, 309-310
  cultural influences in, 309, 310f
  dental hygiene considerations of, 311b
  effecting changes in, 310-311
  food budget influence on, 311-316
  during lactation, 257, 258f
  nutritional directions for, 311b
  religious restrictions in, 311
  respecting cultural differences in, 310
  status and symbolic influences in, 309-310
  unusual, in pregnancy, 244-245
Food preparation, 316-323
  dental hygiene considerations of, 323b
  guidelines for preserving nutrients during, 317b
  methods of, 316-317
  nutritional directions for, 323b
  optimal nutrition maintenance in, 316-323
  preserving nutrients during, 317b
  processed, 318-323, 319f
    additives in, 322-323
    convenience in, 319
    fast food, 322
    irradiated foods in, 319-320
    organic, 320-322
    sanitation and safety in, 317-318
Food processing, effect of, 318-319
Food quackery, 325-326
Food record
  checklist for, 414t
  how to keep, 410b
Food-related behaviors, of toddlers and preschool children, 278-279
Food safety, 317, 318b
  Dietary Guidelines recommendations for, 15-16, 317
Food sanitation, 317-318, 318b
Food security, 333
  status, of United States households, 333f-334f
Food selection. *see* Food choice (selection)
Food stamp, usage of, 329-331
Fortification, definition of, 14
Fructose, 68
Fruits
  nutrients in selected, 18t
  recommended, and frequency, 12t
  reduced cariogenic properties of, 367
Fruits group
  in Food Pyramid Guidance System, 97f
  in *MyPyramid Food Guidance System*, 13-14, 18
Full liquid diet, 385-386, 386b
Functional components, examples of, 402t-403t
Functional fiber, 70-71
Functional foods, health application of, 400b-401b
Functional groups, 35-36, 36f
Fungating lesions, 190
Fungiform papillae, of tongue, 191, 191f

G

Galactose, 69
Gastric digestion, 56-57
  dental hygiene considerations of, 57b
  nutritional directions for, 57b
Gastroesophageal reflux disease (GERD)
  and dental erosion, 246
  oral manifestations in, 345
Gastrointestinal disorders, oral manifestations in, 341t, 345-346
Gastrointestinal motility
  dietary fiber and, 72
  in older adults, 295
Gastrointestinal tract
  physiology of, 51
    dental hygiene considerations of, 52b, 64b
    digestive process, 52f
    esophagus, 56
    gastric digestion in, 56-57
    large intestine, 60-61
    nutritional directions, 52b
    nutritional directions for, 52b
    oral cavity, 52-56
    small intestine, 57-59
Gastrostomy, 346-347
Gender, and basal metabolic rate, 127f, 128
Genetic engineering, 377
Genetically modified foods, health application in, 377b-378b

Genetically modified organisms (GMO), 377
Genetics, and susceptibility to caries, 366
Genomics, health application of, 303b-304b
Gestational diabetes, weight gain and, 245-246
Ghrelin, 28b-30b
Gingiva, normal, 190, 190f
Gingivitis, 382f, 383-384
  in ascorbic acid deficiency, 155, 156f
  atrophic, 259
  with heavy calculus present, 383-384, 384f
  and malnutrition, 383, 383f
  nutritional aspects of, 381-392
  plaque biofilm associated with, 383-384
  in pregnancy, 246f
Gingivostomatitis, menopausal, 259
Ginseng, in energy drinks, 218
Glossitis, 192b, 399-400
  dental hygiene considerations in, 400b
  dental hygiene considerations of, 202b
  in folic acid deficiency, 202, 203f
  nutritional directions for, 203b, 400b
  in pyridoxine deficiency, 200, 200f
  in riboflavin deficiency, 195, 195f
  in thiamin deficiency, 193, 193f
Glossodynia, 343
Glossopyrosis, in vitamin B_{12} deficiency, 204
Glucagon, 47, 47t
Gluconeogenesis, 124
Glucose, 68, 70f
Glucose polymers, 70, 70f
Gluten, and malabsorption, 345-346
Gluten-related disorders, health applications of, 62b-63b
Glycemic effect, 123-124
Glycerol, 103
Glycogen, 38, 70, 122
  branched structures of, 39f
Glycogenesis, 123
Glycyrrhiza, anticariogenic properties of, 368
Goal setting, in nutritional counseling, 416-417, 416b
Goat's milk, and infant nutrition, 268
Goiter, 235, 236f
Goitrogens, 235, 350
Grains group
  in Food Pyramid Guidance System, 97f
  in *MyPyramid Food Guidance System*, 18-19
GRAS (generally recognized as safe), 322
Gravidas, 244-245
Growth, vitamin A in physiology of, 141
Guarana, in energy drinks, 218
Gums and mucilages, 71b
Gustatory sensations, 52-53
  loss of, 294

H

Hairy leukoplakia, 356f
Head start, 332
Health, food factors affecting, 308-338
  case study for, 336b
Health and Nutrition Information website, 275
Health Applications
  Alzheimer's disease, 185b-186b
  Antioxidants, 156b
  Childhood and adolescent obesity, 285b-287b
  Diabetes mellitus, 132b-135b
  Fetal alcohol spectrum disorder, 260b-261b
  Food insecurity in the United States, 333b-335b
  Functional foods, 400b-401b
  Genetically modified foods, 377b-378b
  Genomics, 303b-304b
  Gluten-related disorders, 62b-63b
  Health literacy, 419b
  High-fructose corn syrup, 82b-83b
  Human papillomavirus, 360b, 360f
  Hypertension, 236b-237b
  Lactose intolerance, 48b-49b
  Obesity, 28b-30b
  Osteoporosis, 175b
  Supplements, 206b-209b
  Tobacco cessation, 390b
  Vegetarianism, 95b-96b
Health claims, 21, 25
Health history, 407
  screening tools in, 407

Health literacy, 419b
  levels of, 420b
  strategies in, 420b
  substituting simple words for complex words,
    420b
Health status, and basal metabolic rate, 128
Healthcare disparities, 309
Healthcare during pregnancy, 245
Healthy eating, 320t
Healthy Eating Pyramid, 20, 21f
Healthy People 2020, 5
  objectives of, 5, 28b-30b
  oral health goals of, 365, 382
Heat exhaustion, 227
Hematologic disorders, oral manifestations in, 341t,
    344-345
  see also Anemia(s); Neutropenia
Hematopoiesis, 145
Heme iron, absorption of, 230-231
Hemicellulose, 71t
Hemochromatosis, 231-232
Herbicide-resistant soybeans, 377
Herbs, as supplements, 206b-209b
Herbs and spices, as food complements instead of salt,
    227t
Herpetic ulcerations, in HIV therapies, 356
Hiatal hernia
  dental hygiene considerations in, 345b
  nutritional directions for, 345b
  oral manifestations in, 345
High density lipoproteins (HDLs), 105, 105f
High energy phosphate compounds, 127
High fiber diet, guidelines for, 73t
High quality protein, 88
Highly active antiretroviral therapy (HAART), oral
    manifestations in, 356
Hirsutism, 350
Homeopathic medicine, 206b-209b
Homeopathy, 206b-209b
Homeostatic mechanisms, 295
Hormone replacement therapy (HRT), 259
Hormones, 103
Humectants, as additives, 324t-325t
Hunger, 129-130, 333
  hypothalamic influence in controlling, 130
Hydration status, 214
  see also Water
  hyper states and hypo states in, 221
  metabolic regulation and, 214
Hydrogenation, 44, 45f, 103-104
Hydrolysis, 36, 51
Hydrolyzed protein, 268
Hydroxyapatite, 161
Hyper-states and hypo-states, 77-80
  dental hygiene considerations in, 79b-80b
  nutritional directions for, 79b-80b
Hypercalcemia, 165-166
Hypercalciuria, 165-166
Hypercarotenemia, 143, 144f
Hypercarotenosis, 144f
Hypergeusia, 54
Hyperglycemia, 77, 123
  nutritional prevention of, 132b-135b
Hyperkalemia, 229
Hyperkeratosis, 144f
Hyperlipidemia, 113, 116b-117b
  see also Blood lipid levels
  oral manifestations in, 347
Hypernatremia, 226-227
  symptoms of, 227
Hyperparathyroidism, oral manifestations in, 351
Hyperphosphatemia, 167
Hypertension, 11, 236b-237b
  causes of, 238t
  classification of, 238t
  dental hygiene considerations in, 348b
  nutritional directions for, 348b
  oral manifestations in, 347
Hypervitaminosis A, 143
  discoloration of gingiva in, 144f
Hypocalcemia, 166
Hypodipsia, 221
Hypogeusia, 54, 294
Hypoglycemia, 77, 123
  nutritional prevention of, 132b-135b

Hypokalemia, 229
Hyponatremia, 226-227
  symptoms of, 227
Hypophosphatemia, 167-168
Hypopituitarism, oral manifestations in, 350
Hyposalivation, 342
Hypothyroidism, oral manifestations in, 350-351, 350f
Hypotonic saliva, 190-191

I

Iatrogenic condition, 54
Immune response, 89
  in gingivitis and periodontal disease, 382
Immunocompromised patient, 94
Immunoglobulins, 89
Income, and susceptibility to caries, 366
Incontinence, 298
Indirect calorimetry, 127, 127f
Infant formula(s), 267-268
  discontinuation of, 268
Infants
  with cleft lip and cleft palate, oral care of, 273
  community nutrition resources for, 330t
  dental hygiene considerations, 270b
  feeding practices for, 268-270
  fluoride supplementation for, 267
  food introduction to, 269-270
  growth of, 266
  nutritional care of, 266-273
  nutritional directions for, 270b-271b
  nutritional requirements of, 266
    breast milk in, 266-267, 266t
    commercial milk formulas in, 267-268
  oral and neuromuscular development in, 268-269
  oral care of, 271
    dental hygiene considerations in, 272b-273b
    dietary counseling in, 271
    nutritional directions for, 273b
  supplements for, 270
Innate desire, 270
Institute of Medicine (IOM)
  recommendations of
    for biotin, 205, 205t
    for calcium, 163t
    for chloride, 225t, 228
    for chromium, 181t
    for cobalamin (vitamin B_{12}), 203, 203t
    for copper, 179, 179t
    for fluoride, 172t
    for folate/folic acid, 200, 201t
    for iodine, 234, 235t
    for iron, 230, 230t
    for magnesium, 169t
    for manganese, 182, 182t
    for molybdenum, 183, 183t
    for niacin (vitamin B_3), 195-196, 196t
    for pantothenic acid, 197, 198t
    for phosphorus, 168t
    for potassium, 228-229, 228t
    for pyridoxine (vitamin B_6), 198, 199t
    for riboflavin (vitamin B_2), 194, 194t
    for selenium, 180
    for sodium, 223, 225t
    for thiamin (vitamin B_1), 192, 192t
    for vitamin A, 142, 142t
    for vitamin C, 154, 154t
    for vitamin D, 146, 147t
    for vitamin E, 151t
    for vitamin K, 153t
    for water, 214, 215t
    for zinc, 233, 233t
  revised sets of nutrient-based reference values, 5
Insulin, 47, 47t, 123
  in carbohydrate metabolism, 123, 123f
  chromium potentiation of action of, 181
Interesterified fats, 113-114
Interstitial space, 89
Intestinal bacteria, 72
Intracellular fluid (ICF), 214
Intrinsic factor and absorption of vitamin B_{12}, 203
Iodine, 234-235, 252-253
  dental hygiene considerations of, 236b
  hyper states and hypo states of, 235
  nutritional directions for, 236b
  physiological role of, 234

Iodine *(Continued)*
  recommended dietary allowance (RDA) for, 234,
    235t
  requirements for, 234, 235t
    during pregnancy, 224
  sources of, 234
  supplementation of, and birth defects, 253t
Iron, 230-232
  absorption and excretion of, 230-231, 231f
  deficiency symptoms of, 409t
  dental hygiene considerations of, 232b
  hyper states and hypo states of, 231-232
  nutritional directions for, 232b
  physiological roles of, 230
  recommended dietary allowance (RDA) for, 230,
    230t
  requirements for, 230
  requirements for, during pregnancy, 252
  sources of, 231, 232t
  supplementation of, 270
    during pregnancy, 253
Iron deficiency anemia, 232, 252, 342-343
  dental hygiene considerations in, 343b
  nutritional directions for, 343b
  oral manifestations in, 342-343, 342f
Irradiated foods, 319-320
  official package label for, 320f
Ischemia, cerebral, 346-347
  see also Cerebrovascular accident

K

Kaposi sarcoma, oral manifestations in, 354, 355f
Kayser-Fleischer ring, 180, 180f
Keratinized epithelium, 191
Keshan disease, 181
Ketoacidosis, 125
Ketones, 71
  production of, in lipid metabolism, 124-125
Ketonuria, 125
Ketosis, 71, 125
Kidneys, metabolic processes in, 122
Kilocalorie(s) (kcal), 4, 126
  and measurement of potential energy, 127
Krebs cycle, 45-47, 103
Kwashiorkor, and marasmus, 94, 94f

L

Labeling. *see* Nutrition Facts label; Nutrition
  labeling
Laboratory information, 409
Lactase deficiency, 48b-49b
Lactation, 255-257
  community nutrition resources for, 330t
  dental hygiene considerations of, 257b
  dietary patterns during, 257
  nutritional directions for, 257b
  nutritional recommendations during, 256
Lactobacillus, 366
Lactoferrin, 230
Lactose, 36-38, 69
  structures of, 38f
Lactose intolerance
  health application in, 48b-49b
  suggestions for patients with, 49b
Lactovegetarian, 95b-96b
Large intestine, 51, 60-61
  case application for, 63b
  case study, 64b
  dental hygiene considerations of, 61b
  functions of, 60
  health application in, 62b-63b
  microflora of, 60-61
  nutritional directions for, 61b
  peristalsis in, 51, 61
  undigested residue in, 60
Lauric acid, structural representations of, 42f
Lead, 184
Lecithin, 104
Legumes, in Food Pyramid Guidance System, 97f
Leukemia, oral manifestations in, 355
Leukoplakia, 142
  as manifestation of renal disease, 351-352, 351f
  oral hairy, 356, 356f
Levodopa, 352-353
Levulose, 68

Lichen planus, 399, 399f
Lignin, 71t
Linoleic acid, 105
    structure of, 42f
Lip hypertrophy, 356
Lipases, 39
Lipid soluble vitamins, 40
Lipids, 101-120
    chemical structure of, 103-104. *see also* Fatty acids.
    choosing, 111b, 112-113
    classification of, 102
    compound, 104-105
    and dental health, 107
    dental hygiene considerations of, 104b, 107b, 113b-114b
    dietary requirements for, 108
    as energy source, 105, 124-125
    health application of, 116b-117b
    metabolism of, 48, 124-125
    nutritional directions for, 104b, 107b-108b, 113b, 115b
    over-consumption of, and health-related problems, 113-114
    in palatability of foods, 105
    physiological roles of, 105-107, 106t
    protein-sparing, 105
    satiety value of, 105
    sources of, 108-113
    structure and function of, 40-44. *see also* Fatty acids.
    substitutes for, 115, 115t
    under-consumption of, and health-related problems, 114
Lipoatrophy, 356
Lipodystrophy, 356
Lipogenesis, 71, 124
Lipolysis, 124
Lipoproteins, 44, 104-105, 105f
    structure of, 45f
Listeria monocytogenes, 247, 317
Listeriosis, 247
Lithium, 184
Liver metabolism, 122
    and alcohol metabolism, 125
    and carbohydrate metabolism, 123
    and lipid metabolism, 124
    and protein metabolism, 124
Long-chain fatty acids, 103
Low birth weight (LBW), 244
    dietary intake and education in preventing, 254
Low-density lipoproteins (LDLs), 105, 105f
    in reducing risk of cardiovascular disease, 116b-117b
Low-income food budget, 314-315
    see also Food insecurity in the United States
    economical purchasing on, 316t
Low quality protein, 88
Lower esophageal sphincter (LES), 56
Lymphatic system, 59
Lysosome damage, by high concentrations of vitamin A, 143

M
Macrodontia, 365
Macroglossia, 350
Macronutrients, 6
Macular degeneration, and antioxidant intake, 302
Magnesium, 168-170
    in calcified structures, 168-170
        dental hygiene considerations of, 170b
        nutritional directions for, 170b
    hyper-states and hypo-states of, 169-170
    nutritional requirements for, 168, 169t
    physiologic roles of, 168
    recommended dietary allowance (RDA) for, 168, 169t
    sources of, 168-169, 169f, 169t
Maize diet, niacin deficiency with, 197
Malabsorptive conditions
    dental hygiene considerations in, 346b
    nutritional directions for, 346b
    oral manifestations in, 345-346, 346f
Malnutrition
    kwashiorkor and marasmus in, 94
    in older adults, 293

Maltose, 69
    formation of, 36-38, 37f
Manganese, 182
    dental hygiene considerations of, 182b
    hyper-states and hypo-states of, 182
    nutritional directions for, 183b
    nutritional requirements for, 182, 182t
    physiological roles of, 182
    sources of, 182
Manganese madness, 182
Mannitol, 69, 367-368
Manufactured convenience foods, 319
Marasmus, 94
Mastication, 55
Masticatory efficiency, 56
Materia alba, 355
Maturing agents, as additives, 324t-325t
Maxillofacial surgery, 398
    dental hygiene considerations in, 398b-399b
    nutritional directions in, 399b
Meats
    contributions of, in daily nutrition, 19t
    or meat substitutes
        recommended, and frequency, 12t
Mechanically-altered diet, 386, 387b-388b
Medication use, during pregnancy, 246-247
Medium-chain fatty acids, 103
Megadoses, of vitamins, 206b-209b
Megaloblastic anemia, 257-259
    dental hygiene considerations in, 343b-344b
    and folate deficiency, 202, 343
    nutritional directions for, 344b
    oral manifestations in, 343
Menopause
    dental hygiene considerations in, 260b
    nutritional directions for, 260b
    nutritional requirements in, 259-262
Mental health disorders, oral manifestations in, 341t, 357-359
Mental illness, oral manifestations in, 359
Menu creation and planning, 417, 417f
Mercury, 185
Meta-analysis, 156b, 328-329
Metabolic disorders, oral manifestations in, 341t, 348-352
Metabolic pathways, 102f
Metabolism, 122
    anabolic processes in, 122, 124
    of carbohydrates, 47
    case study for, 138b
    catabolic processes in, 122, 124
    energy balance, 121-138
    and energy balance, 129-131
    and energy production, 127
        from alcohol, 125
        basal metabolic rate in, 127-128
        from carbohydrates, 123-124
        dental hygiene considerations of, 126b
        from lipids, 124-125
        nutritional directions for, 126b
        from proteins, 124
    health application in, 132b-135b
    hormonal regulation of, 47t
    of lipid, 48
    and patient health
        dental hygiene considerations of, 123b
        nutritional directions for, 123b
        and satiety center, 130
    of proteins, 47-48
    and role of kidneys, 122-123
    and role of liver, 122
    summary of, 45-48
Microflora, of large intestine, 60-61
Micrognathia, 353
Micronutrients, 6
Microvilli, of small intestine, 57
Milk, analysis of fat content of, 112t
Milk and dairy products
    anticariogenic properties of, 368, 368f
    for children over two years, 277
    daily consumption of, by Americans, 164
    for infants, 266-268, 266t. *see also* Infant formula(s).
    in *MyPyramid Food Guidance System*, 19
    recommended, and frequency, 12t

Mineral electrolytes
    case application in, 239b
    case study in, 240b
    chloride in, 228
    health application in, 236b-237b
    iodine in, 234-235
    iron in, 230-232
    in oral soft tissue physiology, 213-241. *see also* specific mineral electrolyte.
    potassium in, 228-229
    sodium in, 223-227
    zinc in, 232-234
Mineral elements, in body, 162b
Mineralization, 161
Minerals, 160-188
    and calcified structure physiology, 160-177. *see also* Calcium; Fluoride; Magnesium; Phosphorus.
        bone growth in, 161
        case application of, 176b
        case study for, 177b
        health application of, 175b. *see also* Calcium; Fluoride; Magnesium; Phosphorus.
        introduction to, 161-162
        tooth formation in, 161
    as food additives, 324t-325t
    insufficiency of, in older adults, 299
    in pregnancy, recommended dietary allowance (RDA) of, 249t
    supplemental, for older adults, 302
    trace, in calcified structures, 178-188. *see also* Chromium; Copper; Manganese; Molybdenum; Selenium; Ultratrace elements.
Misinformation, about nutrition, 323-329
    dental hygienist's role in combating, 332
    identifying sources of, 327-329, 327b-328b
Molybdenum, 183
    dental hygiene considerations of, 183b
    hyper-states and hypo-states of, 183
    nutritional directions for, 183b
    nutritional requirements for, 183, 183t
    physiological roles of, 183
    recommended dietary allowance (RDA) for, 183, 183t
    sources of, 183
Monosaccharides, 36, 68-69
    linear structures of, 37f
    metabolism of, 123
Monounsaturated fatty acids (MUFAs), 41, 103
    food sources of, 108-113, 110t
    physiologic actions of, 106t
    structure of cis-trans isomers in, 43f
Mucositis, 343
Myelin synthesis, vitamin B_{12} (cobalamin) in, 203
MyPlate
    for children, 274
    for older adults, 300f, 301-302
    for pregnant and lactating women, 251f, 254. *see also MyPlate* for Moms.
MyPlate food record worksheet, 411f
MyPlate for Moms, 257, 258f
MyPyramid Food Guidance System, 7, 16-19, 20f
    dental hygiene considerations of, 19b-20b
    food group representation in, 17f
    food industry promotion of, 16-17
    foundation for, 6-7
    fruits group in, 18
    grains group in, 18-19
    links to *MyPyramid* Tracker on, 17-18
    milk and dairy products in, 19
    nutritional directions for, 20b
    protein foods group in, 19
    vegetables group in, 18

N
National Osteoporosis Foundation, vitamin D intake recommendations, 146
Natural food products, lack of definition of, 322
Naturopathy, 206b-209b
Necrosis, 93-94
Necrotizing enterocolitis, 268
Necrotizing ulcerative gingivitis (NUG), 93-94, 388-392, 389f
    bland diets in, 386, 388b
    dental hygiene considerations in, 389b-390b
    nutritional directions for, 390b

Necrotizing ulcerative periodontitis (NUP), 356, 388-392
Neoplasia, 206b
Neoplastic disorders, oral manifestations in, 341t, 354-355, 355f
Neotame, 368
Neuromuscular disorders
  dental hygiene considerations in, 354b
  nutritional directions for, 354b
  oral manifestations and oral-motor impairment in, 341t, 352-354
Neurotransmitters, 334
  copper and production of, 179
Neutropenia
  dental hygiene considerations in, 345b
  nutritional directions for, 345b
  oral manifestations in, 344
Niacin (vitamin B₃), 195-197
  deficiency symptoms of, 409t
  dental hygiene considerations of, 197b
  hyper states and hypo states of, 196-197
  nutritional directions for, 197b
  nutritional requirements for, 195-196
  physiological roles of, 195
  recommended dietary allowance (RDA) for, 195-196, 196t
  sources of, 196, 196t
Nickel, 183
Nicotinamide. see Niacin
Nicotinamide adenine dinucleotide (NAD+/NADH), 45-47
Nicotinic acid. see Niacin
Night blindness, 141
Nitrogen balance, 88, 88b
Nocturia, 298
Noma, and protein energy malnutrition, 93-94
Non-nutritive suckling, 269
Non-nutritive sweeteners. see Sugar substitutes; Sugar substitutes (sweeteners)
Nondigestible food components, 70
Nonessential amino acids (NEAAs), 47-48, 48t
Nonheme iron, absorption of, 230-231
NSF International, 210b
Nucleic acids, structure and function of, 40
Nutrient absorption, in small intestine, 59
Nutrient content claims, 21
Nutrient dense foods, 7
Nutrient density, 7, 309
  of diet, 77
Nutrients
  adequate, within kilocalorie needs, 10
  adequate intake (AI) of, 6. see also Adequate intake (AI).
  in calcified structures, 178-188
  essential, 4
  and estimated average requirement (EAR), 5
  and estimated energy requirement (EER), 6
  evaluation of patient intake of, 4b
  physiological roles of, 4
  in processed foods, 318-319, 319f
  recommended dietary allowance (RDA) of, 5. see also Recommended dietary allowance (RDA).
  recommended required, 5. see also Dietary Guidelines for Americans; MyPyramid Food Guidance System.
  stable, 319
  tolerable upper intake level (UL) of, 6
Nutrigenomics, 303b-304b
Nutrition
  acceptable macronutrient distribution ranges (AMDRs) in, 6
  in aging, 292-307. see also Older adults.
  basic, 3-4
  basic concepts of, 4
  and calcified structure health, 364-380. see also Dental caries prevention.
  calcified structure health, trace minerals in, 178-188
  and calcified structure health, minerals in, 160-177. see also Minerals.
  dental hygiene considerations in, 4b
  dental hygienist's role in, 3
  and estimated energy requirement (EER), 6. see also Estimated energy requirement (EER).

Nutrition (Continued)
  and food budgets, 311-316. see also Food budget(s).
  food fads and misinformation about, 323-329
  food insecurity in the United States, 333b-335b
  and food insecurity in United States, 333b-335b
  and food patterns, 309-310
  and food preparation, 316-323
  in growth and development, 265-291. see also Adolescents; Children; Infants.
  and health, 2-33
    case application in, 30b-31b
    health application in, 28b-30b
  in lactation, 255-257. see also Lactation.
  lipids in, 101-120. see also Lipids.
  and metabolism, 121-138. see also Metabolism.
  misinformation about, 323-329
    dental hygiene considerations of, 329b
    dental hygienist's role in combating, 332
    identifying sources of, 327-329, 327b-328b
    nutritional directions for, 329b
  nutritional directions for, 5b
  and oral soft tissue health
    fluids and minerals in, 213-241. see also Mineral electrolytes; Water.
    vitamins in, 189-212. see also Vitamin(s).
  in pregnancy, 243-264. see also Pregnancy.
  principle biomolecules in, 4
  referrals to resources in, 329-332, 330t
  required nutrients recommend for proper, 5. see also Nutrients.
  U.S. government focus on, 5. see also Dietary Guidelines for Americans; MyPyramid Food Guidance System.
Nutrition Facts label, 7, 21-25, 24f
  ease of reading, 25-27
  standardization, 21-24
Nutrition labeling, 21-27
  dental hygiene considerations of, 27b
  nutritional directions for, 27b
Nutrition treatment plan, 415-418
  dental hygiene considerations in, 419b
  documentation of, 417-418
  evaluation of, 417, 418f
  follow-up with, 417
  goal setting in, 416-417
  integration and implementation of, 415-417
  menu creation in, 417, 417f
  motivational interviewing, 415-416, 415f-416f, 416b
  nutritional directions for, 419b
  review of, 416f, 417
Nutritional aspects of gingivitis and periodontal disease, 381-392
Nutritional assessment and counseling, 406-422
  case application in, 420b-421b
  case study in, 421b-422b
  communication skills in, 415f, 418-421
  in dental caries prevention, 371-373, 371b
    assessments in, 371-373
    case application in, 378b
    goals of, 373
    patient education in, 373
  listening skills in, 418, 418f
  nonverbal communication in, 418
  nutritional status evaluation in, 408-413
    clinical observation and, 408-409
    diet history and, 410-413
    laboratory information and, 409
  nutritional status identification in, 413-415
  open-ended questioning in, 418-421
  in oral care of infants, 271
  patient evaluation in, 407-408
    dental history and, 408
    health history and, 407
    psychosocial history and, 407-408, 408b
  plan formation in, 415-418. see also Nutrition treatment plan.
Nutritional deficiency, 140
Nutritional genomics, 303b-304b
Nutritional insult, 247-249
  in adolescent bone growth, 283
Nutritional Program for the Elderly, 331
Nutritional resources, referrals for, 329-332
  dental hygiene considerations in, 332b
  nutritional directions in, 332b

Nutritional status evaluation, 408-413
  clinical observation and, 408-409
  dental hygiene considerations in, 409b-410b
  diet history and, 410-413
  laboratory information and, 409
  nutritional directions in, 410b
Nutritional status identification, 413-415
Nutritionist, 3, 329
Nuts, in Food Pyramid Guidance System, 97f
Nystagmus, 193

O
Obese patients, community nutrition resources for, 330t
Obesity, 9-10, 79-80
  childhood and adolescent obesity, 285b-287b
  and chronic disease, 293
  and chronic diseases, 28b-30b
  fat intake, 113
  health application in, 28b-30b
  in older adults, 293
  and soft drink consumption, expert panel findings on, 285b-287b
Observational studies, 328-329
Odontoblasts, 141
Odynophagia, 354
Oils group, in MyPyramid Food Guidance System, 14
  see also Fats
Older adults, 292-307, 293f
  body changes in, 296, 297f
  community nutrition resources for, 330t
  dental hygiene considerations of, 302b
  dietary (eating) patterns of, 301
    deficiencies in, 301
    food safety for, 301
    snacks and nutritional supplements in, 301
  general health status of, 293-294
  MyPlate, 300f, 301-302
  nutritional directions for, 303b
  nutritional requirements of, 298-301
    case application in, 304b-305b
    case study in, 305b
    dietary reference intakes in, 298
    energy and protein in, 298
    fluids in, 298
    functional foods in, 400b-401b
    health application in, 303b-304b
    vitamin-mineral supplements in, 302
    vitamins and minerals in, 298-301
  physiological factors influencing nutritional needs and status of, 294-296
    dental hygiene considerations of, 297b-298b
    gastrointestinal tract in, 295
    hydration status in, 295
    musculoskeletal system in, 295-296
    nutritional directions for, 298b
    oral cavity in, 294-295
  socioeconomic and psychological factors, 297, 297f
Oleic acid, structure of, 42f
Olfactory nerves, 54
Olfactory sensation, loss of, 294
Omega-3 fatty acids, 104, 106
  physiologic actions of, 106t
Omega-6 fatty acids, 104
  physiologic actions of, 106t
Oral cancer, risk factors for, 360b
Oral cavity, 52-56
  see also Calcified structures; Dentition; Oral soft tissues
  nutrition-related complications of, 409t
Oral cavity alterations, and oral health, 393-405
  alveolar bone loss in, 399
  dentition status in, 397-398
  glossitis in, 399-400
  oral and maxillofacial surgery in, 398
  orthodontics in, 394
  root caries and dentin hypersensitivity in, 396-397
  temporomandibular disorder in, 400
  xerostomia in, 394-395
Oral contraceptive agents (OCAs), nutrients affected by, 257-259
Oral development, factors affecting, 247-249
Oral health
  dental caries prevention in, 364-380
  in infants, 266-273

Oral health *(Continued)*
  in older adults, 294
  and oral cavity alterations, 393-405
    alveolar bone loss in, 399
    case application in, 404b
    dentition status in, 397-398
    glossitis in, 399-400
    oral and maxillofacial surgery in, 398
    orthodontics in, 394
    root caries and dentin hypersensitivity in, 396-397
    temporomandibular disorder in, 400
    xerostomia in, 394-395
  in women, 243-264
Oral health care products, selected ingredients in, 210b
Oral hygiene, and susceptibility to caries, 366
Oral manifestations, 190, 340, 341t
  in acquired immunodeficiency disease (AIDS), 355-356
  in anemias, 342-343
  in cardiovascular disease, 346-347
  in chronic disease, 340-342
  in gastrointestinal disorders, 345-346
  health application of, 360b
  in mental health disorders, 357-359
  in metabolic disorders, 348-352
  in neoplastic disorders, 354-355
  in neuromuscular disorders, 352-354
  in neutropenia, 344-345
  in renal disease, 351-352
  in skeletal changes, 348
Oral soft tissues, 189-212
  dental hygiene considerations of, 192b
  health maintenance of, nutritional directions for, 192b
  hydration of, 214-215. *see also* Hydration status; Water.
    dental hygiene considerations of, 221b-222b
    nutritional directions for, 223b
  minerals nutrients for, 190b, 213-241. *see also* Chloride; Iodine; Iron; Potassium; Sodium; Zinc.
  mucosa in, 191
  physiology of, 190-192
  salivary glands in, 190. *see also* Saliva; Salivary glands.
  systemic disease manifestations in, 190. *see also* Oral manifestations.
  tongue in, 191f. *see also* Tongue.
  vitamin nutrients for, 189-212, 190b. *see also* specific vitamin.
    biotin, 205
    cobalamin (vitamin B$_{12}$), 203-204
    folate/folic acid, 200-202
    niacin (vitamin B$_3$), 195-197
    pantothenic acid, 197-198
    pyridoxine (vitamin B$_6$), 198-200
    riboflavin (vitamin B$_2$), 194-195
    thiamin (vitamin B$_1$), 192-193
    vitamin A, 206
    vitamin C, 206
    vitamin E, 206
Oral surgery, 385-388, 398
  dental hygiene considerations in, 388b, 398b-399b
  nutritional directions for, 388b
  nutritional directions in, 399b
  postoperative considerations in, 385-388
  preoperative assessment and nutrition for, 385
Oral ulcers, associated with ulcerative colitis, 346, 346f
Organic foods, 320-322
  USDA definition of, 320, 320f
Orthodontics, 394
  dental hygiene considerations in, 394b
  nutritional directions in, 394b
Osmoreceptors, 215, 216f
Osmosis, 59, 214
Osmotic pressure, 58f, 214
Osteoblasts, vitamin D in physiology of, 145
Osteocalcin, 145
Osteoclasts, 161
  vitamin A and increased activity of, 143
Osteodystrophy, 184
  caused by aluminum, 184
  renal, 351
Osteoids, 161

Osteomalacia, 150
Osteonecrosis, 348, 349f
Osteoporosis, 150, 166, 175b
  in maxillofacial complex, radiography of, 166f
  in older adults, 295
  risk factors for, 48b-49b, 175b
Osteosclerosis, 351
Overconsumption and health related problems, 95
  dental hygiene considerations of, 95b
  nutritional directions for, 95b
Overweight, 9-10, 28b-30b
  development of, portion sizes and, 274-275
Overweight children
  and childhood obesity, 283, 285b-287b
  and weight gain during pregnancy, 245-246
Ovolactovegetarian, 95b-96b
Ovolactovegetarian diet, sample menu, 92f
Ovovegetarian, 95b-96b
Oxidation, of triglycerides, 124-125
Oxidation-reduction, 36
Oxidative phosphorylation, 45-47

P

Palatability of foods, 105
Pancreatic enzyme, 57
Pantothenic acid, 197-198
  dental hygiene considerations of, 198b
  hypo states of, 198
  nutritional directions for, 198b
  nutritional requirements for, 197, 198t
  physiological roles of, 197
  sources of, 198, 198t
Parasympathetic innervation, of salivary glands, 190
Parkinson's disease, oral manifestations in, 352-353
Pathogenic bacteria, 60
Patient evaluation, 407-408
  dental history and, 408
  health history and, 407
  psychosocial history and, 407-408, 408b
Pectin, 71t
Pedometer, 131
Pellagra, 197, 197f
Periapical dentition, 344-345
Perifollicular petechiae, 155, 155f
Perimenopause, 259
Periodontal disease, 202b, 382, 382f
  calcium deficiency in, 166
  necrotizing, 356, 388-392
  nutritional aspects of, 381-392
  in older adults, 294
  periodontitis in, 384
Periodontal health
  case application in, 391b-392b
  case study in, 392b
  dental hygiene considerations for, 384b
  food and physical effects on, 383
  nutritional considerations for, 383, 383b
  nutritional directions for, 384b
Periodontal surgery, 385-388
  dental hygiene considerations in, 388b
  nutritional directions for, 388b
  postoperative considerations in, 385-388
  preoperative assessment and nutrition for, 385
Periodontitis, 150
  chronic, 384-388
Periodontium, 93, 382, 382f
  immunocompetence of, 385
Peripheral edema, 221
Peristalsis, 61
Pernicious anemia
  oral manifestations in, 343, 344f
  and vitamin B$_{12}$ deficiency, 204, 204f, 343
Pesticides, on foods, 320
Petechiae, 153b-154b
  perifollicular, 155, 155f
Phantom taste, 54, 342
Phenobarbital, 353-354
Phenylketonuria, 80
Phenytoin use, hyperplasia associated with, 353, 353f
Phospholipids, 104
Phosphorus, 167-168
  absorption and excretion of, 167
  in calcified structures, 167-168, 368
    dental hygiene considerations of, 168b
  deficiency symptoms of, 409t

Phosphorus *(Continued)*
  hyper-states and hypostates, 167-168
  metabolism of, and vitamin D, 145
  nutritional directions for, 168b
  nutritional requirements for, 168t
  physiologic roles of, 167
  recommended dietary allowance (RDA) for, 167, 168t
  sources of, 165t, 167
Physical activity(ies)
  for children and adolescents, 276, 276f
  energy expenditure during selected, 129t
  and food intake, 131
  health benefits of, 296b
  in-depth information on, in *MyPyramid*, 17-18
  lack of, in older adults, 296
  need for regular, 128
  recommendations of *Dietary Guidelines for Americans*, 10-11
  and weight loss, 28b-30b
Phytochemicals, 156b, 175b
Pica, 244
Plant sterols, 116b-117b
Plaque acid, foods producing little or no, 370, 370b
Plaque biofilm, 67, 366
  composition of, 366
  dental hygiene considerations of, 366b
  nutritional directions for, 366b
Pocketed foods, 347
Polyols, 69
Polysaccharides, 38, 69-71
  reduced cariogenic properties of, 367
  summary of common, 38t
Polyunsaturated fatty acids (PUFAs), 41, 104
  food sources of, 108-113, 110t
  physiologic actions of, 106t
Popular diets, 28b-30b
Portal circulation, nutrient absorption into, 59
Portion sizes, 10
  for children, 276t
  and overweight development, 274-275
Postabsorptive state, 127
Potassium, 228-229
  dental hygiene considerations of, 229b
  hyper states and hypo states of, 229
  nutritional directions for, 229b
  physiological roles of, 228
  regulation of, 228-229
  requirements for, 228-229, 228t
  sources of, 229, 229t
Potassium intake, and protective effect against hypertension, 236b-237b
Potential energy, measurement of, 127
Poultry, contributions of, in daily nutrition, 19t
Prebiotics, 61
  examples of, 60t
  in infant formulas, 268
Precursors, 4
Preeclampsia, 244
Pregnancy, 244-254
  age during, 245
  community nutrition resources for, 330t
  dental hygiene considerations of, 254b-255b
  dietary intake and education during, 254
  drugs and medications during, 246-247
  food safety during, 247
  healthcare during, 245
  and lactation, basal metabolic rate in, 127
  neural tube defects and folic acid deficiency during, 202
  nutrient supplementation during, 254t
  nutritional directions for, 255b
  nutritional requirements during, 249-254
    B vitamins, 251-252
    calcium and vitamin D, 250-251
    energy and kilocalories, 250, 251f
    fat, 250
    iodine, 252-253
    iron, 252
    protein, 250, 251f
    zinc, 252
  oral development of fetus during, 247-249
  oral health during, 246
  recommended dietary allowances of vitamins and minerals in, 249-250, 249t

Pregnancy (Continued)
  safety of artificial sweetener use during, 247
  unusual dietary patterns in, 244-245
  vitamin B6 (pyridoxine) sufficiency during, 199-200
  vitamin-mineral supplements during, 253-254, 253t
  weight gain during, 245-246
Pregnancy gingivitis, 246, 246f
Premature infants, 244
Preschool children, 277-279
  food-related behaviors of, 278-279
  growth of, 277
  nutrient requirements for, 277, 278t
Preservatives, as food additives, 324t-325t
Probiotics, 60
  examples of, 60t
  in infant formulas, 268
Processed food preparation, 318-323, 319f
  additives in, 322-323
  convenience, 319
  effects of, 318-319
  fast food, 322
  irradiation in, 319-320
  nutritional directions for, 323b
  organic, 320-322
Prostaglandins, and vitamin E, 151
Proteases, 39
Protein digestibility corrected amino acid (PDCAA), 89, 89t
Protein-energy malnutrition (PEM), 93
  and development of noma and necrotizing ulcerative gingivitis, 93-94
  in kwashiorkor and marasmus, 93-94
Protein foods
  contributions of, in daily nutrition, 19t
  protein content in, 91t, 92f
Protein foods group, in MyPyramid Food Guidance System, 14, 19
Protein intake, during pregnancy, 250, 251f
Protein metabolism, 124
  protein-sparing carbohydrates in, 71-72
Protein-sparing nutrients, 105
Protein(s), 67f, 86-100, 87f, 89f
  see also Protein foods
  and amino acids, 87-88
  anticariogenic properties of, 368
  costs of, in food budget, 316t
  deficiency, symptoms of, 409t
  high quality, 88
  low quality, 88
  metabolism of, 47-48, 124
  in nutrition and health
    case application for, 99b
    classification of, 88-89
    dietary guidelines related to, 90b
    health application of, 95b-96b
    recommended dietary allowance (RDA) for, 90t
  over-consumption of, and health related problems, 95
  physiological roles of, 89-90
  in sample menu, 92f
  sources of, 91
  structure and function of, 38-40, 40f
  under-consumption of, and health related problems, 93-94
Proteolytic enzymes, 57
Prothrombin levels, and vitamin K, 152
Psychomotor seizures, 353
Psychosocial history, 407-408
Psyllium, 71t
Purging, 357
Purulent exudates, 384
Pyogenic lesions, 190
Pyridoxine (vitamin B6), 198-200
  absorption and excretion of, 199
  deficiency symptoms of, 409t
  dental hygiene considerations of, 200b
  hyper states and hypo states of, 199-200
  nutritional directions for, 200b
  nutritional requirements for, 198
  physiological roles of, 198
  recommended dietary allowance (RDA) for, 198, 199t
  sources of, 199, 199t

Q
Qualified health claims, on food labels, 25
Quercetin, in energy drinks, 218
Quinones, 152
  see also Vitamin K

R
R-binder, 203
Rachitic rosary, 148-150, 149f
Recommended dietary allowance (RDA), 5, 249-250
  see also Institute of Medicine
  for calcium, 162-163
  for cobalamin (vitamin B12), 203, 203t
  for copper, 179, 179t
  for fats, 109t
  for fluoride, 171, 172t
  for folate/folic acid, 200, 201t
  for folate/folic acid, in pregnancy, 252
  for iodine, 234, 235t
  for iron, 230, 230t
  for magnesium, 168, 169t
  for molybdenum, 183, 183t
  for niacin (vitamin B3), 195-196, 196t
  for phosphorus, 167, 168t
  for pyridoxine (vitamin B6), 198, 199t
  for riboflavin (vitamin B2), 194, 194t
  for selenium, 180, 180t
  for thiamin (vitamin B1), 192, 192t
  for vitamin A, 142
  for vitamin C, 154
  for vitamin E, 151
  for vitamin K, 152
  of vitamins and minerals, in pregnancy, 249t
  for zinc, 233, 233t
Redox coenzymes, 45-47
Reference daily intake (RDI), 25, 25t
Referrals, for nutritional resources, 330t
Regional food, of United States, 312t-314t
Registered dietitian (RD), 3
Religious food restrictions, 311
Remineralize, 55
Renal disorders
  dental hygiene considerations in, 352b
  nutritional directions for, 352b
  oral manifestations in, 341t, 351-352
Renal failure, 132b-135b
Renal osteodystrophy, 351
Renin, and water regulation, 215
Residue of digestion, 60
Resistance to change, understanding, 416-417, 416b
Resistant starch, 70
Retinoic acid, 141
Retinol, 141
  see also Vitamin A
Rhodopsin, 141
Riboflavin (vitamin B2), 194-195
  deficiency symptoms of, 409t
  dental hygiene considerations of, 195b
  hypo states of, 195
  nutritional directions for, 195b
  nutritional requirements for, 194
  physiological roles of, 194
  recommended dietary allowance (RDA) for, 194, 194t
  sources of, 194-195, 194t
Rickets, 148-150, 166
  bone metaphyses in, 149f
  bowlegs in, 149f
Root caries, 396-397
  and dental abrasion, 396-397, 397f
  and dental erosion, 396-397, 397f
  dental hygiene considerations in, 397b
  nutritional directions for, 397b
  in older adults, 294

S
Saccharin, 368
Safe sanitary kitchen guidelines, 318b
Saliva, 55
  calcium in, 162
  composition of, 190-191
  digestive functions of, 55t
  flow of, and buffering capacity, in protection against carries, 366
  fluoride ions in, 170

Saliva (Continued)
  hypotonicity of, 190-191
  physiologic role of, 190-191
  production of, and nutritional status, 342. see also Xerostomia.
Salivary glands, 189-212, 191f
  see also Oral soft tissues
  and absorption of vitamin B12, 203
  autonomic innervation of, 190
Salmonella, 317
Sarcopenia, 90
  in older adults, 296
Satiety center, stimulation of, 130
Satiety value of fats, 105
Saturated fatty acids (SFAs), 41, 103
  food sources of, 108-113, 110t
  physiologic actions of, 106t
Scarlet tongue, 197f
School-age children, 281-282
  dental carries in, 281-282
  nutrition for, dental hygiene considerations of, 282b
  nutritional directions for, 282b
School meal programs, 331
Scorbutic changes, in teeth, 155
Scurvy, 155
Sealants, 282
Secondary deficiency, 140
Secretory immunoglobulin A (sIgA), 93
Selenium, 180-181
  dental hygiene considerations of, 181b
  hyper-states and hypo-states of, 181
  nutritional directions for, 181b
  nutritional requirements for, 180
  physiological roles of, 180
  recommended dietary allowance (RDA) for, 180, 180t
  sources of, 181
Sensory neuropathy, severe, in pyridoxine toxicity, 199-200
Sequestrants, as additives, 324t-325t
Serving, what counts as a, 17b
Severe early childhood caries, 271-272
  see also Early childhood caries (ECC)
Short-chain fatty acids, 103
Signs, of disease, 190
Silicon, 184
Sjögren syndrome, 394-395, 395f
Skeletal changes
  dental hygiene considerations of, 348b
  nutritional directions for, 348b
  oral manifestations in, 341t, 348, 349f
Sleep, and basal metabolic rate, 127
Small intestine, 51, 57-59
  dental hygiene considerations of, 59b
  digestion in, 57-59
  fat-soluble nutrient absorption in, 59
  nutrient absorption, 59f
    into portal circulation, 59
  nutrient absorption in, 59
  nutritional directions for, 60b
  wall of, 53f
Smell, sense of, 52-54
  disorders of, 342
  loss of, 294
Snack foods, healthy, 278b
  for older adults, 302
Socialization, and eating habits of, 283
Sodas, 221
  see also Soft drink consumption
Sodium, 223-227
  dental hygiene considerations of, 227b-228b
  hyper states and hypo states of, 226-227
  nutritional directions for, 228b
  physiological roles of, 223
  regulation of, 223, 225t
  requirements for, 223, 225t
  sources of, 224-226, 225t
Sodium density, 226f
Sodium intake
  American Heart Association recommendations, 236b-237b
  Dietary Guidelines for Americans recommendations, 11, 226b
Soft drink consumption, frequent, and promotion of dental caries, 370, 370f

Soluble fiber, 72
Solutes, in body fluids, 214
Solvent, water as, 214
Sorbitol, 69, 367-368
Soups, recommended, and frequency, 12t
Soy-based milk, and infant nutrition, 268
Special Supplement Food Program for Women, Infants, and Children (WIC), 331
Sphincter muscles, 51
Sphingomyelins, 104
Sport drink consumption, frequent, and promotion of dental caries, 370, 370f
Sports drinks, 220-221
Squamous metaplasia, 206
Stabilizers, as food additives, 324t-325t
Stable nutrients, 319
Stannous fluoride, cariostatic activity of, 184
Starch(es), 38, 69-70, 70f
    recommended, and frequency, 12t
    reduced cariogenic properties of, 367
    resistant, 70
Starvation, effects of, 132f
Stearic acid, 113
Stephan curve, 370f
Steroids, 44
Stomach
    digestive process, 52f
    distention of, after meal, 131
Stomatitis, 192b
    uremic, 351-352
Streptococcus mutans, 67, 272, 366
Stroke
    dental hygiene considerations in, 347b
    nutritional directions for, 347b
    oral manifestations in, 341t, 346-347
Structural lipids, 102
Sucking infant, 268-269
Suckling, 268-269
Sucralose, 368
Sucrose, 36-38, 69
    structures of, 38f
Sugar alcohols, 69, 367-368
    and decreased risk of dental caries, 367-368. see also Sorbitol; Xylitol.
Sugar intake, 12
    misconception about, 280
Sugar substitutes (sweeteners), 83f
    dental hygiene considerations of, 82b
    as food additives, 324t-325t
    non-nutritive, 368
    nonnutritive, 80, 81t
        caloric value/relative sweetness/cariogenicity, 68t
    nutritional directions for, 82b
    safety of, during pregnancy, 247
    synergistic effect of, 80
Sugar(s)
    caloric value/relative sweetness/cariogenicity, 68t
    substitutes for. see Sugar substitutes (sweeteners).
Supplemental Nutrition Assistance Program (SNAP), 329
Supplemental Nutrition Program for Women, Infants, and Children (WIC), 254
Supplements, dietary
    ABCD approach to asking patient about, 210b
    health applications in, 206b-209b
    herbs as, 326
    for infants, 270
    for older adults, 302
    during pregnancy, 254, 254t
Suppuration, 382
Surface area, and basal metabolic rate, 127
Sweeteners. see Sugar substitutes (sweeteners)
Sweets
    in Food Pyramid Guidance System, 97f
    recommended, and frequency, 12t
Sympathetic innervation, of salivary glands, 190
Symptoms, of disease, 190
Syrup of ipecac, 357
Systematic reviews, 328-329
Systemic disorder(s), 54, 341t
    case study for, 361b
    effects of, on nutritional status and oral health, 339-362
    oral manifestations of, 190, 340, 341t

Systemic disorder(s) (Continued)
    in acquired immunodeficiency syndrome (AIDS), 355-356
    in anemias, 342-343
    in cardiovascular disease, 346-347
    case application in, 361b
    in chronic disease, 340-342
    in gastrointestinal disorders, 345-346
    health application of, 360b
    in mental health disorders, 357-359
    in metabolic disorders, 348-352
    in neoplastic disorders, 354-355
    in neuromuscular disorders, 352-354
    in neutropenia, 344-345
    in renal disease, 351-352
    in skeletal changes, 348

T

Tachycardia, 193
Tap water, 215-216
    regulation of contaminant levels in, 216-217
Taste, sense of, 52-54
    disorders of, 342
    loss of, 294
Taste buds, 53, 192
Taste papillae, 53
Taurine, in energy drinks, 218
Teeth, 55-56, 55f
    formation of, 161
Temperature
    basal metabolic rate, 128
    and food intake, 131
Temporomandibular disorder (TMD), 400
Tensional forces, 161
Tetany, 166
Theanine, 218
Thermic effect, of food, 128
Thermogenesis, 95
Thiamin (vitamin B₁), 192-193
    deficiency symptoms of, 409t
    dental hygiene considerations of, 193b
    hypo states of, 193
    nutritional directions for, 194b
    nutritional requirements for, 192
    physiological roles of, 192
    recommended dietary allowance (RDA) for, 192, 192t
    sources of, 192-193, 193t
Thiaminase, microbial, 193
Thickeners, as food additives, 324t-325t
Three D's (symptoms of pellagra), 197, 197f
Thrombus, arterial, 346-347
    see also Cerebrovascular accident
Thyroxine
    and basal metabolic rate, 128
    and enhanced use of vitamin A, 143
Tin, 184
Tinnitus, 400
Tobacco cessation, 390b
    pharmacotherapy for, 391b
    questions for, 391b
Tobacco products, 391b
Tocopherol, 151
    see also Vitamin E
Tocotrienols, 151
    see also Vitamin E
Toddlers, 277-279
    food-related behaviors of, 278-279
    growth of, 277
    nutrient requirements for, 277, 278t
Tolerable upper intake level (UL), of nutrients, 6
Tongue, 191, 191f
    see also Glossitis
    dehydration and longitudinal fissures in, 221, 222f
    regions of taste on, 54f
Tooth development. see Dentition, development of
Total energy requirements, 128
Total parenteral nutrition (TPN), copper deficiency in, 180
Toxoplasmosis, 247
Trabecular bone, 55
Trace mineral(s), 178-188
    see also Ultratrace elements
    case application in, 187b
    chromium in, 181-182

Trace mineral(s) (Continued)
    copper in, 179-180
    in enamel and dentin, 179t
    health application in, 185b-186b
    manganese in, 182
    molybdenum in, 183
    selenium in, 180-181
    upper intake levels of, 179
Trans fat levels in products, 112f
trans fatty acids, 103-104
    and food labeling, 112
    physiologic actions of, 106t
    and risk of heart disease, 113
Transferrin, 230
Tricarboxylic acid (TCA) cycle, 45-47, 103
Triglycerides, 43-44, 44f, 102
    composition of, 103
    formation and structure of, 103f
    oxidation of, 124-125
Twenty-four hour recall, of food intake, 410-412, 410b, 411f

U

Ultratrace elements, 183-185
    dental hygiene considerations for, 185b
    nutritional directions for, 185b
Underconsumption and health related problems, 93-94
    dental hygiene considerations in, 94b
    nutritional directions for, 95b
Undigested residue, in large intestine, 60
Unsaturated fatty acids, 41, 103
    oxidation of, 44
Unusual dietary patterns, 244-245
Upper intake level (UL), of nutrients, 6
Uremic stomatitis, 351-352
U.S. Department of Agriculture (USDA), Dietary Guidelines for Americans, 6-16, 7f
U.S. Department of Health and Human Services (USDHHS), 5
    Dietary Guidelines for Americans, 6-7
U.S. Food and Drug Administration (FDA)
    nutrition labeling promotion by, 21
    qualified health claim permission by, 25, 26b
    standardized serving portions determined by, 21-24
U.S. Pharmacopeia (USP), 210b

V

Valve, gastrointestinal, 51
Vanadium, 184-185
Vegans, 95b-96b, 98f
    and children with vitamin B₁₂ deficiency, 204
Vegetables
    nutrients in selected, 18t
    recommended, and frequency, 12t
Vegetables group
    in Food Pyramid Guidance System, 97f
    in MyPyramid Food Guidance System, 18
Vegetables oils, in Food Pyramid Guidance System, 97f
Vegetarian diets, meal planning tips for, 99b
Vegetarian food guide rainbow, modifications of, for children, adolescents, pregnant and lactating women, 97t
Vegetarian food pyramid, 97f
Vegetarians, 90
Very low-density lipoproteins (VLDLs), 105, 105f
Vipeholm study, 368
Viscous fiber, 72
Vision, vitamin A in physiology of, 141
Vitamin A (carotene)
    absorption and excretion of, 143
    in calcified structures, 141-145
        dental hygiene considerations of, 145b
        nutritional directions for, 145b
    deficiency symptoms of, 409t
    fat solubility of, 141
    hyper-states and hypo-states of, 143-145, 143f
    nutritional deficiency of, and resulting conditions, 144-145
    nutritional requirements for, 142
    in oral soft tissue physiology, 206, 206b
    physiological roles of, 141-142
    recommended dietary allowance (RDA) for, 142t

Vitamin A (carotone) *(Continued)*
  sources of, 142-143, 143t
  supplementation of, and birth defects, 253t
  toxicity of high concentrations of, 143
    symptoms of, 143
Vitamin B₁₂ (cobalamin), 203-204
  absorption and excretion of, 203
  absorption and excretion of, in older adults, 300
  deficiency symptoms of, 409t
  dental hygiene considerations of, 204b-205b
  hyper states and hypo states of, 204
  nutritional directions for, 205b
  nutritional requirements for, 203
  physiological roles of, 203
  recommended dietary allowance (RDA) for, 203, 203t
  sources of, 203, 204t
Vitamin B₃ (niacin), 195-197
  deficiency symptoms of, 409t
  dental hygiene considerations of, 197b
  hyper states and hypo states of, 196-197
  nutritional directions for, 197b
  nutritional requirements for, 195-196
  physiological roles of, 195
  recommended dietary allowance (RDA) for, 195-196, 196t
  sources of, 196t
Vitamin B₆ (pyridoxine), 198-200
  absorption and excretion of, 199
  deficiency symptoms of, 409t
  dental hygiene considerations of, 200b
  hyper states and hypo states of, 199-200
  nutritional directions for, 200b
  nutritional requirements for, 198
  physiological roles of, 198
  recommended dietary allowance (RDA) for, 198, 199t
  sources of, 199, 199t
Vitamin B₂ (riboflavin), 194-195
  deficiency symptoms of, 409t
  dental hygiene considerations of, 195b
  hypo states of, 195
  nutritional directions for, 195b
  nutritional requirements for, 194
  physiological roles of, 194
  recommended dietary allowance (RDA) for, 194, 194t
  sources of, 194-195, 194t
Vitamin B₁ (thiamin), 192-193
  deficiency symptoms of, 409t
  dental hygiene considerations of, 193b
  hypo states of, 193
  nutritional directions for, 194b
  nutritional requirements for, 192
  physiological roles of, 192
  recommended dietary allowance (RDA) for, 192, 192t
  sources of, 192-193, 193t
Vitamin C (ascorbic acid)
  in calcified structures, 154-157
    dental hygiene considerations of, 155b
    nutritional directions for, 156b
  deficiency symptoms of, 409t
  hyper-states and hypo-states of, 155-157, 156f
  nutritional requirements for, 154, 154t
  in oral soft tissue physiology, 206
  physiological roles of, 154
  recommended dietary allowance (RDA) for, 154
  sources of, 143t, 155, 155t
  supplementation of, and birth defects, 253t
  water solubility of, 141
Vitamin D (calciferol)
  absorption of, 148
  in calcified structures, 145-150
    dental hygiene considerations of, 150b
    nutritional directions for, 151b

Vitamin D (calciferol) *(Continued)*
  deficiency of, 148-150
  deficiency of, in older adults, 299
  deficiency symptoms of, 409t
  fat solubility of, 141
  food sources of, 147-148, 148t
  hormonal characteristics of, 145
  hyper-states and hypo-states of, 148-150
  metabolism of, 146f
  nutritional requirements for, 145-147, 147t
  physiological roles of, 145
  production of, using UV rays of sunlight, 147
  requirements for, during pregnancy, 250-251
  sources of, 147-148
  supplementation of, and birth defects, 253t
  toxicity of, at high levels, 148
Vitamin D fortified foods, 147
Vitamin deficiency(ies), 140-141
  group at risk of, 140b
Vitamin E (tocopherol)
  absorption and excretion of, 152
  in calcified structures, 151-152
    dental hygiene considerations of, 152b
    nutritional directions for, 152b
  and enhanced use of vitamin A, 143
  fat solubility of, 141
  hyper-states and hypo-states of, 152
  nutritional requirements for, 151, 151t
  in oral soft tissue physiology, 206, 206b
  physiological roles of, 151
  recommended dietary allowance (RDA) for, 151
  sources of, 151, 152t
  supplementation of, and birth defects, 253t
Vitamin K
  absorption and excretion of, 153
  in calcified structures, 152-153
    dental hygiene considerations of, 153b-154b
    nutritional directions for, 154b
  deficiency symptoms of, 409t
  fat solubility of, 141
  hyper-states and hypo-states of, 153
  nutritional requirements for, 152
  physiological roles of, 152
  recommended dietary allowance (RDA) for, 152
  sources of, 153, 153t
  supplementation of, and birth defects, 253t
Vitamin(s), 140, 190b
  and calcified structures, 139-159, 140b. *see also*
      Vitamin A; Vitamin C; Vitamin D; Vitamin E.
    case application in, 157b
    deficiency in, 140-141
    dental hygiene considerations of, 141b
    health application in, 156b
    nutritional directions for, 141b
    requirements for, 140, 140b
  fat soluble, 59
  fat-soluble, 141
  as food additives, 324t-325t
  insufficiency of, in older adults, 299
  lipid soluble, 40, 41t
  in oral soft tissue and salivary gland physiology,
      189-212. *see also* B-complex vitamins; Biotin;
      Pantothenic acid; Vitamin A; Vitamin C;
      Vitamin E.
    case application in, 211b
    case study in, 211b
    health application in, 206b-209b
  in pregnancy, recommended dietary allowance
      (RDA) of, 249-250, 249t
  supplemental, for older adults, 302
  water soluble, 40, 41t
  water-soluble, 141

W

Washing fruits and vegetables, safe-practice in,
  319-320

Water deprivation, 227
Water fluoridation, 172
  safety of, 174
Water intoxication, 227
Water loss, 227
Water soluble vitamins, 40, 141
Watery diarrhea, 227
Weight
  distribution of, and disease risk, 28b-30b
  hunger and appetite affecting, 130
  maintaining healthy, 28b-30b
Weight gain
  during pregnancy, 245-246
  recommendation for total and rate of, during
      pregnancy, 245t
Weight loss
  equation for, 130b
  unintentional, 408
Weight management
  in children, 287b
  and kilocalorie intake, 130
  recommendations of *Dietary Guidelines for
      Americans*, 9-11
Weight reduction diet, criteria of, 28b-30b
Wernicke-Korsakoff syndrome, associated with
  alcoholism, 193
Whole grains
  definition of, 14
  and enriched products, nutrient values of, 14t
Wilson disease, 180
  cornea in, 180f
Women's nutritional status, 243-264
  case application in, 261b-262b
  case study in, 262b
  health application in, 260b-261b
  in lactation, 255-257. *see also* Lactation.
  in menopause, 259-262
  oral health and, 246
  preconceptional, 244. *see also* Oral contraceptive
      agents.
  in pregnancy, 244-254. *see also* Pregnancy.
World Health Organization (WHO), 74, 90-91

X

Xeroderma, 144-145
Xerophthalmia, 144, 144f
Xerostomia, 54, 342, 395f
  dental hygiene considerations in, 396b
  factors contributing to, 395b
  nutritional directions for, 396b
  and nutritional status, 342, 395b
  in older adults, 294
  and oral health, 394-395
Xylitol, 69, 368

Z

Zinc, 232-234
  absorption and excretion of, 233
  dental hygiene considerations of, 234b
  hyper states and hypo states of, 233-234
  nutritional directions for, 234b
  physiological roles of, 232 233
  recommended dietary allowance (RDA) for, 233, 233t
  requirements for, 233, 233t
  requirements for, during pregnancy, 252
  sources of, 233, 234t
  supplementation of, and birth defects, 253t
Zinc deficiency
  causes of, 233
  symptoms of, 409t

everything but textbook

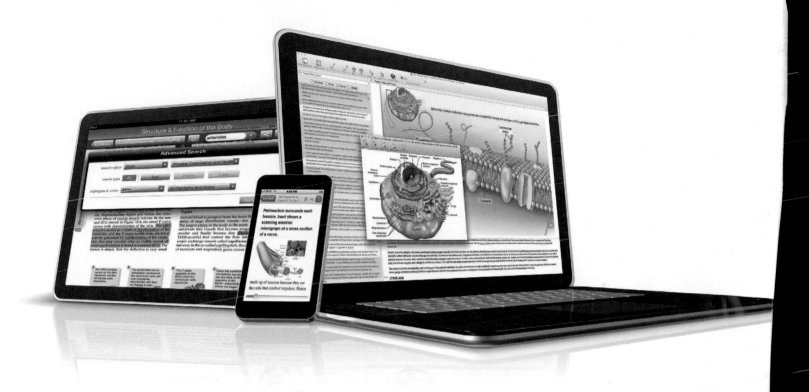

If you've never considered ebooks before, now may be the time.
More than just words on a screen, Pageburst comes with an arsenal
of interactive functionality and time-saving study tools that allow you to:

- access your entire course load from one portable device

- instantly swap notes with your instructors and classmates

- quickly search for topics and key terms

- watch videos and animations

- get the same Elsevier content for a lot less money

Discover more at **pageburst.com**.

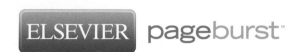